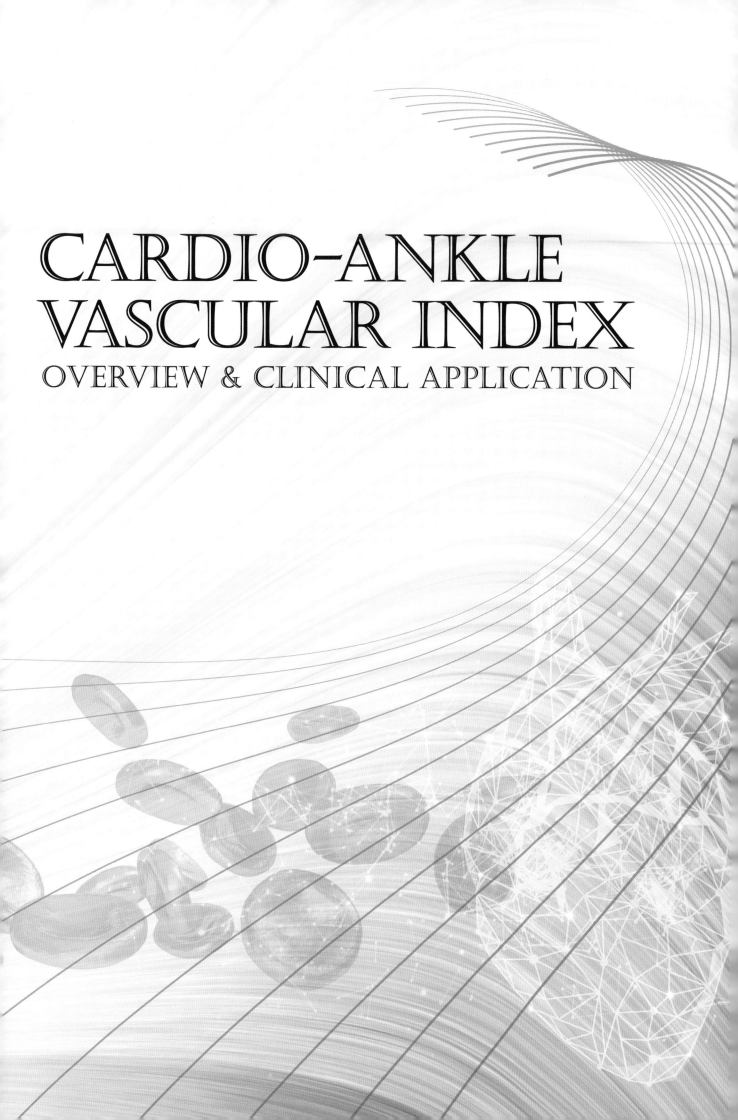

CARDIO-ANKLE VASCULAR INDEX
OVERVIEW & CLINICAL APPLICATION

Foreword

Hajime Orimo[1,2]

It is well known that "A man is as old as his artery." The early detection and prevention of vascular aging or arteriosclerotic diseases was urgently required all over the world, and a marker for the early stages of arteriosclerosis or vascular aging had long been sought. Arterial stiffness was recommended as a good index, and several indices for it had been proposed. The cardio-ankle vascular index (CAVI) was presented as an index reflecting arterial stiffness in 2006. Its noble feature is its independence from blood pressure at measuring time, and that it enables the evaluation of the proper stiffness of the arterial tree from the origin of the aorta to the ankle. Over 700 papers dealing with CAVI have been published by many researchers in the last 15 years.

At the first stage, the role of CAVI as an index for the degree of arteriosclerosis and its relationship with various coronary risk factors was nearly established. The predictive role of CAVI for cardiovascular events was also mostly established.

At the second stage, the role of CAVI as an index for vascular functions co-relating with ventricular functions was presented, and the new field of vascular functions has recently begun using the CAVI.

Important works on the CAVI by researchers from all over the world can be gathered and included in this book. This book can inspire the use of CAVI to contribute to the development of the new field of vascular function, and can lead to the promotion of a better, happier life for people all over the word in the future.

[1]President of Japanese Society of Promoting Vascular Health.
[2]President Emeritus of Tokyo Metropolitan Geriatric Hospital and Institute of Gerontology

Contents

New Field of Arterial Stiffness Developed with New Index

Roland Asmar

Atherosclerosis and cardiovascular diseases constitute a public health problem and remain among the first causes of morbidity and mortality worldwide. The prevalence of their risk factors increases with age in both developed and even more in developing countries. Experts agree to designate the artery, particularly the arterial wall, as the common denominator, the target and the site of almost all the risk factors, complications, the associated cardiovascular conditions and other diseases (kidney, brain, heart, Alzheimer's, etc.).

In recent decades, medical research has made considerable progress, particularly in the identification and management of risk factors and associated cardiovascular diseases, both in primary and secondary prevention. At the same time, while technological advances have made it possible to better assess some diseases, in particular **cardiac conditions**, they have not yet succeeded in making **non-invasive arterial assessment** a practical examination carried out on a daily basis in medical offices. Indeed, although the evaluation of atherosclerosis and the artery are the topics of much research in hemodynamic labs, bioengineering and medical device manufacturers, it is progressing slowly in small steps. In fact, we are now able to assess mainly the geometry, the lumen and some other aspects of the **arterial structure** using invasive examinations (MRI, Scanner, angiography, etc.) and non-invasive investigations (ultrasound, IMT, ABI, etc.); but the evaluation of **arterial function** by non-invasive method, to allow its application, repetition, and dissemination, remains limited to certain specialized centres.

Factors mentioned hereabove give some explanations on why up-to-date, the evaluation of the arterial risk continues to be performed indirectly by assessing risk factors, calculating scores to estimate the global cardiovascular risk or even by using partial and indirect investigations to explore arterial conditions. All this highlights the absolute need of having a direct method to assess the arterial hemodynamics, structure and function, in a non-invasive, reliable and repetitive way since the artery constitutes the site of most the cardiovascular diseases and therefore the target of the treatment.

For better positioning of the subject of this book, it is interesting to have a historical review on the methods and techniques dedicated for the arterial evaluation:

Before the 80s, assessment of the cardiovascular hemodynamics was mainly focused on the heart function and structure. Few resources were devoted to access the hemodynamics of the central and, even less, to the peripheral vascular system. Indeed, cardiologists being interested mainly by the heart, gave little attention to the vascular hemodynamics.

The arterial investigations were mainly performed using invasive methods such as angiography to assess the arterial structure and some functional parameters (diameter, pressure, flow, impedance, compliance...). Several non-invasive methods were available, but their use was not popular within the cardiologists. Among these techniques we may consider the following:

1. The Ankle/Brachial systolic blood pressure index (ABI): This index evaluates the global arterial hemodynamics between the brachial and the ankle arteries; ABI is used according to clinical guideline for diagnosing of the peripheral artery disease (PAD) or arteriosclerosis obliterans (ASO).

2. The Carotidogram: In addition to the use of the carotidogram for the cardiac function assessment, some of its features allow also indirect evaluation of the carotid artery hemodynamics.

3. The Pulse wave velocity: The Pulse wave velocity (PWV) between two arterial sites is directly related to the arterial distensibility; therefore, measurement of PWV allows the determination of the distensibility of a peripheral arterial segment or even of the aorta when considered between the carotid and the femoral arteries.

4. The plethysmograph: This technique uses either mercury gauge or photoelectric sensor to record changes in pulsatile blood flow. When applied to an arterial segment some devices transfer measured changes of volume into changes of pressure using specific algorithms.

5. The Continuous Doppler: This technique was used to evaluate the blood flow in the vessels.

Thus, historically cardiologists were little interested in the arterial function, considered mainly as a conduit function; Their approach was based on the calculation from invasive methods, of systemic parameters such as impedance, total peripheral resistance, blood flow, etc. To assess the arterial hemodynamics, few techniques often time-consuming were available, reflecting the lack of interest of the community in this area.

Chairman, Foundation-Medical Research Institutes – (F-MRI®), Geneva, Switzerland.

Important Conceptual Developments

In the late 70s and early 80s we witnessed an important conceptual shift in the vascular, mainly arterial, hemodynamic approach. Indeed, while most cardiologists considered the arteries as simple passive pipes conducting blood from the heart to the periphery, experts reported the arterial system as an active system with several functions that vary according to the concerned arteries. Thus, arteries have been described with several classifications according to their anatomy (large and small arteries), histology (elastic and muscular arteries) and function (buffering or cushioning, conduit, resistive) with correspondence between these classifications. The large arteries being mainly elastic with the buffering function; the small arteries being mainly muscular with distribution and resistive functions. Therefore, evaluation of the arterial hemodynamics shifted from its systemic evaluation (total peripheral resistance, ...) to its regional segmental and local hemodynamic assessments. Moreover, the crosstalk between large and small arteries, as well as between large arteries and the heart, have been described in the pathophysiology of several cardiovascular and renal conditions. Thus, the vascular system with its various compartments (artery, arteriole, capillary, venule, vein) was considered as a single closed system with specific hemodynamic properties to each of its compartments. The hemodynamic properties of each of them being assessed using specific methods. Considering this approach, assessment of the vascular hemodynamics was performed by different techniques and expressed as tonicity, hysteresis, compliance, distensibility... for veins; density, number, diameter for capillary; resistance, diameter, flow for small arteries; diameter, thickness, compliance, distensibility for large arteries.

There is no doubt that this approach has allowed a better understanding of the physiology and pathophysiology of the vascular and more particularly of the arterial system. In terms of hemodynamic, full distinction of the pulsatile component of the pulse wave from its steady component was made. Comprehensive description of the determinants of each of steady and pulsatile components was reported in various normal and pathological conditions.

In the late 80s and early 90s, assessment of pressure signal at different arterial sites (central and peripheral) was reactivated, first using invasive and then non-invasive techniques. Comprehensive description of the different arterial pressures and the amplification phenomena as well as other derived parameters were reported in normal and various disease conditions.

Thus, a particularly important conceptual changes of the arterial hemodynamics took place. Arteries were considered as a full active system with various functions. Arteries were classified according to their characteristics. Arterial hemodynamics was described as a steady and pulsatile component as well as a peripheral and central aspects with its amplification phenomenon. Assessment of arterial hemodynamics shifted from the systemic to the local and regional evaluations.

Important Technical Developments

In parallel to the conceptual development, the 80s and 90s witnessed an extraordinary technical development of several techniques and methods to assess the arterial hemodynamics. We will mention hereafter only those that seem to have marked this area.

I. Local determination of the arterial hemodynamics

Coupling Continuous Doppler + Bi-dimensional Echography

This duplex system combined a continuous Doppler beam to a bidimensional echography at a fixed angle. The objective of this system was to measure the arterial diameter and the blood flow simultaneously. This device was used for a short time and remained as prototype.

Bi- dimensional pulsed Doppler system

This system incorporates a double transducer probe set at 120°. This device measures the arterial internal diameter and its cross-sectional blood flow velocity. This system was applied mainly on the brachial artery but also on other superficial arteries. This system known as the "ALVAR" system was used in the 80s for many years in limited number of research labs and was not marketed on a larger scale.

The Wall-Track System

This was a high-resolution echo-tracking device that measures internal diameter at diastole, the pulsatile changes of the arterial diameter and the intima-media thickness (IMT). The device provides also the arterial elastic modulus. Despite the use of this device in several research studies it remained reserved for some research Laboratories.

The Non-Invasive Ultrasound System (NIUS)

This Device measures the pressure/diameter curves resulting in estimates for the compliance and the incremental elastic modulus given as isobaric for a definite BP value. The use of this device was reserved for some research Laboratories.

Second Derivative of the Finger Plethysmograph (SDPTG)

The amplitude ratios of the second derivative of the peripheral pulse waveform obtained by finger plethysmography is associated to the arterial stiffness. The use of this device remained limited to research mainly in Japan.

II. Regional / segmental determination of the arterial hemodynamics

Proximal and Distal Compliance

This technique was based on the arterial pulse recording of the radial artery using tonometer sensor strapped at the wrist and a modified Windkessel model allowing determination of proximal "Capacitive" (C1) and distal "Oscillometry" (C2) compliance. The distribution of this technique was extremely limited.

Automatic Measurements of Pulse Transit Time

Until 1990s, the measurement of pulse wave transit time was performed by few specialized teams, mainly in Paris, because its calculation was done manually and time-consuming. Regional PWV is considered up to date as the gold standard for arterial stiffness assessment. It is usually measured at the aortic level (carotid - femoral arteries) or other arterial segments such as the upper and lower limbs. Development of devices for automatic recording and calculation of the PWV has considerably facilitated the examination and its application on a larger scale. Among the most popular devices, we may consider the following:

- *The Complior System*

The Complior system was the first device designed for the automatic measurement of the PWV. It was developed by R. Asmar in collaboration with Artech Medical (Pantin, France) using dedicated specifically designed mechano-transducers. This device was the first one used in several international clinical trials; thus, greatly contributed to the dissemination of the arterial stiffness concept and the PWV measurements worldwide. In fact, its implementation in large clinical trials allowed to initiate many KOLs to the arterial stiffness concept.

- *The Automated Doppler Recording of PWV*

The transit time between flow pulses recorded simultaneously using continuous Doppler probes was recorded between the left subclavian artery and the abdominal aorta bifurcation.

- *The Sphygmocor System*

This device developed in the mid-1990s was originally designed to calculate central BP and to perform the pulse wave analysis. Later, this device incorporated automatic measurement of PWV, using one lead ECG signal and a single applanation tonometer.

- *The Pulse Pen Device*

This device allows automatic measurement of regional PWV, determination of Central BP as well as the pulse wave analysis. This device has been used in few studies; its use remains limited in some specialized centers.

- *The brachial-ankle PWV*

This device was developed by Colin medical technology (Komaki, Japan) in 2002. It allows automatic calculation of brachial-ankle (ba) PWV using a Colin Waveform Analyzer. This device has been used in clinical studies performed mainly in Japan; its use remained restricted mainly in Asia.

- *The Cardio-Ankle Vascular Index (CAVI) - The VaSera System*

Recently, a novel arterial parameter developed in 2004 by K. Shirai et al., the Cardio-Ankle Vascular Index (CAVI) measured by the automatic VaSera device (Fukuda Denshi, Japan) appeared on the market. CAVI assesses arterial mechanical and elastic properties by means of the beta index which is relatively independent of blood pressure levels at the time of the measurement. The use of CAVI for cardiovascular assessment was first introduced in Japan and then in Asia, where it became extremely popular and received institutional and governmental awards. This device is now used in several clinical trials in Asia and Europe; its increasing popularity during the last 5 years, mainly in Europe, seems to be related, at least in part, to its ease of use, its relative independency from blood pressure levels, and other advantages.

Future Perspectives

While many things have been achieved during the last 3 decades, many other important aspects need to be done to establish the arterial stiffness in daily practice:

- *Choice of the arterial parameter:* Even though PWV is considered as the reference method for arterial stiffness assessment, many other parameters measuring or calculating other arterial parameters exist or have been developed. Therefore, a choice among these techniques would be mandatory to establish a gold standard method to be considered in the future large trials.
- *Reimbursement of the arterial stiffness examination:* Arterial stiffness measurement remains not reimbursed by the health system in most countries. This reimbursement issue constitutes a major obstacle for its implementation in daily practice and should be considered as a necessity for the upcoming years.
- *Need for future studies:* More studies are still needed to show that diagnosis and therapeutic strategies, based on arterial stiffness, are effective and of added values.
- *Development of Arterial Stiffness Specific Therapy:* It is necessary to develop specific drugs whose main properties would be to improve arterial stiffness through different mechanisms specific to the arterial hemodynamics. Unfortunately, to date no such drugs are available.

The need of the CAVI book

The increasing popularity of the latest method, the CAVI during the past five years in Asia, Europe and elsewhere is reflected by the number of published papers on CAVI which is increasing year by year and reached more than 630 in 2020. This extra ordinary development of CAVI justifies the publication of a book dedicated to this new and promising arterial parameter.

This book initiated by Pr Shirai, is intended to be a textbook which resumes in details a large part of the CAVI aspects going from its conception, principles, measurement method, to its many clinical applications. This book resumes the present knowledge on all the aspects of CAVI including its principles, measuring method, the VaSera system, its association with the cardiovascular risk factors and diseases, its impact in terms of prognosis (morbidity and mortality) in different populations as well as its role as a pharmacological tool to evaluate the effect of non-pharmacological and pharmacological treatments and finally the impact of its improvement on the patient prognosis. A total of 57 chapters written by outstanding experts, familiar with CAVI have contributed to this extraordinary achievement. This book aims to guide clinicians in the optimal applications of CAVI and to stimulate researchers in filling the gaps in knowledge by performing further studies.

Cardio-Ankle Vascular Index (CAVI) as an index of vascular function

Kohji Shirai[1,2]

The Cardio-ankle vascular index (CAVI) was developed as an index that reflects arterial stiffness in 2004. Since then, over 700 papers dealing with CAVI have been published in the last 15 years. The prominent feature of the index is its independence from blood pressure at measuring time. The meaning, role, and utility of CAVI seemed to be nearly established. Main epoch-making works by researchers all over the world were intended to be summarized in this book. The research presented in this book implies that the CAVI can be used to contribute to the development of the new field of vascular function beyond a marker of arteriosclerosis, and help promote the vascular health of humankind.

Why was CAVI born?

Arteries are not only a conduit for the blood; they also play a role in transporting the blood efficiently to peripheral organs, along with buffering and smoothing functions. The latter function is called the "Windkessel function" or vascular function, and arterial stiffness can influence this function. In case of cardiac functions, there are many established indices, but, for arterial stiffness, there had not been suitable indices, although many parameters were proposed. The reason for this may be due to that arterial stiffness is affected not only by the complex structure of arterial wall, but also by blood pressure changes and contractional state of the smooth muscles. Moreover, diameter of the arterial wall is not elongated linearly as a rubber. The pulse wave velocity (PWV) reflects arterial stiffness, and has been widely used for an index of arterial stiffness, but it is essentially dependent on blood pressure at measuring time. Thus, the real co-relationship between arterial stiffness and blood pressure could not be evaluated.

Hayashi et.al. presented the stiffness parameter β, which is essentially independent from blood pressure at measuring time. The cardio-ankle vascular index (CAVI) was developed as an index independent of blood pressure at measuring time by combining the theory of the stiffness parameter β and the Bramwell Hill equation[1]. Its independence from blood pressure was also confirmed experimentally.

Arteriosclerosis and the predictive role of cardiovascular events

CAVI is high in patients with various atherosclerotic diseases, including coronary artery disease and chronic

The roles of CAVI in clinical practice

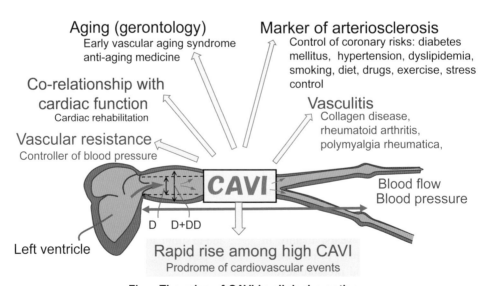

Fig. The roles of CAVI in clinical practice.

[1]Emeritus professor, Medical School, Toho university.
[2]Director, Seijinkai Mihama Hospital, 1-1-5 Utase, Mihama-ku, Chiba-shi, Chiba 261-0013, Japan.

kidney disease[2]. Most coronary risks cause an increase in CAVI and their improvement reduces CAVI. Many prospective studies have investigated the association between CAVI and future cardiovascular disease (CVD), and have proposed a CAVI of 9 as the optimal cut-off value for predicting CVD. These results implied that the significance of CAVI as organic arterial stiffness index was almost established.

Vascular function

Arterial stiffness consists of functional stiffness in addition to organic stiffness. Functional stiffness is derived from contraction and relaxation of the smooth muscle cells in the arterial medial layer. CAVI was shown to reflect this functional stiffness by pharmacological studies in both humans and animals. Nitroglycerin administration to men decreased their CAVI[3]. In animal studies, administration of the vasoconstrictor angiotensin II enhances blood pressure and CAVI[4].

This functional stiffness might be involved in the development of heart failure. It is reported that CAVI decreased during the treatment of patients with heart failure[5]. The CAVI of the patients who suffered from sepsis increased during recovery, suggesting that hypotension during sepsis may be due to relaxation of smooth muscle cell by endotoxins[6].

The above those studies indicated that CAVI reflects the relaxation or contraction of the arterial smooth muscle cells in the acute phase and suggest that it could be a useful index to reflect functional stiffness. Recently, patients with idiopathic pulmonary hypertension showed a high CAVI, which may be involved in the deterioration of the systemic circulation in idiopathic pulmonary hypertension[7].

Thus, CAVI is expected to uncover a new aspect of vascular function coordinating with cardiac function, and helps to develop the new field of vascular function.

Further role of CAVI

A rapid rise of CAVI was observed in patients during big earthquakes, and frequency of cerebrovascular events increased[8]. It has recently been reported that the blood supply of atheromatous lesion of the elastic and muscular arteries is mediated by the vasa vasorum. Considering that vasa vasorum penetrate the medial smooth muscle cell layers, the rapid rise of CAVI, which reflects the contraction of medial smooth muscle cells, induces choking of the vasa vasorum, leading to ischemia of the intimal atheromatous lesion. This may lead necrosis of the intimal plaque. This process could explain the process of plaque rupture, which provokes myocardial infarction. Thus, the rapid rise of CAVI in patients with high basal CAVI may be a warning sign of impending cardiovascular events.

The various proposed utilities of CAVI are shown in the figure. Each item has been described precisely in this book.

We are convinced that CAVI can contribute to the development of the new field of vascular function, and be useful in promoting the vascular health of humankind.

References

1) Shirai K, Utino J, Otsuka K, Takata M. A novel blood pressure-independent arterial wall stiffness parameter; cardio-ankle vascular index (CAVI). J Atheroscler Thromb 2006; 13:101-107.
2) Saiki A, Ohira M, Yamaguchi T, Nagayama D, Shimizu N, Shirai K, Tatsuno I. New Horizons of Arterial Stiffness Developed Using Cardio-ankle Vascular Index (CAVI). J Atheroscler Thromb 2020;27:732-748.
3) Shimizu K, Yamamoto T, Takahashi M, Sato S, Noike H, Shirai K. Effect of nitroglycerin administration on cardio-ankle vascular index. Vasc Health Risk Manag. 2016;12:313-9. doi: 10.2147/VHRM.S106542. eCollection 2016.
4) Sakuma K, Shimoda A, Shiratori H, Komatsu T, Watanabe K, Chiba T, Aimoto M, Nagasawa Y, Hori Y, Shirai K, Takahara A. Angiotensin II acutely increases arterial stiffness as monitored by cardio-ankle vascular index (CAVI) in anesthetized rabbits. J. Pharmacol. Sci. 2019;140:205-209.
5) Zang C, Ohira M, Iizuka T, Nakagami T, Suzuki M, Hirano K, Takahashi M, Shimizu M, Shimizu K, Sugiyama Y, Yamaguchi T, Kawana H, Endo K, Saiki A, Oyama T, Kurosu T, Tomaru T, Wang H, Noike H, Shirai K. Crdioankle vascular index relates to left ventricular ejection fraction in patients with heart failure. Reterospective Study, Int Heart J, 2013,54,216-21.
6) Nagayama D, Imamura H, Endo K, Saiki A, Sato Y, Yamaguchi T, Watanabe Y, Ohira M, Shirai K, Tatsuno I. Marker Of Sepsis Severity Is Associated With The Variation In Cardio-Ankle Vascular Index (CAVI) During Sepsis Treatment Vasc Health Risk Manag 2019;15:509-516.
7) Radchenko G D, Zhyvylo I O, Titov E Y, Sirenko Yuriy M. Systemic Arterial Stiffness in New Diagnosed Idiopathic Pulmonary Arterial Hypertension Patients. Vasc Health Risk Manag 2020;16:29-39.
8) Shimizu K, Takahashi M, Shirai K. A huge earthquake hardened arterial stiffness monitored with cardio-ankle vascular index J Atheroscler Thromb. 2013;20:503-11. doi: 10.5551/jat.16097. Epub 2013 Mar 25.

PART 1

The principle of CAVI and its measuring method

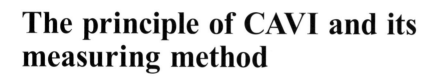

The principle of cardio-ankle vascular index (CAVI) and its features

Kohji Shirai[1,2] and Akira Takahara[3]

Preface

Arteries are not only conduits of the blood, but also play a role in transporting the blood efficiently to peripheral organs by buffering and smoothing against pulsatile blood flow. The latter function is called the "Windkessel function" or vascular function, and arterial stiffness is involved in this function. There had not been adequate indices of arterial stiffness reflecting vascular function itself. One of the reasons for this is the complicated arterial wall structure. It is composed of various materials such as collagen, elastin and hyaluronic acid and smooth muscle cells. Therefore, the diameter of arterial wall is not elongated linearly by intrinsic pressure as a rubber tube[1]. Hooke's law does not apply to the artery. Pulse wave velocity (PWV) is related to arterial stiffness, and has been used as an index of arterial stiffness[2]. However, it is essentially dependent on blood pressure at measuring time[3]. Therefore, PWV is inadequate to evaluate the effect of changes of blood pressure on proper arterial stiffness. Subsequently new index reflecting proper arterial stiffness had been pursued and cardio ankle vascular index (CAVI) was presented[4].

The principle of CAVI

CAVI was defined to reflect arterial stiffness of the arterial tree from the origin of the aorta to the ankle[4]. The specific feature is its independence from the blood pressure at measuring time. The reason for its independence from blood pressure is that CAVI is derived from the stiffness parameter β proposed by Hayashi et al.[1] and Kawasaki et al.[5].

The stiffness parameter β, which indicates the relationship between diameter changes and intrinsic pressure changes, is essentially independent from blood pressure at measuring time. It was applied to segmental artery such as the common carotid artery.

In order to measure the arterial stiffness of the arterial tree from the origin of the aorta to the ankle, CAVI was developed by combining the theory of stiffness parameter β and Bramwell Hill's equation, in which diameter changes in an artery and pulse wave velocity are related[6,7].

Equation of CAVI

The formula for CAVI is defined as follows and is shown schematically in Fig. 1

$$CAVI = a\{(2\rho/\Delta P) \times \ln(Ps/Pd) \, PWV^2\} + b$$
.... CAVI formula

where, Ps is the systolic blood pressure, Pd is the diastolic blood pressure, PWV is the pulse wave velocity from the origin of the aorta to tibial artery at the ankle through the femoral artery, ΔP is Ps - Pd, ρ is blood density, and a and b are constants.

The formula given above is a combination of the stiffness parameter β theory and Bramwell-Hill's equation as shown in Fig. 2; the process is as follows:

Stiffness parameter β equation
$$\beta = \ln (Ps/Pd) \cdot D/\Delta D$$

where D is the diameter of the artery, and ΔD is the change in diameter of the artery according to pressure change.

$D/\Delta D$ can be obtained from a modification of the Bramwell-Hill's equation[7] as follows:

$$PWV^2 = \Delta P/\rho \cdot V/\Delta V \doteqdot \Delta P/\rho \cdot D/2\Delta D \,..........\text{equation 1}$$

where ΔP is the pulse pressure, V is the volume of the blood vessel, ΔV is the change in V, and ρ is blood density

$$
\begin{aligned}
V/\Delta V &= \pi(D/2)^2 \\
&\times L \, / \, [\{\pi((D+\Delta D)/2)^2 - \pi(D/2)^2\} \times L] \\
&= D^2/ \, [D^2 + 2D\Delta D + \Delta D^2 - D^2] \\
&= D^2/ \, [2D\Delta D + \Delta D^2]
\end{aligned}
$$
ΔD^2 is too small and negligible
$$\doteqdot D/2\Delta D$$
$$\therefore PWV^2 = \Delta P/\rho \cdot V/\Delta V \doteqdot \Delta P/\rho \cdot D/2\Delta D$$
$$D/\Delta D = 2 \, \rho/\Delta P \cdot PWV^2$$

Then, $D/\Delta D$ is substituted into Stiffness parameter β equation as shown in Fig. 2

$$
\begin{aligned}
\text{Some length arterial } \beta &= \ln(Ps/Pd) \cdot (D/\Delta D) \\
&\doteqdot \ln(Ps/Pd) \cdot 2\rho/\Delta P \cdot PWV^2
\end{aligned}
$$

$$CAVI = a[\ln(Ps/Pd) \cdot 2\rho/\Delta P \cdot PWV^2] + b$$
a, b: coefficients

[1]Emeritus professor, Medical School, Toho university.
[2]Director, Seijinkai Mihama Hospital, 1-1-5 Utase, Mihama-ku, Chiba-shi, Chiba 261-0013, Japan.
[3]Department of Pharmacology and Therapeutics, Faculty of Pharmaceutical Sciences, Toho University, 2-2-1 Miyama, Funabashi, Chiba 274-8510, Japan.

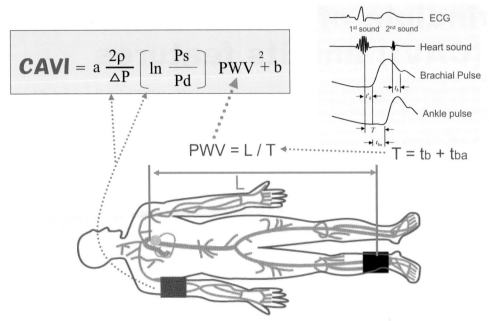

(Shirai K, Utino J, et. al. J Arteriosclerosis Thrombosis, 2006, 13: 101-107[4], modified)

Fig. 1.   Cardio Ankle Vascular Stiffness Index (CAVI).

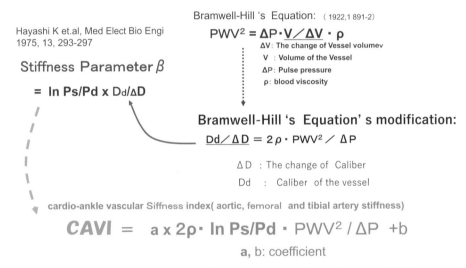

Fig. 2.   CAVI equation derived from stiffness parameter β and Bramwell-Hill's equation.

This new index has been named the cardio-ankle vascular index (CAVI), which reflects the stiffness of the aorta, femoral artery and tibial artery as a whole. Coefficients a and b were adopted to be adjusted to the value of Hasegawa's heart-femoral PWV (hfPWV)※, and were disclosed by Takahashi et al.[8]. The scene of measuring CAVI is shown in Fig. 3.

Ingenuity to obtain the accurate value of haPWV in the VaSera system

Obtaining accurate value of haPWV remains challenging, because it is difficult to detect duration (T) of the time from which the pulse begins at the orifice of the left ventricle to

Table.   Coefficients "a" and "b" in CAVI (Ref. 8).

haβ before transformation	Low Range	Middle Range	High Range
	< 7.34875		10.30372 <
Coefficient a	0.850	0.628	0.432
Coefficient b	0.658	2.103	4.441

Abbreviations: haβ, heart-ankle BETA

the time at which the pulse reaches the ankle; detection of the beginning time of the pulse based on the cardiac sound I is difficult, because the cardiac sound I includes various

---

※ hfPWV is proposed by Hasegawa[9] and had been widely used in Japan. Its main feature differed from other PWV indices such as cfPWV and baPWV, is that for the purpose of blood pressure independency, the value was compensated for at 80 mmHg of diastolic pressure. There were a massive amount of data accumulated during 1970~2000 in Japan.

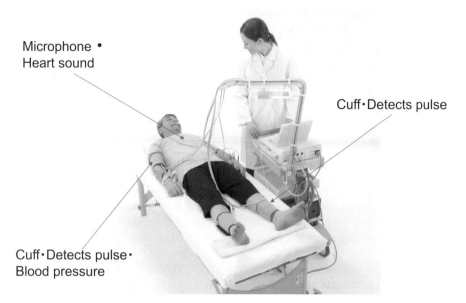

Microphone •
Heart sound

Cuff·Detects pulse

Cuff·Detects pulse·
Blood pressure

Fig. 3. How to Measure CAVI.

sounds such as mitral valve closure. The beginning of the QRS time in ECG does not correspond to the beginning time of the pulse.

To obtain the T in the VaSera system, a slightly complicated method was adopted according to the method of Hasegawa PWV[9] as shown in the right panel in Fig. 1. The T was divided into two parts; the time from assumed beginning of cardiac sound I (opening point of aortic valve) to the rise of a brachial pulse ($t_{b'}$), and the time from the rise of a brachial pulse to a rise of a pulse at the ankle (t_{ba}). While the detection of $t_{b'}$ was difficult, the time from the beginning of the heart sound II to the notch time of the brachial pulse (t_b) was obtained accurately: to calculate T, t_b was used in place of $t_{b'}$.

Thus, an accurate time "T" is obtained by the following equation.

$$T = t_{b'} + t_{ba} \doteqdot t_b + t_{ba}$$

Blood pressure used for CAVI

Equation 1 indicates that CAVI can be calculated by the values of systolic and diastolic blood pressures and haPWV. The values of blood pressures used in this equation should be the mean of the total blood pressure from the origin of the aorta to the tibial artery at the ankle. However, it is impossible to measure the mean of the total blood pressure. In case of CAVI, the blood pressure in the upper brachial artery was adopted for the mean of the total blood pressure. This was based on assumption that the blood pressure in the brachial artery may be representative of the mean of the total blood pressure in the arteries from the origin of aorta to the ankle. The available clinical data supported the rationality of this assumption[8].

Thus, CAVI is obtained non-invasively by measuring the haPWV and the blood pressures. The device 'VaSera' was developed by Fukuda Co., Ltd, Tokyo, Japan, and the measuring scene of CAVI using the VaSera is shown in Fig. 3.

The Length of the arterial tree From the Origin of the Aorta to the Ankle

The length of the artery to obtain pulse wave velocity is defined as follows: L1: from the aortic valve to the femoral artery, L2: from the femoral to the popliteal artery, and L3: from the popliteal artery to the ankle. L1 is calculated as L1 = 1.3 × AF(aorta to femoral) using Nye's method[22], where AF is the direct distance from the sternum at the second intercostal space to the femoral artery at the groin. Thus, the total length of the arteries from the heart to the ankle is calculated as L = L1 + L2 + L3.

When using the VaSera device's automatic measurement mode, L is calculated from the subject's height using the following equation:

$$L = 7.7685 \times \text{body height} - 17.536$$

This formula was obtained from the correlation equation between L and the body height of the 813 subjects at Mihama Hospital[8].

Blood Density ρ

Because the blood density in individuals is generally between 1.045 and 1.05523), the fixed value of 1.05 is used in the CAVI equation[10].

Rationale of CAVI as a stiffness index for a certain length of artery

The question of whether it is acceptable to apply the stiffness parameter β determined at the segment of the artery to an index reflecting the stiffness of a long arterial tree would be raised. One of the answers to this question came from a report that the CAVI value had a strong correlation with the β value measured at a segment of the descending thoracic aorta using ultrasonography[11].

Horinaka et al. also reported that the regional values of

the stiffness parameter β of the ascending and descending aorta were both significantly correlated with CAVI values[12]. Similar results were also obtained on examination of the common carotid artery. In both arteries, the correlation coefficients between CAVI and the stiffness parameter β were 0.67 and 0.39, respectively, with p-values of less than 0.01.

No dependency on heart rate

It is reported that an increase in heart rate causes a small increase in the PWV (measured using the transit-time method) in humans[13]. CAVI is not affected by the changes in heart rate. Ventricular pacing with an AV block under anesthesia showed no change in CAVI.

This has been described by Saiki and Takahara in Chapter 5.

At which blood pressure was the pulse wave velocity measured in the VaSera system?

It is known that pulse wave velocity changes with blood pressure changes from diastolic pressure to systolic pressure[14]. This is very important point to define CAVI. It has been shown that the PWV used for the calculation of CAVI in the VaSera system is at mid-pressure[15]. However, the PWV used for the $CAVI_0$ proposed by Spronck et al.[16] was at diastolic pressure. Thus, the $CAVI_0$ showed erroneous values[15, 17]. This has been described in detail in Chapter 3.

Confirmation of Independency of CAVI on blood pressure at measuring time by clinical and animal experiments

Theoretically, CAVI is independent from blood pressure

at measuring time, because it is derived from the stiffness parameter β, which is not affected by blood pressure at measuring time.

Experimentally, Shirai et al. also[18] showed that CAVI values were not affected by blood pressure when blood pressure was reduced with the administration of a β1 blocker, metoprolol (Fig. 4 left). As is well known, β1 blockers decrease blood pressure by the reduction of heart muscle contractions without affecting arterial smooth muscles. As a result, CAVI remains unchanged even though blood pressure decreases. This result supports the independence of CAVI from blood pressure variations at the measuring time.

As for the independence of CAVI from blood pressure at measuring time, there may be a limited range of blood pressure over which this independence lasts. Hayashi et al.[1] showed that the liner relationship between the distension ratio and log P/Ps is observed between blood pressure values of 60 to 160 mmHg. Therefore, it can be said that CAVI is independent of blood pressure variations between a systolic blood pressure of 63 to 200 mmHg[6].

When an α1 blocker, doxazosin, was administered, CAVI decreased with a decrease in blood pressure as shown in Fig. 4 right[18]. CAVI is apparently dependent on blood pressure. However, in this case, the α1 blocker reduces blood pressure by relaxation of vascular smooth muscles. This reduction of vascular smooth muscle contractions induces a decrease in arterial stiffness, leading to a decrease in CAVI. This result indicates that CAVI reflects the functional arterial stiffness depending on vascular smooth muscle contraction in addition to organic stiffness.

Anyhow, there are some papers describing that CAVI is

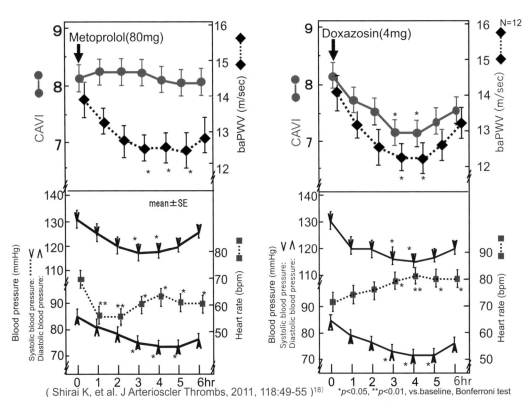

(Shirai K, et al. J Arterioscler Thrombs, 2011, 118:49-55)[18]   *p<0.05, **p<0.01, vs.baseline, Bonferroni test

Fig. 4.   Effects of metoprolol and doxazosin on CAVI.

relatively or less dependent from blood pressure at measuring time. Someone pointed out that CAVI was correlated with blood pressure in epidemiologic studies, and insisted that CAVI is dependent on blood pressure. This is obvious misunderstanding.

Based on above experimental results, it is confirmed that CAVI measured using the VaSera system is independent from blood pressure at measuring time[17].

Reproducibility of CAVI

The results of a reproducibility study on CAVI values measured in the same person (n = 22) 5 times on different days showed that the mean value of the coefficients of variation of different people was 3.8%[4]. This has been described in detail by Kubozono (Chapter 4-3). Here, we must remember that arterial stiffness is composed of organic stiffness and functional stiffness, and the latter essentially changes with blood pressure to maintain general circulatory homeostasis.

Various affecting conditions of CAVI

1) Daily rhythm of CAVI

The daily rhythm of CAVI is not observed in healthy people. However, cases of pathological conditions such as those of hypertensive patients with a morning surge showed higher CAVI values. This has been described in Chapter 5.

2) Room temperature, Smoking and Exercise

The effect of room temperature, food intake, smoking, and exercise on CAVI might be expected. For example, during the cold stress test, CAVI was enhanced, accompanied by enhanced blood pressures (not published). It is recommended that room temperature should be kept at 24°C to 26°C during the measurement of CAVI. Moreover, exercise caused a decrease in CAVI. Smoking immediately raised CAVI in a few minutes. This is described in detail in chapter 4-1. Heavy exercise and smoking should be avoided 3 to 4 hours prior to CAVI measurement.

Limitations of CAVI at a low Ankle Brachial Index

For patients with arteriosclerotic obliteration in the femoral artery, haPWV is apparently low, because stricture of artery delays PWV. Resultantly, lower values of CAVI are observed. CAVI is invalid when Ankle Brachial Index (ABI), which is the ratio of systolic blood pressure in the tibial artery to that in the brachial artery, is less than 0.9.

How to use CAVI in clinical practice

Arterial stiffness itself changes every moment according to the physical and mental states of the individuals. CAVI reflects both organic stiffness and functional stiffness. Therefore, CAVI changes essentially every moment. Measurement of CAVI in clinical practice is recommended at least every 1 to 3 months for coronary risk management such as life style modifications and the administration of various drugs.

In the future, daily measurement of CAVI might be needed just like measurement of blood pressure to control vascular health.

Application of CAVI theory to the measurement of the arterial stiffness of segmental arteries in the future

CAVI reflects the arterial stiffness of the arterial tree from the origin of the aorta to the ankle. The arterial stiffness of segmental arteries such as the aorta and femoral artery can be measured by application of the CAVI theory. Yamamoto et al.[19] reported that the stiffness of the aorta (heart-thigh β (htBeta)) and of the femoral-tibial arteries (thigh to ankle β (taBeta)) could be monitored by applying the CAVI theory, and that a nitroglycerin-induced decrease of arterial stiffness is more prominent in muscular arteries than in elastic arteries; this effect was preserved in arteriosclerotic patients. Katsuta[20] reported that femoral Beta decreased, but aortic Beta was increased during the administration of phentolamine in rabbits. These results suggest that the measurement of arterial stiffness of segmental arteries by applying the CAVI theory is possible, and may contribute to clarification of cross-talk between the elastic and muscular arteries.

References

1) Hayashi K, Handa H, Nagasawa S, Okumura A, Moritake K. Stiffness and elastic behavior of human intracranial and extracranial arteries. J Biomech, 1980;13:175-184.
2) Asmar R. Pulse wave velocity principles and measurement, In: Arterial Stiffness and Pulse Wave Velocity: Clinical Applications (Ed. by Asmar, R., O'Rourke, M.F., Safar, M.). Amsterdam: Elsevier;1999. pp. 25-55.
3) Nye ER, The effect of blood pressure alteration on the pulse wave velocity. Br Heart J, 1964;266,261-265.
4) Shirai K, Utino J, Otsuka K, Takata M. A novel blood pressure-independent arterial wall stiffness parameter; Cardio-ankle vascular index (CAVI). J Atheroscler Thromb, 2006;13,101-107.
5) Kawasaki T, Sasayama S, Yagi S. Noninvasive assessment of the age related changes in stiffness of major branches of the human arteries. Cardiovasc Res,1987; 21:678-687.
6) Hayashi K, Yamamoto T, Takahara A, Shirai K. Clinical assessment of arterial stiffness with cardio-ankle vascular index: theory and applications. J Hypertens. 2015 ;33:1742-57.
7) Bramwell JC, Hill AV. Velocity of the pulse wave in man. Proc Roy Soc, 1922;B:298-306.
8) Takahashi K, Yamamoto T, Tsuda S, Okabe F, Shimose T, Tsuji Y, Suzuki K, Otsuka K, Takata M, Shimizu K, Uchino J, Shirai K. Coefficients in the CAVI Equation and the Comparison Between CAVI With and Without the Coefficients Using Clinical Data. J Atheroscler Thromb. 2019;26:465-475.
9) Hasegawa M. Fundamental research on human aortic pulse wave velocity. Jikei Med J 1970; 85: 742-60. (in Japanese)
10) Nakamori Eizi. An investigation on hematological measurements for screening purpose. Jap J Ind Health, 1971; 13: 191-212 (in Japanese).
11) Takaki A, Ogawa H, Wakeyama T, Iwami T, Kimura M, Hadano Y, et al. Cardio-ankle vascular index is a new noninvasive parameter of arterial stiffness. Circ J 2007; 71: 1710-14.
12) Horinaka S, Yagi H, Ishimura K, Fukushima H, Shibata Y, Sugawara R, et al. Cardio-ankle vascular index (CAVI) correlates with aortic stiffness in the thoracic aorta using

ECG-gated multi-detector row computed tomography. Atheroscler 2014 ;235: 239-45.

13) Mangoni AA, Mircoli L, Giannattasio C, Ferrari AU, Mancia G. Heart rate-dependence of arterial distensibility in vivo. J Hypertens 1996;14:897–901.

14) Hermeling E, Vermeersch SJ, Rietzschel ER, et al. The change in arterial stiffness over the cardiac cycle rather than diastolic stiffness is independently associated with left ventricular mass index in healthy middle-aged individuals. *J Hypertens.* 30:396-402.

15) Shirai K, Suzuki K, Tsuda S, Shimizu K, Takata M, Yamamoto T, Maruyama M, Takahashi K. Comparison of Cardio-Ankle Vascular Index (CAVI) and CAVI $_0$ in Large Healthy and Hypertensive Populations. J Atheroscler Thromb 2019;26:603-615. doi: 10.5551/jat.48314. Epub 2019 May 9.

16) Spronck B, Avolio AP, Tan I, Butlin M, Reesink KD, Delhaas T. Arterial stiffness index beta and cardio-ankle vascular index inherently dependent on blood pressure but can be readily corrected. J Hypertens, 2017; 35: 98-104.

17) Takahashi K, Yamamoto T, Tsuda S, Maruyama M, Shirai K. The Background of Calculating CAVI: Lesson from the Discrepancy Between CAVI and CAVI0. Vasc Health Risk Manag. 2020 ;16:193-201.

18) Shirai K, Song M, Suzuki J, Kurosu T, Oyama T, Nagayama D, et al. Contradictory effects of β1- and α1-aderenergic receptor blockers on cardio-ankle vascular stiffness index (CAVI) - The independency of CAVI from blood pressure. J Atheroscler Thromb 2011; 18: 49-55.

19) Yamamoto T, Shimizu K, Takahashi M, Tatsuno I, Shirai K. The Effect of Nitroglycerin on Arterial Stiffness of the Aorta and the Femoral-Tibial Arteries.J Atheroscler Thromb. 2017 ;24:1048-1057. doi: 10.5551/jat.38646. Epub 2017 Mar 22.

20) Katsuda SI, Fujikura Y, Horikoshi Y, Hazama A, Shimizu T, Shirai K. Different Responses of Arterial Stiffness between the Aorta and the Iliofemoral Artery during the Administration of Phentolamine and Atenolol in Rabbits.J Atheroscler Thromb. 2021;28:611-621.

Background of development of the cardio-ankle vascular index

Masanobu Takata[1], Maiko Ohara[2] and Tsutomu Koike[2]

The use of VaSera (Fukuda Denshi, Tokyo, Japan) measuring the cardio-ankle vascular index (CAVI) and ankle brachial index has increased significantly, and 20,000 units are now deployed in Japan and other countries[1]. CAVI is a simple and accurate measure of the extent of blood pressure-independent arterial stiffness and can be used to estimate the vascular age[2,3]. However, the importance of CAVI is not yet recognized worldwide. In Europe and the United States, the carotid-femoral pulse wave velocity (cfPWV) is used to assess the degree of arteriosclerosis (**Table 1**)[4,5].

In this review, we present the series of steps taken in Japan by Hasegawa and Kawasaki in their search for "an arterial stiffness indicator that is not significantly affected by blood pressure," which was the beginning of the development of CAVI. We describe the development of CAVI and explain how differences in sex and aging affect the results obtained with CAVI, compared to those with cfPWV and the augmentation index (AI), which are conventional vascular stiffness indicators.

1) Is the carotid-femoral pulse wave velocity (cfPWV) the gold standard for artery stiffness?

Before Korotkov developed a method to measure blood pressure, analysis of pulse waves was used to estimate blood pressure. During that time, the PWV was estimated using the difference in distance and time between the muscular blood vessels in the upper or lower limbs. However, since the muscular arteries are affected by blood pressure and sympathetic nerve activity, the degree of arteriosclerosis could not be accurately determined. The cfPWV developed by Frank in 1926 was measured in the elastic blood vessels and provided an approximate estimation of the degree of arteriosclerosis; the measurement methods based on this principle are still used in Europe and the United States (**Fig. 1 left**).

$$cfPWV = D/t$$

D (distance): three segments were measured. A:distance from the heart to the umbilicus; B: distance from the umbilicus to the femoral artery; C: distance from the heart to the carotid artery; and finally, distance D measured as the total of A + B - C.

t: the time lag between the uprise of the carotid artery pulse wave and that of the femoral artery pulse wave

Aortic PWV (aPWV) refers to the PWV of the elastic blood vessels, and the cfPWV and heart-femoral PWV (hfPWV) are also utilized as aPWV[6]. However, aPWV is not simply an indicator of arteriosclerosis. aPWV is an indicator based on intra-aortic pressure, aging, and aortic stiffness; moreover, it is also affected by the heart rate. In particular, the influence of blood pressure makes follow-up observations in the same subject and comparisons between

Table 1. Non-invasive measurement of vascular elasticity.

	BP dependency
I. Pulse wave analysis	
A. Aortic pulse wave velocity (PWV)	
1. Carotid-femoral PWV (cfPWV)(Frank's method) -	+
2. Heart-femoral PWV (hfPWV) corrected by blood pressure (Hasegawa's method) - -	−
B. Brachial-ankle PWV (baPWV). - - - - - - - - - - - - - - - - - -- - - - - - - - - - - - - -	+
C. Augmentation index (AI)- -	+
II. Regional arterial caliber changes analysis	
A. Stiffness parameter β - - - - - - - - - - - - - - - -- -	−
B. Arterial distensibility, arterial compliance, or elastic modulus (Young's modulus) - - -	+
III. Cardio-ankle vascular index (CAVI) -- -- - - - - - - - - - -	−

[1]Department of Internal Medicine, Toyama Nishi General Hospital, 1019 Shimokutuwada, Fuchumachi, Toyama-shi, Toyama, 939-2716, Japan. E mail: masanobutakata@gmail.com
[2]The Second Department of Internal Medicine, University of Toyama, 2630 Sugitani, Toyama-shi, Toyama, 930-0194, Japan.

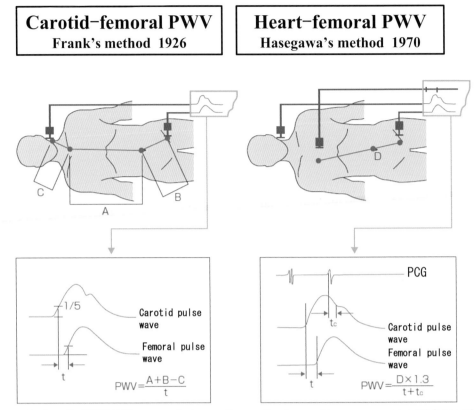

Fig. 1. Measurement of aortic PWV. Differences between the methods used to measure carotid-femoral PWV (cfPWV) and heart-femoral PWV (hfPWV).

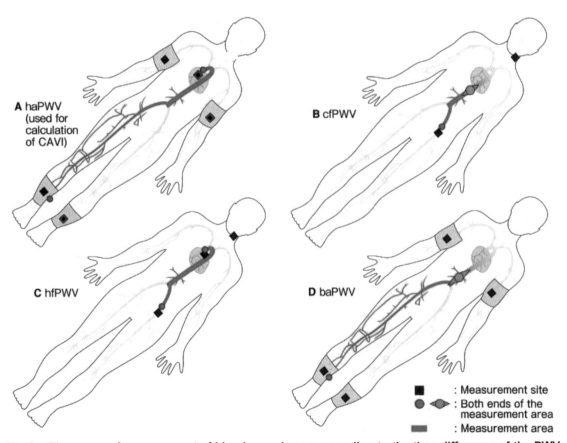

Fig. 2. The scope of measurement of blood vessels corresponding to the time difference of the PWV.

subjects difficult. Statistical analysis is required to determine the degree of severity of atherosclerosis and for follow-up observations after treatment, which limit its clinical usefulness. Therefore, determining arterial stiffness from aPWV depends on how well the impact of blood pressure and aging can be eliminated to evaluate only the stiffness of the artery.

Another challenge with cfPWV is the mismatch between the time difference and the distance. With cfPWV, the time difference is detected by simultaneously recording the carotid pulse wave and the femoral wave, and the PWV is calculated along the distance between a measured "non-specific point" in the descending aorta (the place at which the pulse wave of the descending artery arrives, at the same time when the pulse wave of the carotid artery arrives at the point where the carotid artery is measured) and the point at which the pulse wave of the femoral artery is measured (**Fig. 2**). The central aorta is not considered while measuring cfPWV; hence, the time difference and the distance do not correspond accurately. Nevertheless, this method is used because the measurement is performed in elastic blood vessels, although the degree of blood vessel elasticity and PWV vary at different distances from the aortic arch (**Fig. 3**). This discrepancy cannot be ignored because the PWV in the aorta varies in each region[7, 8]. In addition, the measured length of the aorta is not the same as that in Frank's original method and varies between commercial cfPWV instruments[9]. An expert consensus document determined that the measured cfPWV should be 80% of the direct carotid-femoral distance. Furthermore, the recommended cut-off value was changed from 12 m/s to 10 m/s in 2012[9]. However, the lengths measured by instruments manufactured by different companies have not been standardized.

2) The pressure-corrected "heart-femoral PWV (hfPWV)" as the gold standard in Japan

In the cfPWV reported by Frank, measurements did not include the central portion of the ascending aorta and aortic arch. In 1970, Hasegawa and his associates measured aPWV (hfPWV) over a fixed distance from the aortic valve to the femoral artery, by simultaneously recording the carotid artery pulse wave, femoral artery pulse wave, and heart sounds[10, 11]. Here, tc is the time for pulse transmission from the aortic valve area (point A) to the carotid artery (point C)[12]. When a pulse is transmitted to point X on the descending aorta, tc indicates the time for pulse transmission between point A and point X. Similarly, the time of pulse transmission between point X and point F (femoral artery) corresponds to t. Based on these values, the time of pulse transmission from point A to point F is determined (t + tc). The length of the arterial path between the second intercostal space at the right sternal margin and the groin is calculated as 1.3 times the distance between point A and point F as the anatomical modification value (**Fig. 1 right**)[13].

$$hfPWV = (D \times 1.3)/(t + tc)$$

D: the straight distance between the second intercostal space at the right sternal margin and the pulsatile part of the femoral artery

t: the time lag between the uprise of the carotid artery pulse wave and that of the femoral artery pulse wave

tc: the time lag between the precomponent of the cardiac II sound and the dicrotic notch of the carotid artery pulse wave

The cfPWV does not consider the central aorta and uses an ambiguous measurement interval, whereas, with hfPWV, the time difference and distance are accurately matched. Simultaneously, they confirmed that the hfPWV of an alive

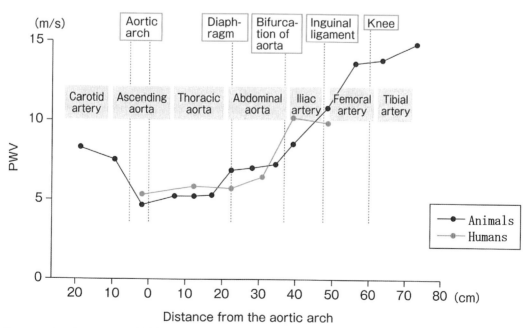

Fig. 3. Progressive increase in PWV with increasing distance from the heart in animals and humans.
Cited from ref.7 【with permission of Elsevier】

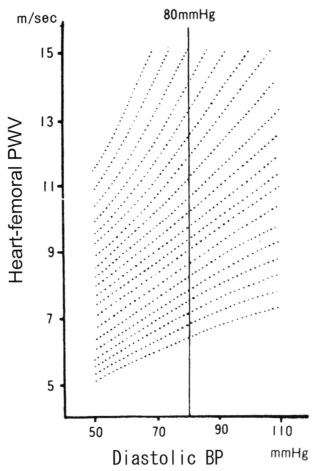

Fig. 4. Nomogram for correction of hfPWV measured to hfPWV at a given constant blood pressure.

individual showed a very strong dependence on the internal pressure. Through basic experiments using isolated aorta, they showed that an important factor affecting hfPWV is the diastolic blood pressure, and they compared subjects by using a nomograph corrected for a diastolic blood pressure of 80 mmHg (**Fig. 4**). Hasegawa's PWV, namely the hfPWV corrected for diastolic blood pressure, was incorporated into aPWV measurement devices by Fukuda Denshi in 1985. Many reports have confirmed the usefulness of the original PWV (Hasegawa's PWV or hfPWV) method in long-term prognostic studies of cardiovascular disease events. In a meta-analysis of aortic PWV[6], 3 of the 19 studies cited examined hfPWV corrected for diastolic blood pressure, while one examined hfPWV not corrected by blood pressure. Hasegawa's PWV was the gold standard to assess arterial stiffness for a long time in Japan. However, this method has been rarely used in other countries.

3) Pressure- independent "stiffness parameter β"

Aortic PWV evaluates the stiffness of a large blood vessel from the longitudinal aspect. In contrast, with the development and spread of ultrasonography, it has become common to examine vascular stiffness based on the caliber changes in a blood vessel. However, the disadvantage of this method is that the measurements are greatly affected by

the intra-aortic pressure (blood pressure); hence, a variety of pressure corrections have been attempted[14]. Of these, the stiffness parameter β, proposed by Hayashi et al.[15] and clinically applied by Kawasaki et al.[12,16,17], has been regarded as the arterial stiffness indicator least affected by the blood pressure for many years. The stiffness parameter β is derived from a correction of the logarithmic pressure ratio animals such as dogs and rabbits, as well as humans.

The β value is obtained by substituting the relevant readings into Kawasaki's equation[17], which is derived from Hayashi's equation[16], as follows:

$$\beta = \ln (Ps/Pd)/[(Ds - Dd)/Dd]$$

Ps: systolic blood pressure
Pd: diastolic blood pressure
Ds: arterial diameter at systole
Dd: arterial diameter at diastole

With the internal pressure/diameter relationship of an artery in a physiological state, assuming the internal pressure to be 100 mmHg, standardizing the diameter to correspond to an internal pressure of 100 mmHg, and expressing the internal pressure parameter as a logarithm and re-plotting, they obtained a linear relationship within the physiological range of 60 to 160 mmHg (**Fig. 5**). In other words, the stiffness parameter approximates the pressure/caliber relationship of the artery within the range of physiological pressures with a simple index function, quantifying the non-linearity.

The caliber of the abdominal aorta or the common carotid artery, and the caliber displacement corresponding to the blood pressure fluctuation in a single heartbeat, are determined accurately (within 0.01 mm) using a phase-tracking ultrasonic displacement meter interlocked with a real-time linear array scanner. However, the measurement device used in this method (Hitachi Healthcare, Chiba, Japan) is very expensive, and the measurements require technical skill; hence, it has not been widely used.

4) The brachial-ankle PWV (baPWV): easily measured, but inaccurate

The Form PWV/ABI, which measures the brachial-ankle pulse PWV (baPWV) (Colin Co. Ltd., Komaki, Japan), was developed in Japan in 1999. Measurements with this method are easy to perform compared to the conventional aortic PWV[18]. Calculation of the distance is based on estimates based on the height of the Japanese population. The baPWV extends the cfPWV's pulse wave area from the carotid artery to the brachial artery and from the femoral artery to the ankle, eliminating the disadvantages of measuring pulse waves in the inguinal region; the measurements usually require 3 to 4 minutes.

1) The PWV between the heart and the arm (brachium) (hbPWV)

hbPWV = Lb/Tb

Lb: the path length from the aortic valve area to the brachial artery

Tb: the time lag between the precomponent of the cardiac II sound and the dicrotic notch of the brachial artery pulse

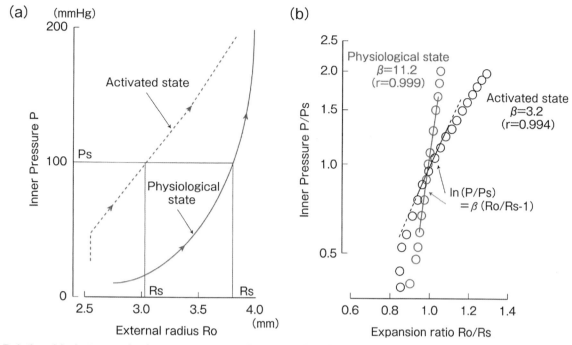

Fig. 5. Relationship between the inner pressure and outer radius (a) and relationship between the inner pressure ratio and expansion ratio (b) under the physiological state and activated state.

wave

2) The haPWV is the PWV between the heart and the ankle.

haPWV = La/(Ta + Tb)

La: the path length from the aortic valve area to the ankle

Ta: the time lag between the uprise of the pulse wave of the brachial artery and that of the posterior tibial artery

3) The baPWV is defined as follows

baPWV = (La − Lb)/Ta

This method avoids the need to detect the dicrotic notch of the brachial artery pulse wave to measure the hbPWV. The measurement of Ta is very simple and accurate. Both aortic PWV (cfPWV and hfPWV) methods involve elastic vessels, whereas baPWV is a PWV that includes the muscular vessels of the upper and lower limbs. Since the PWV is different for each arterial segment, the last equation is incorrect[19]. When using this equation, the distance corresponding to the difference in the time between the brachial and ankle pulse waves will vary widely depending on the degree of stiffness of the aortic walls. As the measured Ta is shorter than the actual value, the values of baPWV are approximately twice as high as the known aPWV[20]. The use of antihypertensive drugs reduces the baPWV, because decreased blood pressure lowers the PWV, even without a change in the intrinsic arterial stiffness.

5) Augmentation index (AI)

Pressure pulsations generated by the left ventricle are propagated by the arterial walls to the periphery (ejection wave). As the arterial tree branches toward the periphery, the arterial lumen narrows, thus increasing the vascular resistance, resulting in backpropagation (reflected wave). Increased aortic stiffness increases the reflected waves

because it accelerates the PWV. The AI is the ratio of the reflected wave to this ejection wave[21]. As a non-invasive measurement method, the pulse wave of the carotid artery was initially used as a surrogate of the central aorta. The aortic root blood pressure waveform is estimated using the generalized transfer function (GTF) from the radial arterial blood pressure waveform, and the ejection wave and reflected wave are conveniently obtained by automatic calculation. The method of obtaining the GTF is complicated[22]. Compared with PWVs, the AI has the disadvantage of smaller changes in the elderly or patients with advanced atherosclerosis (**Fig. 6**)[23]. There are also inconsistencies, such as higher values in females due to the differences in height. In Japan, the equipment for measuring AI utilizes the fact that the second systolic peak pressure of the radial artery blood pressure waveform matches the systolic maximum blood pressure of the central aortic blood pressure waveform. This is unlike the measurements used in the GTF method, which was once commercially available but was discontinued (Omron Healthcare Co. Ltd., Kyoto, Japan)[24].

Both methods could estimate the central aortic pressure simultaneously with AI measurement. However, in the upper arm, systolic blood pressure values obtained by the indirect method using Korotkoff sounds are lower than the intra-brachial arterial pressure values[25]. Hence, central blood pressure estimates using the GTF showed values approximately 10 mmHg lower than the catheter values[26] and this ambiguity might have caused confusion, limiting the widespread uptake of AI and central blood pressure measurement equipment[27]. Recent reports show that central pulse pressure is not more closely associated with cardiovascular events than peripheral pulse pressure[28].

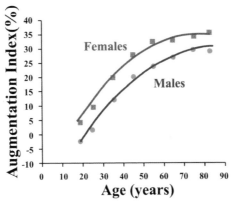 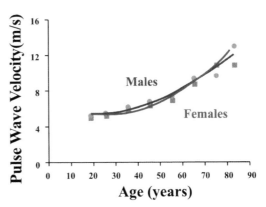

Fig. 6.   Differences of age and gender in AI and cfPWV.
Cited from ref.23 【with permission of Elsevier】

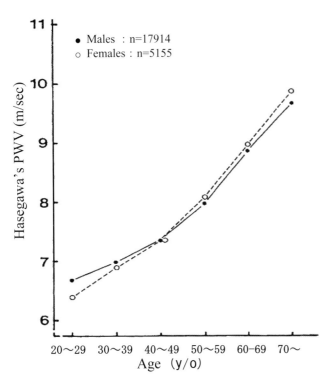

● Males : n=17914
○ Females : n=5155

Fig. 7. Gender differences in Hasegawa's PWV.
Cited from ref.31

6) Blood pressure correction application in the principles of CAVI

CAVI quantifies the stiffness of blood vessels based on the stiffness parameter β theory by applying the Bramwell-Hill formula and applies a scale conversion to Hasegawa's hfPWV (pressure-corrected hfPWV). (see chapter 1-1)[29]. The reason for using a scale conversion to the "pressure-corrected hfPWV" was that there were already many users of the pressure-corrected hfPWV. In Japan, Hasegawa's PWV was considered the gold standard for measuring arterial stiffness for a long period. Many users could therefore easily switch from aPWV to CAVI. The challenge for Hasegawa and his associates was to eliminate the effect of blood pressure from aPWV and the culmination of this approach was the development of CAVI. CAVI is completely different from the concept of PWV. Of course, when CAVI

is measured, both baPWV and haPWV are calculated simultaneously.

7) Gender difference and aging: different effects on arterial stiffness parameters

Several investigators have examined the effect of age and sex on AI and cfPWV. The arterial pressure waveform is a composite of two waveforms, namely a forward pressure wave and a backward wave. Therefore, the reflected waves increase as the aPWV increases or if the person is short, and as a result, the AI values are affected by height. Generally, AI values are higher in females than in males (**Table 2**). Furthermore, there is a tendency for the rate of change to decrease with aging and an increase in the severity of arteriosclerosis. In other words, AI depends on PWV and BP and is inversely proportional to the heart rate and height. In contrast, with cfPWV (**Fig. 6**), the differences are small in younger people and large in older people[30]. Furthermore, no sexual differences are seen with cfPWV. It has been reported that Hasegawa's aPWV is higher in males than in females until their 40s, and conversely is higher in females than in males from their 50s onward (17,914 males, 5,155 females) (**Fig. 7**)[31].

The standardization of CAVI in healthy subjects was conducted among subjects undergoing routine health checks[32]. Analysis of results in healthy subjects, excluding those with hypertension, dyslipidemia, or diabetes, showed that CAVI values increase almost linearly with age for both males and females by approximately 0.5 every ten years. Furthermore, the CAVI values in males are approximately 0.2 higher than in females in each age group, corresponding to an age difference of approximately four to five years (See the Figure, shown in Chapter 6. Fig. 1). This gender difference and effect of aging observed with CAVI is quite different from the results obtained with AI and cfPWV, the conventional indicators of arteriosclerosis. In clinical practice, arteriosclerosis is known to progress with aging, and the progress is faster in males than in females, indicating that the above results with CAVI are reliable. There are no factors related to gender difference or aging in the mathematical formula for CAVI; thus, we can conclude that we have now entered a new era as the extremely fundamental

Table 2. Differences according to gender and aging in AI, cfPWV, and CAVI.

	Gender difference	Aging	Other factors
✓ Augmentation Index	F > M	Non-linear	Height, heart rate, blood pressure
✓ Carotid-femoral PWV	F = M	Non-linear	Blood pressure, heart rate
✓ CAVI	F < M	Linear	

challenges with indicators of arteriosclerosis that have been a major subject for debate for a long time, have now been solved with the development of CAVI.

The CAVI value of a healthy subject can be predicted from their gender and age. From this predicted value and the actual CAVI measurements, we can estimate the vascular age of each individual. Broadly speaking, vascular age is the sum of the physiological age and disease-related aging.

In conclusion, most clinicians are keen to have an easy method to determine accurate arterial stiffness and/or vascular age. For the development of an arterial stiffness parameter that excludes the impact of blood pressure, the pioneering research of Hasegawa was applied to the blood pressure-corrected hfPWV. Following Hayashi's theory, Hasegawa's associate Kawasaki developed the stiffness parameter β, which remains an excellent pressure-independent local arterial stiffness indicator. Hasegawa also contributed to the early development of CAVI. CAVI can be regarded as the final version of all previous blood pressure-corrected parameters. It inherits their accuracy, and is simple to measure by anyone. The advantage of reproducibility, with little disparity between the institutions, has opened the possibility for multicenter studies.

References

1) Shirai K, Utino J, Otsuka K, Takata M. A novel blood pressure-independent arterial wall stiffness parameter; cardio-ankle vascular index. J Atheroscler Thromb. 2006;13:101-107.
2) Shirai K, Hiruta N, Song M, et al. Cardio-ankle vascular index as a novel indicator of arterial stiffness: theory, evidence and perspectives. J Atheroscler Thromb 2011;18:924-933.
3) Hayashi K, Yamamoto T, Takahara, Shirai K. A clinical assessment of arterial stiffness with cardio-ankle vascular index: theory and applications. J Hypertens 2015;33:1742-1757.
4) Laurent S, Cockcroft J, Van Bortel L, et al. Expert consensus document on arterial stiffness: methodological issues and clinical applications. Eur Heart J 2006;27:2588-2605.
5) Urbina EM, Williams RV, Alpert BS, et al. Noninvasive assessment of subclinical atherosclerosis in children and adolescents. Hypertension 2009;54:919-950.
6) Vlachopoulos C, Aznaouridis K, Stefanadis C. Prediction of cardiovascular events and all-cause mortality with arterial stiffness: a systematic review and meta-analysis. J Am Coll Cardiol 2010;55:1318-1327.
7) Asmar R. Pulse wave velocity and prognosis 135-142, in Arterial stiffness and pulse wave velocity edit. by Asmar R, O'Rourke MF, Safar M, Elsevier Amsterdam, 1999.
8) Rogers WJ, Hu YL, Coast D, et al. Age-associated changes in regional aortic pulse wave velocity. J Am Coll Cardiol 2001;38:1123-1129.
9) Van Bortel LM, Laurent S, Boutouyrie P, et al. Expert consensus document on the measurement of aortic stiffness in daily practice using carotid-femoral pulse wave velocity. J Hypertens 2012;30:445-448.
10) Yoshimura S, Sugai J, Hashimoto H, et al. An estimation of arteriosclerosis by the measurement of pulse wave velocity and analysis of the clinical effects of therapeutic agents on arteriosclerosis. Cor Vasa 1968;10:173-182.
11) Hasegawa M. A fundamental study on human aortic pulse wave velocity. J Jikei Med Coll 1970;85:742-760. (in Japanese)
12) Hasegawa M, Arai C. Clinical estimation of vascular elastic function and practical application. Connective Tissue 1995;27:149-157.
13) Nye ER. The effect of blood pressure alteration on the pulse wave velocity. Br Heart J 1964;26:261-265.
14) O'Rourke MF, Staessen JA, Vlachopoulos et al. Clinical applications of arterial stiffness; definitions and reference values. Am J Hypertens 2002;15:426-444.
15) Hayashi K, Handa H, Nagasawa S, et al. Stiffness and elastic behavior of human intracranial and extracranial arteries. J Biomech 1980;13:175-184.
16) Kawasaki T, Sasayama S, Yagi S, et al. Non-invasive assessment of the age related changes in stiffness of major branches of the human arteries. Cardiovasc Res 1987;21:678-687.
17) Hirai T, Sasayama S, Kawasaki T, Yagi S. Stiffness of systemic arteries in patients with myocardial infarction. A noninvasive method to predict severity of coronary atherosclerosis. Circulation 1989;80:78-86.
18) Yamashina A, Tomiyama H, Takeda K et al. Validity, reproducibility, and clinical significance of noninvasive brachial-ankle pulse wave velocity measurement. Hypertens Res 2002;25:359-364.
19) Takata M, Kawasaki T. The clinical significance of pulse wave velocity in patients with hypertension. Rinsho kouketsuatsu (Clinical Hypertension) 2003;8:256-264. (in Japanese)
20) Sugawara J, Hayashi K, Tanaka H. Arterial path length estimation on brachial-ankle pulse wave velocity: validity of height-based formulas. J Hypertens 2014;32:881-889.
21) Kelly R, Hayward C, Avolio A, et al. Noninvasive determinant of age-related changes in the human arterial pulse. Circulation 1989;1652-1659.
22) Hope SA, Meredith IT, Cameron JD. Arterial transfer functions and the reconstruction of central aortic waveforms: myths, controversies and misconceptions. J Hypertens 2008;26:4-7.
23) McEniery CM, Yasmin, Hallet IR, et al. Normal vascular aging: differential effects on wave reflection and aortic pulse wave velocity: the Anglo-Cardiff Collaborative Trial (ACCT). J Am Coll Cardiol 2005;46:1753-1760. https://doi.org/10.1016/j.jacc.2005.07.037

24) Takazawa K, Kobayashi A, Kojima I, et al. Estimation of central aortic systolic pressure using late systolic inflection of radial artery pulse and its application to vasodilator therapy. J Hypertens 2012; 30:908-916.

25) Picone DS, Schultz MG, Otaha P, et al. Accuracy of cuff-measured blood pressure: systematic reviews and meta-analyses. J Am Coll Cardiol 2017;70:572-586.

26) Ding FH, Li Y, Zhang RY, Zhang Q, Wang JG. Comparison of the SphygmoCor and Omron devices in the estimation of pressure amplification against the invasive catheter measurement. J Hypertens 2013;31:86-93.

27) Sharman JE, Avolio AP, Baulmann J, et al. Validation of non-invasive central blood pressure devices: ARTERY Society task force consensus statement on protocol standardization. Eur Heart J 2017;38:2805-2812.

28) Huang QF, Aparicio LS, Thijs L, et al. Cardiovascular end points and mortality are not closer associated with central than peripheral pulsatile blood pressure components. Hypertension 2020;76:350-358.

29) Takahashi K, Yamamoto T, Tsuda S, et al. Coefficients in the CAVI equation and the comparison between CAVI with and without the coefficients using clinical data. J Atheroscler Thromb 2019;26:465-475.

30) Reference Values for Arterial Stiffness' Collaboration. Determinants of pulse wave velocity in healthy people and in the presence of cardiovascular risk factors: 'establishing normal and reference values'. Eur Heart J. 2010;31:2338-2350.

31) Arai, C, Abe N, Takeuchi M, et al. The relationship between aorta pulse wave velocity and each type of serum lipid: Doumyakukouka (Arteriosclerosis) 1984;12:781-787. (in Japanese)

32) Namekata T, Suzuki K, Ishizuka N, et al. Establishing baseline criteria of cardio-ankle vascular index as a new indicator of arteriosclerosis: a cross-sectional study. BMC Cardiovasc Disord 2011;11:51.

CAVI behind the formula

Koji Takahashi, Tomoyuki Yamamoto, Shinichi Tsuda and Mitsuya Maruyama

Introduction

Arterial stiffness is deeply involved in vascular functions and has been well studied for centuries[1-3]. It is physically expressed by an elastic modulus. As it is not easy to measure in vivo, an alternative method of measuring, pulse wave velocity (PWV)[2,3], has been used widely because of its relative easiness. However, PWV is essentially dependent on the blood pressure at the time of measurement[3], and it is difficult to determine the inherent arterial stiffness.

The stiffness parameter β[4] was derived to overcome this limitation, and based on that, together with the Bramwell-Hill equation[2], the cardio–ankle vascular index (CAVI) was developed[5]. CAVI represents the inherent stiffness of the arterial tree from the origin of the aorta to the ankle arteries, independent of the blood pressure at the measuring time; its usefulness has been reported in many studies[6].

The purpose of this chapter is to review the implications of CAVI behind the mathematical formula, return to the origin of the theory and verify its validity. Also, the controversial feature of the recently proposed variant index is reviewed.

Stiffness, Elastic Modulus and PWV

First, let us look back to the meaning of the stiffness. To say simply, it is the difficulty of deformation by an applied stress, and physically, it can be represented by the elastic modulus[1] as follows:

Elastic modulus = Stress / Strain

In the case of a tubular vessel with pressurized fluid inside, the bulk modulus (K), a type of elastic moduli, is appropriate to apply for the overall stiffness of the vessel and it is expressed as follows.

K = Pressure change / Relative volume change
More precisely, it can be formulated in eq.1.

$$K = \Delta P / \frac{\Delta V}{V} = \Delta P \times \frac{V}{\Delta V} \qquad \text{eq.1}$$

[K: bulk modulus, ΔP: pressure change, V: volume, ΔV: volume change]

If volume change of the vessel is caused only by radial change as shown in Fig. 1, it can be substituted by the area change; when the change is small, K can be described using the diameter of the vessel (D) instead of volume as eq.2.

$$K = \Delta P \times \frac{D}{2\Delta D} \qquad \text{eq.2}$$

[K: bulk modulus, ΔP: pressure change, D: diameter, ΔD: diameter change]

Next, we review the relationship between PWV and K. The propagation velocity of a wave, such as a sound wave, is determined generally by the elastic modulus[1], and PWV is also given by the formula eq.3.

$$PWV^2 = \frac{K}{\rho} = \frac{\Delta P}{\rho} \times \frac{D}{2\Delta D} \qquad \text{eq.3}$$

[PWV: pulse wave velocity, K: bulk modulus, ρ: blood density, ΔP: blood pressure change, D: vessel diameter, ΔD: vessel diameter change]

This equation is a general expression of wave velocity based on Newton physics, and in the case of PWV, it is called the Bramwell-Hill equation[2] named after the researchers' valuable experimental study.

Since ρ is nearly constant, PWV is proportional to the square root of K, and as PWV can be measured relatively easily, it has been widely used as a measure of arterial stiffness[3].

Blood Pressure Dependency of Arterial Stiffness

If the artery was made of a plain single component

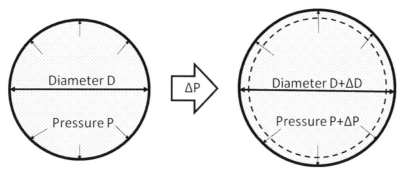

Fig. 1. Schematic of the bulk modulus.
Abbreviations: D, diameter of the blood vessel; ΔD, change of diameter; P, blood pressure; ΔP, change of blood pressure.

Fukuda Denshi Co., Ltd., Tokyo, Japan.

material like rubber, calculations would be simple, but real artery has a multi-layer structure with different compositions. Blood pressure (P) has an exponential relationship to D, and K changes with P. This is the blood pressure dependency of arterial stiffness[3], which renders it difficult to assess the inherent arterial stiffness.

In order to overcome this problem, Hayashi et al[4] experimentally confirmed the exponential relationship of D and P of human arteries within the physiological range and defined the β formula in eq.4, thus providing an index of inherent arterial stiffness independent of P.

$$\beta = (\ln P - \ln P_0) \times \frac{D_0}{D - D_0} \qquad \text{eq.4}$$

[β: stiffness parameter, P: blood pressure, P_0: reference blood pressure, D: vessel diameter, D_0: reference vessel diameter]

From eq.2 and eq.4, the relationship between β and K is obtained as eq.5 (Supplement 1, Seq.1-5).

$$\beta = \frac{2K}{P} \times \frac{D_0}{D} \qquad \text{eq.5}$$

Fig. 2 (a) is an example of the theoretical relationship between D and P, when P_0=100 mmHg (13.3KPa), D_0=10 mm and β=10, and Fig. 2 (b) shows the resultant relationship between P and K. Interestingly, when D and P have an exponential relationship, P and K show almost a linear relationship, since D_0/D is nearly equal to 1 and it can be disregarded as in eq.6.

$$K \approx \frac{\beta}{2} \times P \qquad \text{eq.6}$$

Therefore, β is naturally independent of blood pressure as a proportional constant of the stiffness obtained by dividing K by P. Also, eq.6 can be expressed as in eq.7 by using PWV in place of K of eq.3.

$$PWV \approx \sqrt{\frac{\beta}{2\rho} \times P} \qquad \text{eq.7}$$

Therefore, PWV is nearly proportional to the square root of P, as shown in Fig. 2 (c). This is the essence of the blood pressure dependency in PWV[3].

Using PWV and P instead of K and D, eq.8 is introduced (Supplement 1, Seq.6-8)

$$\beta = \frac{2\rho \times PWV^2}{P} - \ln \frac{P}{P_0} \qquad \text{eq.8}$$

Since $\ln \dfrac{P}{P_0}$ is small and negligible in the physiological range, eq.8 can be approximated by eq.9 as follows:

$$\beta \approx \frac{2\rho \times PWV^2}{P} \qquad \text{eq.9}$$

Meaning of CAVI

Here, we review the formula of CAVI[5] to clarify its meaning.

With the clinically measurable parameters, CAVI is defined as eq.10.

$$CAVI = a \times \left(2\rho \times \frac{\ln \dfrac{Ps}{Pd}}{\Delta P} \times PWV^2 \right) + b \qquad \text{eq.10}$$

[ρ: blood density, Ps: systolic blood pressure, Pd: diastolic blood pressure, ΔP: Ps−Pd, PWV: pulse wave velocity of the arterial tree from the origin of the aorta to the ankle, a, b: coefficients].

The essence of CAVI is inside the parentheses of eq.10, and we define it as 'CAVI' in eq.11, which is the value without coefficients "a" and "b"[7].

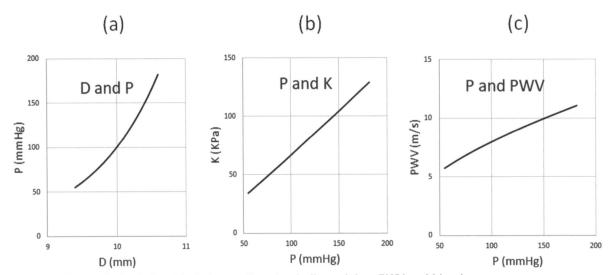

(a)   (b)   (c)

Fig. 2. Theoretical relationship between diameter, bulk modulus, PWV and blood pressure.
(a) Diameter and Blood pressure, (b) Blood pressure and Bulk modulus, (c) Blood pressure and PWV
Abbreviations: D, diameter of the blood vessel; P, blood pressure; K, bulk modulus; PWV, pulse wave velocity.

$$CAVI' = 2\rho \times \frac{\ln \dfrac{Ps}{Pd}}{\Delta P} \times PWV^2 \qquad \text{eq.11}$$

$$= 2\rho \times \frac{\ln Ps - \ln Pd}{Ps - Pd} \times PWV^2$$

In eq.11, $\dfrac{\ln Ps - \ln Pd}{Ps - Pd}$, a blood pressure term, is mathematically proven to be nearly equal to $\dfrac{1}{Pm}$, where Pm is the mid-pressure between Ps and Pd, defined by $Pm = \dfrac{Ps + Pd}{2}$ (Supplement 2).

Thus, the important attribute of CAVI is introduced in eq.12.

$$CAVI' \approx \frac{2\rho \times PWV^2}{Pm} \qquad \text{eq.12}$$

This equation has same form as eq.9, and P in the denominator is specified with Pm. If the blood pressure level of the K or $\rho \times PWV^2$ corresponds to Pm, eq.12 yields the correct β value, and we confirm that hereafter.

Corresponding blood pressure of PWV in CAVI calculation

As stated, PWV changes according to the blood pressure, and it also changes in the cardiac cycle, from Pd to Ps. For example, in the theoretical model shown in Fig. 2, when Pd = 80 mmHg and Ps = 120 mmHg, the corresponding PWV values at Pd (PWVd) and Ps (PWVs) are 7.0 m/s and 8.8 m/s respectively. PWVs is larger than PWVd as illustrated in Fig. 3, and the differences in the PWV values in the cardiac cycle and their significance have been reported in many recent studies[8,9].

Now we assess the corresponding blood pressure of PWV measured in CAVI. As shown in Fig. 4, haPWV, which is the PWV from the heart to the ankle, is measured. It is obtained by dividing the length of the arterial tree by the transit time of the pulse from the heart to the ankle

(haTime). In general, it is not so easy to identify the accurate time for the pulse to start at the origin of the aorta, and CAVI offers some ingenuity. The pulse propagation time from heart to ankle is divided into two time periods, one is the time from the heart to brachium (hbTime), and the other is the time between the brachium and ankle (baTime). The hbTime is measured as the time from heart sound II to the dicrotic notch of the pulse at the brachium. Since hbTime is measured at the blood pressure level of the dicrotic notch, the heart to brachium PWV (hbPWV) corresponds to PWV at the end-systolic phase of the cardiac cycle. On the other hand, since baTime is measured at the foot level of the pulse waves, the brachial-ankle PWV (baPWV) corresponds to PWV at the early-systolic phase. As a result, haPWV corresponds to PWV at blood pressure level of Pm between Pd and Ps. The important fact here is that the corresponding blood pressure of haPWV in CAVI is not Pd but rather Pm, and here the consistency of eq.11 is confirmed.

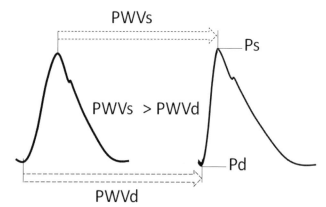

Fig. 3.   Difference of PWV in the cardiac cycle.
Abbreviations: Ps, systolic blood pressure; Pd, diastolic blood pressure; PWV, pulse wave velocity; PWVs, PWV at Ps; PWVd, PWV at Pd.

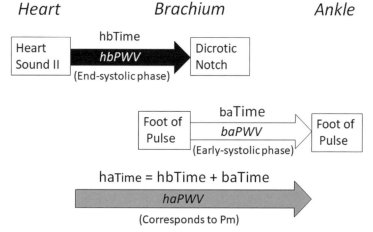

Fig. 4.   Schematics of the PWV from the heart to ankle measured in CAVI.
Abbreviations: PWV, pulse wave velocity; CAVI, cardio-ankle vascular index; hbTime, time from heart to brachium; hbPWV, heart to brachium PWV; baTime, time from brachium to ankle; baPWV, brachium to ankle PWV; haTime, time from heart to ankle; haPWV, heart to ankle PWV.

Variant Index CAVI$_0$

Spronck et al[10-12] proposed a variant index CAVI$_0$ defined by eq.13, claiming that CAVI is yet dependent on the blood pressure, but CAVI$_0$ is not.

$$CAVI_0 = \frac{2\rho \times PWV^2}{Pd} - \ln\frac{Pd}{P_0} \qquad eq.13$$

[ρ: blood density, PWV: pulse wave velocity of the arterial tree from the origin of the aorta to the ankle, Pd: diastolic blood pressure, P_0: reference pressure (100mmHg)]

This equation is obtained by substituting Pd for P in the right side of eq.8. Their reason for using Pd is that PWV measured by foot to foot of the pulse waves corresponds to Pd. However, as we have reviewed, PWV in CAVI corresponds to Pm but not Pd[13-16]. Although eq.8 which is the basis of CAVI$_0$ is correct, marked inconsistency occurs in CAVI$_0$ at this point. If only Pm instead of Pd is substituted for P in eq.8, it yields a proper value.

They also asserted that the CAVI equation without the $\ln\frac{P}{P_0}$ is one of the reasons for blood pressure dependency of CAVI. However actually, $\ln\frac{P}{P_0}$ is small in the physiological range and negligible. For example, when P is 80 mmHg, 100 mmHg and 120 mmHg, the values are -0.22, 0 and 0.18, respectively.

As a result, CAVI is stable but CAVI$_0$ fluctuates with blood pressure change because of the mismatch of the equation[13-16]. For example, in the theoretical model of

Fig. 2, when Ps/Pd/Pm is 100/60/80mmHg and 140/100/120mmHg, and PWV corresponds to Pm, the CAVI$_0$ values are 13.5 and 12.2, respectively, though the correct β is 10. CAVI$_0$ is overestimated depending on the blood pressure, and in this case, the lower the blood pressure, the unreasonably higher the value.

Verification with clinical data

Now, we verify the validity of CAVI with the clinical data. In the previous publications, we reported the comparison results between CAVI and CAVI$_0$ based on medical examination data of a large population[15,16]. Here we review those results. The studied populations were two groups: a healthy group (n = 5,293; 3,071 women and 2,222 men) and a hypertensive group (n = 3,338; 1,006 women and 2,332 men).

First, the relationship between Pm and $\frac{Ps - Pd}{\ln Ps - \ln Pd}$, the reciprocal of the blood pressure term of CAVI, was r = 0.997 (p < 0.001) for both groups, indicating that the blood pressure term of CAVI is almost equal to $\frac{1}{Pm}$[16].

Next, we evaluate the influence of the reference blood pressure term $\ln\frac{P}{P_0}$.

When the values with and without $\ln\frac{Pm}{P_0}$ were compared, the coefficients of correlation were r = 0.997 and r = 0.998

Table 1. Simple and multiple regression analyses of CAVI and CAVI$_0$ with Pd in the Healthy group with a pulse pressure of less than 50 mmHg.

CAVI

	Healthy (N = 3,439)						
	Simple Regression		Multiple Regression				
	r	p value	β	B	95% CI		p value
Age	0.601	p < 0.001	0.627	0.048	0.046	0.050	p < 0.001
Sex	-0.184	p < 0.001	-0.192	-0.327	-0.372	-0.282	p < 0.001
BMI	-0.022	NS	-0.199	-0.058	-0.066	-0.050	p < 0.001
Pd	0.203	p < 0.001			NS		

CAVI$_0$

	Healthy (N = 3,439)						
	Simple Regression		Multiple Regression				
	r	p value	β	B	95% CI		p value
Age	0.530	p < 0.001	0.631	0.090	0.086	0.093	p < 0.001
Sex	-0.130	p < 0.001	-0.201	-0.632	-0.719	-0.544	p < 0.001
BMI	-0.074	p < 0.001	-0.178	-0.096	-0.111	-0.081	p < 0.001
Pd	-0.049	p < 0.01	-0.251	-0.045	-0.050	-0.040	p < 0.001

Abbreviations: BMI, body mass index; Pd, diastolic blood pressure; r, correlation coefficient; β, standardized partial correlation coefficient; B, unstandardized correlation coefficient; CI, confidence interval.

Table 2. Factors which change arterial stiffness.

Element of Arterial stiffness	Term to change	Factors which change arterial stiffness	Participating tissues
Structural	Long term	Aging, hypertension and diseases	Elastic tissues
Functional	Acute	Autonomic nerves, agents and drugs	Muscular tissues

(p < 0.001 for both) for the healthy group and hypertensive group, respectively, indicating that the influence of the reference blood pressure term is small and negligible[16].

Here, we review the comprehensive comparison data.

We reported the negative relationship of $CAVI_0$ with Pd in the healthy group by both simple and multiple regression analysis[15]; in contrast, CAVI had a slightly positive relationship.

The result of CAVI is acceptable because it is considered to have an increase in arterial stiffness due to the long-term exposure of blood pressure. On the contrary, $CAVI_0$ had a negative relationship with Pd[15,16], and this is obviously unreasonable.

Moreover, it was observed that $CAVI_0$ values in hypertensive women aged 30–39 years were significantly lower than the values of healthy women[15]. The reason for these questionable results is the mismatch of the calculation where PWV^2 is divided by Pd instead of Pm.

Against this observation, Spronck et al[17] claimed that the negative correlation of $CAVI_0$ with Pd can be explained by the possibility that subjects with "high pulse pressure" were included in the healthy group. To test this hypothesis, we reanalyzed the data in the same article, and obtained the results shown in Table 1.

Again, there was a negative correlation between CAV_0 and Pd, even in a healthy group with a pulse pressure of less than 50 mmHg; multiple regression analyses showed that the standardized partial coefficient of regression of $CAVI_0$ with Pd was -0.251 (p < 0.001), while CAVI had no significance. Thus, it is not because there were subjects with "high pulse pressure" in the healthy group. This relationship, the lower the blood pressure, the higher the value, is as the same as that seen in the theoretical model, and those unnatural results of $CAVI_0$ are simply due to the mismatch of the calculation.

Major factors to change arterial stiffness

Naturally, blood pressure is not the only factor that changes the arterial stiffness. As shown in Table 2, arterial stiffness is composed of structural and functional elements, each of which changes due to various factors. Structural stiffness changes over the long term with aging, hypertension, or diseases, and primarily elastic tissues are involved. On the other hand, functional stiffness changes are acutely due to the enhancement of autonomic nerves caused by agents or drugs, and mainly muscular tissues are involved. These changes in arterial stiffness are independent of the changes due to blood pressure fluctuations and are different from the blood pressure dependency excluded by β and CAVI.

In this regard, an article[18] was published claiming that CAVI is blood pressure dependent because of the changes in CAVI, based on the results of the Cold pressor test (CPT) and Hand grip test (HGT). It is an off-target discussion, and the fact is that with stimulated sympathetic nerves by CPT or HGT, the stiffness of the artery including smooth muscles increases, as well as the change in blood pressure. This mechanism has been explained in numerous articles[19,20]. CAVI correctly shows the increase of stiffness, and this result does not mean that CAVI is blood pressure dependent

at the time of measurement.

In this association, it was reported[21] that the response of arteries to the vasodilating agents such as nitroglycerin is different between central and peripheral arteries, suggesting that the meaning and role of arterial stiffness differ depending on the segments. As a perspective, more useful information will be obtainable in the future if blood pressure independent arterial stiffness for both central and peripheral segments can be measured separately and more easily.

Conclusion

The conceptual meaning of CAVI is reconfirmed and verified to be as follows: Arterial stiffness is represented by bulk modulus of the blood vessel, which is approximately proportional to blood pressure. When it is divided by blood pressure, a proportionality constant is obtained, representing arterial stiffness independent of blood pressure, and it is the essence of β and CAVI.

CAVI and $CAVI_0$ are compared in recent reports and the claim that $CAVI_0$ is less blood pressure dependent than CAVI has been shown to be suspicious, although the proposition of $CAVI_0$ has contributed to deeper discussions on the blood pressure independency of CAVI.

We conclude that CAVI is a reliable and useful index of blood pressure independent arterial stiffness, in both structural and functional components.

References

1) Young T. The Croonian Lecture: on the functions of the heart and arteries. *Phil Trans R Soc Lond.* 1809 ; 99: 1-31.
2) Bramwell JC, Hill AV. The velocity of the pulse wave in man. *Proc R Soc Lond B Biol Sci.* 1922; 93: 298-306.
3) Bramwell JC, McDowali RJS, McSwiney BA. The variation of arterial elasticity with blood pressure in man. (Part I). *Proc R Soc Lond B.* 1923; 94: 450-454.
4) Hayashi K, Handa H, Nagasawa S, Okumura A, Moritake K. Stiffness and elastic behavior of human intracranial and extracranial arteries. *J Biomech.* 1980; 13: 175-184.
5) Shirai K, Utino J, Otsuka K, Takata M. A novel blood pressure-independent arterial wall stiffness parameter; cardio-ankle vascular index (CAVI). *J Atheroscler Thromb.* 2006; 13: 101-107.
6) Saiki A, Ohira M, Yamaguchi T, Nagayama D, Shimizu N, et al. New Horizons of Arterial Stiffness Developed Using Cardio-Ankle Vascular Index (CAVI). *J Atheroscler Thromb.* 2020; 27: 732-748.
7) Takahashi K, Yamamoto T, Tsuda S, et al. Coefficients in the CAVI equation and the comparison between CAVI with and without the coefficients using clinical data. *J Atheroscler Thromb.* 2019; 26: 465-475.
8) Hermeling E, Vermeersch SJ, Rietzschel ER, et al. The change in arterial stiffness over the cardiac cycle rather than diastolic stiffness is independently associated with left ventricular mass index in healthy middle-aged individuals. *J Hypertens.* 2012; 30: 396-402.
9) Mirault T, Pernot M, Frank M, et al. Carotid stiffness change over the cardiac cycle by ultrafast ultrasound imaging in healthy volunteers and vascular Ehlers-Danlos syndrome. *J Hypertens.* 2015; 33: 1890-1896.
10) Spronck B, Avolio AP, Tan I, Butlin M, Reesink KD, Delhaas T. Arterial stiffness index beta and cardio-ankle vascular index inherently dependent on blood pressure but

can be readily corrected. *J Hypertens*, 2017; 35: 98-104.

11) Spronck B, Avolio AP, Tan I, Butlin M, Reesink KD, Delhaas T. Reply: physics cannot be disputed. *J Hypertens.* 2017; 35: 1523-1525.

12) Spronck B, Avolio AP, Tan I, Butlin M, Reesink KD, Delhaas T. Medical science is based on facts and evidence. *J Hypertens*. 2018; 36: 960-962.

13) Shirai K, Shimizu K, Takata M, Suzuki K. Independency of the cardio-ankle vascular index from blood pressure at the time of measurement. *J Hypertens*. 2017; 35: 1521-1523.

14) Shirai K, Shimizu K, Takata M, Suzuki K. Medical science is based on evidence (answer to Spronck et al's refutation: physics cannot be disputed). *J Hypertens*. 2018; 36: 958-960.

15) Shirai K, Suzuki K, Tsuda S, et al. Comparison of cardio-ankle vascular index (CAVI) and $CAVI_0$ in large healthy and hypertensive populations. *J Atheroscler Thromb*. 2019; 26: 603-615.

16) Takahashi K, Yamamoto T, Tsuda S, Maruyama M, Shirai, K. The background of calculating CAVI: Lesson from the discrepancy between CAVI and $CAVI_0$. *Vasc. Health Risk. Manag*. 2020;16: 193-201.

17) Spronck B, Jurko A, Mestanik M, Avolio AP, Tonhajzerova I. Reply to Comments: Using the Cardio-Ankle Vascular Index (CAVI) or the Mathematical Correction Form ($CAVI_0$) in Clinical Practice. *Int. J. Mol. Sci.* **2020**; 21: 2647.

18) Mestanik M, Spronck B, Jurko AJ, Mestanikova A, Jurko T, Butlin M, *et al*. Assessment of novel blood pressure Corrected Cardio-ankle Vascular Index in Response to Acute Blood Pressure Changes. *Artery Res* 2019; 25(Suppl 1): S173.

19) Antony I, Aptecar E, Lerebours G, Nitenberg A. Coronary artery constriction caused by the cold pressor test in human hypertension. *Hypertension*. 1994; 24: 212-219.

20) Lafleche AB, Pannier BM, Laloux B, Safar ME. Arterial response during cold pressor test in borderline hypertension. *Am J Physiol*. 1998; 275: H409-H415.

21) Yamamoto T, Shimizu K, Takahashi M, Tatsuno I, Shirai K. The Effect of Nitroglycerin on Arterial Stiffness of the Aorta and the Femoral-Tibial Arteries. *J Atheroscler Thromb*. 2017; 24: 1048-1057.

Supplement 1

The β formula eq.4 can be described in Seq.1

$$\ln P - \ln P_0 = \beta \times \frac{D - D_0}{D_0} \qquad \text{Seq.1}$$

[β: stiffness parameter, P: blood pressure, P_0: reference blood pressure, D: vessel diameter, D_0: reference vessel diameter]

When P and D change to $P + \Delta P$ and $D + \Delta D$, Seq.1 yields Seq.2

$$\ln(P + \Delta P) - \ln P_0 = \beta \times \frac{D + \Delta D - D_0}{D_0} \qquad \text{Seq.2}$$

(ΔP: change of P, ΔD: change of D)

Taking the difference between both sides of Seq.1 and Seq.2, Seq.3 is derived.

$$\ln(P + \Delta P) - \ln P = \beta \times \frac{\Delta D}{D_0} \qquad \text{Seq.3}$$

Seq.3 can be transformed to Seq.4.

$$\beta = \frac{\ln(P + \Delta P) - \ln P}{\Delta P} \times \left(\Delta P \times \frac{D}{\Delta D} \right) \times \frac{D_0}{D} \qquad \text{Seq.4}$$

Since $\lim_{\Delta P \to 0} \dfrac{\ln(P + \Delta P) - \ln P}{\Delta P} = \dfrac{1}{P}$ and $\Delta P \times \dfrac{D}{\Delta D} = 2K$, Seq.5 is introduced.

$$\beta = \frac{2K}{P} \times \frac{D_0}{D} \qquad \text{Seq.5}$$

Applying the Bramwell-Hill equation eq.3, Seq.5 is expressed in Seq.6 with PWV.

$$\beta = \frac{2\rho \times PWV^2}{P} \times \frac{D_0}{D} \qquad \text{Seq.6}$$

Again, from the β formula Seq.1, $\dfrac{D_0}{D}$ is described in Seq.7.

$$\frac{D_0}{D} = \frac{\beta}{\beta + \ln P - \ln P_0} \qquad \text{Seq.7}$$

Substituting Seq.7 for Seq.6 and organizing for β, Seq.8 is obtained.

$$\beta = \frac{2\rho \times PWV^2}{P} - \ln \frac{P}{P_0} \qquad \text{Seq.8}$$

Supplement 2

By defining $Pm = \dfrac{Ps + Pd}{2}$, $\Delta P = Ps - Pd$ and $x = \dfrac{\Delta P}{2Pm}$

$$\frac{\ln Ps - \ln Pd}{Ps - Pd} = \frac{\ln\left(Pm + \dfrac{\Delta P}{2}\right) - \ln\left(Pm - \dfrac{\Delta P}{2}\right)}{\Delta P}$$

$$= \frac{1}{\Delta P} \times \left(\ln\left(Pm \times \left(1 + \frac{\Delta P}{2Pm}\right)\right) - \ln\left(Pm \times \left(1 - \frac{\Delta P}{2Pm}\right)\right) \right)$$

$$= \frac{1}{\Delta P} \times \left(\ln Pm + \ln(1 + x) - \left(\ln Pm + \ln(1 - x) \right) \right)$$

$$= \frac{1}{\Delta P} \times \left(\ln(1 + x) - \ln(1 - x) \right)$$

Since in the Maclaurin expansion, $\ln(1 + x) = x - \dfrac{x^2}{2} + \dfrac{x^3}{3} - \dfrac{x^4}{4} + \dfrac{x^5}{5} + \dots$

$$\frac{\ln Ps - \ln Pd}{Ps - Pd} = \frac{1}{\Delta P} \times \left(2x + \frac{2}{3}x^3 + \frac{2}{5}x^5 + \dots \right)$$

As values from the second term are small in the physiological range,

$$\frac{\ln Ps - \ln Pd}{Ps - Pd} \approx \frac{1}{\Delta P} \times (2x) = \frac{1}{Pm}$$

A Comparison between Cardio Ankle Vascular Index (CAVI) and the variant CAVI$_0$ among Community Dwelling Individuals

Javad Alizargar[1] and Elaheh Alizargar[2]

Introduction

Cardio-ankle vascular index (CAVI) has been proposed as an index reflecting arterial stiffness of the arterial tree from the origin of the aorta to the ankle[1]. The feature is its independence from blood pressure at measuring time. It can provide some information about the level and severity of atherosclerosis in the patient. However, CAVI$_0$ (Equation (2)) is presented by Spronck et al. as the mathematically corrected formula that has been obtained from the CAVI formula[2]. This marker is claimed to be less dependent on the blood pressure changes at the time of measurement. However, the utility in clinical practice was not fully verified. We tried to compare both indices for about 163 individuals in Taipei.

Equations of CAVI and CAVIo

Cardio-ankle vascular index (CAVI) (equation (1)) has been proposed by Shirai et al. in 2006[1]. It is considered as a method that can be used to evaluate the overall stiffness of arteries. It can provide some information about the level and severity of atherosclerosis in patients especially patients that are at risk for major adverse cardiovascular events[3]. CAVI$_0$ (Equation (2)) is the mathematically corrected formula that has been obtained from the CAVI formula and was introduced in 2017 as a better substitute for CAVI and Spronck et al.[2] had claimed that this marker is less dependent on the blood pressure changes at the time of measurement. In another paper they also provided a tool to easily convert CAVI into CAVI$_0$ values[4].

$$(1) \quad CAVI = a \left[(2\rho/\Delta P) \times \ln (Ps/Pd) \, PWV^2 \right] + b$$

$$(2) \quad CAVI_0 = 2\rho \times (PWV^2/Pd) - \ln (Pd/P_0)$$

SBP and DBP are systolic and diastolic blood pressure. $\Delta P = SBP-DBP$ and ρ is the blood density. a and b are the constants automatically measured by the device to match

Table 1. Characteristics of study participants stratified by sex. Source: Lin et al.[20]

Variable	Mean ± SD	Sex		P value	Pearson Correlation with CAVI		Pearson Correlation with CAVI$_0$	
	Number (%)	Male	Female		r	P value	r	P value
CAVI	8.64 ± 1.08	8.69 ± 1.15	8.60 ± 1.04	0.614	1	-	0.95	<0.001
CAVI$_0$	13.33 ± 2.68	13.37 ± 2.88	13.30 ± 2.56	0.877	0.95		1	-
Age	63.06 ± 9.40	63.36 ± 9.77	62.86 ± 9.19	0.739	0.57	<0.001	0.61	<0.0001
BMI	24.76 ± 3.60	25.24 ± 3.29	24.44 ± 3.77	0.165	-0.06	0.41	-0.06	0.451
WC	80.53 ± 9.90	85.78 ± 8.55	77.05 ± 9.20	<0.001	-0.03	0.673	-0.03	0.684
HC	93.92 ± 6.93	94.81 ± 5.93	93.33 ± 7.49	0.183	-0.1	0.18	-0.11	0.170
SBP	130.10 ± 17.37	134.09 ± 16.57	127.45 ± 17.47	0.016	0.3	<0.001	0.33	<0.0001
DBP	80.74 ± 10.40	84.16 ± 10.29	78.46 ± 9.89	<0.001	0.18	0.016	0.06	0.461
HR	69.01 ± 9.38	69 ± 9.04	69.02 ± 9.65	0.989	-0.09	0.216	-0.13	0.092
MBP	97.19 ± 12.04	100.81 ± 11.82	94.79 ± 11.63	0.001	0.25	0.001	0.19	0.014

BMI, body mass index; WC, waist circumference; HC, hip circumference; SBP, systolic blood pressure; DBP, diastolic blood pressure; HR, heart rate; MBP, mean blood pressure.

[1]Research Center for Healthcare Industry Innovation, National Taipei University of Nursing and Health Sciences, Taipei City, Taiwan.
[2]Department of Public Health, National Yang Ming Chiao Tung University, Taipei City, Taiwan.

aortic PWV. P_0 is the reference pressure (100 mmHg).

There are some differences between CAVI and $CAVI_0$ as is apparent from their formulas. Unlike CAVI which uses P_d and P_s in its formula $CAVI_0$, only uses P_d, not P_s. The use of P_0 in the formula of $CAVI_0$ is another difference. Although CAVI and $CAVI_0$ can be considered as proper stiffness indices from the origin of the aorta to the ankle, there are some important points that should be considered before using them. PWV is the basis for CAVI and $CAVI_0$ calculation. Differences in PWV in different people arise from the pressure dependency of PWV and/or the intrinsic or actual differences in arterial stiffness between those people. CAVI and $CAVI_0$ are only correct for the pressure dependency of PWV and have no effect on the intrinsic differences due to the atherosclerosis and arterial stiffness e.g age, hypertensive remodeling, obesity, etc. as these differences have already been reflected in the value of CAVI and $CAVI_0$. All these risk factors can influence CAVI and $CAVI_0$ in clinical practice.

Properties of CAVI

Various atherosclerotic diseases have been shown to increase CAVI. Coronary artery disease, cerebral infarction, chronic kidney disease and thickening of carotid intima-media thickness have been evaluated in relation to CAVI in various studies[5]. CAVI increases according to the number of stenotic vessels[6, 7] and CAVI is associated with the presence of carotid and coronary arteriosclerosis[8]. It is also an independent determinant of coronary atherosclerosis severity[7]. CAVI shows high correlations with coronary artery calcification[9-11]. Studies have showed that CAVI increases in patients with large artery atherosclerosis and small vessel occlusion[12, 13]. CAVI is high in patients receiving hemodialysis[14, 15]. CAVI also shows high correlations with estimated glomerular filtration rate,

urinary albumin creatinine ratio and cystatin C[14, 16, 17]. Carotid-femoral PWV (cfPWV) is currently used in early vascular ageing (EVA) syndrome. CAVI can replace cfPWV as CAVI has an advantage over cfPWV for its independence of blood pressure at the time of measurement. CAVI can also be used to evaluate vascular aging effects of anti-aging supplements and super-normal vascular aging (SUPERNOVA) which is the opposite phenotype of EVA[5]. Antiaging supplements such as Resveratrol and S-equol[18, 19] have been shown to lower CAVI.

Comparison between CAVI and $CAVI_0$ among 163 individuals

Knowing which one of the risk factors has the most independent effect on CAVI and $CAVI_0$ measurement can be also necessary for the researchers who may use these indices and clinicians who want to interpret these values for patients at risk of cardiovascular disease. So, studies to evaluate the factors that should be considered if we are dealing with CAVI and $CAVI_0$ in clinical practice seem to be important. For this goal, the participants from a prospective cohort study have been recruited and CAVI and $CAVI_0$ were measured for them. They were excluded if they were younger than 30, had prior history of chronic kidney disease, cancer, admission due to stroke or cardiovascular disease or had hepatitis B or C infection. Finally, the data of 163 individuals were analyzed in the study. Known risk factors for atherosclerosis were assessed in the individuals and the relationship between CAVI and $CAVI_0$ was also assessed[20]. The characteristics of the important variables studied can be found in Table 1 and their correlations with CAVI and $CAVI_0$ can be seen in Fig. 1.

CAVI and $CAVI_0$ has a high correlation with each other as reflected in the Pearson's $r = 0.95$ ($p < 0.001$). There is a sound rationale for this correlation as PWV can be

Table 2. Logistic regression analysis of CAVI and $CAVI_0$ greater than median cut-off point. Source: Lin et al.[20]

			Model 1	Model 2	Model 3	Model 4
CAVI	Age	OR (CI)	**1.14 (1.09-1.19)**	**1.13 (1.08-1.19)**	**1.14 (1.09-1.20)**	**1.14 (1.09-1.19)**
		P value	**<0.001**	**<0.0001**	**<0.0001**	**<0.0001**
	SBP	OR (CI)	-	1.01(0.99-1.03)	-	-
		P value	-	0.1368	-	-
	DBP	OR (CI)	-	-	1.09 (0.99-1.06)	-
		P value	-	-	0.1540	-
	MBP	OR (CI)	-	-	-	1.02 (0.99-1.05)
		P value	-	-	-	0.1260
$CAVI_0$	Age	OR (CI)	**1.17 (1.11-1.23)**	**1.16 (1.10 - 1.22)**	**1.16 (1.11- 1.23)**	-
		P value	**<0.0001**	**<0.0001**	**<0.0001**	-
	SBP	OR (CI)	-	1.01 (0.99-1.03)	-	-
		P value	-	0.1517	-	-
	MBP	OR (CI)	-	-	1.007 (0.97-1.03)	-
		P value	-	-	0.6457	-

Age [years]; SBP = Systolic Blood Pressure [mmHg]; DBP = Diastolic Blood Pressure [mmHg]; MBP = Mean Blood Pleasure [mmHg], CAVI: Model 1 = age; Model 2 = age, SBP; Model 3 = age, DBP; Model 4 = age, MBP, $CAVI_0$: Model 1 = age; Model 2 = age, SBP; Model 3 = age, MBP.

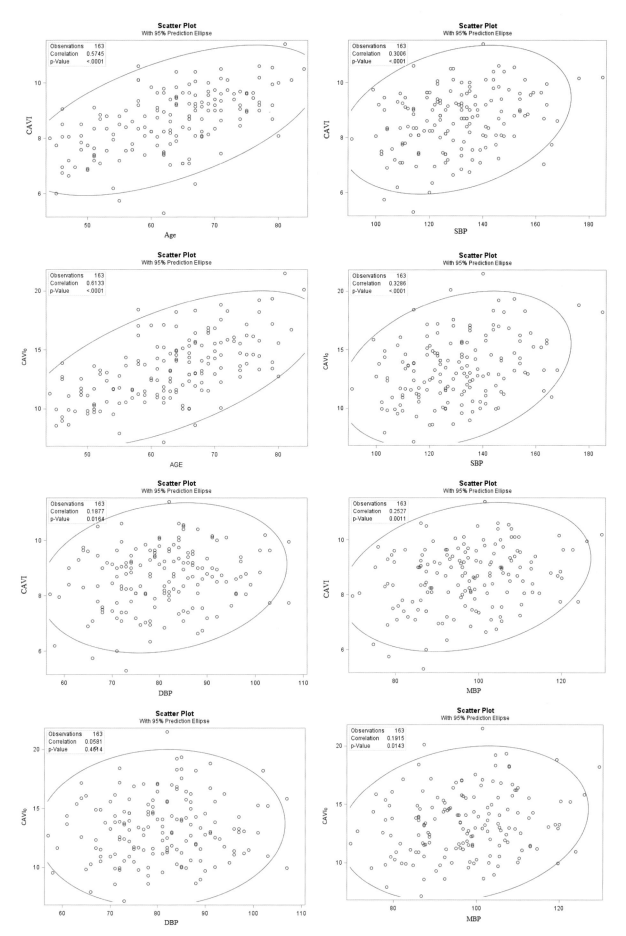

Fig. 1. Scatter plots and 95% prediction eclipse of CAVI and CAVI$_0$ with Systolic Blood Pressure, Diastolic Blood Pressure, Mean Blood Pressure and age. Source: Lin et al.[20]

considered as the main factor which affects the measurements in both CAVI and $CAVI_0$. Another finding shows that CAVI and $CAVI_0$ are associated significantly and independently only to age after adjusting for other risk factors (Table 2). This fact that it is only age that has an independent effect on these indices can help scientists to build reliable models to define individuals at risk of atherosclerosis and cardiovascular events.

SBP and DBP are both important in the evaluation of the risk assessment of hypertension complications. CAVI was related to both SBP and DBP, but $CAVI_0$ was related to SBP and not to DBP. From these results, we should consider that $CAVI_0$ may not be reflective of DBP in the patient. This might be derived from the equation of $CAVI_0$, in which only DPB was in the denominator.

How to treat high CAVI

The effect of different treatments and behavior modifications on CAVI have been studied in the literature. Body weight reduction as calorie restriction in metabolic syndrome and obesity with diabetes has shown to decrease CAVI[21, 22]. Glucose control by using Rapid-acting insulin analogs, Dipeptidyl peptidase 4 inhibitors, Sulfonylurea, Pioglitazone, α-glucosidase inhibitors and Sodium-glucose Cotransporter-2 Inhibitors have been shown to decrease CAVI[23-29]. Blood pressure control by using Calcium blocker (T-type calcium channel blocker), Renin-angiotensin-aldosterone system inhibitors, Mineralocorticoid receptor blocker and Direct renin inhibitor[30-37] have also been shown to decrease CAVI. Lipid control by using Statins, Eicosapentaenoic acid and Fibrates[38-40], smoking cessation and exercise as well as small amount of alcohol are also among the factors which decrease CAVI[41-43].

Conclusion

All these results show that CAVI is a reliable index in differentiating people with a high risk of CVD. The fact that should be taken into account is that SBP and DBP are both important in the evaluation of the risk assessment of hypertension complications, as uncontrolled DBP is associated with a greater risk of CVD events and uncontrolled SBP is more associated with poorer prognosis. When evaluating the results of $CAVI_0$, we should consider that this index maybe not reflective of DBP in the patient.

References

1) Shirai K., et al. A novel blood pressure-independent arterial wall stiffness parameter; cardio-ankle vascular index (CAVI). J Atheroscler Thromb 2006; **13**: 101-107.

2) Spronck, B., et al. Direct means of obtaining CAVI(0)-a corrected cardio-ankle vascular stiffness index (CAVI)-from conventional CAVI measurements or their underlying variables. Physiol Meas 2017; **38**: N128-n137.

3) Alizargar, J., et al. Using the Cardio-Ankle Vascular Index (CAVI) or the Mathematical Correction Form (CAVI(0)) in Clinical Practice. Int J Mol Sci 2020; **21**.

4) Spronck, B., et al. Easy conversion of cardio-ankle vascular index into CAVI0: influence of scale coefficients. J Hypertens 2019; **37**: 1913-1914.

5) Saiki, A., et al. New Horizons of Arterial Stiffness Developed Using Cardio-Ankle Vascular Index (CAVI). J Atheroscler Thromb 2020; **27**: 732-748.

6) Horinaka, S., et al. Comparison of atherosclerotic indicators between cardio ankle vascular index and brachial ankle pulse wave velocity. Angiology. Aug-Sep 2009; **60**: 468-476. doi: 10.1177/0003319708325443

7) Nakamura, K., et al. Cardio-ankle vascular index is a candidate predictor of coronary atherosclerosis 2007; **72**: 598-604.

8) Izuhara, M., et al. Relationship of cardio-ankle vascular index (CAVI) to carotid and coronary arteriosclerosis 2008; 0809160082-0809160082.

9) Chung, S.-L., et al. Coronary artery calcium score compared with cardio-ankle vascular index in the prediction of cardiovascular events in asymptomatic patients with type 2 diabetes 2015; **22**: 1255-1265.

10) Mineoka, Y., et al. Relationship between cardio-ankle vascular index (CAVI) and coronary artery calcification (CAC) in patients with type 2 diabetes mellitus 2012; **27**: 160-165.

11) Park, J.-B., et al. Relation between cardio-ankle vascular index and coronary artery calcification or stenosis in asymptomatic subjects 2013: 15149.

12) Suzuki, J., et al. Stroke and cardio-ankle vascular stiffness index 2013; **22**: 171-175.

13) Saji, N., et al. Comparison of arteriosclerotic indicators in patients with ischemic stroke: ankle–brachial index, brachial–ankle pulse wave velocity and cardio–ankle vascular index 2015; **38**: 323-328.

14) Kubozono, T., et al. Association between arterial stiffness and estimated glomerular filtration rate in the Japanese general population 2009; **16**: 840-845.

15) Ueyama, K., et al. Noninvasive indices of arterial stiffness in hemodialysis patients 2009; **32**: 716-720.

16) Nakamura, K., et al. Association between cardio-ankle vascular index and serum cystatin C levels in patients with cardiovascular risk factor 2009: 0908100064-0908100064.

17) Yamashita, H., et al. Association between cystatin C and arteriosclerosis in the absence of chronic kidney disease 2013: 13193.

18) Imamura, H., et al. Resveratrol ameliorates arterial stiffness assessed by cardio-ankle vascular index in patients with type 2 diabetes mellitus 2017; **58**: 577-583.

19) Usui, T., et al. Effects of natural S-equol supplements on overweight or obesity and metabolic syndrome in the Japanese, based on sex and equol status 2013; **78**: 365-372.

20) Lin, L.-J., et al. Factors Associated with Cardio Ankle Vascular Index (CAVI) and its Mathematically Corrected Formula (CAVI0) in Community Dwelling Individuals 2020.

21) Satoh, N., et al. Evaluation of the cardio-ankle vascular index, a new indicator of arterial stiffness independent of blood pressure, in obesity and metabolic syndrome 2008; **31**: 1921-1930.

22) Nagayama, D., et al. Effects of body weight reduction on cardio-ankle vascular index (CAVI) 2013; **7**: e139-e145.

23) Ohira, M., et al. Improvement of postprandial hyperglycemia and arterial stiffness upon switching from premixed human insulin 30/70 to biphasic insulin aspart 30/70 2011; **60**: 78-85.

24) Akahori, H.J.D.i., Clinical evaluation of thrice-daily lispro 50/50 versus twice-daily aspart 70/30 on blood glucose fluctuation and postprandial hyperglycemia in patients with type 2 diabetes mellitus 2015; **6**: 275-283.

25) Shigiyama, F., et al. Linagliptin improves endothelial function in patients with type 2 diabetes: a randomized study of linagliptin effectiveness on endothelial function 2017; **8**: 330-340.

26) Nagayama, D., et al. Improvement of cardio-ankle vascular

index by glimepiride in type 2 diabetic patients 2010; **64**: 1796-1801.

27) Ohira, M., et al. Pioglitazone improves the cardio-ankle vascular index in patients with type 2 diabetes mellitus treated with metformin 2014; **7**: 313.

28) Uzui, H., et al. Acarbose treatments improve arterial stiffness in patients with type 2 diabetes mellitus 2011;**2**:148-153.

29) Bekki, M., et al. Switching dipeptidyl peptidase-4 inhibitors to tofogliflozin, a selective inhibitor of sodium-glucose cotransporter 2 improve arterial stiffness evaluated by cardio-ankle vascular index in patients with type 2 diabetes: a pilot study 2019; **17**: 411-420.

30) Sasaki, H., et al. Protective effects of efonidipine, a T-and L-type calcium channel blocker, on renal function and arterial stiffness in type 2 diabetic patients with hypertension and nephropathy 2009: 0909110090-0909110090.

31) Bokuda, K., et al. Blood pressure-independent effect of candesartan on cardio-ankle vascular index in hypertensive patients with metabolic syndrome 2010; **6**: 571.

32) Miyashita, Y., et al. Effects of olmesartan, an angiotensin II receptor blocker, and amlodipine, a calcium channel blocker, on Cardio-Ankle Vascular Index (CAVI) in type 2 diabetic patients with hypertension 2009: 0911060106-0911060106.

33) Miyoshi, T., et al. Effect of azilsartan on day-to-day variability in home blood pressure: a prospective multicenter clinical trial 2017; **9**: 618.

34) Kiuchi, S., et al. Addition of a renin-angiotensin-aldosterone system inhibitor to a calcium channel blocker ameliorates arterial stiffness 2015; **7**: 97.

35) Shibata, T., et al. Effects of add-on therapy consisting of a selective mineralocorticoid receptor blocker on arterial stiffness in patients with uncontrolled hypertension 2015; **54**: 1583-1589.

36) Miyoshi, T., et al. Comparable effect of aliskiren or a diuretic added on an angiotensin II receptor blocker on augmentation index in hypertension: a multicentre, prospective, randomised study 2017; **4**.

37) Bokuda, K., et al. Greater reductions in plasma aldosterone with aliskiren in hypertensive patients with higher soluble (Pro) renin receptor level 2018; **41**: 435-443.

38) Miyashita, Y., et al. Effects of pitavastatin, a 3-hydroxy-3-methylglutaryl coenzyme a reductase inhibitor, on cardio-ankle vascular index in type 2 diabetic patients 2009: 0911060105-0911060105.

39) Satoh, N., et al. Highly purified eicosapentaenoic acid reduces cardio-ankle vascular index in association with decreased serum amyloid A-LDL in metabolic syndrome 2009; **32**: 1004-1008.

40) Yamaguchi, T., et al. Bezafibrate ameliorates arterial stiffness assessed by cardio-ankle vascular index in hypertriglyceridemic patients with type 2 diabetes mellitus 2018: 45799.

41) Noike, H., et al. Changes in cardio-ankle vascular index in smoking cessation 2010: 1003080197-1003080197.

42) Nishiwaki, M., N. Kora, and N.J.P.r. Matsumoto, Ingesting a small amount of beer reduces arterial stiffness in healthy humans 2017; **5**: e13381.

43) Alonso-Domínguez, R., et al. Acute effect of healthy walking on arterial stiffness in patients with type 2 diabetes and differences by age and sex: a pre-post intervention study 2019; **19**: 1-9.

Conditions of measuring CAVI
-Check points and the effects of smoking-

Takaaki Shoda[1,2,3]

Introduction

The cardio-ankle vascular index (CAVI) is an index of stiffness of the arterial tree from the origin of the aorta to the ankle, and the measuring device, VaSera, is used to measure the same[1]. VaSera is equipped with a pulse wave detector at the upper brachium and the ankle to detect the pulse wave velocity from the origin of the aorta to those and measure the brachial blood pressure; additionally, it also has a detector for heart sounds. Furthermore, it must be noted that arterial stiffness itself changes according to various conditions of the subjects[2,3]. There are several precautions to be followed before and during measurement to obtain a correct value of CAVI. These precautions are described in this chapter. We also studied the effect of smoking just before measuring CAVI and showed how the CAVI value was acutely affected by smoking.

I.   Instructions to be followed by the patients

The day before and on the day of examination: Avoid heavy drinking (sake, beer, wine, other hard drinks.)
1. The day before and on the day of examination: Please avoid excessive exercise.
2. Sleeping pills and daily medications: Please consult your doctor.
3. The day before examination: Please avoid lack of sleep as much as possible.
4. The day before examination: Please refrain from drinking coffee after 6 pm.
5. The day of examination: Please avoid walking for more than 30 minutes before coming to the hospital.
6. The day of examination: Please avoid eating and drinking on the way to the hospital (2 hours prior).
7. The day of examination: Please stop smoking 2 hours before the scheduled examination.

II.   Explanation of the patient at testing

Make sure you provide the patient with an overview of the procedure to ensure that he or she will remain still and not be surprised during the procedure.

III.   Explain the test procedure
1. CAVI measurement: Application of 50 mmHg (weak) pressure to the four limbs
2. CAVI measurement (right side) Right brachial, right ankle blood pressure measurement
3. CAVI measurement (left side) Left brachial, left ankle blood pressure measurement

The test takes approximately five minutes.

Provide the patient with details of the test to avoid unnecessary stress.

Get the patient to take two or three deep breaths before starting the measurement.

Make sure you inform the patient just before starting the test.

IV.   Confirmation before measurement
1. Clothing at time of measurement

Please perform the test with the patient wearing light clothes (T shirt, shirt, and other light clothing., are acceptable). If the patient is wearing a light shirt, there is no problem with wrapping the cuffs over the shirt. Ideal clothing is an examination gown.

2. Room temperature of the examination room

Keep the room temperature at approximately $22-26\,^{\circ}\mathrm{C}$ for the patient to relax.

3. Resting time before the measurement

Ensure that the patient rests for at least 10 minutes.

Avoid measurement of CAVI immediately after exercise or running.

4. Confirmation of bed size

Have the patient lie face up on a wide bed for examination. If a person with a large body has to squeeze their arms up against their body because the bed is too small and excessive effort is made to hold the arms and legs in place, the blood pressure and pulse wave cannot be measured accurately.

5. Attachment of the medical equipment
1) How to select and wrap the cuffs
   a) Range of cuffs used

Use only cuffs that fit the brachia and ankles of the patient. The cuffs used can be considered as the proper size if the INDEX mark (▲) is within the RANGE zone when the cuffs are wrapped over the brachium or ankle.

---

[1]EHIME Medical Coordinating CO (EMC).
[2](Formerly) Department of Internal Medicine III, Ehime University School of Medicine.
[3]Minami Matsuyama Clinic, Jinyukai Medical Corporation.

b) How to wrap the cuffs and set the air tubes

i) How to wrap the cuffs on the brachia

Ensure that the air hose outlet of the cuff lies over the center of the brachial artery blood vessels on the inside of the brachium. The cuff is positioned so that the lower edge of the cuff is immediately above the elbow joint (the line when the elbow is bent).

ii) How to wrap the cuffs on the ankles

Position the cuff so that its lower edge is 1 cm above the malleolus. Make sure that the hose outlet extends upward from the medial malleolus. If the cuff is wrapped correctly, the arrow on the label points to the malleolus. The ankle cuffs are easier to wrap if the patient bends his/her knees. Firmly attach both the upper and lower edges of the cuff applying the same strength so that there are no gaps. The cuff is firmly wrapped while ensuring that it does not constrict the ankle; confirm that a finger cannot be inserted between the cuff and the ankle. In addition, it needs to be ensured that both the upper and lower edges of the cuff have no gap. The air tube may become buried underneath the body (Fig. 1).

2) Attachment of the heart sound microphone

The heart sound microphone is firmly attached over the sternum in the second intercostal space using double-sided tape (DA-30). The precise procedure and precautions are described in the next section.

6.   Check point of measurement data

1) Waveform check during CAVI measurement

Check the waveforms immediately after pressing the start button and commencing the measurement. Confirm that each type of waveform is accurately recorded on the screen. It is important to confirm that the heart sound, brachial notch, and rise of the pulse wave are detected without any problems. If arrhythmia occurs, the CAVI cannot be accurately measured. Repeat the measurement and ensure that there is no arrhythmia before measuring CAVI. Sometimes, when there is valvular insufficiency (AS, AR), noise enters the heart sound or the notch disappears.

2) Data check after CAVI measurement

If the patient has stenosis or insufficiency of the femoral artery, the inflection point of the pulse wave at the ankle becomes dull. In this case, the notch and rise cannot be recognized; thus, the measurement cannot be taken.

The variation of each heartbeat can be confirmed with the detailed measurement values.

Symbols that prefix the measurements indicate measurement quality, a value that depends on the number of measurements not prefixed by

×: Inadequate △: Almost adequate ○: Good ◎: Excellent

a) Example of good quality

The symbol ◎ next to the mean value of CAVI indicates that there is little variation in the value per heartbeat.

b) Example of bad quality

The symbol △ next to the mean value of CAVI

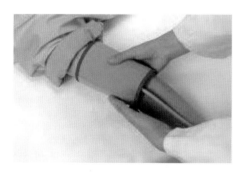

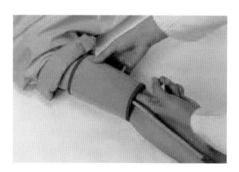

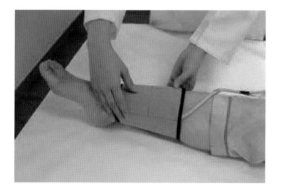

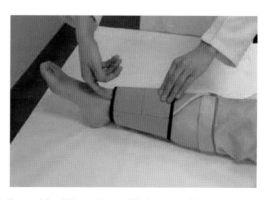

Fig. 1.   How to set and wrap the cuffs around the brachium and at the ankle: Wrap the cuffs firmly without spaces such that a finger cannot be inserted.

indicates that there is a large variation in the value per heartbeat. Thus, the figures are marked as an ×.

V. Acute effect of smoking just before measuring CAVI

The acute effects of smoking on CAVI have not been fully evaluated[4]. We studied the acute changes in CAVI among five smokers (age 29 to 71 years, mean number of cigarettes smoked = 20 per day). After smoking, CAVI was measured immediately. The results are shown in Fig. 2. The mean CAVI increased from 5 to 120 min. Significant differences were observed at 60 min and 120 min with the maximum increase being 0.5-0.7 ΔCAVI. These results suggest that smoking transiently increases CAVI values. Based on these results, we recommend that smoking must be prohibited for more than 3 h before the CAVI measurement.

This study also suggested that smoking might contract the arterial smooth muscle cells, leading to contraction of the

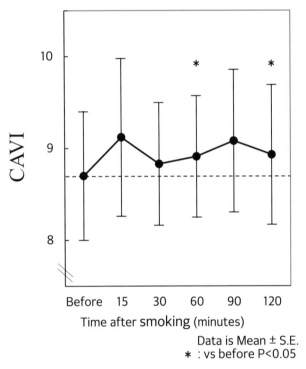

Data is Mean ± S.E.
∗ : vs before P<0.05

Fig. 2. The effects of smoking just before measuring on CAVI.

vasa vasorum in arteries with advanced atherosclerosis. This might induce ischemia of the plaque and cause a rupture, as described in Chapter 57.

Afterward

We nostalgically remember the days when we observed the flexibility and shape of the manchette fabric. Currently, CAVI is recognized by specialists in most of the world, and its utility is nearly established. We believe that CAVI reflects the correct value of arterial stiffness with proper handling of VaSera and will contribute to maintaining the vascular health of the people.

Acknowledgments

We would like to thank Mr. Maki Miyazaki and Ms. Namiko Sakuoka (maiden name: Takeda) of the Ehime University Hospital Test Department, who have cooperated with us since the beginning of the development of VaSera and CAVI, for their cooperation with measurement problems, data organization, and so on.

We would like to express our sincere gratitude to Dr. Hiroshi Matsuoka, Deputy Director of Ehime Prefectural Central Hospital, for the literature and explanations regarding smoking.

We would like to thank Mr. Kotaro Fukuda, Chairman of Fukuda Denshi, Mr. Takahashi and Mr. Maruyama in the Development Department, and Mr. Ozaki and Mr. Sato in the Sales Department.

References

1) Shirai K, Utino J, Otsuka K, Takata M. A novel blood pressure-independent arterial wall stiffness parameter: cardio- ankle vascular index (CAVI). J Atheroscler Thromb. 2006;13:101-107.
2) Shoda T. Arteriosclerosis. 99-115, in JSLM2018, Japanese Society of Laboratory Medicine Guidelines, Editorial Committee, Japan Society of Laboratory Medicine 2018 (in Japanese).
3) Shoda T, Watanabe S, Higaki M. Pulse wave/limb blood pressure test in patients with renal failure and renal dialysis (CAVI-Vasera) value dynamics. Medical and testing equipment. 2005;28:551-557 (in Japanese).
4) Matsuoka H. Prevention and treatment of cardiovascular disease due to quitting smoking from the viewpoint of smoking risk. Heart. 2007;39:510-514 (in Japanese).

Points of confirmation for obtaining correct measurements

Takashi Miki

Preface

The cardio-ankle vascular index (CAVI) is considered an indicator of stiffness of the arterial tree from the origin of the aorta to the ankle. The Vasera system was developed to calculate the value of the CAVI. This system measured the pulse wave velocity (PWV) from the origin of the aorta to the ankle by detecting the time of initiation of the PWV. However, this method is somewhat complicated, and blood pressure at the upper brachial artery on behalf of that of the whole arterial tree. Therefore, there are several prerequisites while using this method. We present these prerequisites below to obtain the correct values of the CAVI using the Vasera system.

1. Body position during measurement

The position of the patient at the time of measurement should be supine, in which the heart and the upper and lower limbs are at the same horizontal level. It has been reported that the ABI (ankle brachial pressure index) values are significantly elevated in the semi-Fowler's (the patient's upper body raised at 30 degrees) and the orthopneic position with both legs hanging down compared to those in the supine position (horizontal position). It has also been reported that the PWV values showed a significant difference when measured in the supine position compared with those in the other positions in which the upper body is raised. This is because raising the upper body changes the diameter and wall thickness of the blood vessels and the peripheral vascular resistance of the lower limbs. When measuring the ABI and PWV, it is important to maintain the patient in the supine position (horizontal position) to ensure the validity and precision of the measurements (Fig. 1).

However, in some cases, when a patient with a bent back tries to lie in the supine position (horizontal position), the entire body might be strained. In such cases, the measurement must be taken in the position in which the patient can feel relaxed, by using pillows to adjust the height at which he or she is comfortable without changing the horizontal level of the heart and the upper and lower limbs.

2. Precautions for accurate monitoring of the heart sound

Since the calculation of the CAVI uses the heart-ankle PWV (haPWV), the distance between the heart and the ankle (L) and the pulse transit time between the heart and the ankle (T) are required. The distance can be obtained by measuring the height of the patient. To obtain the transit time, the duration of propagation of the pulse wave from the opening of the aortic valve until it reaches the ankle is required. However, since the time of opening of the aortic

valve cannot be detected, the accepted principle that the duration between the first component of the second heart sound (S2) (sound of closure of the aortic valve) and the

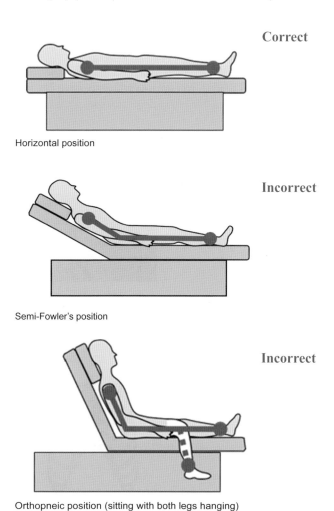

Correct

Horizontal position

Incorrect

Semi-Fowler's position

Incorrect

Orthopneic position (sitting with both legs hanging)

Fig. 1. The heart, brachium, and ankle must be measured in the horizontal position.

Tohoku university hospital Clinical Physiology Center, 1-1 Seiryomachi, Aoba-ku, Sendai City, Miyagi 980-8574, Japan.

notch of the brachial pulse wave is the same as the duration between the opening of the aortic valve and the rise of the brachial pulse wave can be used as shown below.

S2 - notch of brachial pulse wave + rise of the brachial pulse wave - rise of the ankle pulse wave = aortic valve opening - propagation time from the aortic valve to the ankle.

As seen in the above equation, S2 plays an important role in the measurement of the CAVI.

- The possible causes of noise while listening to the heart sounds
① Noise from the external environment
② Incorrect location of the microphone
③ Detachment of the microphone
④ The patient speaking, snoring, or making respiratory noises.
⑤ Heart murmur

3. Attachment of the heart sound microphone

The normal position of the microphone for listening to the heart sounds is over the sternum at the level of the second intercostal space. The microphone for listening to the heart sounds transmits the heart sound to the sensor via bone conduction; however, this procedure is often difficult to perform.

① When the microphone for listening to the heart sounds is placed over an area with excessive fat, such as a large breast in a female patient and a patient with obesity, the heart sounds could be masked, and the microphone may fail to detect the heart sound.
② When the microphone for listening to the heart

sounds is placed on the hairy chest of a male patient, the microphone may get detached from the body and may not be able to detect the heart sound.

The microphone for listening to the heart sounds must be attached firmly with a thin double-sided adhesive tape (Fig. 2). When the heart sound cannot be detected over the sternum or attaching the microphone is difficult, the microphone for listening to the heart sounds can be positioned over the sternal end of the left clavicle (near the sternoclavicular joint) (Fig. 2). Before starting the measurement, it needs to be ensured that the microphone for listening to the heart sounds is not detached from the patient's body due to movement.

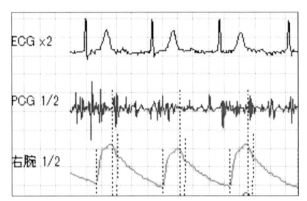

Fig. 3. Severe aortic stenosis (AS) causes a systolic ejection murmur that occurs between the first heart sound (S1) and the second heart sound (S2) and affects the onset of aortic valve closure sounds during S2.

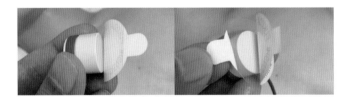

Attaching the microphone for listening to the heart sounds: double-sided tape

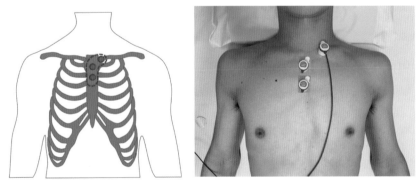

Position of the microphone for listening to the heart sounds

Fig. 2. Place the microphone for listening to the heart sounds over the sternum at the level of the second intercostal space, at the level of the first intercostal space, or the sternal end of the left clavicle (near the sternoclavicular joint), avoiding the spots with excessive fat. The microphone for listening to the heart sounds should be firmly attached with double-sided adhesive tape to prevent the microphone from lifting off from the patient's body.

4. Diseases or conditions affecting detection of the pulse wave

Effect of heart murmurs

As the CAVI measures the haPWV, it is not possible to obtain accurate measurements when there is an influential murmur between the first heart sound (S1) and second heart sound (S2). The CAVI value measured in such cases can be treated only as a reference value or it cannot be measured. The cardiac murmurs that can affect the sound of closure of the aortic valve during S2 include systolic ejection murmurs, systolic regurgitant murmurs, and continuous murmurs. When there is a murmur between S1 and S2 and the recognition of the first component of the S2 becomes irregular, the measurement becomes invalid (Fig. 3).

5. Effect of arrhythmia

Both the PWV and CAVI are affected by arrhythmias. Atrial fibrillation often inhibits an accurate evaluation because it leads to irregular heartbeats, irregular pulse wave amplitude, irregular S2 to brachial notch (tb) duration, and irregular shape of the pulse wave shape (Fig. 4). Other arrhythmias that occur frequently also make it difficult to perform the evaluations.

6. Effect of peripheral arterial diseases

Arteriosclerosis obliterans (ASO) is a condition in which adequate blood flow cannot be maintained due to stenosis or occlusion of blood vessels in the lower extremities. In severe cases, the pulse transit time between the brachium and ankle (tba) becomes irregular due to decreased blood pressure in the lower limbs and sluggish rise of the pulse waveform. When ABI is 0.9 or less, as a recognition of the lower extremity pulse waveforms become irregular (Fig. 5) In such cases, the PWV and CAVI are considered as reference values.

Effect of aortic disease

Aortic diseases that affect the PWV and CAVI include coarctation of the aorta and Takayasu arteritis. When stenosis or occlusion is present in the aorta, the PWV and CAVI serve as reference values, similar to that in cases of ASO.

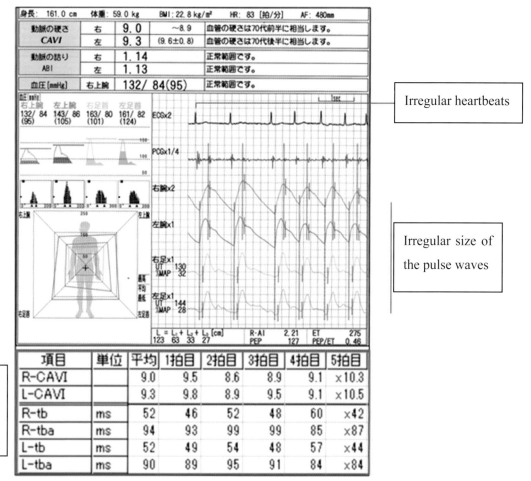

Fig. 4. In atrial fibrillation, the amplitude of pulse waves are inconsistent because of irregular heartbeats. tbs and tba for both right and left sides are in consistent.

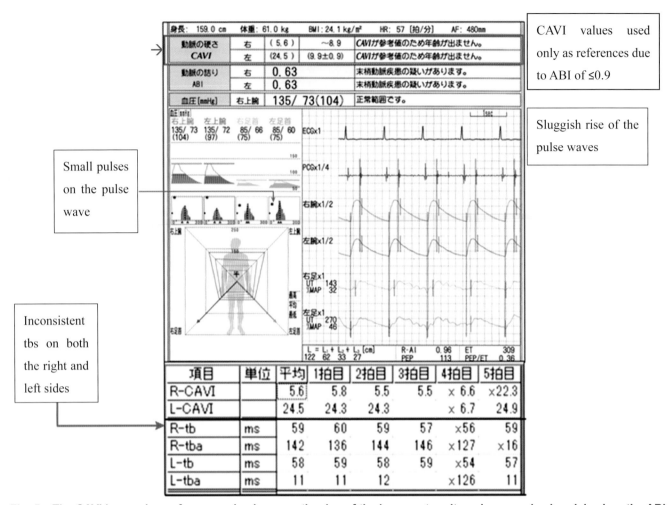

Small pulses on the pulse wave

Inconsistent tbs on both the right and left sides

CAVI values used only as references due to ABI of ≤0.9

Sluggish rise of the pulse waves

項目	単位	平均	1拍目	2拍目	3拍目	4拍目	5拍目
R-CAVI		5.6	5.8	5.5	5.5	× 6.6	×22.3
L-CAVI		24.5	24.3	24.3		× 6.7	24.9
R-tb	ms	59	60	59	57	×56	59
R-tba	ms	142	136	144	146	×127	×16
L-tb	ms	58	59	58	59	×54	57
L-tba	ms	11	11	12		×126	11

Fig. 5. The CAVI is merely a reference value because the rise of the lower extremity pulse wave is sluggish when the ABI value is 0.9 or less.

Reproducibility

Takuro Kubozono

Introduction

The cardio-ankle vascular index (CAVI) is used to assess arteriosclerosis based on the stiffness parameter β, which is not influenced by blood pressure. It has recently become a popular tool to evaluate the arterial stiffness because of its simplicity and non-invasiveness. This article reviews the reproducibility and accuracy of CAVI.

Reproducibility of CAVI

Numerous papers on the reproducibility of CAVI have been reported. CAVI measured twice over a 2-week interval in 22 healthy participants showed a good association with R = 0.93 as shown in Fig. 1[1]. Furthermore, the mean coefficient of variation was found to be 3.8% with good reproducibility when CAVI was measured five times at the same time on different days for 22 participants[2]. In addition, in 105 Caucasians, the mean coefficient of variation of CAVI measurements taken three times was 4.38%, indicating that CAVI is highly reproducible and useful for cardiovascular disease risk assessment[3]. In a study of 50 participants, both inter-and intra-examiner reproducibility were reported to be high[4]. The coefficient of variation was 2.8% when CAVI was measured three times in 25 sleep apnea patients[5]. This result indicates a high reproducibility of CAVI, considering that the coefficients of variation of carotid-femoral pulse wave velocity (PWV) in hypertensive patients and brachial-ankle PWV (baPWV) in patients with coronary artery disease have been reported to be 7 to 14% and 4 to 10%, respectively.

CAVI and blood pressure (BP) during measurement

In distinction to PWV, CAVI is a parameter that is independent of the changes in BP during measurement. We investigated the effect of BP changes on CAVI and baPWV in 1033 consecutive subjects undergoing health checkups[1]. Although both parameters were significantly associated with BP at the time of the measurements, baPWV had a higher coefficient value. Additionally, in multivariate analysis, systolic BP was an independent factor for baPWV in both men and women, whereas CAVI showed an independent association for systolic BP in men but not in women. In a study of changes in CAVI and baPWV using antihypertensive drugs, beta-blockers reduced baPWV but not CAVI, while alpha-blockers reduced both baPWV and CAVI as shown in Chapter1 Fig. 4[6]. Beta-blockers decreased the BP by affecting the cardiac contraction, whereas alpha-blockers decreased BP by acting on the vascular smooth muscles. Therefore, alpha-blockers may affect the arterial stiffness and reduce the CAVI.

Conclusion

CAVI is a highly reproducible and accurate device for the non-invasive assessment of arterial stiffness. Several studies have been reported its usefulness so far, and it is expected to make a significant contribution to clinical practice in the future.

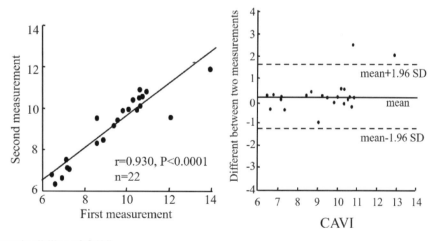

Fig. 1. Reproducibility of CAVI.
When CAVI was measured twice in the same case, a good correlation was observed with R = 0.93. Brant-Altman analysis also revealed that it was highly reproducible (cited from ref. 1).
CAVI, cardio-ankle vascular index

Department of Cardiovascular Medicine and Hypertension, Graduate School of Medical and Dental Sciences, Kagoshima University, 8-35-1 Sakuragaoka, Kagoshima City, Kagoshima 890-8544, Japan.

References

1) Kubozono T, Miyata M, Ueyama K, et al. Clinical significance and reproducibility of new arterial distensibility index. Circ J. 2007; 71: 89-94 https://doi.org/10.1253/circj.71.89.

2) Shirai K, Utino J, Otsuka K, Takata M. A novel blood pressure-independent arterial wall stiffness parameter; cardio-ankle vascular index (CAVI). J Atheroscler Thromb. 2006; 13: 101-7.

3) Endes S, Caviezel S, Dratva J, et al. Reproducibility of oscillometrically measured arterial stiffness indices: Results of the SAPALDIA 3 cohort study. Scand J Clin Lab Invest. 2015; 75: 170-6.

4) Lim J, Pearman ME, Park W, Alkatan M, Machin DR, Tanaka H. Impact of blood pressure perturbations on arterial stiffness. Am J Physiol Regul Integr Comp Physiol. 2015; 309: R1540-5.

5) Kumagai T, Kasai T, Kato M, Naito R, Maeno KI, Kasagi S, Kawana F, Ishiwata S, Narui K. Establishment of the cardio-ankle vascular index in patients with obstructive sleep apnea. Chest. 2009; 136: 779-86.

6) Shirai K, Song M, Suzuki J, et al. Contradictory effects of β1- and α1- aderenergic receptor blockers on cardio-ankle vascular stiffness index (CAVI)--CAVI independent of blood pressure. J Atheroscler Thromb. 2011; 18: 49-55 https://doi.org/10.5551/jat.3582.

PART 2

Basic properties of CAVI

CAVI and other physiological parameters: Changes of CAVI with heart rate and diurnal variation

Atsuhito Saiki[1] and Akira Takahara[2]

Summry
- CAVI was not affected by heart rate changes within the normal range.
- Diurnal changes in CAVI were observed in some but not most individuals. This difference might be dependent on autonomic rhythms. Further studies are needed for more detailed elucidation.

Introduction

To use the cardio-ankle vascular index (CAVI) in clinical practice, it is necessary to remember some of several physiological factors affecting CAVI. Among those factors, blood pressure, heart rate, and diurnal rhythm are candidates. The effects of blood pressure on CAVI been discussed previously, and are essentially negligible[1,2]. Heart rate can potentially influence CAVI during measurement, given that it is debated whether pulse wave velocity (PWV), which is an element of the CAVI equation, is influenced by heart rate itself. Additionally, it is possible that CAVI has a diurnal rhythm, since blood pressure, another element of the CAVI equation, is known vary diurnally. This chapter summarizes the current knowledge on the impact of heart rate on, and the diurnal variation of CAVI.

Does CAVI depend on changes in pulse rate?

The effect of pulse rate on PWV remains controversial. Recently, Vasiliki et al. reported a significant heart rate effect on **carotid-femoral** PWV (cf-PWV), when blood pressure was left free to vary with heart rate[3]. Su et al. evaluated the effects of heart rate on brachial-ankle PWV (baPWV)[4]. Patients without significant organic heart disease underwent elective cardiac catheterization or electrophysiological study, and as heart rate increased, baPWV also increased significantly. Those reports suggested that baPWV is heart rate-dependent.

On the other hand, no report to date has examined whether CAVI is dependent on heart rate in humans. We examined the relationship between heart rate and CAVI in halothane-anesthetized rabbits treated with atrioventricular block. CAVI did not increase with an increase in heart rate from 90 to 300 beats/min (Fig. 1, unpublished). This result suggests that CAVI was not dependent on heart rate. However, further precise studies on the relationship between CAVI and heart rate might be required.

Diurnal variation of CAVI

We observed that there was no diurnal variation in the mean CAVI at 6 time-points (7:30, 10:00, 11:30, 14:00, 17:30, and 20:00) in 30 hospitalized patients with at least one risk factor (Fig. 2). CAVI did not change before or after a meal, and was not associated with changes in blood pressure or blood glucose. On the other hand, Li et al. stated that there was a significant diurnal variation in CAVI, with the highest values at 09:00 h. After adjusting for age, sex, and mean arterial pressure, CAVI maintained significantly higher values at 09:00: these values were 4% higher than those at 13:00 and 5% higher than those at 17:00[5]. However, evidence for the diurnal variability of CAVI is

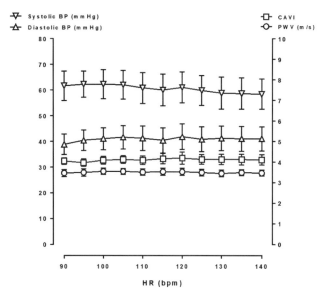

Fig. 1. CAVI was not affected by changes in the ventricular pacing rate in halothane-anesthetized rabbits in which atrioventricular block was induced (n = 5) (unpublished data).

[1]Center of Diabetes, Endocrine, and Metabolism, Toho University Sakura Medical Center, 564-1, Shimoshizu, Sakura-City, Chiba, 285-8741, Japan.
[2]Department of Pharmacology and Therapeutics, Faculty of Pharmaceutical Sciences, Toho University, Funabashi, Chiba, 274-8510, Japan.

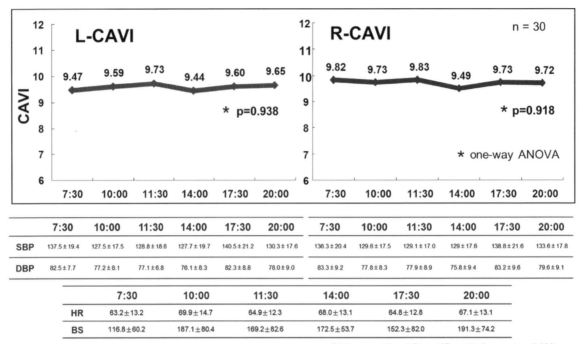

Fig. 2. Effect of blood pressure, diet, and exercise on the diurnal variability of CAVI in 30 patients with one or more risk factor including obesity, dyslipidemia, hypertension, and type 2 diabetes mellitus. CAVI, blood pressure, pulse rate, and blood glucose were measured at 6 time-points: 7:30, 10:00, 11:30, 14:00, 17:30, and 20:00 (unpublished data).

still not sufficient.

Blood pressure (BP) is also reported to display various diurnal patterns. Kario et al. proposed that there are two types of morning hypertension[6]. The nondipper/riser (nocturnal hypertension) type is associated with risk for damage to all target organs (brain, heart, and kidneys) and cardiovascular events[7]. The other type, the morning BP surge type, is associated in part with the extreme dipping of nocturnal BP, which is associated with stroke risk[8]. The mechanisms for those patterns remain controversial. CAVI is an index of arterial stiffness, which comprises organic stiffness and functional stiffness. Both functions might be involved in the regulation of blood pressure, and might contribute to blood pressure diurnal variations.

In principle, there is no diurnal variation in CAVI per se. Further investigation is required to determine whether there are various types of diurnal variation in CAVI, and to define their relationships with various cardiovascular events. The underlying mechanism for these variations should also be clarified by measuring the diurnal CAVI profile.

Future Perspective

Further investigations are required to determine:
- whether CAVI depends on the change in pulse rate in various pathological conditions.
- whether there is diurnal variation in CAVI.
- what conditions or diseases affect the diurnal variability of CAVI.

References

1) Hayashi K, Yamamoto T, Takahara A, Shirai K. Clinical assessment of arterial stiffness with cardio-ankle vascular index: Theory and applications. J Hypertens, 2015; 33: 1742-1757 https://doi.org/10.1097/hjh.0000000000000651.

2) Shirai K, Song M, Suzuki J, et al. Contradictory effects of β1- and α1-aderenergic receptor blockers on cardio-ankle vascular stiffness index (CAVI): The independency of CAVI from blood pressure. J Atheroscler Thromb, 2011; 18: 49-55.

3) Bikia V, Stergiopulos N, Rovas G, et al. The impact of heart rate on pulse wave velocity: an in-silico evaluation. J Hypertens. 2020; 38: 2451-2458.

4) Su HM, Lee KT, Chu CS, et al. Effects of heart rate on brachial-ankle pulse wave velocity and ankle-brachial pressure index in patients without significant organic heart disease. Angiology 2007; 58: 67-74.

5) Li Y, Cordes M, Recio-Rodriguez JI, et al. Diurnal variation of arterial stiffness in healthy individuals of different ages and patients with heart disease. Scand J Clin Lab Invest 2014; 74: 155-162.

6) Kario K. Time for focus on morning hypertension: pitfall of current antihypertensive medication. Am J Hypertens 2005; 18: 149-151.

7) Kario K, Shimada K, Pickering TG. Abnormal nocturnal blood pressure falls in elderly hypertension: clinical significance and determinants. J Cardiovasc Pharmacol 2003; 41 Suppl 1: S61-S66.

8) Kario K, Pickering TG, Matsuo T, et al. Stroke prognosis and abnormal nocturnal blood pressure falls in older hypertensives. Hypertension 2001; 38: 852-857.

Changes in CAVI values by aging, sex, and CVD risk factors

Kenji Suzuki[1], Tsukasa Namekata[2] and Kohji Shirai[3,4]

Background and Purpose

A cardio-ankle vascular index (CAVI) has been developed to represent the extent of arteriosclerosis throughout the aorta, femoral artery, and tibial artery, independent of blood pressure. For practical use of CAVI as a diagnostic tool for determining the extent of arteriosclerosis, our study objectives were (1) to establish the baseline CAVI scores by age and sex among cardiovascular disease (CVD) risk-free persons, (2) to compare CAVI scores between the sexes to test the hypothesis that the extent of arteriosclerosis in men is greater than that in women, and (3) to compare CAVI scores between the CVD risk-free group and the CVD high-risk group, in order to test the hypothesis that the extent of arteriosclerosis in the CVD high-risk group is greater than that in the CVD risk-free group.

Subjects and Methods

In 2005 and 2006, 32,627 urban workers and their families were screened.

The inclusion criteria for healthy individuals were: (1) systolic blood pressure $\leq$ 139 mmHg and diastolic blood pressure $\leq$ 89 mmHg, (2) total cholesterol $\leq$ 219 mg/dL, high-density lipoprotein cholesterol = 40- 99 mg/dL, and triglycerides $\leq$ 149 mg/dL, (3) fasting blood glucose $\leq$ 109 mg/dL and HbA1c (JDS) $\leq$ 5.8%, (4) creatinine $\leq$ 1.10 mg/dL in men, $\leq$ 0.80 mg/dL in women, (5) uric acid $\leq$ 7.0 mg/dL, (6) white blood cell count 3.2–8.5 $\times$ $10^3/\mu L$, (7) exclusion of carriers of Minnesota code: 1-1-1 to 1-3-6, 3-1 to 4, 5-1 to 5, 9-2, (8) normal small artery changes in the retina (based on Scheie's classification): no arteriosclerotic changes and no hypertensive changes, and (9) a medical history without heart disease, hypertension, stroke, diabetes mellitus, kidney disease, gout, and dyslipidemia. Consequently, 2,239 men and 3,730 women were extracted as healthy individuals.

Results and Discussion

As shown in Fig. 1, the CAVI scores (or values) increased essentially linearly with age, and men showed about 0.5 higher CAVI values than women, in all age groups. This corresponds to an age difference of approximately 10 years in terms of advancement of arteriosclerosis. Our results are consistent with the fact that men are biologically more susceptible to arteriosclerosis than women[1].

Fig. 2 shows differences in the average CAVI scores by age between the CVD risk-free group and the CVD high-risk group for men and for women[1]. After the age of 40 years, the difference in age-specific average CAVI scores became statistically significant between the two groups, with borderline significance in men aged 70–74 years (p = 0.054), and also became wider as age advanced for both men and women. We conclude that the overall arteriosclerosis status of the CVD high-risk group was significantly worse than that of the CVD risk-free group. Because no difference in average CAVI scores was detected between the two groups before the age of 40 years, effective CAVI screening might be recommended for people aged 40 years and older.

Pressure dependence was studied by measuring simultaneously aortic pulse-wave velocity (PWV) values and blood pressure among 282 individuals[2]. To eliminate (or minimize) the pressure dependency of the aortic PWV value, the table of the pressure-adjusted PWV values at a diastolic pressure of 80 mmHg was developed based on an experiment by Hasegawa[3] using a postmortem extracted

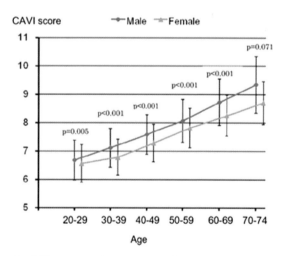

Fig. 1. **Differences in average CAVI scores by age between males (blue line) and females (green line) among cardiovascular disease risk-free individuals. Vertical bars indicate standard deviation.**

Cited from ref.1 【by permission from Springer Nature】

[1]Japan Health Promotion Foundation, 1-24-4 Ebisu, Shibuya-ku, Tokyo, 150-0013, Japan.
[2]Pacific Rim Disease Prevention Center, P.O.Box 25444, Seattle, WA 98165-2344, USA.
[3]Emeritus professor, Toho university, Sakura Hospital.
[4]Seijinkai Mihama Hospital.

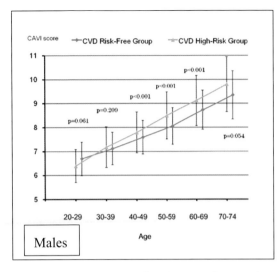
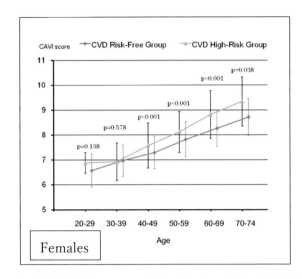

Fig. 2. Differences in average CAVI scores by age between the CVD risk-free group (blue line) and the CVD high-risk group (green line) for males and for females. Vertical bars indicate standard deviation.
Adapted from ref.1 【by permission from Springer Nature】

aorta. We obtained a Spearman's correlation coefficient (r) of 0.307 (p < 0.05) between PWV values adjusted for diastolic blood pressure of 80 mmHg and diastolic blood pressure among the 282 subjects, whereas r = 0.276 (p > 0.05) was obtained between CAVI and diastolic blood pressure among the same subjects. Thus, CAVI values are not dependent on blood pressure. On the other hand, the pressure-adjusted PWV values are not completely independent of blood pressure at the time of measurement, because although the correlation coefficient (r = 0.307) was small, it was statistically significant.

We examined the association of CAVI scores with the established CVD risk factors and coronary heart disease (CHD)[4]. After converting CAVI scores to binary variables (normal or abnormally high CAVI scores), logistic regression analysis was conducted. There was a significant association between CHD and abnormally high CAVI scores [odds ratio (OR) = 3.87, p < 0.001, for men, and OR = 1.45, p < 0.01, for women], after adjusting for CVD risk factors. Our results confirmed that CAVI scores are a reliable indicator of arteriosclerosis, reflecting the extent of arterial stiffness and atherosclerosis in the major artery.

Summary

CAVI clearly showed an aging tendency, and in addition, there were differences in age-specific averages of CAVI scores between the sexes.
   1. CAVI scores (values) increased as age advances. In addition, men showed an average of 0.5 CAVI value (which is equivalent to about a 10-year advance in arteriosclerosis) higher than in women.
   2. After converting CAVI scores to binary variables

(normal or abnormally high CAVI scores ≥ mean + 1 standard deviation), logistic regression analysis revealed a significant association between CHD and abnormally high CAVI scores: OR = 3.87, p < 0.001, for men, and OR = 1.45, p < 0.01, for women, after adjusting for CVD risk factors.
   3. We conclude that the overall arteriosclerosis status of the CVD high-risk group was significantly worse than that of the CVD risk-free group.

References

1) Namekata T, Suzuki K, Ishizuka N, Shirai K. Establishing baseline criteria of cardio-ankle vascular index as a new indicator of arteriosclerosis: a cross-sectional study, BMC Cardiovascular Disorders 2011;11:51. https://bmccardiovascdisord.biomedcentral. com/track/pdf/10.1186/1471-2261-11-51, https://doi. org/10.1186/1471-2261-11-51

2) Ishizuka N, Moriyama H, Suzuki K, Arai K. Comparison of CAVI with PWV (Hasegawa Method) —Pressure dependence and interconversion— 84-89 in All of the new arterial stiffness index CAVI. Nikkei BP Publishing Center Tokyo 2009 (in Japanese).

3) Hasegawa M. Fundamental research on human aortic pulse wave velocity. Jikei Medical Journal 1970;85:742-760 (in Japanese).

4) Namekata T, Suzuki K, Ishizuka N, Nakata M, Shirai K. Association of cardio-ankle vascular index with cardiovascular disease risk factors and coronary heart disease among Japanese urban workers and their families. J Clinical Experimental Cardiology 2012; S1: 003. http:// dx.doi.org/10.4172/2155-9880.S1-003

Regional and racial differences

Masaaki Miyata

Summary

1. Regional differences of CAVI within Japan have been reported, suggesting that environmental factors may affect the arterial stiffness.
2. The CAVI in healthy individuals has been reported to be different among various countries, suggesting that racial differences and environmental factors may influence the arterial stiffness.

Arterial stiffness and atherosclerosis are considered to be influenced by the genetic factors of races and environmental factors, such as diet, lifestyle, and climate. There are several reports which investigated the regional differences between an isolated island and the mainland in Japan or country-specific differences using cardio-ankle vascular index (CAVI), and these are reviewed in this chapter.

1) Regional differences in Japan

Hirasada et al.[1] measured the CAVI, an index of arterial stiffness, in 4,523 individuals (1,853 men and 2,670 women) who received a general medical examination in Amami islands, the isolated island located in the south of Kagoshima Prefecture, and 440 individuals (240 men and 200 women) who underwent health checkups in the

mainland Kagoshima Prefecture; additionally, they investigated the regional differences of CAVI values between the individuals in the isolated island and the mainland in Japan. As a result of comparing the incidences of a high value of CAVI over 9.0 among the subjects of age 40–69 years in both regions, the ratio of a high value of CAVI was significantly higher in the mainland than that in Amami islands in the age ranges of 40-49, 50-59, and 60-69 years in both men and women (Fig. 1).

Furthermore, comparing the CAVI value among the subjects in Amami islands, the mainland Kagoshima Prefecture, and all of Japan by age groups, the CAVI value in the mainland Kagoshima Prefecture was significantly higher than that in Amami islands and all of Japan in both men and women in the age ranges of 40-49, 50-59, and

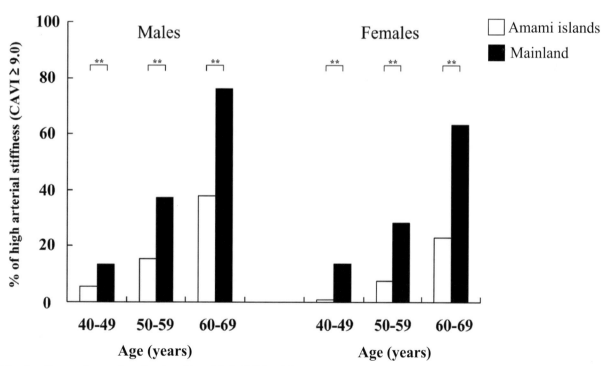

Fig. 1. Percentage of patients with a high CAVI of 9 or higher: comparison between Amami Oshima and the mainland.

**P＜0.01, adapted from reference 1.

School of Health Sciences, Faculty of Medicine, Kagoshima University, 8-35-1 Sakuragaoka, Kagoshima City Kagoshima 890-8544, Japan.

60-69 years. Although the populations from Amami islands and all of Japan showed no significant differences in the CAVI value between the two groups in men in their 40's, 50's, and 60's, and in women in their 60's, the individuals in Amami islands showed a significant lower CAVI compared with healthy adults in women in their 40's and 50's (Fig. 2)[1]. The heart rate was significantly lower in the individuals in Amami islands than the mainland (men: Amami 63.2/min, mainland 71.4/min; women: Amami 65.8/min, mainland 72.0/min), suggesting that environmental factors, such as warmer weather and less mental stress seem to influence the CAVI. Moreover, BMI was significantly higher in Amami islands than in the mainland in both men and women, which may affect this result, because CAVI is negatively associated with BMI[1]. We believe that environmental factors can be clarified by comparing the regional differences among the country, and even among different countries if their populations have a homogeneous race.

2) Comparison of CAVI among various countries

Wang et al.[2] reported the results of comparing the CAVI levels between healthy Japanese and Chinese individuals. They compared the CAVI values by age groups in 1,245 healthy Chinese (524 men and 721 women) and 1,274 Japanese (534 men and 740 women) individuals. As a result, in men, the CAVI values were significantly lower in the Chinese individuals of the age group of 30 years and older compared with Japanese individuals of the same age groups. In women, the values were significantly lower in the Chinese individuals of the age group of 30-60 years compared with the Japanese individuals of the same age group (Fig. 3).

In addition, CAVI was measured in 1,347 healthy Czech individuals (619 men and 728 women)[3], and it was compared with healthy Japanese men and women separately[4]. The CAVI values in the Czech individuals were reported to be significantly lower than those in Japanese individuals from the age range of 20-50 years in men and

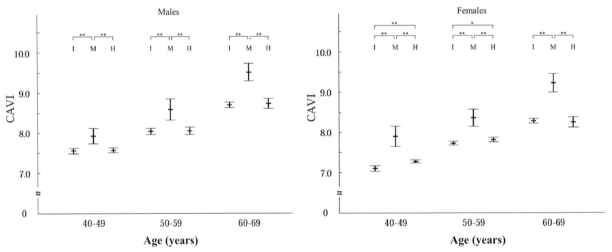

Fig. 2. **CAVI values in age groups: a comparison among the subjects in Amami Oshima and the mainland and healthy adults in Japan.**

The values are expressed as mean and 95% confidential interval of CAVI, I: Amami Oshima Islands, M: Mainland, H: Healthy Adults in Japan, *P<0.05, **P<0.01, cited from reference 1.

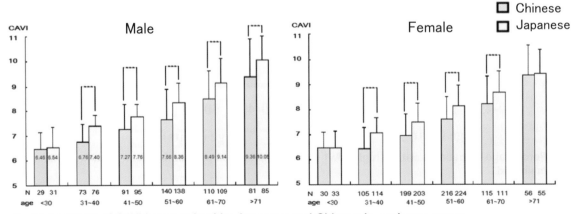

Fig. 3. **Comparison of CAVI between healthy Japanese and Chinese in each age group.**

The values are expressed as mean ± standard deviation, ***P<0.001, adapted from reference 2. 【by permission of Taylor & Francis Ltd】

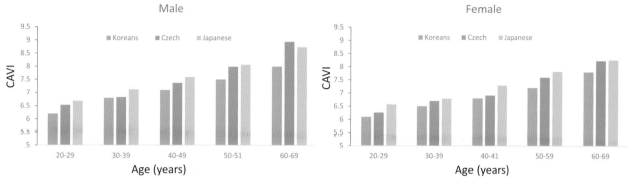

Fig. 4. Comparison of CAVI among healthy Japanese, Czech, and Korean individuals.
Made by the author using data of references 3, 4, and 5.

from the age range of 20-60 years in women. Moreover, the average CAVI values for each age group were reported in 1,380 healthy Koreans (608 men and 772 women) by sex[5]. When the CAVI values of three countries were compared, the CAVI values were observed to increase in the order of Korean, Czech, and Japanese populations (Fig. 4).

In a comparison between 100 Mongolian university students (average age: 20.9 years, 39% men) and 115 Japanese university students (average age 20.9 years, 39% men), the CAVI values in Mongolian students were significantly higher compared with the Japanese students[6]. Although it is a result of small subjects and gender mixing, this finding is notable because of the data from a younger age before atherosclerosis appears. Ulaanbaatar is 1,350 m above the sea level, and the living environment at high altitudes is considered to be one of the factors influencing this difference in the CAVI values.

According to the differences in the countries, not only genetic factors, such as the race, but also environmental factors, such as diet, lifestyle, and climate, seem to be associated with arterial stiffness. Accumulating data from healthy adults in different countries will promote the studies on various aspects and factors affecting the vascular health worldwide. In addition, in countries with more than one race, such as the United States, racial differences can be evaluated by comparing the CAVI values among races in the same region. Further studies in these fields are warranted.

Future challenges

1. It is necessary to compare the CAVI in the region of a multiethnic country or to accumulate and compare the CAVI from healthy subjects by countries to examine racial disparities.

2. Large-scale studies comparing the regional differences of CAVI in Japan are required to investigate the environmental factors for CAVI.

References

1) Hirasada K, Niimura H, Kubozono T, et al. Values of cardio-ankle vascular index (CAVI) between Amami islands and Kagoshima mainland among health checkup examinees. J Atheroscler Thromb. 2012; 19: 69-80. https://doi.org/10.5551/jat.6627

2) Wang H, Shirai K, Liu J, et al. Comparative study of cardio-ankle vascular index between Chinese and Japanese healthy subjects. Clin Exp Hypertens. 2014; 36: 596-601. https://doi.org/10.3109/10641963.2014.897715, http://www.tandfonline.com

3) Wohlfahrt P, Cífková R, Movsisyan N, et al. Reference values of cardio-ankle vascular index in a random sample of a white population. J Hypertens. 2017; 35: 2238-2244.

4) Namekata T, Suzuki K, Ishizuka N, Shirai K. Establishing baseline criteria of cardio-ankle vascular index as a new indicator of arteriosclerosis: a cross-sectional study. BMC Cardiovasc Disord. 2011; 11: 51.

5) Choi SY, Oh BH, Bae Park J, et al. Age-associated increase in arterial stiffness measured according to the cardio-ankle vascular index without blood pressure changes in healthy adults. J Atheroscler Thromb. 2013; 20: 911-923.

6) Uurtuya S, Taniguchi N, Kotani K, et al. Comparative study of the cardio-ankle vascular index and ankle-brachial index between young Japanese and Mongolian subjects. Hypertens Res. 2009; 32: 140-144.

7) Uurtuya S, Kotani K, Taniguchi N, et al. Comparative study of atherosclerotic parameters in Mongolian and Japanese patients with hypertension and diabetes mellitus. J Atheroscler Thromb. 2010; 17: 181-188.

The cut off value of CAVI for Evaluation

Atsuhito Saiki

Summary

- The CAVI is an independent predictor of future cardiovascular (CV) events in patients with hypertension, diabetes, obesity, CKD, and/or a history of cardiovascular disease (CVD).
- In cross-sectional studies, the cut-off value of the CAVI for the presence of CAD is considered to be 8 or 9, depending on the severity of coronary artery stenosis.
- Many prospective studies have proposed a CAVI of 9 as the optimal cut-off value for predicting CVD.

Introduction

Previous studies have demonstrated the significance of arterial stiffness as an indicator of arteriosclerosis and a predictor of CV events[1]. The cardio-ankle vascular index (CAVI) has been widely used in clinical medicine for the last 15 years as an index for the evaluation of CVD and their risk factors. Increased CAVI is seen in persons with CVD and associated risk factors, and several studies have

Table 1. Cross-Sectional Studies on the Association of the CAVI with the Presence of Cardiovascular Disease.

Author	Country	Subjects	Mean Age (years)	Mean CAVI	Multivariate Analysis	What is Cut-off Value of CAVI for?	Cut-off Value	NRI
Nakamura et al. 2008[16]	Japan	109 participants who underwent coronary angiography	58.0-67.6	Not described	CAVI was an independent indicator of the severity of coronary atherosclerosis, unlike mean IMT, maximum IMT and plaque score	Presence of CAD (Significant coronary stenosis defined as ≥ 75% stenosis of the coronary arteries)	**8.81**	Not described
Takenaka et al. 2008[38]	Japan	68 patients with end-stage renal disease	60	7.8	Not available.	Presence of CVD.	**7.55**	Not described
Park et al. 2012[22]	Korea	158 normoglycemic subjects and 373 subjects with abnormal glucose metabolism	56-58	7.5-7.9	Adjusted CAVI ≥8.0 was independently associated with significant coronary artery stenosis (OR 3.143).	Predicting ≥ 50% coronary artery stenosis.	**8.0**	Not described
Yingchoncharoen et al. 2012[21]	Thailand	1391 patients with a moderate to high risk for CAD	59	Not described	There was a correlation between CAVI and the prevalence of coronary stenosis after adjusting for the traditional risk factors for CAD (OR 3.29).	Presence of CAD (Significant coronary stenosis defined as ≥ 50% stenosis of the coronary arteries)	**8.0**	0.277 (p < 0.0001)
Gomez-Sanchez et al. 2015[29]	Spain	500 subjects with intermediate level of CV risk	60.3	8.59	IMT and PWV maintained a positive association with the adjusted CAVI.	Detecting mean IMT > 0.90 mm and maximum IMT > 0.90 mm.	**8.95 (mean IMT > 0.90)** **8.85 (maximum IMT > 0.90)**	Not described
Hitsumoto et al. 2019[39]	Japan	405 patients with CV risk factors	64	8.7	CAVI was as independent factor for the pulsatility index of the common carotid artery, as a subordinate factor.	High pulsatility index of common carotid artery (> 1.60) as a risk value of stroke incidence.	**9.1**	Not described

CAVI, cardio-ankle vascular index; NRI, net reclassification improvement; IMT, intima-media thickness; CAD, coronary artery disease; CVD, cardiovascular disease; OR, odds ratio; CV, cardiovascular; PWV, pulse wave velocity, Cited from ref.40

Center of Diabetes, Endocrine and Metabolism, Toho University Sakura Medical Center 564-1, Shimoshizu, Sakura-City, Chiba, 285-8741, Japan.

investigated the association between the CAVI and the occurrence of CV events[2]. In the last decade, many prospective studies to determine the optimal cut-off values of the CAVI for predicting CVD have been conducted[3-13]. In this chapter, we summarize the cross-sectional studies on the association of the CAVI with the presence of CVD and the prospective studies that aimed to determine the cut-off CAVI values for CV events.

Cross-sectional studies on the association between the CAVI and the presence of CVD

Several cross-sectional studies have verified that numerous factors, including arteriosclerotic diseases, affect the value of the CAVI. The CAVI is known to be high in patients with various atherosclerotic diseases. The cut-off values of the CAVI for the presence of coronary artery disease (CAD) are summarized in Table 1.

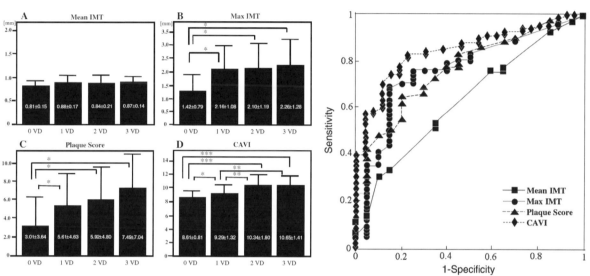

Fig. 1. Relationship between coronary angiographic findings and cardio-ankle vascular index (CAVI) or carotid atherosclerosis parameters. (left side) Mean intima-media thickness (IMT), max IMT, plaque score, and CAVI are shown. 0VD, no lesion; 1VD, 1-vessel disease; 2VD, 2-vesel disease; 3VD, 3-vessel disease. Data are shown as mean ± SD, adjusted for age. *p < 0.05, **p < 0.01, ***p < 0.001. (right side) Curves represent the receiver-operating-characteristic (ROC) curves for discriminating the probability for coronary atherosclerosis. Each curve is defined by mean IMT (■), max IMT (●), plaque score (▲) or CAVI (◆). The ROC area defined by CAVI is the largest among these 4 parameters. Adapted from ref.16

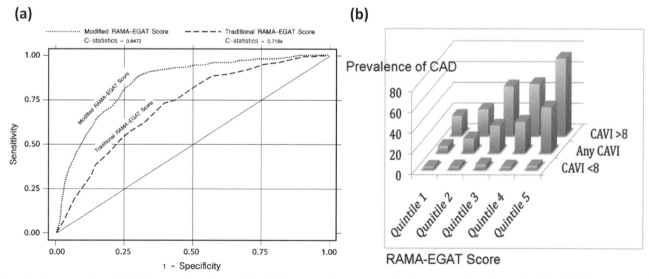

Fig. 2. The study of CAVI and the Ramathibodi-Electric Generating Authority of Thailand (RAMA-EGAT) score. (a) Comparison of receiver operating characteristic (ROC) curve of the modified RAMA-EGAT score (EGAT + CAVI) and traditional RAMA-EGAT score (EGAT score). (b) The CAVI provides additional diagnostic value at all levels of the RAMA-EGAT score. Reproduced from ref.21 [with permission from BMJ Publishing Group Ltd]

(a) CAD

Many researchers have reported that the CAVI is high in patients with CAD[14-17]. The CAVI increases with an increase in the number of stenotic vessels[16,17]. Izuhara et al.[18] reported that the CAVI, but not baPWV, is associated with carotid and coronary arteriosclerosis. In addition, Nakamura et al. reported that the area under the receiver operating characteristic curve defined by the CAVI was the largest, and the CAVI was an independent parameter indicating the severity of coronary atherosclerosis, while mean intima-media thickness (IMT), maximum IMT, and plaque score were not independent parameters[16] (Fig. 1). The CAVI is correlated with coronary artery calcification, which occurs as the CAVI increases above 8.0[12,19,20]. Several cross-sectional studies have determined the cut-off value of the CAVI for the presence of CAD (Table 1). CAVI $\geq$ 8.0 is associated with $\geq$ 50% stenosis of the coronary arteries[21,22], and CAVI $\geq$ 9.0 is associated with $\geq$ 75% stenosis of the coronary arteries[18]. Nakamura et al. reported that the optimal cut-off level of the CAVI indicative of CAD with a 75% narrowing of the coronary arteries was 8.81[16]. In a study from Thailand, the cut-off value of the CAVI indicative of the presence of CAD was considered as 8.0, and adding the CAVI into the traditional risk score (RAMA-EGAT) calculator improves the prediction for the incidence of CAD, increasing the C-statistics from 0.72 to 0.85 and resulting in a net reclassification improvement of 27.7% (p < 0.0001)[21] (Fig. 2).

These findings suggest that the CAVI is an independent variable for the presence of CAD and is more strongly associated with the presence of CAD than baPWV and IMT. The probable cut-off value is considered to be 8 or 9, depending on the severity of coronary artery stenosis (Fig. 4).

(b) Cerebral infarction

CAVI values are high in patients with cerebral infarction[23]. The CAVI was found to be higher in patients with large artery atherosclerosis and small-vessel occlusion than in normal controls with no CVD[23,24]. In the study by Saji et al.[24], the CAVI cut-off value indicative of silent brain infarct was reported to be 9.2, and that for hyperintensities of the white matter was reported to be 8.9.

The And CAVI may also reflect cognitive decline. Patients with lower Mini-Mental State Examination (MMSE) scores have a higher value of the CAVI[25], and the annual decrease in the MMSE score is significantly larger in patients with high CAVI[26]. CAVI $\geq$ 10.0 is associated with future cognitive dysfunction[26]. Elderly people with

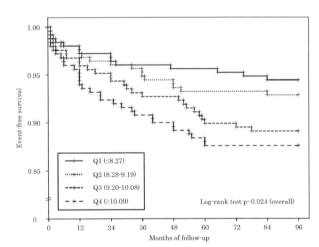

Fig. 3.   Kaplan-Meier survival curves showing CV events according to the quartiles of the CAVI. Overall, 1080 subjects with metabolic disorders including diabetes mellitus, hypertension and dyslipidemia were screened and followed up prospectively[7].

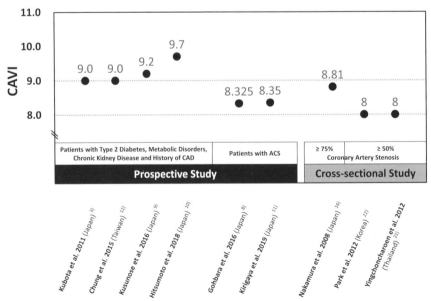

Fig. 4.   Summary of the optimal cut-off values of the CAVI for coronary artery disease reported by prospective and cross-sectional studies. CAD, coronary artery disease; ACS, acute coronary syndrome. Cited from ref.40

Table 2. Summary of the Association of CAVI with Cardiovascular Outcomes in Prospective Studies. Cited from ref.40

Author	Country	Subjects	Mean Age (years)	Baseline CAVI	Duration of Follow-up	CV Outcomes	Incidence (%) (1000 person-years)	Prognostic Value	Cut-off Value	NRI
Kubota et al. 2011[3]	Japan	400 patients with metabolic disorders or past history of CAD	63.2-73.9	Not described	27.2 months	Coronary artery disease, stroke and death	54.0	Hazard ratio of CVD was significantly higher in the group with CAVI ≥ 10.0 (HR 2.25).	**9.0**	Not described
Kato et al. 2012[4]	Japan	135 patients on hemodialysis	60	9.7	63 months	Primary outcome: All-cause and CV mortalities. Secondary outcome: Fatal and non-fatal CV events.	52.2	Not significant.	**Not described**	Not described
Otsuka et al. 2014[5]	Japan	211 CAD patients	65	9.87-10.05	2.9 years	Cardiac death, non-fatal MI, unstable angina pectoris, recurrent angina pectoris requiring coronary revascularization or stroke.	45.8	Persistently impaired CAVI was a significant independent predictor of CV events compared with improved CAVI at 6 months (HR 3.3).	**Not described**	Not described
Laucevičius et al. 2015[13]	Lithuania	2106 patients with metabolic syndrome	53.83	7.92	3.8 years	MI, stroke or transient ischemic attack, and sudden cardiac death.	11.6	CAVI was significantly associated with the occurrence of total CV events (p = 0.045) and MI (p = 0.027).	**7.95**	Not described
Satoh-Asahara et al. 2015[6]	Japan	425 patients with obesity	51.5	7.6	5 years	Angina pectoris, myocardial infarction, stroke and arteriosclerosis obliterans.	15.8	CAVI was a significant predictor of CV events (HR 1.44 per 1 unit increase).	**Not described**	0.164 (p = 0.066)
Sato et al. 2015[7]	Japan	1003 subjects with CV risk factor	62.5	9.25	6.7 years	Myocardial infarction and stable/unstable angina pectoris.	13.4	CAVI was independently associated with the future risk of CV event (HR 1.126 per 1 unit increase).	**Not described**	Not described
Chung et al. 2015[12]	Taiwan	626 patients with type 2 diabetes	64	8.8	4.1 years	Death, ACS, ischemic stroke and any coronary revascularization for coronary artery disease.	38.2	Patients with CAVI ≥ 9.0 had greater CV events than those with CAVI < 9.0 (OR 1.23).	**9.0**	Not described
Gohbara et al. 2016[8]	Japan	288 patients with ACS	58-71	Not described	1.25 years	CV death, non-fatal MI, non-fatal ischemic stroke.	52.8	CAVI > 8.325 was an independent predictor of CV events (HR 18.0) and nonfatal ischemic stroke (HR 9.37).	**8.325**	Not described
Kusunose et al. 2016[9]	Japan	114 patients with at least 2 risk factors for CVD	69	8.5	4.25 years	Cardiac death, non-fatal myocardial infarction/coronary revascularization, acute pulmonary edema and stroke.	72.2	CAVI was not a significant predictor of CV events. CAVI was associated with a 5% per year decline in kidney function (HR: 1.52 per 1 SD increase).	**9.2**	Not described
Hitsumoto et al. 2018[10]	Japan	460 patients with chronic kidney disease	74	9.7	60.1 months	Cardiovascular death, nonfatal myocardial infarction, nonfatal ischemic stroke and hospital admission for heart failure.	39.5	MACE was significantly higher in the group with CAVI > 10 than in the group with CAVI < 10 (HR 2.04).	**9.7**	Not described
Kirigaya et al. 2019[11]	Japan	387 patients with ACS	64	8.4-9.0	62 months	CV death, recurrence of ACS, heart failure requiring hospitalization, or stroke.	31.0	CAVI was an independent predictor of MACE (HR 1.496) and cardiovascular death (HR 2.204), unlike baPWV. The addition of CAVI to the GRACE score enhanced the NRI (0.337).	**8.35**	0.337 (p = 0.034)

CAVI, cardio-ankle vascular index; CV, cardiovascular; CAD, coronary artery disease; CVD, cardiovascular disease; NRI, net reclassification improvement; MI, myocardial infarction; HR, hazard ratio; ACS, acute coronary syndrome; OR, odds ratio; SD, standard deviation; MACE, major adverse cardiovascular events; GRACE, global registry for acute coronary events

high CAVI may be at a greater risk of cognitive decline.

(c) Thickening of carotid intima-media

IMT is associated with the CAVI[14,20,27], and patients with carotid plaque have a higher value of the CAVI[28]. Spanish researchers have shown that IMT and PWV correlate positively with the CAVI, and the cut-off CAVI values indicative of the mean and maximum IMT > 0.90 mm are 8.95 and 8.85, respectively[29].

CAVI as a predictor of CV events

Sato et al. studied 1080 subjects with metabolic disorders, such as diabetes mellitus, hypertension, and dyslipidemia and reported that CAVI was an independent predictor of future CV events[7] (Fig. 3). In the Cox proportional hazards regression analysis, every 1.0-point increase in the CAVI was one of the factors independently associated with a higher risk of future CV events (hazard ratio, 1.126, p = 0.039). Several studies have investigated the association between the CAVI and future CV events (Table 2). The participants in all the studies were at high risk for CVD and had conditions such as hypertension, diabetes, obesity, CKD, and a history of CVD. Nine studies were from Japan[3-11], and the other two were from Taiwan[12] and Lithuania[13]. In most studies, the baseline CAVI was a predictor of future CV events. However, the CAVI did not predict the CV events in patients on hemodialysis in one study[4]. The CAVI is higher in patients with CKD than in those with normal kidney function[30,31] and is especially high in patients undergoing hemodialysis[30,32]. Further investigations are required to determine whether the CAVI predicts CV events in patients on hemodialysis. In the meta-analysis by Matsushita et al.[33], the pooled hazard ratio for composite CVD events per 1 standard deviation increment in CAVI was 1.20 (95% confidence interval 1.05-1.36) in four prospective studies[6,7,9,13]. Otsuka et al.[5] reported that the incidence of CV events after 2.9 years was significantly higher in the group with no improvements in the CAVI at 6 months than in the group that showed an improvement in the CAVI. Furthermore, Saiki et al.[34] reported that the CAVI decreased significantly following the administration of pitavastatin, and the change in the CAVI was an independent predictor of the 3-point major cardiac adverse events in a multicenter randomized controlled trial, TOHO-LIP. These seem to be useful reports that elucidate the relationship between changes in the CAVI over time and the

occurrence of CV events.

Optimal cut-off values of the CAVI for predicting the risk of CAD

Many of the above studies determined the cut-off values of the CAVI for CV events[3,8-12], and they are summarized in Fig. 4. In patients with type 2 diabetes, metabolic disorders, CKD, and/or a history of CAD, the cut-off values for CVD events were 9.0-9.7[3,9,10,12]. Chung et al.[12] reported that patients with CAVI ≥ 9.0 had a greater risk of CV events than those with CAVI < 9.0 (odds ratio 1.23). Therefore, CAVI ≥ 9.0 seems to indicate a higher CV risk. The reported cut-off values for CV events were 8.325-8.35 in patients with acute coronary syndrome[8,11]. Gohbara et al.[8] reported that CAVI > 8.325 was an independent predictor of CV events (hazard ratio 18.0). Kirigaya et al.[11] reported that unlike baPWV, CAVI was an independent predictor of major adverse CV events. Therefore, an optimal CAVI cut-off value of 8 may be recommended for the prevention of secondary CV events.

In several cross-sectional studies, the cut-off value of the CAVI for the presence of CAD defined as coronary artery stenosis ≥ 50% was 8.0, as described earlier[21,22]. In addition, a few studies reported that coronary artery stenosis or calcification occurred as the CAVI increased above 8.0[12,15,18-20]. These findings suggest that CAVI ≥ 8.0 may be associated with subclinical or asymptomatic atherosclerosis.

The Physiological Diagnosis Criteria for Vascular Failure Committee proposed cut-off CAVI values of 8.0 and 9.0 (< 8 for normal, ≥ 8 and < 9 for borderline, ≥ 9 for abnormal) (Fig. 5)[35]. We agree with these values. In Japan, two large multicenter longitudinal studies, CAVI-J and Coupling Registry, that have enrolled 3000-5000 high-risk patients are currently ongoing[36,37]. These studies may reveal whether adding CAVI to the CV risk scoring systems improves the accuracy of the prediction of CV risk.

Conclusions

Since its development in 2004, a large volume of evidence has validated CAVI as a parameter for the clinical evaluation of arterial stiffness. In recent years, an increasing number of studies have investigated the association between the CAVI and future CV events. Based on several cross-sectional studies and prospective studies, a CAVI of 9 has been proposed as the optimal cut-off value for predicting

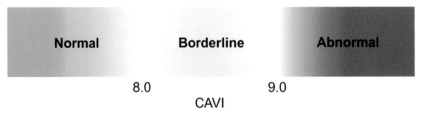

Fig. 5. **Estimated criteria for the medial layer dysfunction and its border zone of the CAVI. CAVI cut-off values of 8.0 and 9.0 (< 8 for normal, ≥ 8 and < 9 for borderline, ≥ 9 for abnormal) are proposed by the Physiological Diagnosis Criteria for Vascular Failure Committee. Cited from ref.35 [with permission from Wolters Kluwer Health, Inc.]**

CVD, including CAD and cerebral infarction. Future investigations might reveal that the CAVI is an excellent predictor of CV events.

Future Perspective

- Two large multicenter longitudinal studies, CAVI-J and Coupling Registry, may reveal whether adding the CAVI to the CV risk scoring systems improves the accuracy of the prediction of CV risk.
- The optimal cut-off value of the CAVI for predicting CVD should also be validated in patients with various diseases and conditions.
- Future studies are required to determine whether the changes in the CAVI after various therapeutic interventions reflect a reduced risk of CVD.

References

1) Oliver JJ, Webb DJ: Noninvasive assessment of arterial stiffness and risk of atherosclerotic events. Arterioscler Thromb Vasc Biol, 2003; 23: 554-566.

2) Saiki A, Sato Y, Watanabe R, et al.: The role of a novel arterial stiffness parameter, cardio-ankle vascular index (CAVI), as a surrogate marker for cardiovascular diseases. J Atheroscler Thromb, 2016; 23: 155-168.

3) Kubota Y, Maebuchim D, Takei M, et al.: Cardio-Ankle Vascular Index is a predictor of cardiovascular events. Artery Res, 2011; 5: 91-96.

4) Kato A, Takita T, Furuhashi M, et al.: Brachial-ankle pulse wave velocity and the cardio-ankle vascular index as a predictor of cardiovascular outcomes in patients on regular hemodialysis. Ther Apher Dial, 2012; 16: 232-241.

5) Otsuka T, Fukuda S, Shimada K, Suzoshikawa J: Serial assessment of arterial stiffness by cardio-ankle vascular index for prediction of future cardiovascular events in patients with coronary artery disease. Hypertens Res, 2014; 37: 1014-1020.

6) Satoh-Asahara N, Kotani K, Yamakage H, et al.: Japan Obesity and Metabolic Syndrome Study (JOMS) Group:. Cardio-ankle vascular index predicts for the incidence of cardiovascular events in obese patients: A multicenter prospective cohort study (Japan Obesity and Metabolic Syndrome Study: JOMS). Atherosclerosis, 2015; 242: 461-468

7) Sato Y, Nagayama D, Saiki A, et al.: Cardio-ankle vascular index is independently associated with future cardiovascular events in outpatients with metabolic disorders. J Atheroscler Thromb, 2016; 23: 596-605. https://doi.org/10.5551/jat.31385

8) Gohbara M, Iwahashi N, Sano Y, et al.: Clinical impact of the cardio-ankle vascular index for predicting cardiovascular events after acute coronary syndrome. Circ J, 2016; 80: 1420-1426.

9) Kusunose K, Sato M, Yamada H, et al.: Prognostic implications of non-invasive vascular function tests in high-risk atherosclerosis patients. Circ J, 2016; 80: 1034-1040.

10) Hitsumoto T: Clinical Usefulness of the cardio-ankle vascular index as a predictor of primary cardiovascular events in patients with chronic kidney disease. J Clin Med Res, 2018; 10: 883-890.

11) Kirigaya J, Iwahashi N, Tahakashi H, et al.: Impact of cardio-ankle vascular index on long-term outcome in patients with acute coronary syndrome. J Atheroscler Thromb, 2019; 18. [Epub ahead of print]

12) Chung SL, Yang CC, Chen CC, et al.: Coronary artery calcium score compared with cardio-ankle vascular index in the prediction of cardiovascular events in asymptomatic patients with type 2 diabetes. J Atheroscler Thromb, 2015; 22: 1255-1265.

13) Laucevičius A, Ryliškytė L, Balsytė J, et al.: Association of cardio-ankle vascular index with cardiovascular risk factors and cardiovascular events in metabolic syndrome patients. Medicina, 2015; 51: 152-158.

14) Takaki A, Ogawa H, Wakeyama T, et al.: Cardioankle vascular index is a new noninvasive parameter of arterial stiffness. Circ J, 2007; 71: 1710-1714.

15) Namekata T, Suzuki K, Ishizuka N, Shirai K: Establishing baseline criteria of cardio-ankle vascular index as a new indicator of arteriosclerosis: a cross-sectional study. BMC Cardiovasc Disord, 2011; 11: 51.

16) Nakamura K, Tomaru T, Yamamura S, et al.: Cardio-ankle vascular index is a candidate predictor of coronary atherosclerosis. Circ J, 2008; 72: 598-604. https://doi.org/10.1253/circj.72.598

17) Horinaka S, Yabe A, Yagi H, et al.: Comparison of atherosclerotic indicators between cardio ankle vascular index and brachial ankle pulse wave velocity. Angiology, 2009; 60: 468-476.

18) Izuhara M, Shioji K, Kadota Y, et al.: Relationship of cardiovascular index to carotid and coronary arteriosclerosis. Circ J, 2008; 72: 1762-1767.

19) Mineoka Y, Fukui M, Tanaka M, et al.: Relationship between cardio-ankle vascular index (CAVI) and coronary artery calcification (CAC) in patients with type 2 diabetes mellitus. Heart Vessels, 2012; 27: 160-165.

20) Park JB, Park HE, Choi SY, et al.: Relation between cardio-ankle vascular index and coronary artery calcification or stenosis in asymptomatic subjects. J Atheroscler Thromb, 2013; 20: 557-567.

21) Yingchoncharoen T, Limpijankit T, Jongjirasiri S, et al.: Arterial stiffness contributes to coronary artery disease risk prediction beyond the traditional risk score (RAMA-EGAT score). Heart Asia, 2012; 4: 77-82. http://dx.doi.org/10.1136/heartasia-2011-010079

22) Park HE, Choi SY, Kim MK, Oh BH: Cardio-ankle vascular index reflects coronary atherosclerosis in patients with abnormal glucose metabolism: assessment with 256 slice multi-detector computed tomography. J Cardiol, 2012; 60: 372-376.

23) Suzuki J, Sakakibara R, Tomaru T, et al.: Stroke and cardio-ankle vascular stiffness index. J Stroke Cerebrovasc Dis, 2011; 22: 171-175.

24) Saji N, Kimura K, Yagita Y, et al.: Comparison of arteriosclerotic indicators in patients with ischemic stroke: ankle-brachial index, brachial-ankle pulse wave velocity and cardio-ankle vascular index. Hypertens Res, 2015; 38: 323-328.

25) Yukutake T, Yamada M, Fukutani N, et al.: Arterial stiffness determined according to the cardio-ankle vascular index(CAVI) is associated with mild cognitive decline in community-dwelling elderly subjects. J Atheroscler Thromb, 2014; 21: 49-55.

26) Yamamoto N, Yamanaka G, Ishikawa M, et al.: Cardio-ankle vascular index as a predictor of cognitive impairment in community-dwelling elderly people: four-year follow-up. Dement Geriatr Cogn Disord, 2009; 28: 153-158.

27) Kim KJ, Lee BW, Kim HM, et al.: Associations between cardio-ankle vascular index and microvascular complications in type 2 diabetes mellitus patients. J Atheroscler Thromb, 2011; 18: 328-336.

28) Wang H, Liu J, Zhao H, et al.: Arterial stiffness evaluation by cardio-ankle vascular index in hypertension and diabetes mellitus subjects. J Am Soc Hypertens, 2013; 7: 426-431.

29) Gomez-Sanchez L, Garcia-Ortiz L, Patino-Alonso MC, et

al.: MARK Group: The association between the cardio-ankle vascular index and other parameters of vascular structure and function in Caucasian adults: MARK Study. J Atheroscler Thromb, 2015; 22: 901-911.

30) Kubozono T, Miyata H, Uegama K, et al.: Association between arterial stiffness and estimated glomerular filtration rate in the Japanese general population. J Atheroscler Thromb, 2009; 16: 840-845.

31) Nakamura K, Iizuka T, Takahashi M, et al.: Association between cardio-ankle vascular index and serum cystatin C levels in patients with cardiovascular risk factor. J Atheroscler Thromb, 2009; 16: 371-379.

32) Ueyama K, Miyata M, Kubozono T, et al.: Noninvasive indices of arterial stiffness in hemodialysis patients. Hypertens Res, 2009; 32: 716-720.

33) Matsushita K, Ding N, Kim ED, et al.: Cardio-ankle vascular index and cardiovascular disease: Systematic review and meta-analysis of prospective and cross-sectional studies. J Clin Hypertens, 2019; 21: 16-24.

34) Saiki A, Watanabe Y, Yamaguchi T, et al.: CAVI-lowering Effect of Pitavastatin may be Involved in Prevention of Cardiovascular Disease: Subgroup Analysis of the TOHO-LIP. J Atheroscler Thromb, 2020, in press.

35) Tanaka A, Tomiyama H, Maruhashi T, et al.: Physiological Diagnosis Criteria for Vascular Failure Committee: Physiological diagnostic criteria for vascular failure. Hypertension, 2018; 72: 1060-1071. https://doi.org/10.1161/hypertensionaha.118.11554 https://www.ahajournals.org/journal/hyp

36) Miyoshi T, Ito H, Horinaka S, et al.: Protocol for evaluating the cardio-ankle vascular index to predict cardiovascular events in Japan: a prospective multicenter cohort study. Pulse, 2017; 4: 11-16.

37) Kabutoya T, Kario K: Comparative assessment of cutoffs for the cardio-ankle vascular index and brachial-ankle pulse wave velocity in a nationwide registry - a cardiovascular prognostic coupling study. Pulse, 2018; 6: 131-136.

38) Takenaka T, Hoshi H, Kato N, et al.: Cardio-ankle vascular index to screen cardiovascular diseases in patients with end-stage renal diseases. J Atheroscler Thromb, 2008; 15: 339-344.

39) Hitsumoto T: Relationships between the cardio-ankle vascular index and pulsatility index of the common carotid artery in patients with cardiovascular risk factors. J Clin Med Res, 2019; 11: 593-599.

40) Saiki A, Ohira M, Yamaguchi T, et al.: New Horizons of Arterial Stiffness Developed Using Cardio-Ankle Vascular Index (CAVI). J Atheroscler Thromb. 2020; 27: 732-748. https://doi.org/10.5551/jat.rv17043

PART 3

CAVI in Arteriosclerotic diseases

Brain arteriosclerotic diseases and CAVI

Ryuji Sakakibara[1], Jun Suzuki[2], Fuyuki Tateno[1] and Yosuke Aiba[1]

Abstract

Stroke and white matter diseases (WMD) in older individuals (collectively referred to as *brain arteriosclerotic diseases*) are the most common cause of neurological disability. These conditions impair quality of life, resulting in early institutionalization. Atherosclerosis is a major contributor to stroke, which can be prevented by early recognition and management. The cardio-ankle vascular stiffness index (CAVI) was introduced clinically as a novel, simple, and non-invasive measure for the assessment of atherosclerosis. CAVI is easily measured and has adequate reproducibility for clinical use. As compared with healthy control subjects, CAVI is statistically significantly greater in patients with ischemic cerebrovascular diseases, particularly in WMD in older individuals, large-artery atherosclerosis, and small-vessel occlusion, but not in patients with transient ischemic attack. CAVI showed a clear relationship with the carotid ultrasound plaque score. CAVI can also be an ideal marker for monitoring "de-stiffening" therapy to prevent stroke/WMD in future.

Keywords: atherosclerosis, cardio-ankle vascular stiffness index, cerebrovascular disease, stroke, white matter disease

Introduction

Stroke and white matter diseases (WMD) in older individuals (collectively referred to as *brain arteriosclerotic diseases*) are the most common cause of neurological disability. These conditions impair quality of life, resulting in early institutionalization. Atherosclerosis is a major contributor to both stroke and WMD in older individuals, but can be prevented by early recognition and management. The cardio-ankle vascular stiffness index (CAVI) was introduced clinically by Shirai et al.[1] as a novel, simple, and non-invasive measure for the assessment of atherosclerosis. The CAVI is easily measured, and has adequate reproducibility for clinical use[1]. In many cases, brain stroke is thought to be a sequel of advanced systemic arteriosclerosis, particularly in the carotid, vertebral, and intra-cranial arteries. Recently, a relationship was found between abnormal CAVI and stroke[2-4]. Here, we discuss the clinical use of CAVI in the management of stroke and WMD in older individuals.

Application of CAVI to stroke and WMD in older individuals

Application of CAVI to stroke and WMD in older individuals has been studied recently[5]. Saji et al.[2,6] studied 220 older subjects (mean age 69 years) in whom CAVI was determined, and found that subjects with WMD showed significantly higher CAVI than those without WMD (increase in CAVI: 0.7). Saji et al.[7] also studied 842 older subjects (mean age: 70 years) who underwent CAVI, and

found that subjects with large infarcts (with WMD) and those with lacunar infarcts plus (presumably up to 20 mm in diameter) (with WMD) showed significantly higher CAVI than control individuals (increase of CAVI: 1.5 and 0.8, respectively), suggesting that infarct size might result in an increase in CAVI.

Shimoyama et al.[8] studied 105 older stroke/transient ischemic attack (TIA) subjects (mean age 70 years), whose CAVI was measured. They found that subjects with silent microbleeds (with more severe WMD) showed significantly higher CAVI (increase in CAVI: 1.9) than those without silent microbleeds (with less severe WMD). The grade of stroke/TIA were the same in both groups. (increase of CAVI, 1.9). Cerebral microbleeds are mostly silent, while WMD can present clinical symptoms. Consequently, this study indicates that CAVI also increases with WMD.

Choi et al.[4] studied 484 middle-aged subjects (mean age 50 years) whose CAVI was measured, and found that subjects with WMD showed significantly higher CAVI than those without WMD (increase in CAVI: 0.3).

We have previously studied 939 older subjects (mean age 69 years) whose CAVI was measured[3]. We described the methods and results elsewhere in detail[4]. We enrolled 854 healthy control subjects, which included 487 men and 367 women (mean age 65.1 ± 9.4 years). During the same 3-year period, we enrolled 85 subjects diagnosed with ischemic cerebrovascular disease, which included 63 men and 22 women (mean age 70.0 ± 10.8 years). The patients included 17 with large-artery atherosclerosis, 30 with small-

[1]Neurology, Internal Medicine, Sakura Medical Center, Toho University, 564-1, Shimoshizu, Sakura, Chiba, 285-8741, Japan.
[2]Clinical Physiology Unit, Sakura Medical Center, Toho University, 564-1, Shimoshizu, Sakura, Chiba, 285-8741, Japan.

vessel occlusions (lacunes), and 12 with TIA. We added a group of 26 patients with white matter ischemic lesions (WML), grade ≥ 2 by magnetic resonance imaging MRI scan. All patients showed one of the following clinical features: cerebrovascular parkinsonism, dementia, and urinary frequency/ urgency. CAVI was measured in the above 854 healthy control subjects and 85 subjects with ischemic cerebrovascular disease. CAVI of the control groups and each cerebrovascular disease group were stratified by 1) 10-year layers into 5 subgroups (40–49, 50–59, 60–69, 70–79, 80–89 years), and 2) by sex into 2 subgroups (male, female). We also performed carotid ultrasound sonography with ischemic cerebrovascular disease with 7.5-MHz, linear-array transducers (EUB-525, Hitachi, Inc, Tokyo, Japan; SSA-260A, Toshiba, Inc, Tokyo, Japan), and measured intima-media thickness (IMT).

Compared with healthy control subjects, CAVI was statistically significantly larger in patients with ischemic cerebrovascular diseases, particularly in those with WML, large-artery atherosclerosis, and small-vessel occlusions ($p < 0.001$) (**Fig. 1**); the grand average of CAVI in ischemic cerebrovascular diseases was as follows: TIA, 9.3 ± 1.5; WML, 10.3 ± 1.3; large-artery atherosclerosis, 10.2 ± 1.2; and small-vessel occlusions, 10.0 ± 1.6. Therefore, the differences in CAVI between the ischemic cerebrovascular disease and control groups were as follows: TIA, 0.492 (no statistical significance); WML, 0.733 ($p < 0.001$ by Fisher's PLSD, Bonferroni–Dunn test, and $p = 0.002$ by Scheffe's test); large-artery atherosclerosis, 0.838 ($p < 0.001$ by Fisher's PLSD, Bonferroni–Dunn test, and $p = 0.005$ by Scheffe's test); and small-vessel occlusions, 1.034 ($p < 0.001$ by Fisher's PLSD, Bonferroni–Dunn test, and

Scheffe's test). Linear regression analysis of CAVI and plaque-score showed that there was a weak but statistically significant relationship between CAVI and plaque score in ischemic cerebrovascular disease patients ($p = 0.045$) (**Fig. 2**). In contrast, there was no significant difference in CAVI between patients with TIA and control subjects. The results agreed with the concept that TIA is the mildest form among the 4 subgroups of ischemic cerebrovascular diseases.

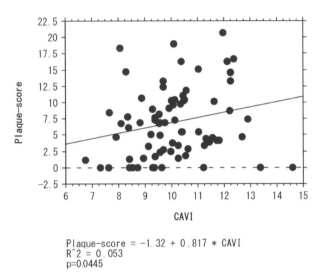

Plaque-score = -1.32 + 0.817 * CAVI
R^2 = 0.053
p=0.0445

Fig. 2. Linear regression analysis of CAVI and plaque-score.

There was a weak but statistically significant relationship between CAVI and the plaque score in ischemic cerebrovascular disease patients ($p = 0.0445$).
Cited from ref. 3 【with permission of Elsevier】

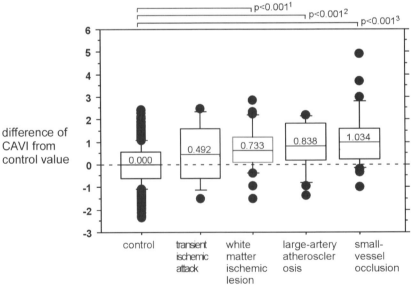

Fig. 1. Difference in CAVI between cerebrovascular disease and control groups.

Note that horizontal bars and values in the box plot indicate the grand average (not the median, in order to visualize the objects of statistics). CAVI: cardio-ankle vascular stiffness index. P values 1, 2, and 3 are driven by three different statistical methods: Fisher's protected least significant difference (all $p < 0.001$), Bonferroni-Dunn test (all $p < 0.001$), and Scheffe's test (WML, $p = 0.002$, infarction [other than lacunes], $p = 0.005$, lacunar infarction, $p < 0.001$). The TIA group was not significantly different from controls by any method.
Cited from ref. 3 【with permission of Elsevier】

Hayashi et al.[9] studied 284 mainly older subjects (mean age 72 years) whose CAVI was measured, and found that subjects with a history of stroke was significantly more common in the high-CAVI group (> 8.0) than in the low-CAVI group (< 8.0) (incidence of stroke, 31% and 0%, respectively).

The above reports indicate that CAVI might predict stroke/WMD and possibly also TIA. This is because the majority of stroke/WMD cases are related to systemic arteriosclerosis (which CAVI measures), and to some extent, on the pulse wave/heart-beat (termed the "shock wave," as it is regarded as being harmful to the brain[10]), of which CAVI is a relative measure, as described below.

Pulse wave and brain
Increased cerebral pulsatility-induced microvascular damage[11,12]

Cerebral blood flow (CBF) is maintained constant within a pressure range of 50–150 mmHg. Below 50 mmHg,

hypoxia dilates cerebral blood vessels, but the brain is hypoperfused; above 150 mmHg, blood vessels are passively dilated and CBF rises dangerously. A normal pulse pressure (50–150 mmHg) does not affect CBF "autoregulation." In extreme hypertension, the amplitude of the pulse pressure is markedly increased, CBF autoregulation is disrupted, which may further augment the risk of stroke and increase mortality. In other cases, an increase in pulse pressure itself could induce brain microvascular damage. In mice, aging combined with hypertension is associated with a deregulation of pressure-induced myogenic tone[13], cerebral microvascular injury, oxidative stress, neuroinflammation, and cerebral microhemorrhages[11]. In humans, it has been reported that a similar mechanism as in the aged brain is involved in pulse-wave encephalopathy[10], a tsunami-effect in the brain[7], destruction of the brain by the pulse in Alzheimer's disease (AD)[14]. Epidemiological data have demonstrated an association of increased CAVI and pulse wave velocity (PWV) with microvasculature-

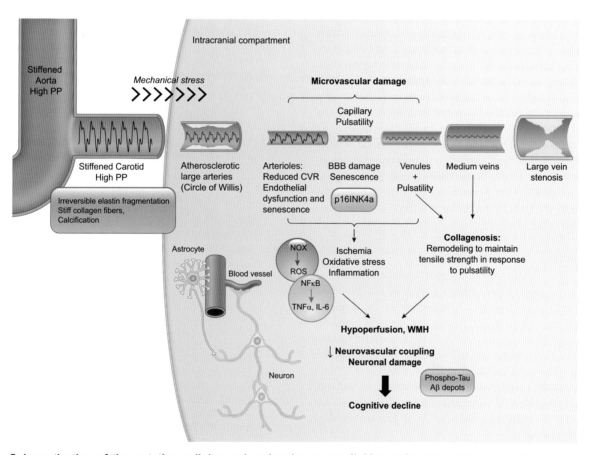

Fig. 3. Schematization of the putative cellular and molecular events linking pulse pressure penetration in the cerebral microcirculation and the development of cognitive decline.

Age-associated stiffening of large elastic arteries, such as the aorta and carotids, is due to irreversible elastin fragmentation induced by the lifelong exposure of the vascular wall to the mechanical stress inherent to the heart beat. Stiff collagen, which replaces elastin, and calcification of the vascular wall significantly reduce arterial elasticity and augment the amplitude of the pulse pressure (PP) that penetrates into the fragile, low-resistance cerebral microcirculation. Arteriolar, venular, and capillary pulsatility is associated with endothelial nitric oxide synthase dysfunction and possibly endothelial senescence (p16INK4a expression), reduced cerebrovascular reactivity (CVR), and blood–brain barrier (BBB) disruption. The latter permits the infiltration of inflammatory cells and toxic molecules, leading to inflammation (through NF-κB), oxidative stress (via NADPH oxidase [NOX] activation], and ischemia. In the venules and medium-size veins, pulsatility promotes collagenosis that contributes to cerebral hypoperfusion. Altogether, this deleterious ischemic and inflammatory environment favors parenchymal damage (including white matter hyperintensity [WMH]), neurovascular uncoupling, and neuronal damage (phospho-tau and amyloid-β [Aβ] depots), ultimately leading to cognitive decline and dementia. ROS, reactive oxygen species. Cited from ref. 24.

related WMD[15,16].

Increased cerebral pulsatility-induced neuronal damage

In humans, WMD alone is associated with some extent of cognitive decline[17], and contributes to the development of AD pathology (a combination of WMD and AD)[18]. By these mechanisms, increased PWV is associated with memory loss and dementia[19]. In contrast, a recent meta-analysis showed that arterial stiffening was significantly associated with cerebral vascular diseases, but only weakly associated with cognition[20]. This is because WMD comprises only a part of dementia in older individuals, whereas the major source of dementia in older individuals is AD. In mice, "neurovascular coupling" significantly contributes to the maintenance of neural function. This is defined by anatomic proximity between arterioles, neurons, astrocytes, glia, and complex signaling mechanisms, permitting the local adjustment of blood flow to local neuronal activity in which endothelium-derived nitric oxide (NO) plays a central role[20]. Vascular stiffness is also known to be regulated by the brain. Steroid receptor coactivator-1 (SRC-1) protein[21] is distributed in the central amygdala, medial amygdala, supraoptic nucleus, arcuate nucleus, ventromedial, dorsomedial, paraventricular hypothalamus, and solitary tract nucleus, i.e., the area overlapping the circulation regulatory area. SRC-1 is known to regulate blood pressure and aortic stiffness[22]. Therefore, there might be a crosstalk between the brain and the periphery in order to prevent abnormal systemic/cranial vascular stiffness and resultant stroke/WMD. Collectively, experimental studies have suggested that both cerebral microvascular damage, disruption of the blood–brain barrier, and parenchymal damage induced by the penetrating pulse pressure could contribute to the association between arterial stiffening and memory loss (**Fig. 3**).

Conclusion

Stroke and WMD are the most common cause of neurological disability and impairs quality of life, resulting in early institutionalization. Atherosclerosis is a major contributor to stroke/WMD, but it can be prevented by early recognition and management. CAVI is a useful routine test at the early suspicion of ischemic cerebrovascular disease, particularly in clinical practice. CAVI is a simple and non-invasive indicator of atherosclerosis in patients with stroke/WMD. CAVI can also be an ideal marker for monitoring "de-stiffening" therapy[23], to prevent stroke/WMD in future.

References

1) Shirai K, Utino J, Otsuka K, Takata M. A novel blood pressure independent arterial wall stiffness parameter; Cardio-Ankle Vascular Index(CAVI). J Atheroscler Thromb. 2006; 13: 101-107.

2) Saji N, Kimura K, Shimizu H, Kita Y. Silent brain infarct is independently associated with arterial stiffness indicated by cardio-ankle vascular index (CAVI). Hypertens Res. 2012; 35: 756-760.

3) Suzuki J, Sakakibara R, Tomaru T, et al. Stroke and cardio-ankle vascular stiffness index. J Stroke Cerebrovasc Dis. 2013; 22: 171-175.

4) Choi SY, Park HE, Seo H, et al. Arterial stiffness using cardio-ankle vascular index reflects cerebral small vessel disease in healthy young and middle aged subjects. J Atheroscler Thromb. 2013; 20: 178-185.

5) Sakakibara R, Suzuki J, Tsuyusaki Y, et al. Stroke and cardio-ankle vascular stiffness index: A clinical use. J Stroke Neurological Disorders 2014; 2: 1037.ePuB.

6) Saji N, Kimura K, Yagita Y, et al. Comparison of arteriosclerotic indicators in patients with ischemic stroke: ankle-brachial index, brachial-ankle pulse wave velocity and cardio-ankle vascular index. Hypertens Res. 2015; 38: 323-328.

7) Saji N, Toba K, Sakurai T. Cerebral small vessel disease and arterial stiffness: Tsunami effect in the brain? Pulse 2015; 3: 182-189.

8) Shimoyama T, Iguchi Y, Kimura K, et al. Stroke patients with cerebral microbleeds on MRI scans have arteriolosclerosis as well as systemic atherosclerosis. Hypertens Res. 2012; 35: 975-979.

9) Hayashi S. Useful method to monitor cerebral infarction in atherosclerotic patients without atrial fibrillation by the combination of carotid intima-media thickness, cardio-ankle vascular index, and plasma d-dimer. Atheroscler Open Access 2017; 2:113.

10) Bateman GA. Pulse-wave encephalopathy: a comparative study of the hydrodynamics of leukoaraiosis and normal-pressure hydrocephalus. Neuroradiology. 2002; 44: 740-748.

11) Thorin-Trescases N, de Montgolfier O, Pinçon A, et al. Impact of pulse pressure on cerebrovascular events leading to age-related cognitive decline. Am J Physiol Heart Circ Physiol. 2018;314:H1214-H1224.

12) Levin RA, Carnegie MH, Celermajer DS. Pulse pressure: an emerging therapeutic target for dementia. Front Neurosci. 2020 14:669.

13) Toth P, Csiszar A, Tucsek Z, et al. Role of 20-HETE, TRPC channels, and BKCa in dysregulation of pressure-induced Ca^{2+} signaling and myogenic constriction of cerebral arteries in aged hypertensive mice. Am J Physiol Heart Circ Physiol. 2013; 305: H1698-H1708.

14) Stone J, Johnstone DM, Mitrofanis J, O'Rourke M. The mechanical cause of age-related dementia (Alzheimer's disease): the brain is destroyed by the pulse. J Alzheimers Dis. 2015; 44: 355-373.

15) Balestrini CS, Al-Khazraji BK, Suskin N, Shoemaker JK. Does vascular stiffness predict white matter hyperintensity burden in ischemic heart disease with preserved ejection fraction? Am J Physiol Heart Circ Physiol. 2020; 318: H1401-1409.

16) Badji A, de la Colina AN, Boshkovski T, et al. A cross-sectional study on the impact of arterial stiffness on the corpus callosum, a key white matter tract implicated in Alzheimer's disease. J Alzheimers Dis. 2020; 77: 591-605.

17) Levit A, Hachinski V, Whitehead SN. Neurovascular unit dysregulation, white matter disease, and executive dysfunction: The shared triad of vascular cognitive impairment and Alzheimer disease. Geroscience. 2020; 42: 445-465.

18) Sakakibara R, Tateno F, Aiba Y, et al. Prevalence of triple/dual disease (Alzheimer's disease, Lewy body disease, and white matter disease). Neurol Clin Neurosci. 2020; 8: 171-176.

19) Rabkin SW. Arterial stiffness: detection and consequences in cognitive impairment and dementia of the elderly. J Alzheimers Dis. 2012; 32: 541-549.

20) van Sloten TT, Protogerou AD, Henry RM, et al. Association between arterial stiffness, cerebral small vessel disease

and cognitive impairment: a systematic review and meta-analysis. Neurosci Biobehav Rev. 2015; 53: 121-130.

21) Toth P, Tarantini S, Davila A, et al. Purinergic glio-endothelial coupling during neuronal activity: Role of P2Y1 receptors and eNOS in functional hyperemia in the mouse somatosensory cortex. Am J Physiol Heart Circ Physiol. 2015; 309: H1837-H1845.

22) Hinton Jr AO, Yang Y, Quick AP, et al. SRC-1 regulates blood pressure and aortic stiffness in female mice. PLoS

One. 2016; 11: e0168644.

23) Chen Y, Shen F, Liu J, Yang GY. Arterial stiffness and stroke: De-stiffening strategy, a therapeutic target for stroke. Stroke Vasc Neurol. 2017; 2: 65-72.

24) Nathalie T-T, Olivia de M, Anthony Pinçon, et al. Impact of pulse pressure on cerebrovascular events leading to age-related cognitive decline.Am J Physiol Heart Circ Physiol. 2018; 314:H1214-H1224. doi: 10.1152/ajpheart.00637.2017. Epub 2018 Feb 16.

Coronary Artery Disease and Cardio-ankle Vascular Index (CAVI)

Shigeo Horinaka

Introduction

In recent years, people's lifestyles and diets have become more fast-paced, and the incidence of lifestyle-related diseases such as metabolic syndrome is increasing rapidly. Modification in the lifestyle and controlling diseases such as hypertension, diabetes, and dyslipidemia can prevent the development of acute coronary syndrome, which is a critical endpoint of coronary atherosclerosis. The presence of these risk factors induces vascular endothelial dysfunction and increases the arterial stiffness. Progression of coronary atherosclerosis causes tearing of the thin fibrous cap, leading to rupture of the plaque[1], and the lipid plaque components leak into the lumen of the vessel, inducing thrombus formation, which is followed by acute coronary artery occlusion[2]. Although monitoring the risk factors of atherosclerosis (i.e., age, blood pressure, smoking, and serum glucose and cholesterol levels) has been recommended to evaluate the risk of mortality due to coronary artery disease[4], it is difficult to predict the corrected risk in a person, since the effect of each risk factor differs in each individual patient.

In our country, one-fourth of the deaths are due to cerebral and myocardial infarctions caused by atherosclerosis[4]. These diseases are difficult to predict using investigations such as brain computed tomography or electrocardiogram; hence, a convenient and simple test that can measure atherosclerosis itself is necessary. In recent times, an examination for evaluating the vascular function has been clinically used, and this new examination can not only estimate the risk of cardiovascular events but also assess the therapeutic effects of drugs[5-7].

The cardio-ankle vascular index (CAVI) is used for evaluating atherosclerosis because it is not dependent on the blood pressure at the time of measurement and is derived from the arterial stiffness parameter β[8], which is calculated based on the brachial blood pressure and pulse wave velocity (PWV) from the heart to the ankle[9,10]. This chapter reviews the clinical implications of the CAVI for estimating the risk of the coronary artery disease (CAD).

1. The CAVI correlates with the stiffness of the thoracic aorta using electrocardiographic (ECG)-gated multi-detector row computed tomography (MDCT)

Forty-nine patients suspected to have CAD were assessed using pulsatility-related cross-sectional area (CSA) changes in the aortic lumen constructed by the ECG-gated MDCT. The largest and smallest luminal CSAs during the RR-interval in the ascending or descending aorta at the pulmonary bifurcation level, brachial systolic and diastolic blood pressures, and CAVI were simultaneously measured. Subsequently, the regional PWV and stiffness parameter β were calculated using the following formulas.

$$\text{Regional PWV (cm/s)} = \sqrt{CSAmin \times (SBP - DBP) \times 133 / \rho (CSAmax - CSAmin)} \quad [11\text{-}13]$$

where mmHg $= 133$ dyne/cm^2, ρ is blood density (1.059 g/cm^2)

$$\text{Regional stiffness parameter } \beta = \ln (SBP/DBP)/((Dmax\text{-}Dmin)/Dmin) \quad [8]$$

where ln is the natural logarithm, D is the diameter $= 2\sqrt{CSA/\pi}$, Dmax and Dmin are the maximum and minimum lumen diameter, respectively.

Determinant of the CAVI using the multiple regression model.

Multiple regression analysis revealed that age was the common determinant for the CAVI ($R^2 = 0.245$, $P < 0.0003$), regional stiffness parameter β (ascending aorta: $R^2 = 0.383$, $P < 0.0001$; descending aorta: $R^2 = 0.336$, $P < 0.0001$), and regional PWV (ascending aorta: $R^2 = 0.372$, $P < 0.0001$; descending aorta: $R^2 = 0.287$, $P < 0.0001$) (Table 1). Since age was a confounding factor for these indices, we performed a multiple stepwise regression analysis excluding age. The regional stiffness parameter β in the ascending aorta was the only independent determinant of the CAVI ($R^2 = 0.235$, $P = 0.0004$; Table 1)[14]. This finding was in line with previous reports[15,16]. These data support the potential role for the CAVI as part of an integrated approach to evaluate central arterial stiffness in the aorta.

2. Comparing the stiffness of the heart–thigh and thigh–ankle arteries with heart–ankle arterial segments for detecting the presence of CAD

The main drawback of the CAVI is that it is calculated from the PWV, which includes the measurement of the lower limb segment (from the femoral to the posterior tibial arteries), which has no predictive value for the risk of

Department of Cardiovascular Medicine, Dokkyo Medical University, 880 Kitakobashi, Mibu-cho, Tochigi, 321-0293, Japan.

Table 1. Determination of the Regional stiffness parameter β and Regional pulse wave velocity (PWV) in the ascending or descending aortas and Cardio-ankle vascular index (CAVI) using multiple regression models including and excluding age.

Regional stiffness parameter β	β	P value
Ascending aorta		
Age	0.619	<0.0001
Descending aorta		
Age	0.580	<0.0001

Regional stiffness parameter β on the ascending and descending aortas included variable is age ($R^2 = 0.383$; $P < 0.0001$, $R^2 = 0.336$; $P < 0.0001$), respectively.

Regional PWV	β	P value
Ascending aorta		
Age	0.610	<0.0001
SBP	0.415	0.0013
Descending aorta		
Age	0.536	<0.0001
SBP	0.496	<0.0001

Regional PWVs on the ascending and descending aortas included variables are age and SBP status (age: $R^2 = 0.372$; $P < 0.0001$, $R^2 = 0.287$; $P < 0.0001$, SBP: $R^2 = 0.172$; $P < 0.0001$, $R^2 = 0.246$; $P < 0.0001$), respectively.

CAVI	β	P value
Age	0.495	0.0003
Ascending aorta		
Regional PWV	0.483	0.0705
Regional stiffness parameter β	0.485	0.6006
Descending aorta		
PWV	0.327	0.8400
Stiffness parameter β	0.304	0.8003

CAVI included variable age ($R^2 = 0.245$; $P < 0.0003$).

CAVI without age	β	P value
Ascending aorta		
Regional PWV	0.485	0.2497
Regional stiffness parameter β	0.304	0.0004
Descending aorta		
Regional PWV	0.483	0.7363
Regional stiffness parameter β	0.327	0.9541

CAVI included variable stiffness parameter β of the ascending aorta status without age ($R^2 = 0.235$; $P = 0.0004$).

This table was modified from Fig. 3 of the following literature (Ref.14: S. Horinaka et al./Atherosclerosis 235 (2014) 239–245).
【with permission of Elsevier】

cardiovascular events or mortality[17]. The CAVI equation includes the coefficients "a" and "b" for adjustment of the value of Hasegawa's PWV, which is compensated for a diastolic pressure of 80 mmHg[18]. Recently, Takahashi et al. demonstrated that the CAVI could interpret the heart–ankle β (haBETA) in epidemiological and clinical studies[19]. Thus,

Table 2. htBETA, taBETA, and haBETA in healthy subjects and patients with CAD.

	Healthy Subjects (n = 90)	Patients with CAD (n = 41)	P-value
haBETA	9.22 ± 2.20	10.52 ± 1.58	<0.01
htBETA	7.04 ± 1.95	8.65 ± 1.76	<0.01
taBETA	21.27 ± 8.68*	21.14 ± 8.36*	n.s.

Notes: Data are shown as mean ± standard deviation. Student's *t*-test, *p < 0.01 vs haBETA and htBETA.

Abbreviations: CAD, coronary artery disease; haBETA, heart–ankle β; htBETA, heart–thigh β; taBETA, thigh–ankle β; n.s., non-significant.

This table was modified from Table 3 of the following literature (Ref. 21: Watahiki M. et al. Vascular Health and Risk Management 2020:16 561-570. Originally published by and used with permission from Dove Medical Press Ltd.

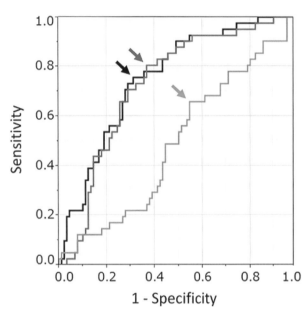

Fig. 1. Receiver operating characteristic (ROC) curves of haBETA, htBETA, and taBETA in coronary artery disease (CAD).

haBETA: cutoff value 9.20 (black arrow), sensitivity 80.5, specificity 63.3%. htBETA: cutoff value 7.72 (dark gray arrow), sensitivity 75.6, specificity 68.9%. taBETA: cutoff value 21.0 (gray arrow), sensitivity 65.6, specificity 45.6%. Each arrow indicates the optimal threshold (cutoff value) of haBETA, htBETA, and taBETA for the detecting of the presence of CAD.

This figure was modified from Figure 5 of the following literature (Ref. 21: Watahiki M. et al. Vascular Health and Risk Management 2020:16 561-570. Originally published by and used with permission from Dove Medical Press Ltd.

the segmental stiffness parameter β was applied using an additional new thigh cuff in the CAVI measurement apparatus (VaSera)[20]. The impact of the stiffness of elastic aorta [heart-thigh β (htBETA)] and the medium-sized muscular artery [thigh-ankle β (taBETA)] on the heart–ankle β (haBETA) was investigated; further, it was evaluated whether the htBETA (haBETA-taBETA) improved the power of diagnosis of CAD. Ninety healthy subjects who underwent periodic health examinations and 41 patients with CAD were included. In both groups, haBETA and htBETA, but not taBETA, correlated with age, and taBETA was similar between the healthy subjects and

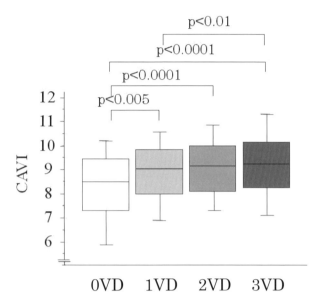

Number of major vessels involved

Fig. 2. The box and whisker plots show the CAVI in the 0, 1, 2, and 3 vessel diseases.

CAVI: cardio-ankle vascular index; VD: vessel disease; 0VD: no significant stenosis; 1 VD: single VD; 2 VD: double VD; 3 VD: triple VD.

This figure was modified from Figure 2 of the following literature (Ref. 28: Horinaka S. et al. Angiology 2009 Apr;60:468–476).

patients with CAD; its value was three times higher than htBETA (P < 0.01), as shown in Table 2. The area under the ROC curve (AUC) for CAD in taBETA (0.493, P = not significant) was smaller than that for haBETA (0.731, P < 0.01) or htBETA (0.757, P <0.01); no difference was observed in the AUC between haBETA and htBETA (Fig. 1). Therefore, the AUC of haBETA could be replaced by that of htBETA, thus extending the measurement segment without affecting the diagnostic power for CAD[21]. This finding was in line with previous reports[22-25].

In our study, the cutoff value of haBETA for CAD was 9.2. To convert the value of haBETA to CAVI using the conversion formula[9], the cutoff value of CAVI for detecting CAD was 8.2[21].

3. Association between the CAVI and plaque burden in the coronary artery and aortic sclerosis

The association between the CAVI and the plaque burden measured by intravascular ultrasound (IVUS) in the left main coronary artery (LMCA) was evaluated in patients with CAD who had normal LMCA on angiography (n = 70). The CAVI was significantly correlated with the percentage plaque area (R = 0.649, P < 0.0001) measured by IVUS in the most diseased segment of LMCA. The CAVI remained a significant factor among the risk factors for cardiovascular disease included in the multiple regression analysis for predicting the percentage plaque area[26]. Furthermore, to examine the relationship between the CAVI and aortic atherosclerosis on MDCT, patients with (n = 49) or without (n = 49) CAD who underwent MDCT for suspected CAD were studied. The CAVI was an independent predictor of the thickness of the wall of the descending aorta at the level of pulmonary bifurcation, based on multiple stepwise regression analysis[27]. These data suggest that the CAVI, a simple and convenient index, is useful for evaluating atherosclerosis of the coronary arteries and thoracic aorta.

4. Diagnostic accuracy and evaluating severity of CAD using the CAVI

The CAVI was measured and compared in 696 patients who had chest pain and underwent coronary angiography (Mean age: 60 ± 5 years). The average CAVI value was significantly greater in the group of patients with 1-, 2-, or 3- vessel diseases (VD) than in the group of participants without vascular disease (P < 0.005, P < 0.0001, P < 0.0001, respectively). The average value of the CAVI was also significantly greater in the group of patients with 3 VDs than in patients with 1 VD (P < 0.01; Fig. 2). The average values of CAVI did not differ between the group of patients with 1 and 2 VDs and those with 2 and 3 VDs, as shown in Fig. 2[28].

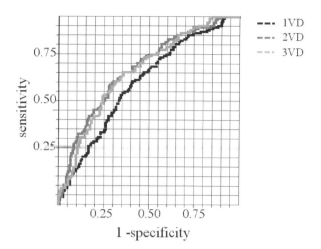

Fig. 3. The receiver operating characteristic (ROC) curve of the CAVI in the 1, 2, and 3 vessel diseases.

The area under the receiver operating characteristics curve (AUC ± SE) of the CAVI was 0.648 ± 0.029 in 1 VD (black line), 0.722 ± 0.030 in 2 VD (dark gray line), and 0.710 ± 0.032 in 3 VD (gray line). SE: standard error; VD: vessel disease
This figure was modified from Figure 3 of the following literature (Ref. 27: Horinaka S. et al. Angiology 2017 Apr;68(4):330–338).

Table 3. CAVI in coronary artery disease.

	CAVI cutoff value or CAD- vs. CAD+	Reference
Detection of coronary artery disease		
	8.5	Sakaguchi M et al.[31]
	8.81	Nakamura et al.[32]
	9.0	Izuhara M et al.[33]
	8.67	Horinaka S et al.[28]
	8.7 vs. 9.1	Miyoshi T et al.[34]
	8.0	Yingchoncharoen T et al.[29]
	8.0	Park HE et al.[35]
	8.0	Park JB et al.[36]
	8.6*	Gökdeniz et al.[37]

Cardiovascular prognosis					
Author	Subjects	Mean age (years)	Follow-up period	Outcome	Prognostic value
Kubota et al.[38]	400 with MS or CVD history	63.2-73.9	26.8-27.7 months	Cardiovascular events	Significant CAVI > 10.0 vs. < 9.0
Laucevičius et al.[39]	2,106 with MS	53.83 ± 6.18	3.8 ± 1.7 years	Cardiovascular events	Significant CAVI > 7.95
Satoh-Asahara et al.[40]	425 with obesity	51.5	5 years	Cardiovascular events	Significant CAVI > 7.825
Sato Y et al.[41]	1,003 with MS	62.5 ± 1.61	6.7 ± 1.6 years	Cardiovascular events	Significant CAVI > 10.09
Gohbara M et al.[42]	288 with STMI	58 ± 11, 71 ± 9	15 months	Cardiovascular events	Significant CAVI > 8.325
Otsuka K et al.[43]	211 with CAD and impaired CAVI	64 ± 11, 66 ± 8	2.9 ± 1.0 years	Cardiovascular events	Significant Persistently impaired vs. improved CAVI at baseline and 6 months
Chung SL et al.[44]	626 with DM	64 ± 9	4 years	Cardiovascular events	Significant CAVI ≥ 9.0
Kirigaya J et al.[45]	387 with ACS	64 ± 11	62 months	MACE and CV death	Significant CAVI > 8.35

* for prediction of intermediate-high SYNTAX score,
MS: metabolic syndrome; STEMI: ST-segment elevation myocardial infarction; CAD: coronary artery disease; impaired CAVI was defined as greater than the mean plus 1 SD of the age- and gender-specific normal CAVI values, according to results obtained in 5188 healthy subjects; DM: diabetes mellitus; MACE: Major adverse cardiac events (CV death, recurrence of ACS, heart failure requiring hospitalization); CV death: cardiovascular death (death from acute myocardial infarction; heart failure; stroke; or documented sudden death without apparent cardiovascular cause).

ROC curve of the CAVI based on the all number of major vessels involved were computed. Using the threshold of 8.67 for the CAVI, the sensitivity and specificity were 66.5% and 65.8%, respectively. In the subgroup analysis, the AUC ± SE of the CAVI was 0.648 ± 0.029 for 1 VD, 0.722 + 0.030 for 2 VDs (P< 0.05 vs. 1 VD), and 0.710 ± 0.032 for 3 VDs (P< 0.05 vs. 1 VD), respectively as shown in Fig. 3[28]. Data about the CAVI value in patients with CAD showed a discrepancy in some studies[29-31], such as no increase in the CAVI with an increase in the number of vessels involved, while in other studies[32-34], increasing CAVI was associated with an increase in the number of vessels involved. This discrepancy may be explained that multivessel disease usually associated with severe coronary atherosclerosis, but severe coronary atherosclerosis did not necessary cause significant coronary stenosis.

It has been reported that the CAVI was a better predictor of CAD than brachial-ankle PWV[29]. In 809 individuals from the Czech post-MONICA study, BETA derived from the carotid-femoral PWV (cfPWV) and carotid-ankle PWV (caPWV) was less dependent on blood pressure, while it was more closely correlated with the presence of CAD compared to cfPWV and caPWV[25].

Thus, the CAVI can be clinically useful as a predictive marker of the extent of CAD as assessed by the number of major vessels involved.

5. Coronary risk factors and the CAVI

The cutoff value of the CAVI to detect the presence of CAD has been reported (Table 3). The relationships between the coronary risk factors and CAVI have also been reported. Moreover, the CAVI was useful as a predictor for the onset of cardiovascular events in high-risk patients with metabolic syndrome, obesity, and/or ST-elevation myocardial infarction, and CAD (Table 3).

A systematic review revealed that the CAVI was higher in patients with CVD than in those without. In terms of the prospective prognostic value of the CAVI, a limited number of studies have been conducted, but they indicated a modest association between the CAVI and CVD outcome[46].

In our country, the CAVI-J study, which was a multicenter, prospective, observational cohort study to evaluate the CAVI for the prediction of the onset of cardiovascular events, has been completed, and results showing the usefulness of the CAVI for secondary prevention in patients with CAD has been reported[47,48].

In summary

The CAVI reflects the degree of coronary atherosclerosis regardless of the classical risk factors for CAD, even in the absence of symptoms. Considering age, it is possible to evaluate the severity of CAD, and it can be a predictor for the onset of a cardiovascular event such as acute coronary syndrome. Therefore, the CAVI is a useful screening tool for latent coronary atherosclerosis as well as for evaluating the risk for CAD, which might be useful in predicting major adverse cardiovascular events.

References

1) van der Sijde JN, Karanasos A, Villiger M, Bouma BE, Regar E. First-in-man assessment of plaque rupture by polarization-sensitive optical frequency domain imaging in vivo. Eur Heart J. 2016;37:1932.
2) Bentzon JF, Otsuka F, Virmani R, Falk E. Mechanisms of plaque formation and rupture. Circ Res. 2014;114:1852-1866.
3) Brown JC, Gerhardt TE, Kwon E. Risk Factors for coronary artery disease. 2020 Jun 6. In: StatPearls [Internet]. Treasure Island (FL): StatPearls Publishing; 2020 Jan.
4) Ministry of Health, Labour and Welfare. The Ministry of Health Population Movement Statistics 2010. http://www.mhlw.go.jp/toukei/saikin/hw/jinkou/kakutei10/ (accessed March 2, 2016).
5) Laurent S, Cockcroft J, Van Bortel L, Boutouyrie P, et al. European Network for Non-invasive Investigation of Large Arteries. Expert consensus document on arterial stiffness: methodological issues and clinical applications. Eur Heart J. 2006;27:2588-2605.
6) Mitchell GF, Hwang SJ, Vasan RS, et al. Arterial stiffness and cardiovascular events: the Framingham Heart Study. Circulation. 2010;121:505-511.
7) Vlachopoulos C, Aznaouridis K, Stefanadis C. Prediction of cardiovascular events and all-cause mortality with arterial stiffness: a systematic review and meta-analysis. J Am Coll Cardiol. 2010;55:1318-1327.
8) Hayashi K, Handa H, Nagasawa S, et al. Stiffness and elastic behavior of human intracranial and extracranial arteries. J Biomech. 1980;13:175-184.
9) Shirai K, Utino J, Otsuka K, Takata M. A novel blood pressure-independent arterial wall stiffness parameter Cardio-ankle vascular index (CAVI) J Atheroscler Thromb. 2006;13:101-107.
10) Shirai K, Utino J, Saiki A, et al. Evaluation of blood pressure control using a new arterial stiffness parameter, cardio-ankle vascular index (CAVI). Curr Hypertens Rev. 2013;9:66-75.
11) Bramwell JC, Hill AV. The velocity of the pulse wave in man. Proc R Soc Lond B. 1922;93:298,e306.
12) Dogui A, Kachenoura N, Frouin F, et al. Consistency of aortic distensibility and pulse wave velocity estimates with respect to the Bramwell-Hill theoretical model: a cardiovascular magnetic resonance study. J Cardiovasc Magn Reson. 2011;13:11.
13) Westenberg JJ, van Poelgeest EP, Steendijk P, et al. Bramwell-Hill modeling for local aortic pulse wave velocity estimation: a validation study with velocity-encoded cardiovascular magnetic resonance and invasive pressure assessment. J Cardiovasc Magn Reson. 2012;14:2.
14) Horinaka S, Yagi H, Ishimura K, et al. Cardio-ankle vascular index (CAVI) correlates with aortic stiffness in the thoracic aorta using ECG-gated multi-detector row computed tomography. Atherosclerosis. 2014;235:239-245 https://doi.org/10.1016/j.atherosclerosis.2014.04.034.
15) Tomochika Y, Tanaka N, Ono S, et al. Assessment by transesophageal echography of atherosclerosis of the descending thoracic aorta in patients with hypercholesterolemia. Am J Cardiol. 1999;83:703-709.
16) Takaki A, Ogawa H, Wakeyama T, et al. Cardioankle vascular index is a new noninvasive parameter of arterial stiffness. Circ J. 2007;71:1710-1714.
17) Pannier B, Guérin AP, Marchais SJ, et al. Stiffness of capacitive and conduit arteries: prognostic significance for end-stage renal disease patients. Hypertension. 2005;45:592-596.
18) Hasegawa M, Arai C. Clinical estimation of vascular elastic function and practical application. Connective Tissue. 1995;27:149-157.

19) Takahashi K, Yamamoto T, Tsuda S, et al. Coefficients in the CAVI equation and the comparison between CAVI with and without the coefficients using clinical data. J Atheroscler Thromb. 2019;26:465-475.

20) Yamamoto T, Shimizu K, Takahashi M, et al. The effect of nitroglycerin on arterial stiffness of the aorta and the femoral-tibial arteries. J Atheroscler Thromb. 2017;24:1048-1057.

21) Watahiki M, Horinaka S, Ishimitsu T, et al. Comparing the Heart-Thigh and Thigh Ankle Arteries with the Heart-Ankle Arterial Segment for Arterial Stiffness Measurements. Vasc Health Risk Manag. 2020;16:561-570 https://doi.org/10.2147/vhrm.s284248.

22) van der Heijden-Spek JJ, Staessen JA, Fagard RH, et al. Effect of age on brachial artery wall properties differs from the aorta and is gender dependent: a population study. Hypertension. 2000;35:637-642.

23) Boutouyrie P, Laurent S, Benetos A, et al. Opposing effects of ageing on distal and proximal large arteries in hypertensives. J Hypertens. 1992;10:S87-S91.

24) Wohlfahrt P, Krajčoviechová A, Seidlerová J, et al. Lower-extremity arterial stiffness vs. aortic stiffness in the general population. Hypertens Res. 2013;36:718-724.

25) Wohlfahrt P, Krajčoviechová A, Seidlerová J, et al. Arterial stiffness parameters: how do they differ? Atherosclerosis. 2013;231:359-364.

26) Horinaka S, Yabe A, Yagi H, et al. Cardio-ankle vascular index could reflect plaque burden in the coronary artery. Angiology. 2011;62:401-408.

27) Horinaka S, Yagi H, Fukushima H, et al. Associations Between Cardio-Ankle Vascular Index and Aortic Structure and Sclerosis Using Multidetector Computed Tomography. Angiology 2017;68:330-338.

28) Horinaka S, Yabe A, Yagi H, et al. Comparison of atherosclerotic indicators between cardio ankle vascular index and brachial ankle pulse wave velocity. Angiology 2009;60:468-476 https://doi.org/10.1177/0003319708325443. SAGE as the original publissher. https://journals.sagepub.com/home/ang

29) Yingchoncharoen T, Limpijankit T, Jongjirasiri S, et al. Arterial stiffness contributes to coronary artery disease risk prediction beyond the traditional risk score (RAMA-EGAT score). Heart Asia. 2012;4:77-82.

30) Kanamoto M, Matsumoto N, Shiga T, et al. Relationship between coronary artery stenosis and cardio-ankle vascular index (CAVI) in patients undergoing cardiovascular surgery. J Cardiovasc Dis Res 2013;4:15-19.

31) Sakaguchi M, Hasegawa T, Ehara S, et al. Cardio-ankle vascular index associated with coronary plaque burden not plaque morphology. Osaka City Med J. 2016;62:47-57.

32) Nakamura K, Tomaru T, Yamamura S, et al. Cardio-ankle vascular index is a candidate predictor of coronary atherosclerosis. Circ J. 2008;72:598-604.

33) Izuhara M, Shioji K, Kadota S, et al. Relationship of cardio-ankle vascular index (CAVI) to carotid and coronary arteriosclerosis. Circ J. 2008;72:1762-1767.

34) Miyoshi T, Doi M, Hirohata S, et al. Cardio-ankle vascular index is independently associated with the severity of coronary atherosclerosis and left ventricular function in patients with ischemic heart disease. J Atheroscler Thromb.

2010;17:249-258.

35) Park HE, Choi SY, Kim MK, Oh BH. Cardio-ankle vascular index reflects coronary atherosclerosis in patients with abnormal glucose metabolism: assessment with 256 slice multi-detector computed tomography. J Cardiol. 2012;60:372-376.

36) Park JB, Park HE, Choi SY, et al. Relation between cardio-ankle vascular index and coronary artery calcification or stenosis in asymptomatic subjects. J Atheroscler Thromb. 2013;20:557-567.

37) Gökdeniz T, Turan T, Aykan AÇ, et al. Relation of epicardial fat thickness and cardio-ankle vascular index to complexity of coronary artery disease in nondiabetic patients. Cardiology. 2013;124:41-48.

38) Kubota Y, Maebuchim D, Takei M, et al. Cardio-ankle vascular index is a predictor of cardiovascular events. Artery Res. 2011;5:91-96.

39) Laucevicius A, Ryliškyte L, Balsyte J, et al. Association of cardio-ankle vascular index with cardiovascular risk factors and cardiovascular events in metabolic syndrome patients. Medicina (Kaunas). 2015;51:152-158.

40) Satoh-Asahara N, Kotani K, Yamakage H, et al. Japan Obesity and Metabolic Syndrome Study (JOMS) Group. Cardio-ankle vascular index predicts for the incidence of cardiovascular events in obese patients: a multicenter prospective cohort study (Japan Obesity and Metabolic Syndrome Study: JOMS). Atherosclerosis. 2015;242:461-468.

41) Sato Y, Nagayama D, Saiki A, et al. Cardio-Ankle Vascular Index is Independently Associated with Future Cardiovascular Events in Outpatients with Metabolic Disorders. J Atheroscler Thromb. 2016;23:596-605.

42) Gohbara M, Iwahashi N, Sano Y, et al. Clinical Impact of the Cardio-Ankle Vascular Index for Predicting Cardiovascular Events After Acute Coronary Syndrome. Circ J. 2016;80:1420-1426.

43) Otsuka K, Fukuda S, Shimada K, et al. Serial assessment of arterial. stiffness by cardio-ankle vascular index for prediction of future cardiovascular events in patients with coronary artery disease. Hypertens Res. 2014;37:1014-1020.

44) Chung SL, Yang CC, Chen CC, et al. Coronary artery calcium score compared with cardio-ankle vascular index in the prediction of cardiovascular events in asymptomatic patients with type 2 diabetes. J Atheroscler Thromb. 2015;22:1255-1265.

45) Kirigaya J, Iwahashi N, Tahakashi H, et al. Impact of cardio-ankle vascular index on longterm outcome in patients with acute coronary syndrome. J Atheroscler Thromb, 2020;27:657-668.

46) Matsushita K, Ding N, Kim ED, et al. Cardio-ankle vascular index and cardiovascular disease: Systematic review and meta-analysis of prospective and cross-sectional studies. J Clin Hypertens (Greenwich) 2019;21:16-24.

47) Miyoshi T, Ito H, Horinaka S, et al. Protocol for Evaluating the Cardio-Ankle Vascular Index to Predict Cardiovascular Events in Japan: A Prospective Multicenter Cohort Study. Pulse (Basel). 2017;4:11-16.

48) Miyoshi T, Ito H. Assessment of Arterial Stiffness Using the Cardio-Ankle Vascular Index. Pulse (Basel). 2016;4:11-23.

Renal Diseases and CAVI

Satoshi Morimoto and Atsuhiro Ichihara

Introduction

Chronic kidney disease (CKD) is associated with an increased risk of cardiovascular disease. Arteriosclerosis progression is one of the major causes of cardiovascular disease in patients with CKD. This chapter reviews the association between the cardio-ankle vascular index (CAVI), an indicator of arterial stiffness, and renal function and CKD progression as well as that between CAVI and cardiovascular diseases in CKD.

The relationship between CAVI and kidney function

A significant negative association between CAVI and the estimated glomerular filtration rate (eGFR) was reported in a study involving 881 subjects undergoing health checkups (**Fig. 1**)[1]. This association was independent of other risk factors for arteriosclerosis. In another study in 206 patients with cardiovascular risk factors and/or coronary artery diseases, cystatin C was independently associated with CAVI[2]. The association between CAVI and renal tissue, eGFR, and urinary albumin excretion was examined in 55 patients undergoing renal biopsies[3]. The results showed an association between CAVI and eGFR or urinary albumin excretion. However, CAVI was not associated with renal arteriosclerosis[3]. These results indicate that CAVI may be associated with renal function.

CAVI is associated with future decreases in renal function

The renal function of 369 patients without CKD who underwent CAVI was followed up for ≥ 1 year. CAVI was positively associated with a decrease in eGFR (**Fig. 2**), and high CAVI was significantly associated with CKD incidence (eGFR < 60 ml/min/1.73 m^2)[4]. In addition, high CAVI was independently associated with an eGFR decrease as observed in 352 patients with a high risk of cardiovascular disease with or without CKD[5]. These results suggest that a high CAVI may predict future decreases in renal function.

Relationship between CAVI and indices of atherosclerosis in CKD patients

Since patients with end-stage kidney disease undergoing maintenance hemodialysis (HD) have a high incidence of– and mortality associated with–cardiovascular diseases caused by accelerated arteriosclerosis, an accurate evaluation of the extent of arteriosclerosis in these patients is extremely important. In a clinical study investigating 103 HD patients, we found that CAVI was positively associated with the degree of arterial fibrosis in the brachial artery (**Fig. 3**)[6]. Interestingly, this association was stronger than that between the brachial-ankle pulse-wave velocity (baPWV), another index of arterial stiffness, and arterial fibrosis (**Fig. 3**)[6]. Similarly, CAVI and baPWV were associated with carotid maximum intima-media thickness in 160 HD patients[7]. These findings suggest the usefulness of CAVI as an index of arterial stiffness in HD patients.

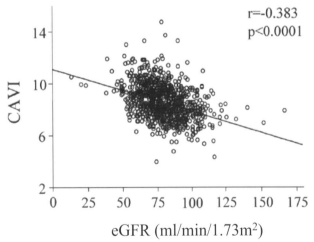

Fig. 1. **Relationship between the cardio-ankle vascular index (CAVI) and estimated glomerular filtration rate (eGFR) in the general population.**
Cited from Ref. 1.

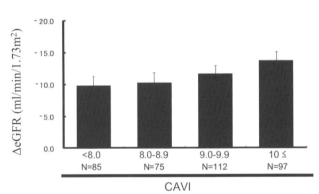

Fig. 2. **Relationship between the cardio-ankle vascular index (CAVI) and decreasing estimated glomerular filtration rate (ΔeGFR).**
P < 0.04 for the trend.
Cited from Ref. 4. 【with permission of Elsevier】

Department of Endocrinology and Hypertension, Tokyo Women's Medical University, 8-1 Kawada-cho, Shinjuku-ku, Tokyo 162-8666, Japan.

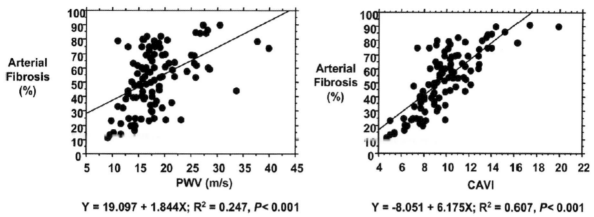

Fig. 3. Significant association of arterial fibrosis with the pulse wave velocity (PWV) and cardio-ankle vascular index (CAVI) in patients with kidney failure treated with hemodialysis. Cited from Ref. 6. [with permission of Elsevier]

Relationship between CAVI and cardiovascular diseases in CKD patients

In 68 HD patients, CAVI was markedly elevated in patients with a history of cardiovascular diseases[8]. An analysis using a receiver operating characteristic curve determined a CAVI of 7.55 as cut-off value for the presence of cardiovascular diseases, with an equal sensitivity and specificity of 0.79[8]. CAVI may be used as a screening tool to detect cardiovascular diseases in HD patients. On the other hand, in a study examining the association between baPWV or CAVI and cardiovascular outcomes in 135 HD patients, baPWV, but not CAVI, showed an association with cardiovascular deaths or events[9].

Conclusion

A high CAVI value has been shown to be associated with renal dysfunction and may predict deterioration of renal function and suggest the existence of cardiovascular diseases in CKD patients. The evolution of CKD clinical practice is expected to be marked by advances in CAVI's clinical applications and an increase in the knowledge of kidney diseases and CAVI.

References

1) Kubozono T, Miyata M, Ueyama K, Nagaki A, Hamasaki S, Kusano K, et al. Association between arterial stiffness and estimated glomerular filtration rate in the Japanese general population. *J Atheroscler Thromb*, 2009; **16**: 840-5. https://doi.org/10.5551/jat.1230

2) Nakamura K, Iizuka T, Takahashi M, Shimizu K, Mikamo H, Nakagami T, et al. Association between cardio-ankle vascular index and serum cystatin C levels in patients with cardiovascular risk factor. *J Atheroscler Thromb*, 2009; **16**: 371-9.

3) Namikoshi T, Fujimoto S, Yorimitsu D, Ihoriya C, Fujimoto Y, Komai N, et al. Relationship between vascular function indexes, renal arteriolosclerosis, and renal clinical outcomes in chronic kidney disease. *Nephrology (Carlton)*, 2015; **20**: 585-90.

4) Maebuchi D, Arima H, Ninomiya T, Yonemoto K, Kubo M, Doi Y, et al. Arterial stiffness and QT interval prolongation in a general population: the Hisayama study. *Hypertens Res*, 2008; **31**: 1339-45. https://doi.org/10.1016/j.artres.2012.11.004

5) Satirapoj B, Triwatana W, and Supasyndh O. Arterial Stiffness Predicts Rapid Decline in Glomerular Filtration Rate Among Patients with High Cardiovascular Risks. *J Atheroscler Thromb*, 2020; **27**: 611-619.

6) Ichihara A, Yamashita N, Takemitsu T, Kaneshiro Y, Sakoda M, Kurauchi-Mito A, et al. Cardio-ankle vascular index and ankle pulse wave velocity as a marker of arterial fibrosis in kidney failure treated by hemodialysis. *Am J Kidney Dis*, 2008; **52**: 947-55. https://doi.org/10.1053/j.ajkd.2008.06.007

7) Ueyama K, Miyata M, Kubozono T, Nagaki A, Hamasaki S, Ueyama S, et al. Noninvasive indices of arterial stiffness in hemodialysis patients. *Hypertens Res*, 2009; **32**: 716-20.

8) Takenaka T, Hoshi H, Kato N, Kobayashi K, Takane H, Shoda J, et al. Cardio-ankle vascular index to screen cardiovascular diseases in patients with end-stage renal diseases. *J Atheroscler Thromb*, 2008; **15**: 339-44.

9) Kato A, Takita T, Furuhashi M, Maruyama Y, Miyajima H, and Kumagai H. Brachial-ankle pulse wave velocity and the cardio-ankle vascular index as a predictor of cardiovascular outcomes in patients on regular hemodialysis. *Ther Apher Dial*, 2012; **16**: 232-41.

Cervical arterial arteriosclerosis and CAVI

Toru Miyoshi

Atherosclerotic changes in the carotid arteries generally reflect systemic atherosclerosis and are predictive of atherosclerotic diseases, such as cerebrovascular and coronary artery disease. Carotid atherosclerosis is measured with ultrasonography as a simple, safe, and reliable method in a clinical setting. The Japanese Society of Hypertension Guidelines for the Management of Hypertension (JSH 2019) recommend carotid ultrasonography for risk stratification in patients with cerebrovascular infarction[1]. The 2018 European Society of Cardiology/European Society of Hypertension guidelines for the management of arterial hypertension state that carotid ultrasonography should be used to predict target organ damage[2]. Carotid intima-media thickness (CIMT), plaque size, and plaque score (based on plaque thickness) are typically measured during the ultrasonic examination of atherosclerosis. These characteristics of carotid ultrasonography are affected by age, smoking status, blood pressure, lipid profile, glycemic control, and medications; these factors are also involved in the CAVI.

A cohort study including 1,014 Japanese adults demonstrated that the mean CIMT had a significant positive correlation with CAVI, and this association retained significance even after adjusting for traditional atherosclerotic risk factors[3]. The MARK study, a cross-sectional study including 500 Caucasian adults, demonstrated that the mean CIMT in subjects with CAVI < 8, 8–9, and > 9 increased stepwise at 0.71 ± 0.09 mm, 0.73 ± 0.09 mm, and 0.77 ± 0.10 mm, respectively[4]. In the MARK study, the cut-off level for detecting a mean CIMT of > 0.90 mm was reported to be a CAVI of 8.95. Carotid ultrasonography is performed in healthy individuals and in patients with a cardiometabolic risk. In 70 patients with hypertension, CAVI was reported to be associated with the mean CIMT, but not with the carotid plaque score, calculated as the sum of the areas of bilateral thickness > 1.1 mm[5]. A study in patients with metabolic syndrome or diabetes showed that the mean CIMT in patients with CAVI < 9 was significantly lower than that in patients with a CAVI > 9 (0.74 ± 0.10 mm and 0.84 ± 0.13 mm, respectively). Another study in 219 patients with diabetes demonstrated that the mean CIMT in patients with a CAVI < 8, 8–9, and > 9 increased

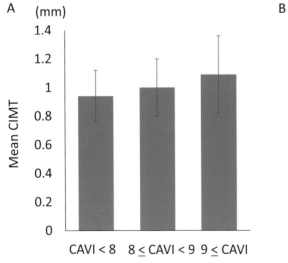
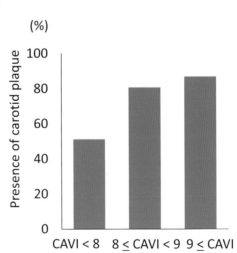

p = 0.001 by ANOVA

p < 0.001 by chi-square test

Fig. 1. Mean CIMT and the presence of carotid plaque according to CAVI.
(A). Mean CIMT. Data are presented as mean ± SD. (B). The proportion of patients with carotid plaque.
CAVI = cardio-ankle vascular index; CIMT = carotid intima media thickness.

Department of Cardiovascular Medicine, Okayama University Graduate School of Medicine, Dentistry and Pharmaceutical Sciences, 2-5-1 Shikata-cho, Kita-ku, Okayama city, Okayama 700-8558, Japan.

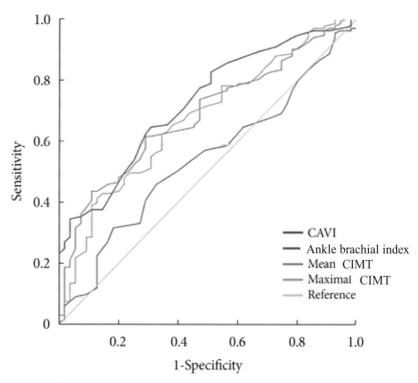

Fig. 2. Predicative ability of 10-year atherosclerotic cardiovascular disease risk.
The utility of the CAVI, ankle-brachial index, the mean CIMT, and the maximum CIMT for predicting the prevalence of atherosclerotic cardiovascular disease is shown.
CAVI = cardio-ankle vascular index; CIMT = carotid intima media thickness.
Adapted from ref.6

stepwise at 0.94 ± 0.18 mm, 1.00 ± 0.20 mm, and 1.09 ± 0.27 mm, respectively (Fig. 1A), and that the proportion of patients with a CAVI < 8, 8–9, and > 9 with carotid artery plaque also increased stepwise at 51.1%, 80.0%, and 86.8%, respectively (Fig. 1B)[6]. In this study, the CAVI value for predicting atherosclerotic cardiovascular disease was compared to that of CIMT. Both the CAVI and CIMT were shown to be independent predictors of atherosclerotic cardiovascular disease, while the area under the curve for predicting atherosclerotic cardiovascular disease was greater for the CAVI than for the mean CIMT (0.66 and 0.64, respectively). Thus, this study suggested that the CAVI may be a sensitive surrogate marker for the detection of subclinical atherosclerosis and for prediction of atherosclerotic cardiovascular disease in diabetic patients (Fig. 2)[6].

These findings indicate that the CAVI is closely associated with the CIMT. The CIMT is a useful modality for evaluating cardiovascular risk; however, serial measurement is not recommended to evaluate the success of a therapy, due to poor reproducibility. Moreover, the CAVI could be used to evaluate therapeutic efficacy. Therefore, the CAVI may be superior to the CIMT. The usefulness of a combination of the CAVI and CIMT for risk assessment and prediction of atherosclerotic cardiovascular disease should be investigated in a future study.

References

1) Umemura S, Arima H, Arima S, et al. The Japanese Society of Hypertension guidelines for the management of hypertension (JSH 2019), *Hypertens Res*, **2019**;42:1235-1481.
2) Williams B, Mancia G, Spiering W, et al. 2018 ESC/ESH guidelines for the management of arterial hypertension, *Eur Heart J*, **2018**;39:3021-3104.
3) Kadota K, Takamura N, Aoyagi K, et al. Availability of cardio-ankle vascular index (CAVI) as a screening tool for atherosclerosis, *Circ J*, **2008**;72:304-308.
4) Gomez-Sanchez L, Garcia-Ortiz L, Patino-Alonso MC, et al. The association between the Cardio-ankle Vascular Index and other parameters of vascular structure and function in Caucasian adults: MARK Study, *J Atheroscler Thromb*, **2015**;22:901-911.
5) Okura T, Watanabe S, Kurata M, et al. Relationship between cardio-ankle vascular index (CAVI) and carotid atherosclerosis in patients with essential hypertension, *Hypertens Res*, **2007**;30:335-340.
6) Park SY, Chin SO, Rhee SY, et al. Cardio-Ankle Vascular Index as a surrogate marker of early atherosclerotic cardiovascular disease in Koreans with type 2 diabetes mellitus, *Diabetes Metab J*, **2018**;42:285–295. https://doi.org/10.4093/dmj.2017.0080

Vasculitis and CAVI: Autoimmune diseases

Takashi Yamaguchi[1] and Kohji Shirai[2]

Significance of the measurement of arterial stiffness in autoimmune diseases and related vasculitis

Vasculitis includes autoimmune diseases, the causes of which remain unspecified. The diagnosis of vasculitis is made based on the concomitant presence of fever, rash, pain, elevation of inflammatory markers, and elevation of disease-specific markers. There are no established diagnostic criteria for each condition.

Meanwhile, it has been reported that atherosclerosis often occur in some of the diseases that cause vasculitis. However, given the absence of any accurate method for diagnosing vascular lesions, the presence of vasculitis remains unnoticed in many cases until the onset of an aneurysm or myocardial infarction. This paper covers Takayasu arteritis, systemic lupus erythematosus, rheumatoid arthritis, Kawasaki disease, and polymyalgia rheumatic as typical autoimmune vasculitis and presents the reports on arterial stiffness, including the cardio-ankle vascular index (CAVI) and describes the role that the CAVI can play in the management of these diseases in the future.

(1) Takayasu arteritis (TA)

TA is a disease that causes chronic inflammation of the carotid, subclavian, and renal arteries and mainly the aorta. It presents with symptoms of systemic inflammation, such as fever, malaise, and weight loss, in the early stage of the pathological condition, while aneurysms and stenosis occur with manifestations of local symptoms of the disorder as the angiopathy progresses. The diagnosis is made based on angiography or clinical findings indicative of systemic inflammation.

In 2006, Ng et al. reported high cfPWV (carotid-femoral pulse wave velocity) in patients with TA[1]. Subsequently, Masugata et al. reported a high CAVI in patients with TA[2] and improvement in inflammation following the administration of steroids and immunosuppressive drugs; a decrease in the CAVI was also seen[3]. In this report, there was no association between changes in the CAVI and blood pressure. The CAVI is an index that does not depend on blood pressure at the time of measurement, suggesting that it may be useful as a diagnostic and therapeutic marker for this disease.

(2) Systemic lupus erythematosus (SLE)

SLE causes various symptoms related to each organ of the body. In addition to fever, various symptoms occur in all the joints and the skin, along with symptoms related to dysfunction of the kidneys, lungs, and central nervous system. These manifestations can occur together or separately. Given the possibility that the main pathophysiology of this disease is vasculitis, measurement of arterial stiffness has been attempted as an index reflective of the diseases in large- and medium-sized arteries.

Shang et al. reported high ha(heart-carotid)PWV in patients with SLE[4], and Sacre et al. reported that cfPWV was high in SLE patients without coronary atherosclerosis risk[5], and that high systolic blood pressure was involved as a factor. Carlucci et al. reported a high CAVI in patients with SLE in 2018[6]. The CAVI, which is unaffected by the blood pressure at the time of measurement, can reflect the pathological condition of angiopathy more accurately. Moreover, elucidating that the vascular lesions are ubiquitous in each organ affected by SLE may change the understanding of these diseases. Furthermore, it is important to verify whether the CAVI is meaningful as an index of the effectiveness of various treatments.

(3) Rheumatoid arthritis (RA)

RA causes joint destruction due to polyarthritis, and the synovium of the joint is the main site of inflammation. Epidemiological studies have shown that cardiovascular events are more frequent in patients with RA. The pathological condition of RA is not associated with the classical cardiovascular risk factors such as diabetes and dyslipidemia and is therefore thought to cause angiopathy directly. However, given the absence of any appropriate method for diagnosing angiopathy, this mechanism has not been clarified so far. Studies have reported the usefulness of evaluating the arterial stiffness using PWV.

In 2006, Mäki-Petäjä et al. reported high PWV in patients with RA, and PWV decreased following the administration of antibodies against the tumor necrosis factor[7]. Subsequently, Cypiene et al. and Wong et al.[8, 9] found no correlation between PWV and blood pressure, which indicates reduced arterial stiffness in RA.

In the future, the pathological condition of angiopathy associated with RA is expected to be further clarified using

[1]Center of Diabetes, Endocrinology and Metabolism, Toho University Sakura Medical Center, 564-1 Shimoshizu, Sakura City, Chiba 285-8741, Japan.
[2]Director, Seijinkai Mihama Hospital, 1-1-5 Utase, Mihama-ku, Chiba-shi, Chiba 261-0013, Japan.

the CAVI. Consequently, it might be necessary to recognize RA as a pathological condition that affects not only the joints but also systemic blood vessels, and a treatment strategy might have to be formulated accordingly.

(4) Kawasaki disease (KD)

KD occurs in children and causes systemic vasculitis; its exact cause remains unknown. It is known to damage the medium vessels, such as coronary arteries, in addition to the iliac arteries, renal arteries, and mesenteric arteries. Some patients with KD may develop coronary aneurysms and stenosis in the later years, and the presence of coronary artery lesions affects the prognosis. Therefore, it is important to evaluate the vascular lesions appropriately, and studies on arterial stiffness are being conducted.

Iwazu et al. reported high PWV in patients with KD[10]. Cheung et al. reported that KD patients with coronary artery lesions have a higher cervical β value and ba(brachial-ankle)PWV than other patients with KD[11]. Vaujois et al. also reported a high β value in the KD group with coronary artery disease[12]. These reports suggest the potential usefulness of measuring arterial stiffness for the non-invasive assessment of the prognosis of this disease. In the future, cross-sectional surveys and follow-up surveys using the CAVI may be useful for selecting the treatment options for KD and predicting the prognosis.

(5) Polymyalgia rheumatica (PMR)

PMR is a systemic inflammatory disease that occurs mainly in the elderly, and its cause and pathophysiology remain unknown. The main site of inflammation in PMR is reportedly the synovial bursae of the joints. However, considering the reports about vasculitis in PMR, studies on vascular stiffness are being conducted.

Schillaci et al. reported high cfPWV in patients with PMR and improvement in inflammation following the administration of steroids, which also decreased the PWV[13]. The relationship between the PWV and blood pressure in PMR has not been reported, suggesting reduced aortic stiffness. Furthermore, there are reports of patients with PMR who developed fever of unknown origin with a

marked increase in the CAVI, which decreased rapidly with steroid therapy (Fig. 1). Given that there are few reports that have examined the pathological condition of angiopathy in PMR, the actual status is not completely clear. In the future, understanding the pathological condition of angiopathy in patients with PMR by measuring the CAVI may change the understanding about the disease.

(6) Other diseases

In addition to the diseases listed above, reduced arterial stiffness based on the measurement of PWV has been reported in Behcet's disease[14], granulomatosis with polyangiitis[15], psoriasis[16], familial Mediterranean fever[17], systemic sclerosis[18], and sarcoidosis[19]. The presence of vasculitis was indicated in the pathological conditions of all these diseases. However, there are few reports, and no studies using the CAVI have been conducted. Thus, further studies are necessary in the future.

The mechanism of impaired arterial stiffness in vasculitis is unknown. The hypothetical mechanisms include the expression of proinflammatory cytokines in the vascular smooth muscle cells, which are the primary pathophysiology of vasculitis, leading to smooth muscle cell contraction and remodeling of the arterial wall, including its interstitial components. The CAVI has been reported to be associated with acute phase reactants such as C-reactive protein, amyloid A, sialic acid, fibrinogen, and leukocytes[20, 21]. However, there are few reports about the mechanisms, and further studies are necessary.

References

1) Ng WF, et al.: Takayasu Arthritis: a cause of prolonged arterial stiffness. Rheumatology (Oxford). 2006; 45:741-745.

2) Masugata H, et al.: Detection of increased arterial stiffness in a patient with early stage of large vessel vasculitis by measuring cardio-ankle vascular index. Tohoku J. Exp. Med. 2009; 219:101-105.

3) Masugata H, et al.: Cardio-ankle vascular index for evaluating immunosuppressive therapy in a patient with aortitis syndrome. Tohoku J. Exp. Med. 2010; 222:77-81.

4) Shang Q, et al.: Increased arterial stiffness correlated with

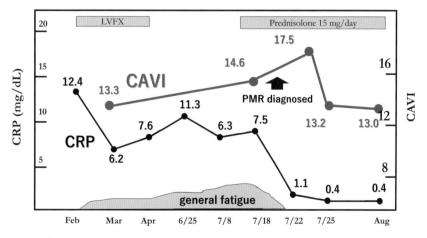

Fig. 1.   Course of C-reactive protein level and CAVI in patients with polymyalgia rheumatica treated with steroids.

disease activity in systemic lupus erythematosus. Lupus. 2008; 17:1096-1102.

5) Sacre K, et al.: Increased arterial stiffness in systemic lupus erythematosus (SLE) patients at low risk for cardiovascular diseases: a cross-sectional controlled study. PLoS One. 2014; 9: e94511.

6) Carlucci P, et al.: Neutrophil subsets and their gene signature associated with vascular inflammation and coronary atherosclerosis in lupus. JCI Insight. 2018; 3: e99276.

7) Mäki-Petäjä KM, et al.: Rheumatoid arthritis is associated with increased aortic pulse-wave velocity, which is reduced by anti-tumor necrosis factor-alpha therapy. Circulation. 2006; 114:1185-1192.

8) Cypiene A, et al.: Non-invasive assessment of arterial stiffness indices by applanation tonometry and pulse wave analysis in patients with rheumatoid arthritis treated with TNF-alpha blocker remicade (infliximab). Proc West Pharmacol Soc. 2007; 50:119-122.

9) Wong M, et al.: Infliximab improves vascular stiffness in patients with rheumatoid arthritis. Ann Rheum Dis. 2009; 68:1277-1284.

10) Iwazu Y, et al.: Pulse wave velocity in Kawasaki disease. Angiology. 2017; 68:189-195.

11) Cheung YF, et al.: Relationship between carotid intima-media thickness and arterial stiffness in children after Kawasaki disease. Arch Dis Child. 2007; 92:43-47.

12) Vaujois L, et al.: The biophysical properties of the aorta are altered following Kawasaki disease. J Am Soc Echocardiogr. 2013; 26:1388-1396.

13) Schillaci G, et al.: Aortic stiffness is increased in polymyalgia rheumatica and improves after steroid treatment. Ann Rheum Dis. 2012; 71:1151-1156.

14) Chang HK, et al.: Arterial stiffness in Behcet's disease: increased regional pulse wave velocity values. Ann Rheum Dis. 2006; 65:415-416.

15) Yildiz M, et al.: Arterial distensibility in Wegener's granulomatosis: a carotid-femoral pulse wave velocity study. Anadolu Kardiyol Derg. 2007; 7:281-285.

16) Gisondi P, et al.: Chronic plaque psoriasis is associated with increased arterial stiffness. Dermatology. 2009; 218:110-113.

17) Yildiz M, et al.: Assessment of aortic stiffness and ventricular functions in familial Mediterranean fever. Anadolu Kardiyol Derg. 2008; 8:395-396.

18) Cypiene A, et al.: The impact of systemic sclerosis on arterial wall stiffness parameters and endothelial function. Clin Rheumatol. 2008; 27:1517-1522.

19) Yildiz M.: Arterial distensibility in chronic inflammatory rheumatic disorders. Open Cardiovasc Med J. 2010; 4:83-88.

20) Wakabayashi I, et al.: Association of acute-phase reactants with arterial stiffness in patients with type 2 diabetes mellitus. Clin Chim Acta. 2006; 365:230-235.

21) Kotani K, et al.: The correlation between the cardio-ankle vascular index (CAVI) and serum amyloid A in asymptomatic Japanese subjects. Heart Vessels. 2012; 27:499-504.

Ophthalmologic diseases and CAVI

Tomoaki Shiba

Introduction

The arterial system is designed to receive the blood bolus from the left ventricle and distributing them as a steady flow through the peripheral capillaries. In older humans, the momentum of the ejected bolus is not absorbed by the large arteries, and thus those pulses extend down into the microcirculation[1]. For instance, the elasticity of large arteries should allow for smooth steady blood flow into the eye's small vessels, but it becomes pulsatile or intermittent with arterial stiffness.

The cardio-ankle vascular index (CAVI), an arterial stiffness parameter, was developed as a marker for arteriosclerosis of vessels from the aorta to the tibial artery[2,3]. A relationship between systemic arteriosclerosis and ocular diseases, such as retinal vein occlusion- and age-related macular degeneration (AMD), has been confirmed[4–6]. Thus, there is a clear overlap in relevant risk factors for cardiovascular, cerebrovascular and ocular vessel disease.

Laser speckle flowgraphy (LSFG), which is a quantitative and noninvasive method for determining the ocular blood flow[7,8], is based on the changes in the speckle pattern of laser light reflected from the eye fundus[9]. We defined blow out time as an index of pulsatile flow gentleness using LSFG. In this chapter, I will introduce novel findings about the relationship among 1) ocular pulsatile blood flow by LSFG, 2) AMD as a typical ocular vessel disease, and 3) CAVI from an ophthalmological viewpoint.

Ocular pulsatile blood flow in the optic nerve head and CAVI

LSFG measurements

LSFG depends on erythrocyte movements in the retina, the choroid, and the optic nerve head; the mean blur rate (MBR) is an indicator of ocular blood flow and a parameter of ocular blood flow velocity[10, 11]. MBR was measured using the LSFG-NAVI™ (Softcare Co., Fukuoka, Japan; Fig. 1), which was approved in 2008 as a medical apparatus by Japan's Pharmaceuticals and Medical Devices Agency and in 2016 by the U.S. Food and Drug Administration.

MBR variations show pulse-wave patterns synchronized with the cardiac cycle. We have focused on the relationship between subjects' systemic conditions and pulse waveform and reported that the blowout time (BOT; see below) in the optic nerve head area is associated with age, brachial-ankle pulse-wave velocity, abnormal carotid intima-media thickening (IMT)[12,13], and systemic vascular resistance[14].

The BOT can be explained as the proportion of time the wave maintains more than half of the mean between maximum and minimum MBR during a beat. A high BOT indicates that high blood flow for a long time during each heartbeat and serves to ensure that the peripheral tissue is supplied with sufficient blood, in short, the proportion of the heart cycle during which organs are well perfused by their capillaries. To evaluate the BOT in the optic nerve head area, a circle surrounding the optic nerve head (ONH) is typically drawn (Fig. 2). Then, 118 MBR images (frames) are recorded from the circle area within a 4-sec period tuned to the cardiac cycle. A gray-scale map of the still images is then built by averaging the MBR images (Fig. 2, upper panel). On the analysis screen, the pulse wave of changing MBR values corresponding to each cardiac cycle is obtained (Fig. 2, middle panel). These data are then normalized to one pulse (Fig. 2, lower panel) and analyzed[11-15]. The scheme for the BOT is shown in Fig. 3.

BOT values were determined by the following formula:

$$BOT = 100 \times W/F^{10-14}$$

W: Time over half of pulse height (half width)
F: Time for one heartbeat

Relationships between CAVI and BOT in the optic nerve head[16]

The purpose of our previous study was to determine whether there are significant correlations between the BOT in the capillary area of the optic nerve head, as shown by LSFG, and the CAVI in patients with a variety of disorders. We studied 130 men (ages 60.5 ± 10.9 yrs) who visited the Vascular Function Section of the Department of

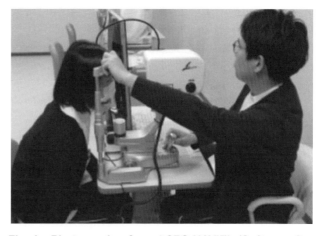

Fig. 1. Photograph of an LSFG-NAVI™ (Softcare Co., Fukuoka, Japan).

Department of Ophthalmology, International University of Health and Welfare Narita Hospital, 852 Hatakeda Narita City, Chiba 286-0124, Japan.

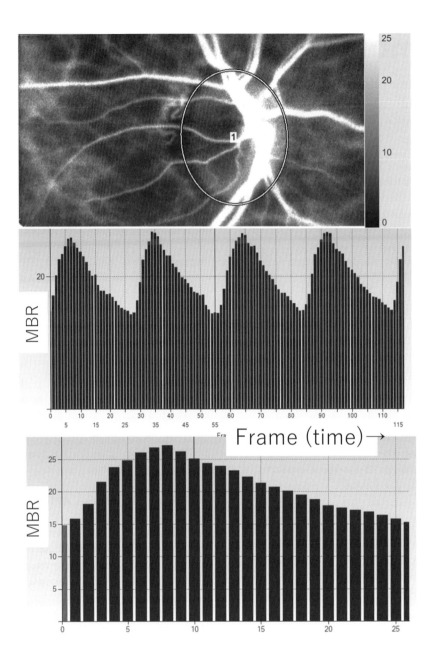

Fig. 2.   Method for analyzing the MBR and pulsatile waveform in the optic nerve head and choroid circulation using LSFG.

Upper panel: Gray-scale map of the total measurement area. The circle designates the area corresponding to the optic nerve head.

Middle panel: Pulsatile waves show changes in the mean blur rate, which is tuned to the cardiac cycle for 4 s. Total frame number: 118.

Lower panel: Single pulse normalization. The pulsatile waveform analysis is calculated on this screen.

Adapted from ref.14 【by permission from Springer Nature】

Cardiovascular Center of Toho University Sakura Medical Center, and we evaluated the BOT in the optic nerve head for each one. The CAVI, the echocardiographic E/e' ratio as measure of diastolic left ventricular function, and the mean IMT were also evaluated as systemic parameters. We performed a Pearson's correlation analysis and a multiple regression analysis to determine independent factors for BOT. Multiple regression analysis revealed that CAVI, heart rate, urinary albumin concentration, mean IMT, spherical refraction, body mass index, and pulse pressure were all factors contributing independently to the BOT (Table 1).

Our study observed that the BOT area in the optic nerve head decreases in parallel with a CAVI increase. In other words, when pulsations are not absorbed in large arteries, they send stronger pulsatile blood flow into the optic nerve head along CAVI's exacerbation (Fig. 4). Our study's findings also revealed that the systemic arterial function described by the CAVI is an important contributor to ocular microcirculation. Microcirculation in the optic nerve head as calculated by LSFG may allow detecting the conditions of systemic large arteries. We believe our findings may provide insight into the relationships between cardio/

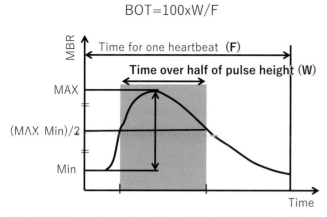

BOT=100xW/F

Fig. 3. Schematic explanation of the BOT obtained from pulsatile waveform analysis in the optic nerve head.

Table 1. Results of multiple regression analysis for factors independently contributing to BOT in the optic nerve head area (Referred from reference no. 15 [by permission from Springer Nature]).

Explanatory variables	β	p
Heart rate	0.32	<0.0001
CAVI	**-0.27**	**0.0002**
UAC	-0.17	0.005
Mean IMT	-0.19	0.007
Spherical refraction	-0.16	0.01
BMI	0.16	0.02
Pulse pressure	-0.15	0.03
HbA1c	-0.10	0.11
Hematocrit	0.07	0.31
E/e' ratio	-0.06	0.39
Cystatin C	-0.02	0.69

Objective variable: BOT, R=0.78, p <0.0001
CAVI, cardio ankle vascular index; UAC, urinary albumin concentration; BMI, body mass index; HbA1c, glycated hemoglobin A1c
The explanatory variables in the table showed a significant correlation with CAVI by Pearson's correlation analysis.

cerebrovascular and ocular diseases, such as normal-tension glaucoma and retinal and choroidal vascular diseases.

Evaluation of CAVI in patients with AMD[17]

AMD is a major cause of blindness and severe visual loss in older people in developed countries[18,19], while exudative choroidal neovascularization (CNV; Fig. 5) is responsible for severe visual loss[20]. Many documented risk factors for exudative AMD are also cardiovascular risks. We evaluated whether the CAVI independently contributes to exudative AMD compared with carotid atherosclerosis parameters obtained from high-resolution B-mode ultrasonography and other risk factors. Eighty-eight consecutive patients with exudative AMD who visited the Department of Ophthalmology of Toho University Sakura Medical Center were enrolled. We also evaluated the control group (40 age-matched men ≥65 years: AMD, 71.5 ± 7.7 y; Control, 70.8 ± 4.5 y, p= 0.61), and compared the parameters of both groups. The CAVI in the AMD group was significantly higher than in the control group, while the mean IMT and carotid plaque score in the AMD group did not differ significantly from those in the control group (Table 2). Logistic regression analysis identified a high CAVI value as

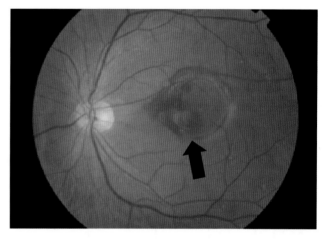

Fig. 5. Fundus photography of typical exudative AMD.
Black arrow shows retinal hemorrhage and retinal pigment epithelium detachment due to choroidal neovascularization.

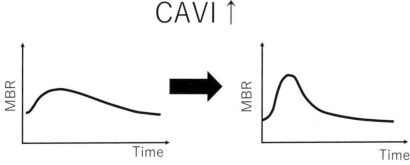

CAVI ↑

Large arteries absorb the pulsatile flow distributing a steady blood flow into the optic nerve head.

In higher CAVI, pulsations are not absorbed in the large arteries, and send a stronger pulsatile blood flow into the optic nerve head.

Fig. 4. Relationship between CAVI and the pulsatile wave of the optic nerve head microcirculation.

Table 2. Results of IMT, plaque score, and CAVI in the AMD and control groups (Referred from reference no. 17).

	AMD Group	Control Group	p
Mean IMT (mm)	0.92 ± 0.15	0.93 ± 0.14	0.74
Carotid plaque score	5.4 ± 3.6	6.4 ± 4.5	0.20
CAVI	**9.9 ± 1.1**	**9.3 ± 0.9**	**0.01**
Range	7.4 to 14.0	7.9 to 11.8	
Median	9.8	9.4	

Unpaired t-test.

Table 3. Results of logistic regression analysis for factors independently contributing to the AMD (Referred from reference no. 17).

Explanatory variables	odds ratio	95% CI	p
CAVI	**1.91**	**1.20-3.04**	**0.007**
Lipid-lowering drugs	0.29	0.10-0.86	0.03
ACE-I or ARB	0.42	0.18-1.02	0.06
Smoking yes = 1, no = 0	1.95	0.81-4.70	0.14
Triglycerides (mg/dl)	1.00	1.00-1.01	0.14
Pulse pressure (mmHg)	1.03	0.99-1.07	0.20
Total cholesterol (mg/dl)	1.00	0.98-1.03	0.85
LDL-C (mg/dl)	1.00	0.97-1.03	0.93

Objective variables: AMD group = 1, Control (without AMD) group = 0
CI, confidence interval; ACE-I, angiotensin-converting enzyme inhibitor; ARB, angiotensin II receptor blockers; LDL-C, low-density lipoprotein-cholesterol

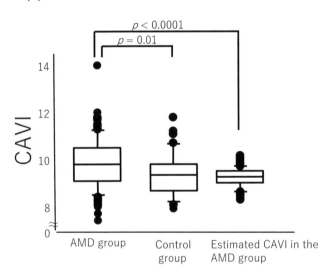

Fig. 6. Box plot representing CAVI values in the AMD and control groups, and the estimated CAVI values of the AMD group, as calculated by the formula: $5.43 + 0.053 \times age^{3)}$.

Statistical differences between groups are calculated using one-way ANOVA, followed by Dunnett's post hoc test.
Cited from ref.17

a risk factor and use of lipid-lowering drugs as a protective factor for AMD (Table 3). Fig. 6 shows the CAVI in the AMD and control groups and the estimated CAVI of the AMD group. Our study confirmed that the CAVI is more significantly associated with exudative AMD than carotid

atherosclerotic parameters. Indeed, the overall arterial stiffness represented by CAVI may correlate with the pathology of exudative AMD. Thus, CAVI may be a useful marker for risk and/or progression of exudative AMD.

Conclusion

From the above findings, large vessel function, as measured by CAVI, has a very important role in the pathology of ocular microvascular conditions and diseases. When large arteries are healthy, microcirculation can enable a smooth, steady blood flow into the eye's small vasculature.

As CAVI increases, pulsations are not absorbed in large arteries, resulting in stronger pulsatile blood flow and a BOT decrease in the eye. These changes in large arterial stiffness and ocular microcirculation may become an important trigger in the onset of AMD. Promoting the understanding of the CAVI and how large-vessel function impacts microvascular function will expand our knowledge on the pathology of ocular micro-vessel diseases.

References

1) O'Rourke MF, Hashimoto J. Mechanical factors in arterial aging: A clinical perspective. *J Am Coll Cardiol* 2007; **50**: 1–13.
2) Shirai K, Utino J, Otsuka K, Takata M. A novel blood pressure-independent arterial wall stiffness parameter; cardioankle vascular index (CAVI). *J Atheroscler Thromb* 2006; **13**: 101–107.
3) Shirai K, Hiruta N, Song M, et al. Cardio-ankle vascular index (CAVI) as a novel indicator of arterial stiffness: theory, evidence and perspectives. *J Atheroscler Thromb* 2011; **18**: 924-938.
4) Wong TY, Larsen EK, Klein R, et al. Cardiovascular risk factors for retinal vein occlusion and arteriolar emboli: the Atherosclerosis Risk in Communities & Cardiovascular Health studies. *Ophthalmology*, 2005;**112**: 540-547.
5) Klein R, Cruickshanks KJ, Myers CE, et al. The relationship of atherosclerosis to the 10-year cumulative incidence of age-related macular degeneration: the Beaver Dam studies. *Ophthalmology*, 2013;**120**: 1012-1019.
6) Olea JL, Tuñón J. Patients with neovascular age-related macular degeneration in Spain display a high cardiovascular risk. *Eur J Ophthalmol*, 2012; **22**: 404-411.
7) Tamaki Y, Araie M, Kawamoto E, et al. Non-contact, two-dimensional measurement of tissue circulation in choroid and optic nerve head using laser speckle phenomenon. *Exp Eye Res* 1995; **60**: 373–383.
8) Isono H, Kishi S, Kimura Y, et al. Observation of choroidal circulation using index of erythrocytic velocity. Arch Ophthalmol 2003; **121**: 225–231.
9) Fujii H. Visualisation of retinal blood flow by laser speckle flow-graphy. *Med Biol Eng Comput* 1994; **32**: 302–304.
10) Takahashi H, Sugiyama T, Tokushige H, et al. Comparison of CCD-equipped laser speckle flowgraphy with hydrogen gas clearance method in the measurement of optic nerve head microcirculation in rabbits. *Exp Eye Res*, 2013; **108**:10-15.
11) Sugiyama T. Basic technology and clinical applications of the updated model of laser speckle flowgraphy to ocular diseases. *Photonics*, 2014; **1**: 220-234. doi:10.3390/photonics1030220
12) Shiba T, Takahashi M, Hori Y, Maeno T. Pulse-wave analysis of optic nerve head circulation is significantly correlated with brachial–ankle pulse-wave velocity, carotid intima-media

thickness, and age. *Graefes Arch Clin Exp Ophthalmol* 2014; **250**: 1275–1281.

13) Rina M, Shiba T, Takahashi M, et al. Pulse waveform analysis of optic nerve head circulation for predicting carotid atherosclerotic changes. *Graefes Arch Clin Exp Ophthalmol* 2015; **253**: 2285–2291.

14) Shiba T, Takahashi M, Hashimoto R, et al. Pulse waveform analysis in the optic nerve head circulation reflects systemic vascular resistance obtained via a Swan-Ganz catheter. *Graefes Arch Clin Exp Ophthalmol* 2016; **254**: 1195 1200. https://doi.org/10.1007/s00417-016-3289-y

15) Shiba T, Takahashi M, Hori Y, Maeno T. Pulse-wave analysis of optic nerve head circulation is significantly correlated with brachial ankle pulse-wave velocity, carotid intima-media thickness, and age. *Graefes Arch Clin Exp Ophthalmol* 2012; **250**: 1275–1281. https://doi.org/10.1007/s00417-012-1952-5

16) Shiba T, Takahashi M, Matsumoto T, et al. Arterial stiffness shown by the cardio-ankle vascular index is an important contributor to optic nerve head microcirculation. *Graefes Arch Clin Exp Ophthalmol* 2017; **255**: 99–105.

17) Taniguchi H, Shiba T, Takahashi M, et al. Cardio-Ankle Vascular Index Elevation in Patients with Exudative Age-Related Macular Degeneration. *J Atheroscler Thromb* 2013; **20**: 903-910. https://doi.org/10.5551/jat.18796

18) Muñoz B, West SK, Rubin GS, et al. Causes of blindness and visual impairment in a population of older Americans: the Salisbury Eye Evaluation Study. *Arch Ophthalmol* 2000; **118**: 819-825.

19) Attebo K, Mitchell P, Smith W. Visual acuity and the causes of visual loss in Australia: The Blue Mountains Eye Study. *Ophthalmology* 1996; **103**: 357-364.

20) Ferris FL 3rd, Fine SL, Hyman L. Age-related macular degeneration and blindness due to neovascular maculopathy. *Arch Ophthalmol* 1984; **102**: 1640-1642.

Combined assessment of ToCA-MCI and CAVI cost-effectively predicts conversion from MCI to dementia in community dwelling elderly

Kuniaki Otsuka[1,2], Germaine Cornelissen[2], Larry A. Beaty[2] and Tsering Norboo[3]

Summary

Elderly people living at high altitude in Ladakh have higher arterial stiffness (estimated by CAVI, which interferes with effects of aging and gender), lower SpO_2, higher systolic blood pressure, and shorter functional reach, which were associated with declined overall cognitive function evaluated by the Kohs block design test and disordered time estimation of 10 and 60 seconds. In another small village in Hokkaido, the combination of a lower ToCA-MCI score (17 or lower) and increased arterial stiffness was a short-term (within 2 years) predictor of cognitive decline in older adults. A lower activity of daily living due to aging, as shown by walking slowly, a weaker handgrip power, or lower SpO_2 may be a long-term (5 years) predictor of cognitive decline in older adults. Hence, lifestyle interventions to improve arterial compliance and prevent frailty should be therapeutic targets to delay or prevent the onset of dementia in community-dwelling citizens.

Keywords: CAVI, ToCA-MCI, Mild Cognitive Impairment (MCI), risk of conversion from MCI to dementia, community-based comprehensive geriatric assessment, citizens in Himalayan valley, community dwelling Japanese elderly

Introduction

Pulse wave velocity (PWV) is a relatively simple, non-invasive and reproducible method to determine arterial stiffness[1, 2, 3, 4]. Arterial stiffness is a measure of brain vascular structure and function, and PWV is considered the gold standard for measuring stiffness of the elastic central arteries[5]. There is mounting evidence implicating arterial stiffness in the pathogenesis of impaired cognitive function and dementia in the elderly[6, 7, 8, 9].

It has been recognized that an elevated PWV is a significant predictor of subsequent cognitive decline that can predict progression from normal cognitive function to mild cognitive impairment, and to Alzheimer's disease (AD) and vascular dementia[10, 11, 12]. Several investigations showed that arterial stiffness may play a central role in association with large brain $A\beta$ deposition[13, 14, 15]. Rouch et al.[16] followed 375 patients with mild cognitive impairment (MCI) yearly for 4.5 years and found conversion from MCI to dementia in 28% patients. Based on their multi-factorial analysis, Rouch et al. argued for an association of higher PWV with a greater risk of conversion from MCI to dementia.

Caution is indicated, however, as follows. First, the AHA/ASA[17] states that arterial hypertension contributes to the development of cognitive impairment and dementia, attributable to both vascular dementia and AD, but PWV essentially depends on blood pressure (BP) at the time of measurement. The cardio-ankle vascular index (CAVI) reflects global arterial stiffness of the aorta to the ankle arteries independently of BP[2, 4]. CAVI can thus be expected to also predict the progression from MCI to dementia independently of BP. Second, the mini-mental state examination (MMSE) is not sufficiently sensitive to detect mild changes in cognitive status, particularly in high functioning populations. In most investigations, cognitive function was assessed based on the non-specific global cognition MMSE test[18]. Japanese studies reported an association between poor cognitive function (defined as < 24 points on the MMSE scale) and the middle tertile of baPWV ($>$ 1750 cm/s) after adjustment for age, education, and indices of atherosclerosis[19, 20]. Scuteri et al.[21] reported inverse cross-sectional relations between PWV, normalized for BP, and MMSE scores in elderly individuals with memory complaints. The Sydney Memory and Aging Study reported no association between PWV and memory and executive functions[22]. Another tool is thus needed as an alternative to the MMSE for evaluating cognitive function in the elderly. The Tokyo Cognitive Assessment of MCI

[1]Executive Medical Center, Totsuka Royal Clinic, Tokyo Women's Medical University, 1-104-19 Totsukamachi, Shinjuku-ku, Tokyo, 169-0071 Japan.
[2]Halberg Chronobiology Center, University of Minnesota, Minneapolis, Minnesota, USA.
[3]Ladakh Institute of Prevention, Founder and Secretary, Dambuchan, Ladakh.

(ToCA-MCI) has been developed and widely used for the early detection of MCI in Japanese community-dwelling elderly citizens[23, 24, 25].

Herein, we propose the combined assessment of CAVI and ToCA-MCI for the early detection of MCI and the risk of conversion from MCI to dementia in elderly Japanese citizens. We examine (1) how CAVI is associated with cognitive function in Ladakhi citizens living in the Himalayan valley; and (2) how ToCA-MCI is able to predict better than the MMSE the conversion from MCI to dementia in elderly Japanese citizens followed-up for 5 years.

All data were analyzed with the Statistical Software for Windows (StatFlex Ver.5.0, Artec, Osaka, http://www.statflex.net). Student's t-tests and one-way analyses of variance (ANOVA) served for the comparison of two or more groups. A P-value below 0.05 was considered to indicate statistical significance.

Elevated CAVI is associated with cognitive decline in Ladakhi citizens living at high altitude

A community-based comprehensive geriatric assessment (CGA) was performed to assess the contribution of arterial stiffness to cognitive decline in two villages. In the first village, we have conducted a chronoecological health-watch in Ladakh[26], one of the most remote regions of India, with the Karakoram to the northwest, the Himalayas in the southwest, and the Trans Himalayas at its core. It was virtually unknown to the West until the 1970s, and it still has limited contacts with the outside world today. The economy is based on subsistence farmers who grow mainly barley but also legumes. Whereas physiological adjustment to high altitude has been studied in resident populations of the Andes, Tibet, Nepal, North America, and Europe, much less is known about high-altitude natives in India. Individuals living permanently at high altitude must contend with chronic hypobaric hypoxia. Several compensatory mechanisms have evolved to enable them to live and work in this inhospitable environment. Herein, we examine particularly how CAVI is associated with cognitive function in older Ladakhi individuals.

CAVI was measured twice on both the right and left sides, using a VaSera instrument (Fukuda Denshi, Tokyo) in 1,858 resting Ladakhi citizens living in 119 villages at altitudes between 2,200 to 4,590 m (1,081 women and 777 men, aged from 13 to 92 years, average 51.4 years). It was also measured in 25,211 Japanese (13,366 men and 11,845 women, aged from 16 to 98 years, average 48.0 years). The

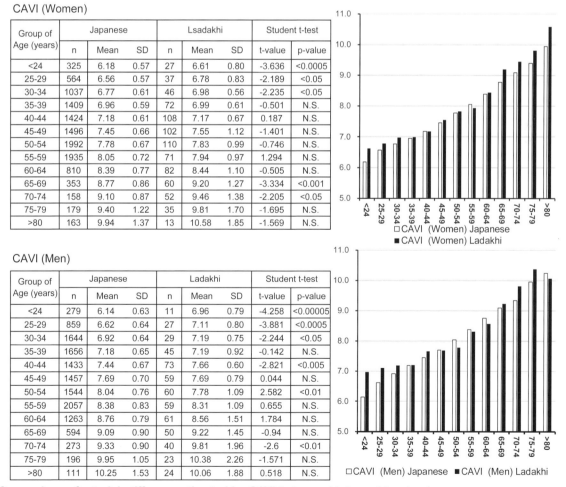

CAVI (Women)

Group of Age (years)	Japanese			Lsadakhi			Student t-test	
	n	Mean	SD	n	Mean	SD	t-value	p-value
<24	325	6.18	0.57	27	6.61	0.80	-3.636	<0.0005
25-29	564	6.56	0.57	37	6.78	0.83	-2.189	<0.05
30-34	1037	6.77	0.61	46	6.98	0.56	-2.235	<0.05
35-39	1409	6.96	0.59	72	6.99	0.61	-0.501	N.S.
40-44	1424	7.18	0.61	108	7.17	0.67	0.187	N.S.
45-49	1496	7.45	0.66	102	7.55	1.12	-1.401	N.S.
50-54	1992	7.78	0.67	110	7.83	0.99	-0.746	N.S.
55-59	1935	8.05	0.72	71	7.94	0.97	1.294	N.S.
60-64	810	8.39	0.77	82	8.44	1.10	-0.505	N.S.
65-69	353	8.77	0.86	60	9.20	1.27	-3.334	<0.001
70-74	158	9.10	0.87	52	9.46	1.38	-2.205	<0.05
75-79	179	9.40	1.22	35	9.81	1.70	-1.695	N.S.
>80	163	9.94	1.37	13	10.58	1.85	-1.569	N.S.

☐ CAVI (Women) Japanese
■ CAVI (Women) Ladakhi

CAVI (Men)

Group of Age (years)	Japanese			Ladakhi			Student t-test	
	n	Mean	SD	n	Mean	SD	t-value	p-value
<24	279	6.14	0.63	11	6.96	0.79	-4.258	<0.00005
25-29	859	6.62	0.64	27	7.11	0.80	-3.881	<0.0005
30-34	1644	6.92	0.64	29	7.19	0.75	-2.244	<0.05
35-39	1656	7.18	0.65	45	7.19	0.92	-0.142	N.S.
40-44	1433	7.44	0.67	73	7.66	0.60	-2.821	<0.005
45-49	1457	7.69	0.70	59	7.69	0.79	0.044	N.S.
50-54	1544	8.04	0.76	60	7.78	1.09	2.582	<0.01
55-59	2057	8.38	0.83	59	8.31	1.09	0.655	N.S.
60-64	1263	8.76	0.79	61	8.56	1.51	1.784	N.S.
65-69	594	9.09	0.90	50	9.22	1.45	-0.94	N.S.
70-74	273	9.33	0.90	40	9.81	1.96	-2.6	<0.01
75-79	196	9.95	1.05	23	10.38	2.26	-1.571	N.S.
>80	111	10.25	1.53	24	10.06	1.88	0.518	N.S.

☐ CAVI (Men) Japanese ■ CAVI (Men) Ladakhi

Fig. 1. Comparison of arterial stiffness estimated by CAVI between high- and low-landers.
Average of 4 CAVI measurements increased with age in both Ladakhi and Japanese people. Highlanders showed higher CAVI than lowlanders in both women and men.

average and maximal values from the four measurements (taken twice on both the right and left sides) were defined as CAVI-mean and CAVI-max, respectively. Overall cognitive function was evaluated by means of the Kohs block design test[27]. It was conducted together with three other tests. One test is the Up & Go test, which measures the time to stand up from a chair, walk a distance of 3 meters, turn, walk back to the chair, and sit down again. Functional Reach is another test measuring the maximal distance a citizen can reach forward beyond arm's length while maintaining a fixed base of support in the standing position. The Button test measures manual dexterity by using a panel with combinations of 10 hooks (hook-on), 10 big buttons (button-on-and-off), and 5 small buttons (button-on-and-off). The total manual dexterity time (in seconds), defined as the button score (Button), was calculated by adding the average times for one hook-on and

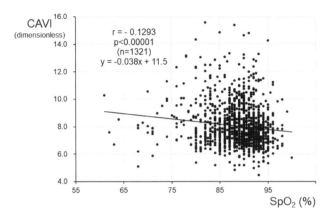

Fig. 2. Relation between CAVI and SpO$_2$ in Ladakhi citizens.

Some Ladakhi residents had low SpO$_2$ readings; CAVI correlated statistically significantly with SpO$_2$; on average, a lower SpO$_2$ was associated with a higher CAVI.

Table 1. Higher arterial stiffness, estimated by CAVI, is associated with lower cognitive function, gauged by the Kohs block design test.

Ladakh Women		Group I			Group II			Group III			Group IV	
	n	Mean	SD	n	Mean	SD	n	Mean	SD	n	Mean	SD
Age (years)	14	65.21	8.14	18	66.06	7.56	8	68.38	6.50	11	70.27	4.84
BMI	14	21.76	3.55	18	22.65	2.91	8	24.58	4.16	11	24.42	4.68
CAVI	14	7.43	0.39	18	8.57 **	0.27	8	9.34 **	0.21	11	10.73 **	0.54
ABI	14	1.05	0.06	18	1.00	0.17	8	1.07	0.10	10	1.08	0.07
Kohs block design test	14	6.79	6.35	18	4.72	3.58	8	7.00	6.21	11	5.27	4.17
Time Estimation 10-s (sec)	13	7.87	1.99	16	8.52	2.18	8	7.37	1.82	10	7.77	2.05
Time Estimation 60-s (sec)	13	38.96	8.06	16	40.29	9.01	8	37.94	11.16	10	41.42	12.57
Up & Go (sec)	13	16.05	6.39	18	14.56	2.69	8	16.77	2.77	10	13.12	1.12
Functional Reach (cm)	12	21.67	8.84	18	19.89	8.74	8	18.88	11.38	10	18.90	9.61
Button test	14	18.74	5.08	18	20.44	6.49	8	19.45	3.56	11	20.00	5.22
SpO$_2$ (%)	14	87.00	3.35	18	87.33	4.07	8	87.63	3.62	10	88.70	3.27
Respiration Rate (breaths/min)	14	19.86	3.96	18	19.67	4.96	8	19.25	3.37	10	19.60	2.95
sitting Systolic BP (mm Hg)	14	122.21	11.64	18	140.33 **	20.12	8	137.63	17.03	11	158.91 **	22.63
sitting Diastolic BP (mm Hg)	14	83.93	12.85	18	83.72	9.78	8	91.88	12.41	11	89.27	15.64
sitting Heart Rate (bpm)	14	75.00	12.90	18	78.72	17.10	8	82.38	12.70	11	75.09	19.31

Ladakh Men		Group I			Group II			Group III			Group IV	
	n	Mean	SD	n	Mean	SD	n	Mean	SD	n	Mean	SD
Age (years)	16	62.06	5.59	16	69.06 **	6.30	6	72.17 *	7.99	12	69.00 **	5.53
BMI	16	23.06	4.10	16	23.06	4.78	6	25.85 *	1.29	12	23.81	4.08
CAVI	16	7.18	0.67	16	8.45 **	0.25	6	9.41 **	0.34	12	11.28 **	1.45
ABI	16	1.08	0.14	16	1.05	0.28	6	1.12	0.05	11	1.10	0.12
Kohs block design test	16	22.81	12.92	16	13.69 *	7.04	6	18.67	13.47	12	13.25 *	5.48
Time Estimation 10-s (sec)	16	6.21	1.80	15	7.47	2.80	5	9.59 **	0.68	12	5.74	1.37
Time Estimation 60-s (sec)	16	41.03	13.55	15	38.20	12.06	5	42.03	9.19	12	29.00 **	4.39
Up & Go (sec)	15	12.16	3.23	15	13.16	2.64	6	13.19	2.88	11	12.74	1.50
Functional Reach (cm)	14	32.14	8.11	14	24.83 *	8.80	6	26.17	8.91	11	25.27 *	7.71
Button test	15	11.73	2.68	16	12.51	3.17	6	13.67	1.62	12	15.60	5.85
SpO$_2$ (%)	16	87.81	3.35	15	86.27	7.36	5	89.40	2.41	12	91.00 **	2.41
Respiration Rate (breaths/min)	16	20.25	2.91	16	22.00	5.56	6	19.67	2.34	12	21.17	5.22
sitting Systolic BP (mm Hg)	16	124.31	14.06	16	136.69 *	15.52	6	155.67 **	11.47	12	168.17 **	23.62
sitting Diastolic BP (mm Hg)	16	86.94	14.48	16	87.75	9.45	6	92.83	5.56	12	93.92	16.82
sitting Heart Rate (bpm)	16	75.75	16.00	16	75.81	18.54	6	71.83	13.75	12	72.33	10.80

*P < 0.05; **P < 0.01: Group II, Group III or Group IV vs. Group I
P-values from Student t-test; SD = standard deviation

one big or small button-on-and-off.

CAVI values increased with age in both Ladakhi and Japanese people. As compared to Japanese living at low altitude, both highland men and women had higher CAVI values, Fig. 1. In Ladakhi people, CAVI regressed negatively with respect to SpO$_2$ (p<0.00001), Fig. 2. Elderly Ladakhi men and women with higher CAVI measures had a higher systolic BP (p<0.01), Table 1. A stronger correlation with systolic BP is seen for baPWV than for CAVI, two surrogate measures of arterial stiffness; baPWV measurements showed a steeper positive slope as a function of systolic BP than CAVI measurements in Ladakh, located at high altitude under environmental conditions of chronic hypobaric hypoxia, Fig. 3.

As overall cognitive function, the Kohs block design test was applied together with an assessment of time estimation and activity of daily living. Elderly residents with higher CAVI measurements had a poorer cognitive function estimated by the Kohs block design test (p=0.00006), Fig. 4; a lower time estimation of 60 seconds and a shorter functional reach were found in elderly men with higher CAVI measurements (p<0.01), Table 1.

In conclusion, elderly people living at high altitude were at a higher risk of cardiovascular disease. Although adverse outcomes have not yet been recorded in follow-up studies, observations herein suggest that higher arterial stiffness, estimated by CAVI, differs between men and women and changes as a function of age (Fig. 1), and depends on SpO$_2$ (Fig. 2) and systolic BP (Table 1 and Fig. 3). It is associated with a shorter functional reach (Table 1), declined overall cognitive function evaluated by the Kohs block design test, and lower time estimation of 10 and 60 seconds. Studies are thus needed to longitudinally follow-up communities to investigate how neurocardiological function affects aging and longevity. Our goal is to examine whether CAVI can cost-effectively predict progression to senile dementia of elderly residents, and whether the combined use of ToCA-MCI may help.

Combined assessment of ToCA-MCI and PWV predicts conversion from MCI to senile dementia in Uraus, Hokkaido, Japan

A chronoecological health watch was performed in another village to assess the contribution of arterial stiffness

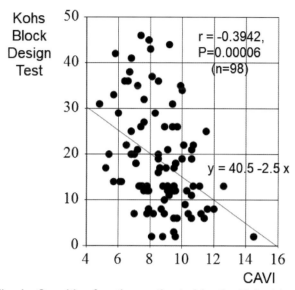

Fig. 4. Cognitive function, estimated by the Kohs block design test depends on CAVI.

The Kohs block design test was used to assess overall cognitive function in 98 Ladakh residents older than 60 years, living at an altitude of 3,300 to 4,600 m. Residents with higher CAVI measurements had a statistically significantly poorer cognitive function.

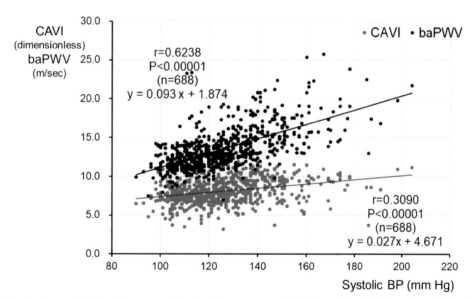

Fig. 3.   Relation between arterial stiffness, estimated by means of CAVI and baPWV, and systolic blood pressure in Ladakhi citizens.

The positive slope of the regression line of baPWV versus systolic BP is steeper than that of CAVI. It also confirms that CAVI, reflecting global arterial stiffness of the aorta to the ankle arteries, is less dependent on blood pressure in highland residents living under environmental conditions of hypobaric hypoxia at high altitude.

to cognitive decline. Community-based CGA started in 2000 in Uraus, Hokkaido, Japan, that has a population of 937 women and 865 men. Uraus has a full-fledged aged population of 37%. The goal of this investigation was to determine how effectively the wellbeing of elderly citizens can be supported with a small investment. Hemodynamics, including BP, ankle brachial index (ABI), and baPWV were measured in 2004, 2005, and 2010; maxima were analyzed.

The community-based CGA study for Mild Cognitive Impairment (MCI) started in 2015. The Tokyo Cognitive Assessment for Mild Cognitive Impairment (ToCA-MCI) was administered in addition to the MMSE, the Revise version of Hasegawa's Dementia Scale (HDS-R), and the Clock Drawing Test (CDT). Since March 2015, we followed-up for 5 years 95 citizens, who were 64 to 95 years of age at start. Originally, 99 elderly entered the study, but 4 of them were excluded because 3 already suffered from senile dementia and another had severe hearing impairment. Based on the scoring of the ToCA-MCI, using cut-off points of 17/18 and 24/25, the 95 elderly citizens were classified into 3 groups. Group A consisted of 27 citizens (64-88 years, average 75.2 ± 6.0 years, 19 women) with a ToCA-MCI score of 25 or higher. Group B consisted of 38 citizens (68-93 years, average 79.2 ± 5.5 years, 27 women) with a ToCA-MCI score between 18 and 24. Group C consisted of 30 citizens (65-95 years, average 79.6 ± 6.2 years, 22 women) with a ToCA-MCI score of 17 or lower. At the 2-year and 5-year follow-ups, the Kaplan-Meier method tested whether the ToCA-MCI score could predict progression to senile dementia. Results are depicted in Fig. 5.

At the 2-year follow-up (lower left quadrant delineated by the dotted lines in Fig. 5), the frequency of occurrence of dementia was statistically significantly higher in Group C as compared to both Groups B and A. As compared to citizens in Group B, elderly in Group C had a lower score and recalled fewer words of the story regeneration on the short-term memory topic: 1.2 ± 1.8 vs. 3.5 ± 2.3 (P < 0.0001), and 2.7 ± 2.3 vs. 5.8 ± 3.1 words (P < 0.0001), respectively. No statistically significant difference was found between them for the Mini-Mental State Examination (MMSE) recall item: 2.10 ± 0.96 vs. 2.00 ± 1.03 (P = 0.6841), suggesting that it was the short-term memory test of long sentences (25 words) that enabled the prediction of progression to dementia. (SDAT: senile dementia of the Alzheimer type, Table 2).

In Group C, the 7 citizens who progressed to dementia were older (84.7 ± 6.7 vs. 78.1 ± 5.2 years, P = 0.0465), had a quicker pulse (83.4 ± 4.8 vs. 72.9 ± 10.0 bpm, P = 0.0012), and a higher pulse wave velocity (PWV) (2367.6 ± 224.1 vs. 1937.1 ± 383.5 cm/s, P = 0.0021) as compared to the other 23 citizens of Group C who maintained cognitive performance, Table 2. As reported previously[9], the combined assessment of ToCA-MCI and PWV is thus useful for the early detection of amnestic MCI in elderly Japanese. These findings, observed after 2-year follow-up, prompted the village's mayor to make available a medical device to measure PWV at the community health center, where citizens can have their PWV measured any time with the help of public health nurses. The 7 citizens who

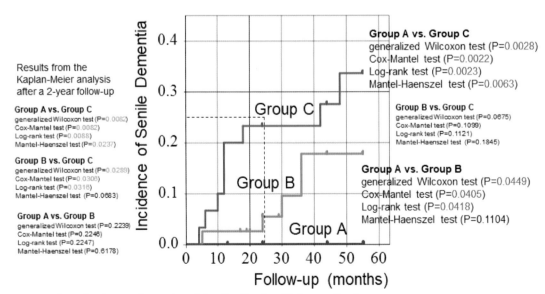

Fig. 5. Incidence of senile dementia analyzed by the Kaplan-Meier method.

After 2-year follow-up (lower left quadrant delineated by the dotted lines), the frequency of occurrence of dementia was statistically significantly higher in Group C as compared to both Groups B and A (left). As compared to citizens in Group B, elderly in Group C had a lower score and recalled fewer words of the story regeneration on the short-term memory topic: 1.2 ± 1.8 vs. 3.5 ± 2.3 (P < 0.0001), and 2.7 ± 2.3 vs. 5.8 ± 3.1 words (P < 0.0001), respectively.

After 5-year follow-up, the frequency of occurrence of dementia was statistically significantly higher in Groups C and B as compared to Group A (right). The occurrence of dementia was statistically significantly higher in Group C (30 citizens; ToCA-MCI score ≤ 17) as compared to Group A (27 citizens; ToCA-MCI score ≥ 25) by generalized Wilcoxon test (P = 0.0028), Cox-Mantel test (P = 0.0022), Log-rank test (P = 0.0023), and Mantel-Haenszel test (P = 0.00634). It was also statistically significantly higher in Group B (38 citizens; ToCA-MCI score between 18 and 24) as compared to Group A by generalized Wilcoxon test (P = 0.0449), Cox-Mantel test (P = 0.0405) and Log-rank test (P = 0.0418), but not by Mantel-Haenszel test (P = 0.1104).

Table 2. Comparison of neurobehavioral function in Group C elderly between the 7 who progressed to dementia and the 23 who maintained cognitive performance: 2-year follow-up.

	Maintained Cognitive Performance (n = 23)		Progressed to SDAT (n = 7)		t-test with Welch's correction	
	Mean	SD	Mean	SD	t-value	p-value
Age (years)	78.1	5.2	84.7	6.7	− 2.403	0.0465
Gender (F; 0, M; 1)	0.26	0.45	0.29	0.49	− 0.120	0.9086
Height (cm)	147.7	7.0	146.7	9.6	0.253	0.8073
Weight (kg)	52.7	7.2	49.2	9.0	0.951	0.3822
Body mass index (kg/m²)	24.1	2.6	22.7	2.1	1.482	0.1647
Systolic BP (mm Hg)	14.75	13.1	145.9	17.4	0.228	0.8271
Diastolic BP (mm Hg)	84.0	12.7	75.0	9.4	2.025	0.0675
Pulse (beats per minute)	72.9	10.0	83.4	4.8	− 3.817	0.0012
baPWV (cm/sec)	1937.1	383.5	2367.6	224.1	− 3.696	0.0021
ABI	1.08	0.06	1.07	0.08	0.313	0.7771
SpO₂ (%)	97.0	1.0	98.1	1.1	− 2.430	0.0402
Hand grip power (kg)	20.9	6.1	15.6	3.2	2.975	0.0075
Walking speed (m/s)	1.482	0.453	1.123	0.257	2.655	0.0168
Clinalcal Dementia Rating Scale (range 0-3)	0.15	0.24	0.14	0.24	0.089	0.9333
MMSE (range 0-30)	25.4	2.4	24.7	5.6	0.334	0.7621
Dalayed Recall of MMSE (range 0-3)	2.3	0.8	1.4	1.1	1.897	0.0947
Clock Drawing Test (range 0-5)	3.7	1.3	4.0	1.4	− 0.436	0.6771
ToCA-MCI (range 0-30)	14.3	3.2	14.1	2.9	0.093	0.9280
ToCA-MCI sub-items 1. short-term memory test of long sentences (25 words) (range 0-7)	1.13	1.52	1.43	2.51	− 0.298	0.7798
2. Word Crossing out test (range 0-2)	0.26	0.69	0.29	0.76	− 0.078	0.9406
3. Figure Reproducing test (range 0-1)	0.57	0.51	0.71	0.49	− 0.701	0.5050
4. Clock Drawing Test (range 0-3)	1.43	1.27	1.86	1.21	− 0.796	0.4522
5. Block design test (range 0-1)	0.13	0.34	0.00	0.00	1.817	0.0829
6. Number Repeating test (range 0-2)	0.78	0.85	0.86	0.38	− 0.327	0.7491
7. Counting backward test from 100 by 7s (range 0-3)	1.35	1.11	2.00	1.00	− 1.471	0.1901
8. Inhibitory control (Go/No-Go) test (range 0-3)	1.26	1.05	0.71	1.25	1.047	0.3463
9. Words recall test (10 or more specific words) (range 0-3)	1.96	0.71	1.00	0.58	3.634	0.0034
10. Orientation (range 0-1)	4.39	0.99	4.43	0.53	− 0.129	0.8993
11. recalled words of the story regeneration (range 0-25)	2.74	2.05	2.43	3.21	0.242	0.8227
Education level (range 0-1)	0.78	0.42	0.86	0.38	− 0.444	0.6805

SDAT: senile dementia of the Alzheimer type

progressed to dementia had a weaker grip strength (15.6 ± 3.2 vs. 20.9 ± 6.1 kg, P = 0.0075) and walked more slowly (1.123 ± 0.257 vs. 1.482 ± 0.453 m/s, P = 0.0168) than the other 23 elderly of group C, Table 2. These results prompted the village health nurses to start an education program at the health center, where they provided guidance to increase muscular strength, and nutritional advice. Small trials such as this one may help yield effective outcomes by decreasing morbidity of dementia[25].

At 5-year follow-up, the occurrence of dementia increased in Group B citizens, Fig. 5. The frequency of occurrence of dementia no longer differed between Groups B and C. It was statistically significantly higher in both Groups C and B than in Group A. As compared to the 29 citizens of Group B who maintained cognitive performance, the 5 citizens who progressed to dementia had a lower SpO₂

(96.6 ± 1.5 vs. 97.7 ± 0.9 &, P = 0.0350), a weaker hand grip power (17.9 ± 4.4 vs. 23.3 ± 6.0 kg, P = 0.0606), and a slower walking speed (1.11 ± 0.40 vs. 1.49 ± 0.31 m/sec, P = 0.0220). Their pulse wave velocity (PWV) did not differ (1829.0 ± 631.3 vs. 1861.3 ± 372.9 cm/s, P = 0.8729), Table 3. The combined assessment of ToCA-MCI and PWV was no longer useful to detect progression to senile dementia in elderly Japanese at 5-year follow-up.

In conclusion, our observations herein indicate that a lower ToCA-MCI score (17 or lower) combined with an elevated arterial stiffness may be a short-term (within 2 years) predictor of the conversion from MCI to dementia. Moreover, a reduced activity of daily living by aging, as shown by walking slowly, weaker hand grip power, or lower SpO₂ may be a long-term (within 5 years) predictor of cognitive decline in the elderly.

Table 3. Comparison of neurobehavioral function in Group B elderly between the 5 who progressed to dementia and the 29 who maintained cognitive performance: 5-year follow-up.

	Maintained Cognitive Performance (n = 29)		Progressed to SDAT (n = 5)		Student t-test	
	Mean	SD	Mean	SD	t-value	p-value
Age (years)	78.8	5.5	80.4	7.5	− 0.945	0.3515
Gender (F; 0, M; 1)	0.31	0.47	0.20	0.45	0.487	0.6296
Height (cm)	151.7	8.1	148.1	5.3	0.956	0.3465
Weight (kg)	54.3	9.0	54.2	12.7	0.036	0.9719
Body mass index (kg/m^2)	23.6	2.8	24.7	5.5	− 0.673	0.5055
Systolic BP (mm Hg)	147.7	21.9	143.8	22.6	0.369	0.7148
Diastolic BP (mm Hg)	76.9	10.9	69.6	17.3	1.269	0.2136
Pulse (beats per minute)	72.8	13.1	73.6	8.2	− 0.128	0.8990
baPWV (cm/sec)	1861.3	372.9	1829.0	631.3	0.161	0.8729
ABI	1.1	0.1	1.1	0.2	0.819	0.4188
SpO$_2$ (%)	97.7	0.9	96.6	1.5	2.202	0.0350
Hand grip power (kg)	23.3	6.0	17.9	4.4	1.945	0.0606
Walking speed (m/s)	1.49	0.31	1.11	0.40	2.407	0.0220
Clinalcal Dementia Rating Scale (range 0-3)	0.0	0.1	0.0	0.0	0.410	0.6846
MMSE (range 0-30)	27.5	1.8	27.2	1.6	0.385	0.7025
Dalayed Recall of MMSE (range 0-3)	2.0	1.1	2.0	1.0	0.000	1.0000
Clock Drawing Test (range 0-5)	4.5	0.7	4.6	0.9	− 0.338	0.7377
ToCA-MCI (range 0-30)	21.6	2.3	21.8	2.3	− 0.227	0.8223
1. short-term memory test of long sentences (25 words) (range 0-7)	3.4	2.3	3.6	2.9	− 0.191	0.8497
2. Word Crossing out test (range 0-2)	0.8	1.0	1.6	0.9	− 1.722	0.0947
3. Figure Reproducing test (range 0-1)	0.7	0.5	0.8	0.5	− 0.345	0.7322
4. Clock Drawing Test (range 0-3)	2.4	0.9	2.6	0.9	− 0.442	0.6616
5. Block design test (range 0-1)	0.2	0.4	0.0	0.0	1.224	0.2300
6. Number Repeating test (range 0-2)	1.3	0.8	1.6	0.9	− 0.869	0.3914
ToCA-MCI sub-items 7. Counting backward test from 100 by 7s (range 0-3)	2.5	0.8	2.4	0.6	0.319	0.7518
8. Inhibitory control (Go/No-Go) test (range 0-3)	2.7	0.6	2.2	1.3	1.277	0.2110
9. Words recall test (10 or more specific words) (range 0-3)	2.1	0.6	2.4	0.6	− 0.938	0.3552
10. Orientation (range 0-1)	5.0	0.7	4.0	0.7	3.122	0.0038
11. recalled words of the story regeneration (range 0-25)	5.8	3.2	5.2	3.6	0.404	0.6887
Education level (range 0-1)	0.7	0.5	0.6	0.6	0.385	0.7029

Because four citizens moved out of town during the 5-year follow-up, Group B only included 34 citizens in this analysis.
SDAT: senile dementia of the Alzheimer type

Discussion

Because of a rapid global increase in population size and life expectancy, the number of people with dementia is estimated to almost double every 20 years, and to reach 65.7 million by 2030 and 115.4 million by 2050[28]. Prevention of dementia is a major public health challenge. Identification of modifiable risk factors is critically important, but it is complex and differs depending on when during the lifespan risk factors are assessed. Many studies showed a positive correlation between PWV and cognitive impairment, but only few explored factors potentially predicting the conversion from MCI to dementia. Hanon et al.[29] showed that higher PWV was associated with poorer cognitive function, and that for a 2 m/s increment in PWV, the adjusted odds ratio (95% CI) was 1.73 (1.27 - 2.47) for

Alzheimer's disease. Several mechanisms have been discussed, and it was noted that arterial stiffness may favor an increase in central pulse pressure, which may influence arterial remodeling at the site of the extracranial and intracranial arteries. Cognitive impairment should be involved with small-vessel diseases, which are associated with small infarcts (lacunae), white matter lesions, and cortical brain atrophy. Alzheimer's disease is also associated with lesions in the cerebral micro-vessels (cerebral amyloid angiopathy, microvascular degeneration affecting the cerebral endothelium and smooth muscle cells, basal lamina alterations, luminal narrowing, hyalinosis, and fibrosis)[30]. Rouch et al.[16] reported very important findings, as follows. In a cohort of elderly subjects with memory complaints attending a memory clinic, 404 consecutive patients with a diagnosis of MCI according to Petersen criteria[31] were selected and followed-up for 6 years. Higher pulse wave velocity was associated with greater risk of conversion to dementia (hazard ratio associated with 1-SD increase in PWV: 1.33; 95% CI: 1.04–1.71; $P = 0.02$), independently of age, sex, educational level, systolic BP, cardiovascular diseases, body mass index, calcium channel blockers intake, Mini–Mental State Examination at start, and apoE ε4 status. It has been shown that structural parameters (intima-media thickness, carotid plaques, and carotid artery diameter) did not predict conversion to dementia, and that functional parameter (arterial stiffness estimated by PWV) should be a therapeutic target to delay or prevent the onset of dementia.

In a small cohort study in Hokkaido county, we also observed that an exacerbating factor related to the conversion from MCI to dementia within 2 years was a higher PWV among cognitive impaired citizens with a ToCA-MCI score below 18 (Table 2). Our findings suggest that a higher PWV should be a unique vascular biomarker to identify MCI patients at higher risk of dementia. PWV reflects arterial stiffness, which is one of the earliest indicators of changes in vascular function[32]. Disturbed neurovascular pathways in the brain induce blood-brain barrier dysfunction, which is associated with the accumulation of several vasculotoxic and neurotoxic molecules, such as β-amyloid peptide, that might initiate and/or contribute to neuronal degeneration, notably Alzheimer's disease[33]. In addition, vessel remodeling and hypoperfusion after arterial stiffness might affect the volume of brain structure. Lilamand et al.[34] showed that higher PWV was associated with medial temporal lobe atrophy in MCI and Alzheimer's disease patients. The medial temporal lobe is particularly known for its sensitivity to ischemia[35]. Atrophy of the medial temporal lobe is characteristic of various neurodegenerative diseases in elderly people, including senile dementia.

In our previous investigation, arterial stiffness estimated by CAVI was a good predictor of longitudinal changes in cognitive function in older individuals in Tosa-town, Shikoku county, Japan[6]. It is noteworthy that the HDS-R was more sensitive than MMSE to reflect longitudinal cognitive decline, i.e., the annual assessments of HDS-R were significantly decreased from reference to 1 and 4 years later in citizens with higher arterial stiffness (p < 0.001), whereas annual changes in MMSE were only significantly decreased from reference to 4 years (p = 0.002). Since the MMSE is not sufficiently sensitive to detect mild changes in cognitive status[21, 22], we used the Kohs block design test for assessing cognitive function in the Ladakh elderly citizens in our Himalayan chronoecological study. Another suitable tool is needed to accurately predict progression to dementia. We have developed ToCA-MCI as an alternative to the MMSE to evaluate cognitive functions in the elderly, particularly focusing on MCI[23, 24, 25]. ToCA-MCI is a 20-minute cognitive screening tool of touch panel type to assist paramedical staff and first-line physicians in the detection of MCI, which correlated highly with the MMSE (r = 0.664, P < 0.0001), HDS-R (r = 0.538, P < 0.0001), Clock Drawing Test (r = 0.437, P < 0.0001), and Clinical

Dementia Rating (r = -0.442, P < 0.0001) scores. The area under the receiver-operator curves (AUC) for predicting MCI by the ToCA-MCI was 0.9581 (odds ratio = 60.9). Using a cut-off point of 17/18, the ToCA-MCI had a sensitivity of 92.3% and a specificity of 83.5% in screening for MCI[23]. ToCA-MCI was superior to MoCA-J for detecting amnestic MCI in elderly Japanese citizens. After examining 34 elders (mean age: 79.3 years; 21 women) complaining of memory disturbances, we clinically diagnosed amnestic mild cognitive impairment (MCI) and Alzheimer's disease in 11 and 1 elderly, respectively. ToCA-MCI correctly diagnosed MCI in 31 (91.2%) cases. MoCA-J had more false positives (14/34) than ToCA-MCI (1/34) (P < 0.05) and it is suggested that ToCA-MCI detects amnestic MCI better than MoCA-J, while MoCA-J may be more suitable to diagnose an overall MCI with or without amnesia[24].

Conclusions

We reported herein on a chronoecological health watch performed in two villages. The frequency of occurrence of dementia was statistically significantly higher in elderly with a ToCA-MCI score of 17 or lower. Such a differentiation was not achieved by the Mini-Mental State Examination (MMSE) recall item. We showed that a low ToCA-MCI score is a short-term predictor of progression to senile dementia within 2 years. ToCA-MCI's 25-word story for the delayed recall test significantly contributes to the prediction. Elderly who progress to dementia had a higher pulse wave velocity (PWV). The combined use of ToCA-MCI and PWV is useful to detect amnestic MCI early in elderly Japanese.

In conclusion, ToCA-MCI combined with CAVI provides a brief cognitive screening tool with high sensitivity and specificity for detecting MCI as currently conceptualized in patients performing in the normal range on the MMSE. The ToCA-MCI could be recommended for geriatric health screening in the community as a multi-player participation type screening tool as well as in a primary clinical setting for the early detection of MCI. Lifestyle interventions for improving arterial stiffness and preventing frailty should be therapeutic targets to delay or prevent the onset of dementia in community-dwelling citizens.

Acknowledgements

The authors thank Ms. Yoshie Saito and the public health nurses from the Health and Welfare Center, Uraus town, Kabato District, Hokkaido, Japan, for cooperation in our study. The authors also acknowledge all elderly participants in the town.

Conflict of Interest

The authors declare no competing financial and non-financial interests in relation to the work described. There is no sponsor's role.

Author Contributions:

K.O. and G.C. designed the study. K.O. and G.C. wrote the first draft of the manuscript and prepared the figures.

L.A.B. and T.N. analyzed the data and contributed to the writing and editing of the manuscript. All authors read and contributed to the final version of the manuscript.

Ethics

This study was approved by the Medical Ethics Committee of Tokyo Women's Medical University as Clinical Study #2912, entitled "Health assessment of community-dwelling elderly in Japan". Written informed consent was obtained from all participants regarding data analysis and the publication of results thereof.

References

1) Yamashina A, Tomiyama H, Takeda K, Tsuda H, Arai T, Hirose K et al. Validity, reproducibility, and clinical significance of noninvasive brachial-ankle pulse wave velocity measurement. Hypertens Res 2002; 25: 359-364.
2) Shirai K, Utino J, Otsuka K, Takata M. A novel blood pressure-independent arterial wall stiffness parameter; cardio-ankle vascular index (CAVI). J Atheroscler Thromb 2006; 13: 101-107.
3) Yoshinaga K, Fujii S, Tomiyama Y, Takeuchi K, Tamaki N. Anatomical and functional estimations of brachial artery diameter and elasticity using oscillometric measurements with a quantitative approach. Pulse (Basel) 2016; 4:1-10.
4) Takahashi K, Yamamoto T, Tsuda S, Okabe F, Shimose T, Tsuji Y et al. Coefficients in the CAVI equation and the comparison between CAVI with and without the coefficients using clinical data. J Atheroscler Thromb 2019; 26: 465-475.
5) Laurent S, Cockcroft J, Van Bortel L, Boutouyrie P, Giannattasio C, Hayoz D et al. European Network for Non-invasive Investigation of Large Arteries. Expert consensus document on arterial stiffness: methodological issues and clinical applications. Eur Heart J 2006; 27: 2588-2605.
6) Yamamoto N, Yamanaka G, Ishikawa M, Takasugi E, Murakami S, Yamanaka T et al. Cardio-ankle vascular index as a predictor of cognitive impairment in community-dwelling elderly people: four-year follow-up. Dement Geriatr Cogn Disord 2009; 28: 153-158.
7) Rabkin SW. Arterial stiffness: detection and consequences in cognitive impairment and dementia of the elderly. J Alzheimers Dis 2012; 32: 541-549.
8) Iulita MF, Noriega de la Colina A, Girouard H. Arterial stiffness, cognitive impairment and dementia: confounding factor or real risk?. J Neurochem 2018; 144: 527-548.
9) Menezes ST, Giatti L, Colosimo EA, Ribeiro ALP, Brant LCC, Viana MC et al. Aortic stiffness and age with cognitive performance decline in the ELSA-Brasil cohort. J Am Heart Assoc 2019; 8: e013248.
10) Carmichael O, Schwarz C, Drucker D, Fletcher E, Harvey D, Beckett L et al. Alzheimer's Disease Neuroimaging Initiative. Longitudinal changes in white matter disease and cognition in the first year of the Alzheimer disease neuroimaging initiative. Arch Neurol 2010; 67:1370-1378.
11) Villemagne VL, Burnham S, Bourgeat P, Brown B, Ellis KA, Salvado O et al. Amyloid β deposition, neurodegeneration, and cognitive decline in sporadic Alzheimer's disease: a prospective cohort study. Lancet Neurol. 2013; 12: 357-367.
12) Hughes TM, Kuller LH, Barinas-Mitchell EJ, Mackey RH, McDade EM, Klunk WE et al. Pulse wave velocity is associated with β-amyloid deposition in the brains of very elderly adults. Neurology 2013; 81: 1711-1718.
13) Langbaum JB, Chen K, Launer LJ, Fleisher AS, Lee W, Liu X et al. Blood pressure is associated with higher brain amyloid burden and lower glucose metabolism in healthy late middle-age persons. Neurobiol Aging 2012; 33: 827. e11-9.
14) Toledo JB, Toledo E, Weiner MW, Jack CR Jr, Jagust W, Lee VM et al. Cardiovascular risk factors, cortisol, and amyloid-β deposition in Alzheimer's Disease Neuroimaging Initiative. Alzheimers Dement 2012; 8: 483-489.
15) Hughes TM, Wagenknecht LE, Craft S, Mintz A, Heiss G, Palta P et al. Arterial stiffness and dementia pathology: Atherosclerosis Risk in Communities (ARIC)-PET Study. Neurology 2018; 90: e1248-e1256.
16) Rouch L, Cestac P, Brigitte Sallerin B, Andrieu S, Bailly H, Beunardeau M et al. Pulse wave velocity is associated with greater risk of dementia in mild cognitive impairment patients. Hypertension 2018; 72: 1109-1116.
17) Gorelick PB, Scuteri A, Black SE, Decarli C, Greenberg SM, Iadecola C et al. Vascular contributions to cognitive impairment and dementia: A statement for healthcare professionals from the AHA/ASA. Stroke 2011; 42: 2672-2713.
18) Folstein MF, Folstein SE, McHugh PR. "Mini-mental state". A practical method for grading the cognitive state of patients for the clinician. J Psychiatr Res 1975; 12: 189-198.
19) Fujiwara Y, Chaves PH, Takahashi R, Amano H, Yoshida H, Kumagai S et al. Arterial pulse wave velocity as a marker of poor cognitive function in an elderly community-dwelling population. J Gerontol A Biol Sci Med Sci 2005; 60: 607-612.
20) Fukuhara M, Matsumura K, Ansai T, Takata Y, Sonoki K, Akifusa S et al. Prediction of cognitive function by arterial stiffness in the very elderly. Circ J 2006; 70: 756-761.
21) Scuteri A, Brancati AM, Gianni W, Assisi A, Volpe M. Arterial stiffness is an independent risk factor for cognitive impairment in the elderly: a pilot study. J Hypertens 2005; 23: 1211-1216.
22) Singer J, Trollor JN, Crawford J, O'Rourke MF, Baune BT, Brodaty H et al. The association between pulse wave velocity and cognitive function: the Sydney Memory and Ageing Study. PLoS One 2013; 8: e61855.
23) Otsuka K, Kubo Y, Yamanaka G, Sasaki J, Kikuchi T, Saito Y et al. Tokyo cognitive assessment for mild cognitive impairment, ToCA-MCI. Validity and utility in elderly Japanese. Ther Res 2017; 38: 579-621.
24) Otsuka K, Cornelissen G, Yamanaka G, Kubo Y, Kikuchi T, Murakami S et al. Combination assessment of ToCA-MCI and Cardio-Ankle Vascular Index (CAVI) is useful for early detection of amnestic MCI in elderly Japanese citizens. In: Orimo H, Shirai K, Takata M et al. (Editors), CAVI and Neuro-Cardiovascular Function (1st Edition), Tokyo, Vascular Health Promotion Society, 2019, pp. 80-86.
25) Otsuka K, Cornelissen G, Kubo Y, Kikuchi T, Yamanaka G, Murakami S. Preventing progression to senile dementia in community-dwelling citizens of a small Japanese village. Am J Biomed Sci Res 2020; 10: 5-7.
26) Otsuka K, Norboo T, Kawasaki T, Ishikawa M, Matsubayashi K, Okumiya K. Impaired cognitive function and increased aortic stiffness, estimated by Cardio-Ankle Vascular Index, in Ladakh, at an altitude of 3250 to 4647 m, compared with Japanese town. Himalayan Study Monographs. 2009; 10: 25-38.
27) Hutt M L. The Kohs block-design tests. A revision for clinical practice. J Appl Psychol 1932; 16: 298-307.
28) Prince M, Bryce R, Albanese E, Wimo A, Ribeiro W, Ferri CP. The global prevalence of dementia: a systematic review and meta analysis. Alzheimers Dement 2013; 9: 63-75. e2.
29) Hanon O, Haulon S, Lenoir H, Seux ML, Rigaud AS, Safar M et al. Relationship between arterial stiffness and cognitive function in elderly subjects with complaints of memory loss. Stroke 2005; 36:2193-2197.
30) Perlmutter LS, Barrón E, Saperia D, Chui HC. Association

between vascular basement membrane components and the lesions of Alzheimer's disease. J Neurosci Res 1991; 30: 673-681.

31) Peterson RC, Lopez O, Armstrong MJ, Getchius TSD, Ganguli M, Gloss D et al. Practice guideline update summary: Mild cognitive impairment. Report of the guideline development, dissemination, and implementation subcommittee of the American Academy of Neurology. Neurology 2018; 90 (3): 126-135.

32) van Sluten TT, Protogerou AD, Henry RM, Schram MT, Launer LJ, Stehouwer CD. Association between arterial stiffness, cerebral small vessel disease and cognitive impairment: A systematic review and meta-analysis.

Neurosci Biobehav Rev 2015; 53: 121-130.

33) Zlokovic BV. Neurovascular pathways to neurodegeneration in Alzheimer's disease and other disorders. Nat Rev Neurosci 2011; 12: 723-738.

34) Lilamand M, Vidal JS, Plichart M, De Jong LW, Duron E, Hanon O. Arterial stiffness and medial temporal lobe atrophy in elders with memory disorders. J Hypertens. 2016; 34: 1331-1337.

35) de Jong LW, Forsberg LE, Vidal JS, Sigurdsson S, Zijdenbos AP, Garcia M et al. Different susceptibility of medial temporal lobe and basal ganglia atrophy rates to vascular risk factors. Neurobiol Aging 2014; 35: 72-78.

PART 4

Cardiovascular risk factors and CAVI

CAVI in hypertensive patients

Takafumi Okura

Summary

1. The CAVI can be used to evaluate arteriosclerosis in hypertensive patients correctly because it is not affected by the blood pressure at the time of measurement.
2. The CAVI is a good indicator of hypertensive organ damage.

Introduction

Aortic stiffness is an independent predictor of all-cause and cardiovascular mortality, fatal and nonfatal coronary events, and fatal strokes in patients with essential hypertension. Arterial stiffness can be evaluated by measuring the pulse wave velocity (PWV). However, the challenge with the clinical use of PWV is that the index itself is closely dependent on the blood pressure. To overcome this disadvantage, a novel diagnostic parameter for stiffness called the cardio-ankle vascular index (CAVI) has been developed in Japan. The CAVI can assess vascular stiffness independent of the blood pressure at the time of measurement in hypertensive patients[1].

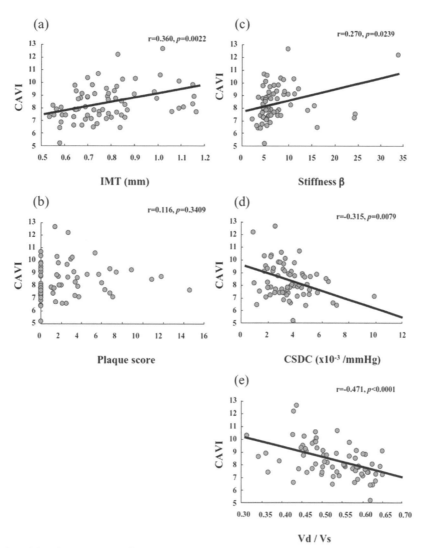

Fig. 1. Relationships between the CAVI and the respective indices derived from the carotid echoes.
(cited from Ref. 3)

Director, Yawatahama City General Hospital, Ohira 638, Yawatahama City, Ehime 796-8502, Japan.

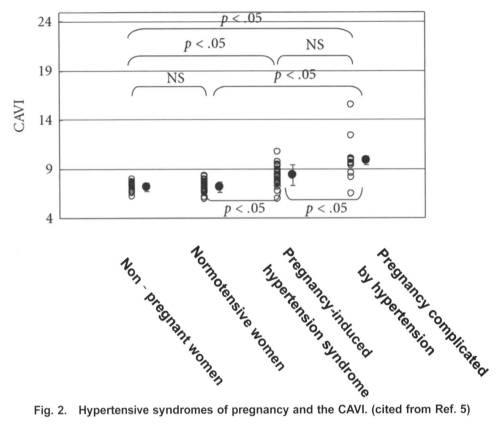

Fig. 2.   Hypertensive syndromes of pregnancy and the CAVI. (cited from Ref. 5)

Indicators of organ damage in hypertensive patients.

The Japanese Society of Hypertension Guideline 2019 recommends evaluating angiopathy, including atherosclerosis and arteriosclerosis, in patients with hypertension using carotid ultrasonography, ankle-brachial index, and PWV (including the CAVI)[2].

We investigated the usefulness of the CAVI as an indicator of hypertensive organ damage in patients with hypertension[3]. Seventy consecutive patients with essential hypertension were enrolled in this study. Patients with congestive heart failure, history of myocardial infarction, angina pectoris, atrial fibrillation, diabetes mellitus (fasting glucose level > 126 mg/dl), chronic renal failure (serum creatinine > 1.5 mg/dl), history of stroke, malignant tumor, or autoimmune diseases were excluded. The intima-media thickness (IMT), cross-sectional distensibility coefficient (CSDC), stiffness parameter β, and mean diastolic (Vd) and mean systolic (Vs) flow velocities were evaluated by carotid ultrasound. The Vd/Vs ratio, an index of peripheral arterial resistance, was also calculated.

The CAVI was positively correlated with age, systolic blood pressure, pulse pressure, and HbA1c. It was not associated with diastolic blood pressure, total cholesterol, triglycerides, HDL, and serum creatinine. The CAVI was significantly correlated with IMT (Fig. 1a), stiffness β (Fig. 1c), CSDC (Fig. 1d), and Vd/Vs (Fig. 1e) but not with the plaque score (Fig. 1b). Among these carotid factors, Vd/Vs was an independent determinant factor estimated by stepwise regression analysis. These results suggested that the CAVI is a useful clinical marker for evaluating

arteriosclerosis in patients with hypertension.

Circadian rhythm in blood pressure and the CAVI

The blood pressure follows a circadian rhythm over 24 hours. Normally, the nocturnal blood pressure decreases by more than 10% compared to the daytime blood pressure (dipper). However, the non-dipper pattern of high blood pressure is associated with an increased risk of organ damage and cardiovascular disease in hypertensive patients. Chen et al. compared the cardiac function and the CAVI between the dipper and non-dipper hypertensive patients[4]. Compared to patients with dipper hypertension, those with non-dipper hypertension had increased left ventricular mass index, higher degree of impairment of the left ventricular diastolic and systolic function, and higher peripheral arterial stiffness estimated by the CAVI. These results suggest that the CAVI is a good indicator of hypertensive organ damage.

Hypertension in pregnancy

Preeclampsia refers to a condition with systolic blood pressure > 140 mmHg and > 300 mg of proteinuria in a 24-hour urine sample after week 20 of pregnancy. Chronic hypertension is defined as hypertension diagnosed prior to conception or within the first 20 weeks of pregnancy. Yoshida et al. examined arterial stiffness using the CAVI and baPWV in patients with preeclampsia and chronic hypertension[5]. No significant difference in baPWV was seen between patients with preeclampsia and chronic hypertension; however, the CAVI was significantly high in patients with chronic hypertension (Fig. 2), indicating that the CAVI can distinguish between the structural differences in the blood vessels in the two diseases.

Conclusions

The objectives of antihypertensive treatment are to prevent target organ damage associated with high blood pressure. Hence, diagnostic tools to evaluate the target organ damage conveniently and accurately are necessary. The CAVI does not depend on the blood pressure at the time of the measurement, thus allowing a simple and accurate assessment of arterial stiffness in patients with hypertension.

By monitoring the CAVI, an appropriate treatment plan for hypertension and improvement of the patient's willingness of the treatment continuation can be obtained.

Future challenges:

1. It is unclear whether the CAVI can predict the risk of development of cardiovascular disease in patients with hypertension.
2. It is unclear which classes of antihypertensive drugs are most effective in improving the CAVI.

References

1) Shirai K, Utino J, Otsuka K, Takata M. A novel blood pressure-independent arterial wall stiffness parameter; cardio-ankle vascular index (CAVI). J Atheroscler Thromb. 2006; 13: 101-107.

2) Umemura S, Arima H, Arima S, et al; The Japanese Society of Hypertension Guidelines for the Management of Hypertension (JSH 2019). Hypertens Res. 2019; 42: 1235-1481.

3) Okura T, Watanabe S, Kurata M, et al. Relationship between cardio-ankle vascular index (CAVI) and carotid atherosclerosis in patients with essential hypertension. Hypertens Res. 2007; 30: 335-340. http://dx.doi.org/10.1291/hypres.30.335

4) Chen Y, Liu JH, Zhen Z et al. Assessment of left ventricular function and peripheral vascular arterial stiffness in patients with dipper and non-dipper hypertension. J Investig Med. 2018; 66: 319-324.

5) Yoshida A, Sugiyama T, Sagara N. Assessment of the cardiovascular index in pregnant women complicated with hypertensive disorders. ISRN Obstet Gynecol 2011; 2011: 919816. https://doi.org/10.5402/2011/919816

CAVI and Cardiovascular Disease Progression in Young Adults

Paul Leeson

Abstract

Cardiovascular disease remains a major cause of morbidity and mortality. To address this disease burden a better understanding of the early stages of disease development within both the blood vessels and the heart during adolescence and young adult life may be required to maintain health. By mapping disease progression across multiple organs, over time, rate of progression of disease in different areas of body can be described. This information may be of value to identify the key times in life when disease accelerates and the optimal points for intervention. Within this type of modelling, measures of arterial stiffness are of particular importance because of the central role of the aorta in maintaining haemodynamic control. CAVI provides a unique biomarker of arterial function that is associated with changes in central aortic function and can differentiate central from peripheral influences on disease. Thereby CAVI can provide information on how arterial function could contribute to disease development in different organs such as the brain, heart and kidneys. Future work will establish whether, in addition, CAVI provides a useful biomarker to guide prevention in younger people.

Cardiovascular disease progression in young adults

Cardiovascular disease remains a major cause of mortality and morbidity in the world despite significant advances in detection and treatment over the last 30 years. In part, this is because the disease originates from very early in life[1-5], and gradually progresses over the lifecourse, with acute events emerging in later life[6]. Therefore complete prevention of disease may require interventions early in life to 'maintain health' rather than 'reverse disease'. There is increasing exposure to lifestyle risk factors, occupation-related risk factors and a rise in sedentary behaviour during adolescence and young adult life[7, 8]. At the same time, traditional risk factors such as adverse lipid profiles and hypertension start to become more prevalent[6, 8] with higher prevalence in those with familial predispositions for cardiovascular disease[9]. Not surprisingly, some of the earliest studies into the natural history of atherosclerotic disease show this period of life corresponds with a rapid progression of disease within the walls of blood vessels[1-5].

Can disease progression be managed in young adults?

How to manage this risk in young people remains unclear. There have been few clinical trials or investigative research that have focused on this age group to identify the optimal interventions[6, 10]. This problem is compounded by the fact young adulthood is a time when interaction with health services tends to be reduced and therefore opportunities for risk interventions can be limited[7, 8, 11]. Cardiovascular risk scores are difficult to implement in this age group as they are usually modelled on mortality or risk of acute events over 5 or 10 year time horizons[10]. Lifetime risk scores or relative risk scoring have more applicability but are still limited by low ability to meaningfully differentiate between individuals. To better understand disease progression during the first decades of life, and identify whether there may be opportunities for targeted interventions, a better understanding of how the vasculature and heart change and remodel during this time may be of value[12] (**Fig. 1**). Traditional cardiovascular risk factors, although providing guidance on state of risk at a particular point in time, do not provide this information. Direct assessment of underlying cardiac and vascular disease therefore provides an alternative approach to risk stratify young people.

Identifying disease progression in young adulthood

Multi-modality imaging provides an opportunity to capture information on cardiovascular structure and function 'from heart to capillary'. This information can be used to establish interrelationships between features of the cardiovascular system and, with longitudinal data, can then be used to model progression of disease over time across the blood vessels and heart[13]. If data capture can be extended to other organs such as brain and liver, a system-wide physiological understanding of disease development can be developed[14]. Multi-modality, multi-organ imaging has the potential to provide this unprecedented insight into disease development[15-17]. Value is also now being extracted from these multi-modality imaging datasets because of the emergence of new computational modelling and statistical approaches. These raise the possibility to apply machine

Oxford Cardiovascular Clinical Research Facility, Division of Cardiovascular Medicine, Radcliffe Department of Medicine, University of Oxford, John Radcliffe Hospital – Oxford University Hospitals, Oxford, UK.

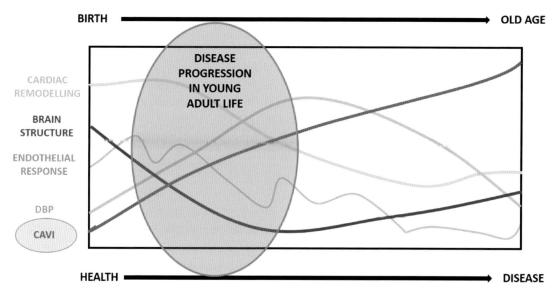

Fig. 1. Diagram to illustrate, hypothetically, how the relation between different characteristics of the cardiovascular system, including CAVI, may change over time as individuals progress from health to disease. Understanding this relationship in early adult life may help identify key points, and the most appropriate interventions, to slow disease progression and maintain health.

Table 1. Correlations between SBP and DBP variability and measures of aortic distensibility and stiffness. Reproduced with permission of Wolters Kluwer from Boardman et al. J Hypertens. 2017;35:513-522[24].

	SD of 24-h SBP – awake period	Weighted SD of 24-h SBP	SBP ARV	SD of 24-h DBP – awake period	Weighted SD of 24-h DBP	DBP ARV
Aortic distensibility						
Global	−0.39***	−0.42***	−0.34***	−0.39***	−0.44***	−0.41***
AA	−0.38***	−0.40***	−0.30***	−0.34***	−0.38***	−0.36***
PDA	−0.33***	−0.31***	−0.24***	−0.33***	−0.35***	−0.33***
DDA	−0.33***	−0.37***	−0.28***	−0.36***	−0.40***	−0.35***
AbA	−0.42***	−0.44***	−0.41***	−0.41***	−0.46***	−0.45***
Peripheral measures of stiffness						
CAVI	0.19*	0.24**	0.17	0.25**	0.31***	0.28***
cf PWV	0.11	0.20*	0.17	0.11	0.21*	0.21*
bf PWV	0.10	0.11	0.10	0.12	0.14	0.10
Peripheral distensibility						
Carotid	0.15	0.17	0.23**	0.19*	0.19*	0.23**
Brachial	−0.07	0.03	0.20	−0.16	−0.16	−0.07

AA, ascending aorta; AbA, abdominal aorta; bf PWV: brachial-femoral pulse wave velocity, Vicorder; CAVI, cardio-ankle vascular index; cf PWV, carotid-femoral pulse wave velocity, SphygmoCor; DDA, distal descending aorta; PDA, proximal descending aorta.
*$P < 0.05$.
**$P \leq 0.01$.
***$P \leq 0.001$.

learning techniques to better define the complex relationships between aspects of the cardiovascular system captured in imaging studies[18, 19]. The phrase 'digital twin' has been coined to describe an approach of *in silico* modelling of health and disease for individuals and patients using such rich phenotype data[18, 20, 21]. Using this approach it may be possible to model impact of disease or treatment across different components of the cardiovascular system including the heart, central vasculature and peripheral vascular beds. As a result deep phenotyping studies have the potential to unravel the heterogeneity in cardiac and vascular changes that are present in young people as cardiovascular disease progresses[12, 22, 23].

Arterial stiffness as a biomarker of disease progression

Arterial stiffness is of particular importance in understanding disease progression during young adult life[12]. Aortic structure and function, as a component of arterial stiffness, holds a particularly pivotal role because of the strategic position of the aorta between cardiac output and other organs. Changes in aortic function influences cardiac afterload and thereby disease progression within the myocardium. Furthermore, the Windkessel function of the aorta, in smoothing pulsatile flow, influences exposure of the peripheral vasculature to changes in pressure that impact disease progression within vascular beds in the kidneys and brain[24]. Arterial stiffness can be monitored in studies investigating disease progression using a range of different techniques. Cardiovascular magnetic resonance can directly image aortic size and geometry as well as wall thickness[24, 25] while cine imaging allows assessment of changes in shape over the cardiac cycle[24]. By linking this variation with blood pressure, indices of central aortic stiffness can be generated. Tonometer and cuff-based measures of pulse arrival time at peripheral vessels such as the carotid, femoral or radial artery[26] can also provide information on speed of pulse wave travel as a measure of arterial wall stiffness. While additional measures can be extracted from the peripheral waveform to inform on features of pulse wave analysis[27]. Cardio-Ankle Vascular Index (CAVI) combines approaches to provide a global measure of arterial pathophysiology using microphone-based identification of aortic valve closure linked to limb cuff-based identification

of both pulse arrival and characteristics peripherally[28, 29]. The measure is independent of blood pressure at time of measurement[29]. Imaging also allows assessment of a further, vascular bed important in determining blood pressure levels, the smaller vessels that extend from resistance arterioles to the capillary bed[30].

What has CAVI explained about arterial disease progression in young adulthood?

Several studies have followed individuals throughout the

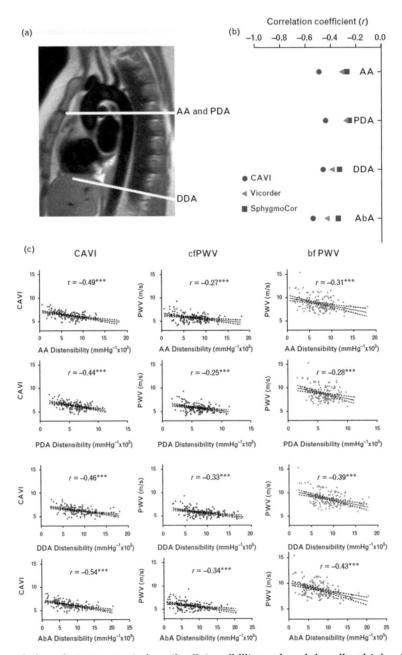

Fig. 2. **Correlations between central aortic distensibility and peripherally obtained measures of arterial stiffness. Cardio-ankle vascular index is most closely correlated with central aortic distensibility with a consistent association across the range of levels of aortic distensibility [part(b) (circle)] with weaker associations between central aortic distensibility and both carotid-femoral pulse wave velocity and brachial-femoral pulse wave velocity (triangle and square, respectively). (***P < = 0.001; **P < = 0.01; *P < 0.05).** Reproduced with permission of Wolters Kluwer from Boardman et al. J Hypertens. 2017;35:513-522[24].

first decades of life with multiple vascular measures to help understand disease progression during this time. They have demonstrated that vascular measures during adolescence can predict progression of cardiovascular phenotype during this period and that the association between cardiac and vascular measures differs between younger people and older individuals[12, 22, 31]. Adolescents with reduced endothelial responses tend to have a more accelerated increase in their blood pressure over this period of time[23]. Furthermore, those with impaired vascular responses have increases in cardiac mass out of proportion to the expected increase seen in young adulthood with a greater degree of endothelial responsiveness[23]. However, relationships are not always predictable and the reductions in arterial compliance, endothelial response and microvascular structure and function, as well as altered cardiac morphology[32], seen in someone with established cardiovascular disease may differ with type of risk factor exposure in younger people[12].

CAVI has proved particularly valuable in understanding the differences in disease progression at this time. Families with a history of pregnancy hypertension or reduced birthweight typically show adverse endothelial responses during childhood before development of overt changes in blood pressure or other risk markers[33]. Whereas, by using CAVI as a global measure of arterial function it has been possible to demonstrate that developmental influences on cardiovascular development, such as preterm birth, can lead to regional changes in aortic function related to use of antenatal steroids[34] or intravenous lipids[25] but without having a clinically significant impact on arterial stiffness[13, 35]. In contrast, physiological changes that drive increases in blood pressure variability, an important risk factor for stroke in later life, can be linked with increases in CAVI. By extending this investigation to incorporate cardiovascular magnetic resonance measures associations between CAVI and changes in central aortic stiffness have been shown to underlie these associations[24]. As demonstrated in **Table 1**, in young people blood pressure variability is significantly related to changes in central aortic distensibility as measured by cardiovascular magnetic resonance and also with CAVI. Whereas simple measures of pulse wave velocity do not show a clear association. **Fig. 2** shows the strong correlation between measures of CAVI in a young population and arterial distensibility at multiple aortic levels from ascending to abdominal aorta.

Future possibilities for clinical understanding and use of CAVI and disease progression modelling in young adults

Multi-modality imaging protocols that incorporate unique indices, such as CAVI, have provided critical insights into complex patterns of vascular disease progression in young adulthood. No single measure provides a complete assessment of cardiovascular risk phenotype in younger people but using a panel of measures that can assess changes in specific vascular beds have helped to define interactions between conventional and novel risk factors and disease progression. Use of disease modelling techniques that incorporate techniques for computational

learning based on application of artificial intelligence approaches provide the opportunity to start to understand how arterial stiffness fits into the landscape of multi-organ changes during the early stages of disease in young adulthood. It is expected that changes in larger artery pathophysiology will emerge as of central importance to particular features or early disease development, such as blood pressure control, including central blood pressure and blood pressure variability. With increased understanding from these models new targets and timings for treatments, whether lifestyle or pharmacological, should be identifiable that may be able to be guided by biomarkers, such as CAVI, measured during early stages of life.

References

1) Relationship of atherosclerosis in young men to serum lipoprotein cholesterol concentrations and smoking. A preliminary report from the Pathobiological Determinants of Atherosclerosis in Youth (PDAY) Research Group. *JAMA*. 1990;264:3018-24.

2) McGill HC, Jr., McMahan CA, Malcom GT, Oalmann MC and Strong JP. Effects of serum lipoproteins and smoking on atherosclerosis in young men and women. The PDAY Research Group. Pathobiological Determinants of Atherosclerosis in Youth. *Arterioscler Thromb Vasc Biol*. 1997;17:95-106.

3) McGill HC, Jr., McMahan CA, Tracy RE, Oalmann MC, Cornhill JF, Herderick EE and Strong JP. Relation of a postmortem renal index of hypertension to atherosclerosis and coronary artery size in young men and women. Pathobiological Determinants of Atherosclerosis in Youth (PDAY) Research Group. *Arterioscler Thromb Vasc Biol*. 1998;18:1108-18.

4) McGill HC, Jr., McMahan CA, Zieske AW, Sloop GD, Walcott JV, Troxclair DA, Malcom GT, Tracy RE, Oalmann MC and Strong JP. Associations of coronary heart disease risk factors with the intermediate lesion of atherosclerosis in youth. The Pathobiological Determinants of Atherosclerosis in Youth (PDAY) Research Group. *Arterioscler Thromb Vasc Biol*. 2000;20:1998-2004.

5) McMahan CA, McGill HC, Gidding SS, Malcom GT, Newman WP, Tracy RE, Strong JP and Pathobiological Determinants of Atherosclerosis in Youth Research G. PDAY risk score predicts advanced coronary artery atherosclerosis in middle-aged persons as well as youth. *Atherosclerosis*. 2007;190:370-7.

6) Lewington S, Clarke R, Qizilbash N, Peto R, Collins R and Prospective Studies C. Age-specific relevance of usual blood pressure to vascular mortality: a meta-analysis of individual data for one million adults in 61 prospective studies. *Lancet*. 2002;360:1903-13.

7) Williamson W, Boardman H, Lewandowski AJ and Leeson P. Time to rethink physical activity advice and blood pressure: A role for occupation-based interventions? *Eur J Prev Cardiol*. 2016;23:1051-3.

8) Williamson W, Foster C, Reid H, Kelly P, Lewandowski AJ, Boardman H, Roberts N, McCartney D, Huckstep O, Newton J, Dawes H, Gerry S and Leeson P. Will Exercise Advice Be Sufficient for Treatment of Young Adults With Prehypertension and Hypertension? A Systematic Review and Meta-Analysis. *Hypertension*. 2016;68:78-87.

9) Davis EF, Lewandowski AJ, Aye C, Williamson W, Boardman H, Huang RC, Mori TA, Newnham J, Beilin LJ and Leeson P. Clinical cardiovascular risk during young

adulthood in offspring of hypertensive pregnancies: insights from a 20-year prospective follow-up birth cohort. *BMJ open*. 2015;5:e008136.

10) Piepoli MF, Hoes AW, Agewall S, Albus C, Brotons C, Catapano AL, Cooney MT, Corra U, Cosyns B, Deaton C, Graham I, Hall MS, Hobbs FD, Lochen ML, Lollgen H, Marques-Vidal P, Perk J, Prescott E, Redon J, Richter DJ, Sattar N, Smulders Y, Tiberi M, van der Worp HB, van Dis I, Verschuren WM and Authors/Task Force M. 2016 European Guidelines on cardiovascular disease prevention in clinical practice: The Sixth Joint Task Force of the European Society of Cardiology and Other Societies on Cardiovascular Disease Prevention in Clinical Practice (constituted by representatives of 10 societies and by invited experts) Developed with the special contribution of the European Association for Cardiovascular Prevention & Rehabilitation (EACPR). *Eur Heart J*. 2016;37:2315-81.

11) Johnson HM, Thorpe CT, Bartels CM, Schumacher JR, Palta M, Pandhi N, Sheehy AM and Smith MA. Antihypertensive medication initiation among young adults with regular primary care use. *Journal of general internal medicine*. 2014;29:723-31.

12) Lewandowski AJ, Pitcher A, Banerjee R and Leeson P. Arterial stiffness: using simple surrogate measures to make sense of a biologically complex phenomenon. *Hypertens Res*. 2012;35:155-6.

13) Boardman H, Birse K, Davis EF, Whitworth P, Aggarwal V, Lewandowski AJ and Leeson P. Comprehensive multi-modality assessment of regional and global arterial structure and function in adults born preterm. *Hypertens Res*. 2016;39:39-45.

14) Boardman H, Birse K, Davis EF, Whitworth P, Aggarwal V, Lewandowski AJ and Leeson P. Comprehensive multi-modality assessment of regional and global arterial structure and function in adults born preterm. *Hypertens Res*. 2015.

15) Petersen SE, Matthews PM, Bamberg F, Bluemke DA, Francis JM, Friedrich MG, Leeson P, Nagel E, Plein S, Rademakers FE, Young AA, Garratt S, Peakman T, Sellors J, Collins R and Neubauer S. Imaging in population science: cardiovascular magnetic resonance in 100,000 participants of UK Biobank - rationale, challenges and approaches. *J Cardiovasc Magn Reson*. 2013;15:46.

16) Littlejohns TJ, Holliday J, Gibson LM, Garratt S, Oesingmann N, Alfaro-Almagro F, Bell JD, Boultwood C, Collins R, Conroy MC, Crabtree N, Doherty N, Frangi AF, Harvey NC, Leeson P, Miller KL, Neubauer S, Petersen SE, Sellors J, Sheard S, Smith SM, Sudlow CLM, Matthews PM and Allen NE. The UK Biobank imaging enhancement of 100,000 participants: rationale, data collection, management and future directions. *Nat Commun*. 2020;11:2624.

17) Coffey S, Lewandowski AJ, Garratt S, Meijer R, Lynum S, Bedi R, Paterson J, Yaqub M, Noble JA, Neubauer S, Petersen SE, Allen N, Sudlow C, Collins R, Matthews PM and Leeson P. Protocol and quality assurance for carotid imaging in 100,000 participants of UK Biobank: development and assessment. *Eur J Prev Cardiol*. 2017;24:1799-1806.

18) Corral-Acero J, Margara F, Marciniak M, Rodero C, Loncaric F, Feng Y, Gilbert A, Fernandes JF, Bukhari HA, Wajdan A, Martinez MV, Santos MS, Shamohammdi M, Luo H, Westphal P, Leeson P, DiAchille P, Gurev V, Mayr M, Geris L, Pathmanathan P, Morrison T, Cornelussen R, Prinzen F, Delhaas T, Doltra A, Sitges M, Vigmond EJ, Zacur E, Grau V, Rodriguez B, Remme EW, Niederer S, Mortier P, McLeod K, Potse M, Pueyo E, Bueno-Orovio A and Lamata P. The 'Digital Twin' to enable the vision of precision cardiology. *Eur Heart J*. 2020.

19) Gevaert AB, Adams V, Bahls M, Bowen TS, Cornelissen V, Dorr M, Hansen D, Kemps HM, Leeson P, Van Craenenbroeck EM and Krankel N. Towards a personalised approach in exercise-based cardiovascular rehabilitation: How can translational research help? A 'call to action' from the Section on Secondary Prevention and Cardiac Rehabilitation of the European Association of Preventive Cardiology. *Eur J Prev Cardiol*. 2020;27:1369-1385.

20) Alsharqi M, Woodward WJ, Mumith JA, Markham DC, Upton R and Leeson P. Artificial intelligence and echocardiography. *Echo Res Pract*. 2018;5:R115-R125.

21) Dey D, Slomka PJ, Leeson P, Comaniciu D, Shrestha S, Sengupta PP and Marwick TH. Artificial Intelligence in Cardiovascular Imaging: JACC State-of-the-Art Review. *J Am Coll Cardiol*. 2019;73:1317-1335.

22) Lazdam M, de la Horra A, Diesch J, Kenworthy Y, Davis E, Lewandowski AJ, Szmigielski C, Shore A, Mackillop L, Kharbanda R, Alp N, Redman C, Kelly B and Leeson P. Unique blood pressure characteristics in mother and offspring after early onset preeclampsia. *Hypertension*. 2012;60:1338-45.

23) Lazdam M, Lewandowski AJ, Kylintireas I, Cunnington C, Diesch J, Francis J, Trevitt C, Neubauer S, Singhal A and Leeson P. Impaired endothelial responses in apparently healthy young people associated with subclinical variation in blood pressure and cardiovascular phenotype. *Am J Hypertens*. 2012;25:46-53.

24) Boardman H, Lewandowski AJ, Lazdam M, Kenworthy Y, Whitworth P, Zwager CL, Francis JM, Aye CY, Williamson W, Neubauer S and Leeson P. Aortic stiffness and blood pressure variability in young people: a multimodality investigation of central and peripheral vasculature. *J Hypertens*. 2017;35:513-522.

25) Lewandowski AJ, Lazdam M, Davis E, Kylintireas I, Diesch J, Francis J, Neubauer S, Singhal A, Lucas A, Kelly B and Leeson P. Short-term exposure to exogenous lipids in premature infants and long-term changes in aortic and cardiac function. *Arterioscler Thromb Vasc Biol*. 2011;31:2125-35.

26) Reference Values for Arterial Stiffness C. Determinants of pulse wave velocity in healthy people and in the presence of cardiovascular risk factors: 'establishing normal and reference values'. *Eur Heart J*. 2010;31:2338-50.

27) Kelly RP, Millasseau SC, Ritter JM and Chowienczyk PJ. Vasoactive drugs influence aortic augmentation index independently of pulse-wave velocity in healthy men. *Hypertension*. 2001;37:1429-33.

28) Shirai K, Hiruta N, Song M, Kurosu T, Suzuki J, Tomaru T, Miyashita Y, Saiki A, Takahashi M, Suzuki K and Takata M. Cardio-ankle vascular index (CAVI) as a novel indicator of arterial stiffness: theory, evidence and perspectives. *J Atheroscler Thromb*. 2011;18:924-38.

29) Shirai K, Utino J, Otsuka K and Takata M. A novel blood pressure-independent arterial wall stiffness parameter; cardio-ankle vascular index (CAVI). *J Atheroscler Thromb*. 2006;13:101-7.

30) Shore AC and Tooke JE. Microvascular function in human essential hypertension. *J Hypertens*. 1994;12:717-28.

31) Nethononda RM, Lewandowski AJ, Stewart R, Kylinterias I, Whitworth P, Francis J, Leeson P, Watkins H, Neubauer S and Rider OJ. Gender specific patterns of age-related decline in aortic stiffness: a cardiovascular magnetic resonance study including normal ranges. *J Cardiovasc Magn Reson*. 2015;17:20.

32) Lee JM, Shirodaria C, Jackson CE, Robson MD, Antoniades C, Francis JM, Wiesmann F, Channon KM, Neubauer S and Choudhury RP. Multi-modal magnetic resonance imaging quantifies atherosclerosis and vascular dysfunction in patients with type 2 diabetes mellitus. *Diabetes Vasc Dis Res*. 2007;4:44-48.

33) Lewandowski AJ and Leeson P. Preeclampsia, prematurity and cardiovascular health in adult life. *Early Hum Dev*.

2014;90:725-9.

34) Kelly BA, Lewandowski AJ, Worton SA, Davis EF, Lazdam M, Francis J, Neubauer S, Lucas A, Singhal A and Leeson P. Antenatal glucocorticoid exposure and long-term alterations in aortic function and glucose metabolism. *Pediatrics*. 2012;129:e1282-90.

35) Lewandowski AJ, Davis EF, Yu G, Digby JE, Boardman H, Whitworth P, Singhal A, Lucas A, McCormick K, Shore AC and Leeson P. Elevated blood pressure in preterm-born offspring associates with a distinct antiangiogenic state and microvascular abnormalities in adult life. *Hypertension*. 2015;65:607-614.

The interest of CAVI measurements in older adults

Athanase Benetos

A- Arterial stiffness: A major risk factor during the aging process

During the aging process, arterial stiffness develops as a result of several structural and functional changes in the large arteries[1,2]: Hypertrophy of the arterial wall, calcium deposits as well as changes in the extracellular matrix, such as increased collagen and fibronectin and fragmentation of the elastin networks are common age-related structural changes in the arterial wall. In addition, enzymatic and non-enzymatic crosslinks, cell-matrix interactions, endothelial dysfunction, characterized by decreased release of vasodilators and increased synthesis of vasoconstrictors and smooth muscle phenotypic changes are major functional age-related arterial changes. The combination of these structural and functional modifications leads to arterial stiffness (arterio-sclerosis), which is the most typical manifestation of arterial aging, and its clinical manifestations i.e. an increase in systolic and a decrease in diastolic blood pressure.

Thus, in older adults, the visco-elastic properties of the arterial wall are the main determinants of blood pressure (BP) levels (Fig. 1): the peak systolic BP (SBP) will be higher if the arterial wall is more rigid. Then, after the aortic valve closes, BP gradually decreases as blood is drained to peripheral vascular networks. Diastolic BP (DBP) at the end of the cardiac cycle is determined by the length of the diastolic interval and the rate at which the pressure decreases. The latter is influenced by the peripheral resistance, and by the arterial stiffness. At a given vascular resistance, the drop in diastolic pressure will be greater if the stiffness of the large arteries is higher and this phenomenon explains the decrease in DBP levels in older individuals.

Large artery stiffness is also a determinant of the speed of propagation of the arterial pressure wave (pulse wave velocity, PWV) and the timing of wave reflections. Thus, the stiffening of the arteries increases the PWV leading to an earlier return of the reflected waves, which are superimposed on the incident pressure wave during the systolic and not as in younger adults during the diastolic-period, thus further contributing to the increase of SBP and the decrease in the DBP[1,2].

Therefore, the amplitude of pulse pressure (SBP-DBP) is a rough indicator of the degree of the large arteries' stiffness. Clinical studies these last 25 years, in various populations, demonstrated that taking account of pulse pressure values

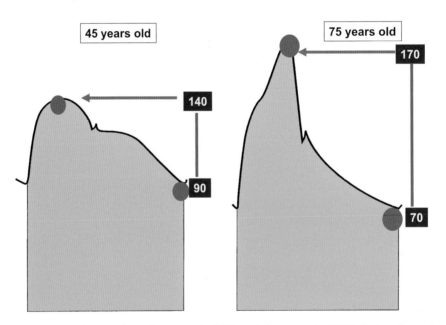

Fig. 1. Changes in the BP waveform (increase in SBP and decrease in DBP) during the aging process are mainly explained by the stiffening of the aorta and the other large arteries. Note that the two mean BP (areas under the curve in grey) are not different.

President of the European Geriatric Medicine Society (EuGMS), Chairman of Geriatric and Clinical Gerontology Dpt., University Hospital of Nancy, Université de Lorraine, Nancy, France

contributes to a better assessment of the risk of cardiovascular morbidity and mortality[3-5]. Interestingly, it has been shown that the relationship between PP and morbidity and mortality was more pronounced in individuals over the age of 60 since, as mentioned above, PP is strongly dependent on arterial stiffness in individuals over 60 years[5]. Thus, over these last 3 decades PP has largely been used in the estimation of CV risk. However, although PP is easily measured, it remains an indirect method for the estimation of arterial stiffness, since both systolic and diastolic BP are influenced by several parameters and age-related diseases such as heart failure, autonomic nervous system function, various neurological diseases, several medications, etc. Under those conditions PP values may not reflect arterial stiffness status and therefore this measurement loses its predictive value (Fig. 2).

This is particularly the case in highly aged populations with several comorbidities, frailty and polymedication. In those subjects, despite a marked arterial stiffness, SBP and therefore PP can remain unchanged or events decrease due to a decrease in cardiac output, dysautonomia, marked frailty, etc. Since these populations have greatly increased over these last few years, the need for direct and if possible, pressure-independent measurements of arterial stiffness become more pronounced.

B- Direct methods for measuring Arterial Stiffness Devices developed for the measurements of arterial stiffness

In the 70s, most measurements of arterial stiffness were performed mainly with invasive methods mostly in animal studies and only occasionally in humans.

In the 80s the non-invasive methods for the evaluation of large artery stiffness were based on measurements of systolic-diastolic changes of the arterial diameter (mainly in carotid, femoral brachial and radial arteries) using Echo-Doppler sophisticated devices[6-8]. During this period, it was shown that arterial stiffening was responsible for the selective increase in systolic pressure in older adults – and that this differed from the increased peripheral vascular resistance observed in mid-life hypertension[7]. Using these methods several studies were able to investigate the mechanisms of action of a variety of antihypertensive drugs, some of which (calcium channel blockers and angiotensin converting enzyme inhibitors) had shown to have more pronounced effects on the arterial wall elastic properties[7,8].

In the early 90s, measuring the pulse wave velocity (PWV) became the most popular method for the assessment of large artery stiffness[9]. This method, defined a century ago by the Bramwell-Hill equation[10], is based on the principle that the speed of the pulse wave between a central (carotid) and a peripheral (femoral) depends on the stiffness in the arterial segments through which this pulse wave travels. In clinical practice, the non-invasive measurements of PWV are performed by recording pulse waves using tonometers placed on superficial large arteries such as carotid, brachial, radial, femoral, etc. Since clinically the stiffness of the aorta is the most important regulator of cardiac afterload and systolic/diastolic BP, thus the PWV between the carotid-femoral arteries (cfPWV) has been considered since that period as the referent method. Beginning in these years, a large number of automatic

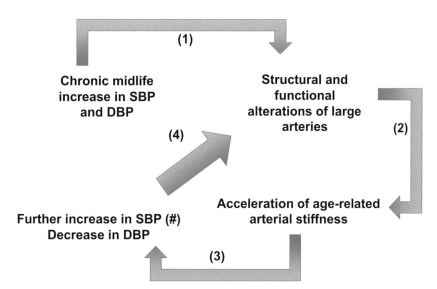

Fig. 2. **Strong Relationship between SBP and arterial stiffness in older adults: High levels of SBP are determinants (1) + (4) but also a consequence of the arterial stiffness (3). Therefore, SBP is strongly related with arterial stiffness as captured by both PWV and stiffness index beta (CAVI) measurements.**
(#) However, in very old adults despite high arterial stiffness, SBP does not increase or even decreases due to several geriatric conditions such as heart failure, dysautonomy, dehydration, malnutrition, etc. Since PWV is strongly related to the SBP levels at the moment of its measurements, we will obtain in this case normal/low PWV. By contrast stiffness index beta (CAVI) is able to capture the intrinsic wall stiffness, which is very little dependent on SBP levels at the moment of its measurement.

devices measuring PWV have been developed, which enabled several laboratories working in the filed to further expand clinical, pharmacological and epidemiological studies showing the usefulness of the cfPWV[12].

In the 90s also some echo-tracking techniques have been developed[13], for high-precision assessment of arterial intima-media thickness, cross sectional distensibility and compliance. While PWV was able to measure arterial stiffness in arterial segments (e.g., between carotid and femoral or between femoral and tibial arteries, etc.), the echo-tracking technique was able to measure cross-sectional elastic properties at precise arterial points (e.g., common carotid, femoral or radial arteries). This method made it possible to directly measure the changes in the pulsatile diameter of peripheral vessels, calculate their compliance and distensibility, and compare the behavior of peripheral arteries such as the femoral artery, with that of a central artery, i.e., the carotid artery[14]. Indeed, the age-related arterial stiffening mainly occurs in the aorta and the other central arteries rather than in the more peripheral arteries such as femoral, brachial and radial arteries.

C- Interest in assessing large artery stiffness in older adults: Role of arterial stiffness on CV frailty and loss of autonomy

In recent years, our group among others extended the study of vascular stiffness in older adults especially in those with increasing frailty, comorbidities and loss of functionality. We have now a large body of evidence showing that even in advanced age the more elevated the arterial stiffness, the higher the risk for CV complications and mortality. Interestingly, there is also increasing evidence that the level of arterial stiffness is associated with the development of conditions other than cardiovascular age-related degenerative diseases and syndromes such as cognitive decline, neurodegenerative diseases, sarcopenia and osteopenia, and renal failure, all together leading to frailty and loss of autonomy[15].

Thus, the extension of arterial aging, which is very variable among older people of the same age, will be a major modulator of the pace of aging by influencing age-related diseases, functional status, and autonomy especially after the age of 80 years. A limited number of studies conducted in very old adults have shown the link between increased arterial stiffness measured by PWV and cognitive decline[16]. This relationship was also observed in the PARTAGE study, a large observational study conducted in very old living in nursing homes (NHs)[17] but in this study cfPWV was not correlated with mortality[18]. Also, several studies in very old and very frail patients reported an inverse relationship between BP (both SBP and DBP) values and cognitive decline, morbidity and mortality, especially in those patients with antihypertensive treatment[19-22]. Interestingly, the PARTAGE study showed that mortality in this very old and frail population living in NHs was related to the ratio of central/peripheral BP[18] which is very weakly related to the absolute BP levels but not to PWV which was strongly related to the BP levels.

These data point out a major limitation of PWV in very

old frail patients, i.e. its strong dependency on blood pressure levels at the moment of the measurement of the PWV. In other words, as we mentioned above, heart failure, frailty, poly-medication and other geriatric conditions lead to significant BP drop and therefore PWV can be low/normal despite presence of high arterial stiffness. In these clinical profiles measuring the Cardio-Ankle Vascular Index (CAVI) has a particular interest since it can much better capture the intrinsic stiffness of the arterial wall which is much less dependent on acute BP variations (see Fig. 2).

D- Differences between PWV and CAVI methodological approaches

Although CF-PWV and CAVI both represent measures of arterial stiffness, their fundamentals differ, primarily for 2 reasons[23,24]:

a- PWV is based on the Moens-Korteweg / Bramwell-Hill equations[25] and measures the velocity of pulse waves between two arterial sites. As we mentioned above PWV depends both on the intrinsic arterial stiffness but also on the distension pressure (i.e. the blood pressure levels) at the time of measurement thus explaining a more pronounced influence of the variations in the BP during the measurement. In contrast, the CAVI corresponds to the index β, which reflects the slope of the relationship between pressure changes and volume changes[25], thus explaining why this index is much less dependent on acute pressure changes at the time of measurement. A triple A large multi-centric study[26] recently confirmed a less pronounced effect of BP levels on CAVI than on cfPWV, in line with previous observations[27]. However, it is important to repeat here that presence of chronic hypertension alters arterial structure and function increasing arterial stiffness (Fig. 2) and therefore the relative "pressure-independence" of CAVI measurements refer to BP at the time of measurement but not to chronic BP levels over time.

b- CF-PWV measures arterial stiffness mainly of the descending aorta while the CAVI estimates the stiffness of a more general area including the ascending aorta, the aortic arch, the descending aorta and the arteries of the lower limbs.

These two differences also explain why the correlation between cfPWV and CAVI, although statistically significant, remains relatively weak in the different studies[26].

In our opinion, these two characteristics make CAVI an interesting approach for the routine assessment of overall aortic stiffness especially in older adults as mentioned above. In addition, the CAVI measured with the VaSera device is easy to use, does not induce significant physical or psychological stress for very old people and allows automatic measurements without significant subjective influence by the operator. These reasons explain the increasing number of studies using this approach for the evaluation of the stiffness status of older adults[26,28].

References

1) Safar ME, Levy BI, Struijker-Boudier. Current perspectives

on arterial stiffness and pulse pressure in hypertension and cardiovascular disease. Circulation 2003;107:2864-9.

2) Lakatta E. Arterial and cardiac aging: major shareholders in cardiovascular disease enterprises: Part III: cellular and molecular clues to heart and arterial aging. Circulation. 2003;107:490-7.

3) Benetos A, Safar M, Rudnichi A, et al. Pulse pressure: A predictor of long-term cardiovascular mortality in a French male population. Hypertension 1997;30:1410-5.

4) Khattar RS, Swales JD, Dore C, Senior R, Lahiri A. Effects of aging on the prognostic significance of ambulatory systolic, diastolic and pulse pressure in essential hypertension Circulation, 2001;104:783-9.

5) Franklin SS, Larson MG, Khan SA, Wong ND, Leip EP, Kannel WB, et al. Does the relation of blood pressure to coronary heart disease risk change with aging? The Framingham Heart Study. Circulation 2001;103:1245-9.

6 Safar ME, Peronneau PA, Levenson JA, Toto-Moukouo J, Simon A. Pulsed Doppler: diameter, blood flow velocity and volumic flow of the brachial artery in sustained essential hypertension. Circulation 1981;63:393-400.

7) Simon AC, Levenson JA, Safar ME. Hemodynamic mechanisms of and therapeutic approach to systolic hypertension. J Cardiovasc Pharmacol 1985;7:S22-S27.

8) Safar ME, Laurent S, Bouthier JA, London G. Comparative effects of captopril and isosorbide dinitrate on the arterial wall of hypertensive human brachial arteries. J Cardiovasc Pharmacol 1986;8:1257-61.

9) Asmar R, Benetos A, Topouchian J, Laurent P, Pannier B, Brisac AM, et al. Assessment of arterial distensibility by automatic pulse wave velocity measurement. Validation and clinical application studies. Hypertension 1995;26:485-90.

10) Bramwell JC, Hill AV. The velocity of the pulse wave in man. Proc R Soc London Series B 1926; 93:298-306.

11) Asmar RG, London GM, O'Rourke M, Safar ME, for the REASON Project Coordinators and Investigators. Improvement in blood pressure, arterial stiffness and wave reflections with a very-low-dose perindopril/ indapamide combination in hypertensive patients: a comparison with atenolol. Hypertension. 2001;38:922-6.

12) The Reference Values for Arterial Stiffness' Collaboration. Determinants of pulse wave velocity in healthy people and in the presence of cardiovascular risk factors. Establishing normal and reference values. Eur Heart J 2010;31:2338-50.

13) Van Bortel LM, Balkestein EJ, van der Heijden-Spek JJ, Vanmolkot FH, Staessen JA, Kragten JA, et al. Non-invasive assessment of local arterial pulse pressure: comparison of applanation tonometry and echo-tracking. J Hypertens. 2001;19:1037-44.

14) Benetos A, Laurent S, Hoeks AP, Boutouyrie PH, Safar ME. Arterial alterations with aging and high blood pressure. A noninvasive study of carotid and femoral arteries. Arterioscler Thromb 1993;13:90-7.

15) Tap L, Kirkham FA, Mattace-Raso F, Joly L, Rajkumar C, Benetos A. Unraveling the Links Underlying Arterial Stiffness, Bone Demineralization, and Muscle Loss Hypertension. 2020;76:629-639.

16) Rouch L, Cestac P, Sallerin B, Andrieu S, Bailly H, Beunardeau M, et al. Pulse Wave Velocity Is Associated With

Greater Risk of Dementia in Mild Cognitive Impairment Patients. Hypertension. 2018;72:1109-1116.

17) Watfa G, Benetos A, Kearney-Schwartz A, Labat C, Gautier S, Hanon O, et al; PARTAGE study investigators. Do arterial hemodynamic parameters predict cognitive decline over a period of 2 years in individuals older than 80 Years living in nursing homes? The PARTAGE Study. J Am Med Dir Assoc 2015;16:598-602.

18) Benetos A, Gautier S, Labat C, Salvi P, Valbusa F, Marino F, et al. Mortality and cardiovascular events are best predicted by low central/periph-eral pulse pressure amplification but not by high blood pressure levels in elderly nursing home subjects: the PARTAGE. J Am Coll Cardiol 2012;60:1503-1511.

19) Aparicio LS, Thijs L, Boggia J, Jacobs L, Barochiner J, Odili AN, et al; International Database on Home Blood Pressure in Relation to Cardiovascular Outcome (IDHOCO) Investigators. Defining thresholds for home blood pressure monitoring in octogenarians. Hypertension. 2015;66:865-873.

20) Benetos A, Labat C, Rossignol P, Fay R, Rolland Y, Valbusa F, et al. Treatment with multiple blood pressure medications, achieved blood pressure, and mortality in older nursing home residents: the PARTAGE study. JAMA Intern Med. 2015;175:989-995.

21) Mossello E, Pieraccioli M, Nesti N, Bulgaresi M, Lorenzi C, Caleri V, et al. Effects of low blood pressure in cognitively impaired elderly patients treated with antihypertensive drugs. JAMA Intern Med. 2015;175:578-585.

22) Streit S, Poortvliet RKE, Gussekloo J. Lower blood pressure during antihypertensive treatment is associated with higher all-cause mortality and accelerated cognitive decline in the oldest-old-data from the Leiden 85-plus Study [published online May 8, 2018]. Age Ageing. 2018;47:545-550.

23) Shirai K, Utino J, Otsuka K, Takata M. A novel blood pressure-independent arterial wall stiffness parameter: cardio-ankle vascular index (CAVI). J Atheroscler Thromb 2006; 13:101–107.

24) Asmar R. Principles & Usefulness of the cardio Ankle vascular index (CAVI). A new global arterial stiffness index. Eur Heart J Suppl 2017; 19: B4-B10.

25) Ogawa T, Shimada M, Ishida H, Matsuda N, Fujiu A, Ando Y, et al. Relation of stiffness parameter beta to carotid arteriosclerosis and silent cerebral infarction in patients on chronic hemodialysis. Int Urol Nephrol 2009; 41:739-745.

26) Topouchian J, Labat C, Gautier S, Bäck M, Achimastos A, Blacher J, et al. Effects of metabolic syndrome on arterial function in different age groups: the Advanced Approach to Arterial Stiffness study. J Hypertens. 2018;36:824-833.

27) Gomez-Sanchez L, Garcia-Ortiz L, Patino-Alonso M, Recio-Rodriguez J, Frontera G, Ramos R, et al for the MARK group. The association between the Cardio Ankle Vascular Index and other parameters of vascular structure and function in Caucasian adults: the MARK study. J Atheroscler Thromb. 2015; 22:901-911.

28) Kirkham FA, Bunting E, Fantin F, Zamboni M, Rajkumar C. Independent Association Between Cardio-Ankle Vascular Index and Sarcopenia in Older U.K. Adults. J Am Geriatr Soc. 2019;67:317-322.

24-hour Blood Pressure Profiles and CAVI

Andrea Grillo[1] and Gianfranco Parati[2]

Introduction

Evaluation of the viscoelastic properties of arteries is becoming increasingly important in clinical medicine. Arterial stiffness is recognized not only as a determinant of blood pressure (BP) regulation, but also as an early marker of subclinical target organ damage in cardiovascular medicine. The assessment of arterial stiffness is helpful as a prognostic marker for cardiovascular events and mortality in several categories of patients even beyond routine biomarkers. In addition to the classic approaches for the assessment of carotid-femoral pulse wave velocity (PWV), another method for the evaluation of arterial stiffness was proposed, through calculation of CAVI (Cardio Ankle Vascular Index)[1], computed by combining the stiffness parameter β and the Bramwell-Hill formula[2, 3]. The PWV included in the equation is the heart-ankle PWV, making CAVI suitable to evaluate global vascular wall stiffness across the aorta, including its segments from the proximal ascending aorta down to the femoral and tibial arteries[4]. The inclusion of the β parameter in the calculation makes CAVI independent from BP values at the time of its measurement[5]. CAVI has been proposed as a suitable candidate for the routine evaluation of vascular organ damage and for the estimation of cardiovascular risk, especially in hypertensive subjects[6], and is emerging as a predictor of future cardiovascular events in longitudinal studies, independently of traditional cardiovascular risk factors[7, 8].

In the clinical management of hypertensive patients, 24 hour ambulatory BP monitoring (ABPM) represents a frequently used methodology for an accurate assessment of BP levels in daily life. ABPM provides clinically relevant information on systolic and diastolic day and night BP profiles, on ambulatory average BP levels, on dipping status (i.e. the fall in pressure between daytime and nightime), as well as on indices of BP variability (BPV) over the same time periods[9]. The latter indices are particularly relevant in relation to arterial wall properties, because BPV has been shown to be related, among other factors, also to the degree of arterial stiffness[10]. The stiffening of aorta affects the ventricular-aortic coupling and the cardiac afterload, by increasing the aortic systolic BP achieved in correspondence to each cardiac contraction. The degree of systolic BP fluctuations with increased aortic stiffness is also influenced by a possible impairment of the carotid and aortic baroreceptors activity, due to their reduced stimulation determined by the altered distensibility of stiffer arteries.

The relationship of CAVI with variables derived from analysis of 24 hour ambulatory BP profiles, and how these parameters may interact in determining the development of vascular organ damage and vascular aging in hypertensive individuals, is an important target for research. This chapter reviews the available evidence on this issue.

1. CAVI and 24-hour ambulatory blood pressure monitoring

The relationship between arterial stiffness and BP levels, and the association of high BP levels with the loss of arterial elastic properties have been widely investigated, although most of the studies have been based only on office BP measurement. On the contrary, the relationship between 24 hour BP profiles and arterial mechanical properties still needs to be explored more in detail. CAVI was indeed shown to be a pressure independent parameter for the evaluation of arterial mechanical properties, when focusing on office or clinic BP values. Since BP is subjected to continuous variations during the 24 hours, however, it would be important to investigate the possible relationship between CAVI and these dynamic features of ambulatory BP. This would also allow to overcome possible biases due to transient variations in BP at the time of office measurement and to the inherent inaccuracy of isolated office BP readings[9, 11].

1.1. Mean ambulatory BP level and arterial stiffness

In the general population as well as in hypertensive patients[12, 13], conventional measures of arterial stiffness, such as carotid-femoral PWV, are significantly related not only to conventional office BP measurements but also to 24 hour ambulatory BP levels, and have been shown to carry prognostic information. Even after adjustment for mean 24 hour BP, arterial stiffness seems to maintain its prognostic significance[12]. Whether a parameter such as CAVI, reported to be independent from office BP values, would correlate with ABPM derived mean BP values and with cardiovascular organ damage in essential hypertensive patients is still an open issue. Data from a population of essential hypertensive patients in the age range from 14 to 90 years confirmed the

[1]Azienda Sanitaria Universitaria Giuliano Isontina, Medicina Clinica, Trieste, Italy.
[2]Istituto Auxologico Italiano, IRCCS, Cardiology Unit, Milan, Italy and Department of Medicine and Surgery, University of Milano-Bicocca, Milan, Italy.

independency of CAVI from actual (office) BP values, while showing a significant relation with ambulatory pulse pressure and systolic BP[14]. The relation between CAVI and ambulatory pulse pressure lost significance after accounting for age, the strongest predictor of CAVI. These observations need however to be confirmed by further studies, which are required to clarify whether, in a hypertensive population, a BP independent measure of arterial stiffness such as CAVI relates with ambulatory BP values, an issue which has both clinical and pathophysiological relevance.

1.2. 24h ambulatory BP profile and arterial stiffness

(1) White coat or isolated office hypertension

The relationship of CAVI not only with average ambulatory BP levels over 24 hours but also with alterations in the 24h ambulatory BP profile, is also an issue that needs to be further explored. It should be emphasized that there might be substantial differences between the BP measured in the doctor's office and the average BP values recorded during the day and night, differences which allow the identification of specific BP phenotypes. When office BP is significantly higher than average ambulatory BP values this may be due to a white coat effect raising BP during a doctor's visit. As a consequence, when office BP is repeatedly above normal reference levels while 24h ambulatory BP remains within a normal range, this condition is defined as "white coat" or "isolated office" hypertension[9, 11]. Evidence is available that such a condition carries a lower risk of organ damage or events than sustained hypertension, i.e. a condition where both office and ambulatory BP are elevated. However, some studies suggest that white coat hypertension might be the sign of an alteration in the arterial tree properties that might not be entirely innocent. Indeed, a strong association was found between a surrogate measure of the white-coat effect, based on the difference between office and ambulatory BP values, and arterial stiffness, with the white-coat effect being suggested to be a clinical manifestation of increased arterial stiffness[15]. How CAVI relates with this commonly found BP phenotype is an important issue that needs to be investigated in future research.

(2) Masked hypertension

An association with an increased risk of organ damage and cardiovascular events has been reported even more clearly for an opposite condition, characterized by the occurrence of normal office BP values associated with elevated ambulatory BP levels, known as "masked hypertension"[9, 11]. This BP phenotype, which is highly prevalent in patients with conditions like obstructive sleep apnea and type-2 diabetes mellitus, has been shown to carry an independent association with arterial stiffness in such patients[16, 17]. Many common pathophysiological mechanisms and risk factors, like obesity and hypertension, are shared between masked hypertension and arterial stiffness, and can interact to increase the probability of vascular damage. As a consequence of these findings, it has been suggested that an early diagnosis of vascular wall alterations by PWV or by CAVI assessment might be helpful for a preventive management of later cardiovascular complications in masked hypertension.

(3) Circadian profile variations

It has been suggested that specific patterns of circadian variation in blood pressure may affect the risk of cardiovascular events, such as acute coronary and aortic syndromes[18-20].

a. Relationship of morning BP surge with arterial stiffness

This is the case for nocturnal BP reduction ("dipping") and for morning BP surge. In particular, the degree of morning BP surge, which can be evaluated using ABPM, has been shown to independently predict cardiovascular outcomes[21]. Evidence is also available that, in hypertensive subjects, morning BP surge is associated with arterial stiffness[22]. Similarly to ambulatory BP, which typically shows circadian BP changes over 24 hours following the wake-sleep cycle, also arterial stiffness, which is modulated by vascular tone and by BP levels, may display circadian variations. However, available studies have shown inconsistent results regarding the possible occurrence of diurnal variations in PWV[23-25], although these inconsistencies could partly reflect lack of standardization in the methodology of data collection in these papers. Interestingly, in one study, CAVI was found to be higher when measured in the morning than at other times over the 24 hours, even after adjustment for mean BP levels[26]. Current guidelines for assessing arterial stiffness[27] already recommend to standardize the time of arterial stiffness measurements in research studies, a suggestion which would apply also to CAVI measurement. Nevertheless, the available evidence on the occurrence of significant circadian variations in CAVI seems to be yet insufficient to recommend any specific time of the day for CAVI assessment in the everyday clinical practice, an issue which thus requires additional investigations to be better clarified.

b. Relationship between nocturnal BP fall and arterial stiffness

Data are also available to support the concept that the BP change from day- to night-time is an important determinant of arterial stiffness, as demonstrated by measuring aortic PWV values[13].

The relationship between arterial stiffness and dipper-status appears to be of some complexity, being characterized by J-shaped nature, with extreme-dippers and reverse-dippers having higher carotid-femoral PWV values than dippers. This relationship remains significant even after multiple adjustment for covariates, with reverse-dippers showing the highest PWV values[28]. Increased sympathetic tone at night has been suggested as a potential mechanism for this altered BP and vascular wall properties profile, being in the end responsible for the reported increase in target organ damage and for a worse cardiovascular prognosis in these patients.

c. CAVI and nocturnal BP fall.

The relationship between dipper/non-dipper pattern and elastic properties of the arterial system, was evaluated using CAVI in a study considering a large population of hypertensive diabetic patients[29]. In this study, a linear correlation between the percentage of BP nocturnal decline and CAVI was found, with considerably elevated values of

CAVI in patients with a reverse-dipping pattern. In another study[30] conducted among 183 hypertensive patients with no history of adverse cardiovascular events, a non-dipper pattern of hypertension was an independent risk factor for LV systolic dysfunction and for impaired arterial properties measured by CAVI. These results were confirmed in a cohort of non-dipper hypertensive elderly patients who showed a significantly higher CAVI[31]. Interestingly, in this latter study Vitamin D levels were independently associated with CAVI, suggesting that deficiency of Vitamin D may contribute to vascular stiffening and increase the risk of cardiovascular disease.

Current overall evidence suggests that, in the hypertensive patients and particularly in the hypertensive diabetic patients, which are already characterized by an increased cardiovascular risk, an altered dipping status and increased arterial stiffness determined by CAVI seem to be frequently associated. This condition should thus be considered by physicians to better enable risk stratification and personalized treatment strategies. The relationship of CAVI with these specific 24 hour BP pattern alterations needs to be more widely investigated in future research.

2. Blood pressure variability and CAVI

Epidemiological and observational clinical studies have repeatedly shown that cardiovascular risk is not only related to an increase in mean arterial pressure values or to alterations in the circadian pattern of BP changes, but also to the degree of short term 24h BPV independently from the contribution of the increased average values of systolic or diastolic BP[32]. Actually the degree of short term BPV has been repeatedly shown to represent an additional correlate of, and a causal factor for hypertension-related cardiovascular complications[32].

BPV consists of different components which can be assessed over different time intervals and with different methods: 1) very short term BPV, assessed by means of continuous beat-to-beat BP recordings, 2) short term BPV, assessed within a 24 hour period, by 24 hour ABPM monitoring, 3) mid-term BPV, assessed day-to-day through home BP monitoring, or 4) long term BPV, assessed visit-to-visit or across different seasons by means of repeated office BP measures or through repeated performance of home or ambulatory BP monitoring. Each of these BPV components, when showing an increase, has been related to the development or the progression of hypertensive target organ damage and to an increased risk of cardiovascular events and mortality[32].

BPV in itself is a physiological expression of spontaneous cardiovascular regulation, and reflects the degree of sympathetic activation[33], the effectiveness of cardiovascular baroreflex modulation[34] as well as the effects of other intrinsic control mechanisms, both at rest and in response to a number of environmental factors[35, 36] including physical exercise and emotional stress. The baroreflex modulation of cardiovascular homeostasis may itself affect changes in sympathetic activity[37], causing reflex changes of arterial tone and modifications of cardiac output (including vagally mediated changes in heart rate), that may affect BPV.

Indeed, a reduced arterial baroreflex sensitivity has been reported to be associated with an increased 24 hour BPV[38, 39].

2.1. Short term BPV, arterial baroreflexes and arterial stiffness

The arterial baroreflex is in fact one of the most important mechanisms for short-term control of BP. This reflex system consists of stretch receptors located in the carotid arteries, at the carotid sinus level in proximity to the origin of the internal carotid artery, as well as in the wall of the aortic arch. Actually, the aortic arch and carotid arteries are prevalently elastic vessels, particularly liable to arteriosclerotic degeneration with advancing age and in case of endothelial alterations due to atherosclerotic processes. It is important to underline that arterial baroreceptors respond to the extent of recurrent stretching/relaxation of carotid/aortic arterial walls in response to changes in pulsatile BP, rather than directly to changes in BP values themselves. Thus, in subjects with increased arterial stiffness, whose vessels are less distensible than in individuals with more elastic arteries in response to BP changes, baroreflex responsiveness will be reduced, and such a baroreflex dysfunction might affect the degree of short term BPV.

This pathophysiological hypothesis is supported by studies showing that, in animals as well as in humans, increased local carotid stiffness is associated with reduced cardiovagal baroreflex sensitivity[40, 41]. Okada et al.[42] clearly demonstrated a significant inverse correlation between the sympathetic baroreflex sensitivity and the degree of carotid stiffness as well as between sympathetic baroreflex sensitivity and aortic stiffness, assessed by carotid-femoral PWV.

Apart from the baroreflex control, BPV may be influenced directly from large artery mechanics. The passive effects of arterial mechanical properties clearly influence BP pulsatile behavior, so that in a stiff arterial system an increased stroke volume variability and an increase in sympathetic activity in response to environmental challenges may produce wider BP fluctuations, compared to what occurs in an elastic arterial system. This phenomenon can be understood by considering the "Windkessel" properties of the large arteries. In a stiffer model, stroke volume cannot be properly cushioned, and an increase in systolic BP is accompanied by a reduction in diastolic BP, resulting in a wider pulse pressure. Considering the physiological variations in stroke volume over 24 hours, short-term systolic BPV will therefore be amplified in the presence of increased large artery stiffness.

Relevant determinants of short-term BPV are therefore both the active mechanisms involved in the reflex closed-loop control of BP (i.e. the arterial baroreflex), and the passive mechanical elastic properties of large conduit arteries. These mechanisms are inextricably intertwined with each other and with other mechanisms influencing BP variations *in vivo*, such as mechanical (e.g. ventilation), neurohumoral and psychological factors, and may contribute to modify BPV in a complex manner.

However, determining the relative contribution to BPV

by large artery stiffness and fluctuations in stroke volume is made difficult by the fact that *in vivo* active and passive mechanisms of BP control are not only influenced by the above mentioned intrinsic mechanical, neurohumoral or psychological factors, but also by external, environmental factors. This has led some authors to develop models of simulated systemic circulation under controlled conditions in a laboratory setting in order to better explore the specific effect of large artery mechanics on BPV. In a recent study, Avolio et al.[43] developed a lumped parameter model of systemic circulation in order to quantify the effects of large artery stiffness on BPV due to changes in vascular (total peripheral resistance) or cardiac (stroke volume and heart rate) properties without the interference of active mechanisms involved in closed loop control (i.e. autonomic reflex modulation). This study showed that BPV is related to the degree of pressure dependency of arterial compliance. Since the stiffness of large arteries is known to increase with age and with increases in BP (i.e. distending pressure), this study also evaluated the relative contribution of these factors to BPV. It was shown that the hemodynamic effect of age-related increases in large artery stiffness is an increase in BPV, which is clearly evident in the elderly as compared to the young, when exposed to the same BP values. In other words, the effect of age-related changes in large artery stiffness seems to increase BPV in the elderly at similar pressures as in young individuals. Interestingly, the study showed that the optimal mean BP value, where BPV is minimal, is also age-dependent due to the known age-related changes of pressure dependency on aortic stiffness[44]. These findings are relevant since this phenomenon might explain the increased risk of vascular events (i.e. small vessel disease in the brain) in subjects with mean BP controlled with antihypertensive treatment, but with a persisting increase in BPV, as reported in several studies[45]. CAVI would ideally provide an easy way to evaluate the pressure-dependency of arterial stiffness, as it is derived from the β parameter, which is a measure of the exponent of the vascular BP-diameter relationship. However, the possibility to estimate the blood-pressure dependency of the arterial system by CAVI, and to relate it to short-term BPV needs to be evaluated in physiological and clinical studies.

Evidence is available that arterial stiffness and short term BPV are closely interrelated phenomena (**Fig. 1**) A reduced baroreflex sensitivity, which is a characteristic feature of the altered autonomic cardiac modulation in hypertension, might thus be one of the factors, together with the accompanying increase in arterial stiffness, responsible not only for the increased BPV typical of hypertensive subjects[46], but also for the higher speed of changes in beat-to-beat systolic BP fluctuations reported to occur in hypertensive patients as compared with normotensive individuals[47]. The effects of changes in baroreflex sensitivity on BPV should be considered in the context of the complex interactions among different mechanisms involved in cardiovascular regulation, including among them chemoreflex influences which may play a major role in conditions of hypoxia exposure.

In two large cohorts of treated and untreated patients we recently demonstrated that short-term 24 hour BPV and large artery stiffness, the latter assessed as carotid-femoral PWV, are significantly related to each other in human hypertension[10]. The relationship between short-term BPV and arterial stiffness was confirmed after excluding multiple confounding factors, and survived after accounting for differences in average BP levels, thus demonstrating the independence of this association from office and 24-h average BP. As it is possible to quantify BPV from ABPM in different ways, various measures of BPV were explored. The stronger association with carotid-femoral PWV was found with measures of BPV focusing on short-term changes of systolic BP, such as those assessed as average real variability (ARV, the average difference between successive BP measurements over 24 hours) and weighted-24 h standard deviation (i.e. the average of daytime and night-time standard deviation separately considered and weighted for the different duration of daytime and night-time, a calculation which therefore excludes the influence exerted on 24 hour standard deviation by the day-night BP changes). Indeed, both these measures of short term BPV are free from any influence by the degree of day-night BP changes. No measure of diastolic BPV was associated with arterial stiffness in this study, which is not surprising if we consider that, with the stiffening of large arteries, diastolic BP is

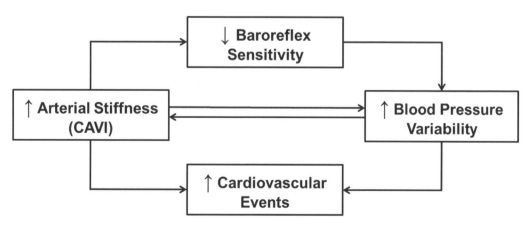

Fig. 1. Relationship between arterial stiffness, blood pressure variability, baroreflex sensitivity and cardiovascular complications.

progressively lower and less modulated.

In a recent clinical study[48] on 152 patients, aged between 20 and 49 years and free from cardiovascular disease, a multimodality investigation of central and peripheral parameters of viscoelastic arterial properties was performed in relation to indices of BPV from ABPM. A significant relationship between CAVI and BPV (measured either as weighted SD of systolic and diastolic BP or as average real variability of diastolic BP) was present. The relationship of BPV with CAVI was closer than that with other measurements of global arterial stiffness (carotid-femoral or brachial-femoral PWV), while it was weaker than the relationship of BPV with measures of central aortic stiffness obtained by magnetic resonance imaging. This is consistent with the notion that the proximal segments of aorta are the most vulnerable to vascular damage and stiffening, and that excluding these segments in the evaluation (as in the assessment of carotid-femoral or brachial-femoral PWV) may preclude obtaining important information.

An association between short-term systolic BPV parameters, obtained from ambulatory BP monitoring and PWV, has been reported also in young healthy volunteers[50].

2.2. Mid-term BPV and arterial stiffness

An association of home day-to-day BPV with PWV was also reported, independent of other known risk factors, in Japanese patients with type 2 diabetes[49]. Within-visit systolic BPV, estimated during a single clinic visit, was also found to have a closer correlation than mean SBP levels with cardiovascular risk factors and with CAVI[42]. CAVI is of particular interest in this context because, as previously discussed, it is affected by changes in wall properties of both elastic and muscular arteries, and because it is independent from mean BP levels.

Conversely, visit-to-visit systolic BPV showed no correlation with arterial stiffness, measured with CAVI, nor with mean systolic BP, in a small cohort of treated Japanese hypertensive patient. On the other hand, it showed a correlation with left ventricular diastolic dysfunction, therefore suggesting a possible role of arterial stiffness in explaining such an alteration[51].

The increasing evidence of a significant association between BPV and arterial stiffness emphasizes the importance of arterial wall property changes in relation to the effectiveness of cardiovascular control mechanisms and to the degree of hemodynamic fluctuations. These findings may suggest that attention to mean BP levels in the management of patients with arterial hypertension may not be enough to achieve cardiovascular protection. The additional assessment of the degree of BPV by ABPM and, at the same time, of the degree of arterial stiffness, appear therefore both to be clinically relevant, and the possibility of their direct association deserves to be further assessed in future studies. These studies should also include assessment of vascular wall properties through CAVI measurement, i.e. through the assessment of a parameter shown to be independent from BP levels.

Conclusions

CAVI has been proposed as a tool for the assessment of atherosclerotic cardiovascular alterations and its ability as independent predictor of cardiovascular events is now emerging[4, 7, 8]. The ability of CAVI to evaluate arterial wall properties independently from BP values at the time of measurement makes this index promising in the perspective of an accurate evaluation of how arterial stiffness translates into an alteration of the 24-hour BP profile. Current data from observational studies investigating the relationship of CAVI with 24-hour ambulatory BP levels, with indices of short-term BPV and with specific alterations in 24-hour BP profiles suggest the predictive ability of CAVI in hypertensive patients. Larger studies with long-term follow up will help to better support this suggestion in future.

References

1) Shirai K, Utino J, Otsuka K, Takata M. A novel blood pressure-independent arterial wall stiffness parameter; cardio-ankle vascular index (CAVI). J Atheroscler Thromb 2006;13:101-107.
2) Kawasaki T, Sasayama S, Yagi SI, Asakawa T, Hirai T. Non-invasive assessment of the age related changes in stiffness of major branches of the human arteries. Cardiovasc Res 1987;21:678-687.
3) Bramwell JC, Hill AV. The velocity of the pulse wave in man. P Roy Soc Lond B Bio 1922;93:298-306.
4) Hayashi K, Yamamoto T, Takahara A, Shirai K. Clinical assessment of arterial stiffness with cardio-ankle vascular index: theory and applications. J Hypertens 2015;33:1742-1757.
5) Miyoshi T, Ito H. Assessment of Arterial Stiffness Using the Cardio-Ankle Vascular Index. Pulse 2016;4:11-23.
6) Saiki A, Sato Y, Watanabe R, Watanabe Y, Imamura H, Yamaguchi T, Ban N, Kawana H, Nagumo A, Nagayama D. The Role of a Novel Arterial Stiffness Parameter, Cardio-Ankle Vascular Index (CAVI), as a Surrogate Marker for Cardiovascular Diseases. J Atheroscler Thromb 2015;23:155-168.
7) Sato Y, Nagayama D, Saiki A, Watanabe R, Watanabe Y, Imamura H, Yamaguchi T, Ban N, Kawana H, Nagumo A. Cardio-ankle vascular index is independently associated with future cardiovascular events in outpatients with metabolic disorders. J Atheroscler Thromb 2016;23:596-605.
8) Gohbara M, Iwahashi N, Sano Y, Akiyama E, Maejima N, Tsukahara K, Hibi K, Kosuge M, Ebina T, Umemura S. Clinical impact of the cardio-ankle vascular index for predicting cardiovascular events after acute coronary syndrome. Circ J 2016;80:1420-1426.
9) Parati G, Stergiou G, O'Brien E, Asmar R, Beilin L, Bilo G, Clement D, de la Sierra A, de Leeuw P, Dolan E. European Society of Hypertension practice guidelines for ambulatory blood pressure monitoring. J Hypertens 2014;32:1359-1366.
10) Schillaci G, Bilo G, Pucci G, Laurent S, Macquin-Mavier I, Boutouyrie P, Battista F, Settimi L, Desamericq G, Dolbeau G, Faini A, Salvi P, Mannarino E, Parati G. Relationship between short-term blood pressure variability and large-artery stiffness in human hypertension: findings from 2 large databases. Hypertension 2012;60:369-377.
11) O'Brien E, Parati G, Stergiou G, Asmar R, Beilin L, Bilo G, Clement D, de la Sierra A, de Leeuw P, Dolan E. European Society of Hypertension position paper on ambulatory blood pressure monitoring. J Hypertens 2013;31:1731-1768.
12) Hansen TW, Staessen JA, Torp-Pedersen C, Rasmussen S,

Thijs L, Ibsen H, Jeppesen J. Prognostic value of aortic pulse wave velocity as index of arterial stiffness in the general population. Circulation 2006;113:664-670.

13) Lekakis JP, Zakopoulos NA, Protogerou AD, Papaioannou TG, Kotsis VT, Pitiriga VC, Tsitsirikos MD, Stamatelopoulos KS, Papamichael CM, Mavrikakis ME. Arterial stiffness assessed by pulse wave analysis in essential hypertension: relation to 24-h blood pressure profile. Int J Cardiol 2005;102:391-395.

14) Giuli V, Lonati L, Guida V, Bilo G, Seravalle G, Vergani C, Parati G. Evaluation of relationship between cardio-ankle vascular index and 24h ambulatory blood pressure variables. J Hypertens, 2016;34 Suppl 2:e70.

15) de Simone G, Schillaci G, Chinali M, Angeli F, Reboldi GP, Verdecchia P. Estimate of white-coat effect and arterial stiffness. J Hypertens 2007;25:827-831.

16) Takeno K, Mita T, Nakayama S, Goto H, Komiya K, Abe H, Ikeda F, Shimizu T, Kanazawa A, Hirose T. Masked hypertension, endothelial dysfunction, and arterial stiffness in type 2 diabetes mellitus: a pilot study. American journal of hypertension 2012;25:165-170.

17) Drager LF, Diegues-Silva L, Diniz PM, Bortolotto LA, Pedrosa RP, Couto RB, Marcondes B, Giorgi DM, Lorenzi-Filho G, Krieger EM. Obstructive sleep apnea, masked hypertension, and arterial stiffness in men. Am J Hypertens 2010;23:249-254.

18) Mehta RH, Manfredini R, Hassan F, Sechtem U, Bossone E, Oh JK, Cooper JV, Smith DE, Portaluppi F, Penn M, Hutchison S, Nienaber CA, Isselbacher EM, Eagle KA. Chronobiological Patterns of Acute Aortic Dissection. Circulation 2002;106:1110-1115.

19) Muller JE, Stone PH, Turi ZG, Rutherford JD, Czeisler CA, Parker C, Poole WK, Passamani E, Roberts R, Robertson T. Circadian variation in the frequency of onset of acute myocardial infarction. N Engl J Med 1985;313:1315-1322.

20) Cohen MC, Rohtla KM, Lavery CE, Muller JE, Mittleman MA. Meta-analysis of the morning excess of acute myocardial infarction and sudden cardiac death. Am J Cardiol 1997;79:1512-1516.

21) Bilo G, Grillo A, Guida V, Parati G. Morning blood pressure surge: pathophysiology, clinical relevance and therapeutic aspects. Integr Blood Press Control 2018;24:47-56.

22) Gelos DFS, Otero-Losada ME, Azzato F, Milei J. Morning surge, pulse wave velocity, and autonomic function tests in elderly adults. Blood Press Monit 2012;17:103-109.

23) Kollias G, Stamatelopoulos K, Papaioannou T, Zakopoulos N, Alevizaki M, Alexopoulos G, Kontoyannis D, Karga H, Koroboki E, Lekakis J. Diurnal variation of endothelial function and arterial stiffness in hypertension. Journal of human hypertension 2009;23:597-604.

24) Drager LF, Diegues-Silva L, Diniz PM, Lorenzi-Filho G, Krieger EM, Bortolotto LA. Lack of circadian variation of pulse wave velocity measurements in healthy volunteers. Hum Hypertens 2011;13:19-22.

25) Ter Avest E, Holewijn S, Stalenhoef AF, de GRAAF J. Variation in non-invasive measurements of vascular function in healthy volunteers during daytime. Clin Sci (Lond) 2005;108:425-431.

26) Li Y, Cordes M, Recio-Rodriguez JI, García-Ortiz L, Hanssen H, Schmidt-Trucksäss A. Diurnal variation of arterial stiffness in healthy individuals of different ages and patients with heart disease. Scand J Clin Lab Invest 2014;74:155-162.

27) Van Bortel LM, Laurent S, Boutouyrie P, Chowienczyk P, Cruickshank JK, De Backer T, Filipovsky J, Huybrechts S, Mattace-Raso FU, Protogerou AD, Schillaci G, Segers P, Vermeersch S, Weber T, Artery S, European Society of Hypertension Working Group on Vascular S, Function, European Network for Noninvasive Investigation of Large

A. Expert consensus document on the measurement of aortic stiffness in daily practice using carotid-femoral pulse wave velocity. J Hypertens 2012;30:445-448.

28) Jerrard-Dunne P, Mahmud A, Feely J. Circadian blood pressure variation: relationship between dipper status and measures of arterial stiffness. J Hypertens 2007;25:1233-1239.

29) Kalaycioglu E, Gökdeniz T, Aykan AÇ, Gül I, Dursun I, Kiris G, Çelik S. The relationship between dipper/nondipper pattern and cardioankle vascular index in hypertensive diabetic patients. Blood Press Monit 2013;18:188-194.

30) Chen Y, Liu JH, Zhen Z, Zuo Y, Lin Q, Liu M, Zhao C, Wu M, Cao G, Wang R, Tse HF, Yiu KH. Assessment of left ventricular function and peripheral vascular arterial stiffness in patients with dipper and non-dipper hypertension. J Investig Med 2018;66:319-324.

31) Gu JW, Liu JH, Xiao HN, Yang YF, Dong WJ, Zhang QB, Liu L, He CS, Wu BH. Relationship between plasma levels of 25-hydroxyvitamin D and arterial stiffness in elderly Chinese with non-dipper hypertension: An observational study. Medicine (Baltimore). 2020;99:e19200.

32) Parati G, Ochoa JE, Lombardi C, Bilo G. Assessment and management of blood-pressure variability. Nat Rev Cardiol 2013;10:143-155.

33) Narkiewicz K, Winnicki M, Schroeder K, Phillips BG, Kato M, Cwalina E, Somers VK. Relationship between muscle sympathetic nerve activity and diurnal blood pressure profile. Hypertension 2002;39:168-172.

34) Parati G, Saul JP, Di Rienzo M, Mancia G. Spectral analysis of blood pressure and heart rate variability in evaluating cardiovascular regulation. A critical appraisal. Hypertension 1995;25:1276-1286.

35) Parati G, Ulian L, Santucciu C, Tortorici E, Villani A, Di Rienzo M, Mancia G. Clinical value of blood pressure variability. Blood Press Suppl 1997;2:91-96.

36) Parati G, Di Rienzo M, Omboni S, Ulian L, Mancia G. Blood pressure variability over 24 hours: its different components and its relationship to the arterial baroreflex. J Sleep Res 1995;4:21-29.

37) Mancia G, Mark A. Arterial baroreflexes in humans. In: Shepherd J, Abboud F, eds. Handbook of Physiology, Section 2 The Cardiovascular System IV, Volume 3, Part 2 Bethesda, MD: American Physiologic Society; 1983. p. 755-793.

38) Parati G, Di Rienzo M, Bertinieri G, Pomidossi G, Casadei R, Groppelli A, Pedotti A, Zanchetti A, Mancia G. Evaluation of the baroreceptor-heart rate reflex by 24-hour intra-arterial blood pressure monitoring in humans. Hypertension 1988;12:214-222.

39) Parati G, Di Rienzo M, Omboni S, Ulian L, Mancia G. Blood pressure variability over 24 hours: its different components and its relationship to the arterial baroreflex. J Sleep Res 1995;4:21-29.

40) Mattace-Raso FU, van den Meiracker AH, Bos WJ, van der Cammen TJ, Westerhof BE, Elias-Smale S, Reneman RS, Hoeks AP, Hofman A, Witteman JC. Arterial stiffness, cardiovagal baroreflex sensitivity and postural blood pressure changes in older adults: the Rotterdam Study. J Hypertens 2007;25:1421-1426.

41) Parati G, Lantelme P. Mechanical and neural components of the cardiac baroreflex: new insights into complex physiology. J Hypertens 2005;23:717-720.

42) Masugata H, Senda S, Inukai M, Himoto T, Hosomi N, Imachi H, Murao K, Okada H, Goda F. Relationship between arterial stiffness and variability in systolic blood pressure during a single clinic visit in patients with hypertension. J Int Med Res 2013;41:325-333.

43) Avolio AP, Xu K, Butlin M. Effect of large arteries on blood pressure variability. Engineering in Medicine and Biology

Society Annual Conference 2013;2013:4078-4081.

44) Wesseling KH, Jansen JR, Settels JJ, Schreuder JJ. Computation of aortic flow from pressure in humans using a nonlinear, three-element model. J Appl Physiol 1993;74:2566-2573.

45) Poels MM, Zaccai K, Verwoert GC, Vernooij MW, Hofman A, van der Lugt A, Witteman JC, Breteler MM, Mattace-Raso FU, Ikram MA. Arterial stiffness and cerebral small vessel disease: the Rotterdam Scan Study. Stroke 2012;43:2637-2642.

46) Mancia G, Ferrari A, Gregorini L, Parati G, Pomidossi G, Bertinieri G, Grassi G, di Rienzo M, Pedotti A, Zanchetti A. Blood pressure and heart rate variabilities in normotensive and hypertensive human beings. Circ Res 1983;53:96-104.

47) Mancia G, Parati G, Castiglioni P, Tordi R, Tortorici E, Glavina F, Di Rienzo M. Daily life blood pressure changes are steeper in hypertensive than in normotensive subjects. Hypertension 2003;42:277-282.

48) Boardman H, Lewandowski AJ, Lazdam M, Kenworthy Y, Whitworth P, Zwager CL, Francis JM, Aye CY, Williamson W, Neubauer S, Leeson P. Aortic stiffness and blood pressure variability in young people: a multimodality investigation of central and peripheral vasculature. J Hypertens 2017;35:513-522.

49) Fukui M, Ushigome E, Tanaka M, Hamaguchi M, Tanaka T, Atsuta H, Ohnishi M, Oda Y, Hasegawa G, Nakamura N. Home blood pressure variability on one occasion is a novel factor associated with arterial stiffness in patients with type 2 diabetes. Hypertens Res 2013;36:219-225.

50) Kotsis V, Stabouli S, Karafillis I, Papakatsika S, Rizos Z, Miyakis S, Goulopoulou S, Parati G, Nilsson P. Arterial stiffness and 24 h ambulatory blood pressure monitoring in young healthy volunteers: the early vascular ageing Aristotle University Thessaloniki Study (EVA-ARIS Study). Atherosclerosis 2011;219:194-199.

51) Masugata H, Senda S, Murao K, Inukai M, Hosomi N, Iwado Y, Noma T, Kohno M, Himoto T, Goda F. Visit-to-visit variability in blood pressure over a 1-year period is a marker of left ventricular diastolic dysfunction in treated hypertensive patients. Hypertens Res 2011;34:846-850.

Antihypertensive Agents and CAVI

Satoshi Morimoto and Atsuhiro Ichihara

Introduction

Hypertension increases the risk of cardiovascular complications owing to the development of arteriosclerosis. Assessment of arterial stiffness is critical in the treatment of hypertension and can be assessed by pulse pressure, augmentation index, and pulse wave velocity (PWV). However, these measures cannot be used to determine whether the improvement in arterial stiffness is due to a blood pressure (BP)-dependent or -independent mechanism. The cardio-ankle vascular index (CAVI) is a novel marker of arterial stiffness that is calculated from the PWV and adjusted according to the BP value; thus, it is independent of the BP effect[1]. Therefore, CAVI is considered extremely useful in the assessment of the efficacy of an antihypertensive treatment. In addition, studies have also revealed the effects of antihypertensive agents on CAVI. In this article, we review the available clinical data on the effect of various antihypertensive agents on CAVI.

Angiotensin-converting enzyme (ACE) inhibitors

Angiotensin II leads to vascular endothelial damage and arteriosclerosis by increasing oxidative stress through the stimulation of angiotensin type I receptors[2]. Therefore, renin-angiotensin system (RAS) inhibitors might improve arterial stiffness. The concomitant administration of perindopril, an ACE inhibitor, was investigated for 6 months in patients with no history of cardiovascular disease who had not met their BP goals with calcium-channel blockers (CCBs)[3]. Both BP and CAVI decreased significantly for these patients (**Fig. 1 A**); moreover, CAVI significantly decreased not only in the responder group with adequate BP reduction (systolic BP reduction > 20 mmHg or diastolic BP reduction > 10 mmHg) (**Fig. 1 C**) but also in the non-responder group (**Fig. 1 B**)[3]. Perindopril has strong tissue ACE inhibitory action that is independent of the BP-lowering effect[4]. Thus, perindopril might decrease CAVI by inhibiting tissue ACE activity.

Angiotensin receptor antagonists (ARBs)

We compared the effect of candesartan, an ARB, with that of CCBs on the CAVI of hypertensive patients with metabolic syndrome who had not been treated with RAS inhibitors[5]. In both groups, BP was significantly decreased, and the degree of BP reduction was not significantly different between the two groups after the 12-month treatment period. Although the CAVI was unchanged in the CCB group, it significantly decreased in the candesartan

group (**Fig. 2**)[5]. We also compared the effect of the ARB telmisartan and CCBs on CAVI in hypertensive patients who were not treated with RAS inhibitors. In both groups, BP was significantly reduced, and the degree of BP decrease was not significantly different between the two groups after the 12-month treatment period. Moreover, CAVI was unchanged in the CCB group, whereas it was significantly

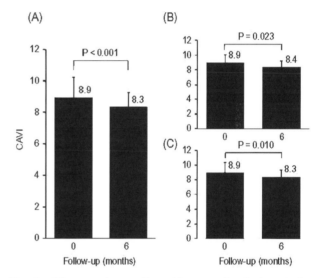

Fig. 1. Changes in cardio-ankle vascular index during the 6-month treatment with perindopril.
(A) Overall, (B) non-responder groups, (C) responder groups. Cited from Ref. 3. 【by permission of Taylor & Francis Ltd】

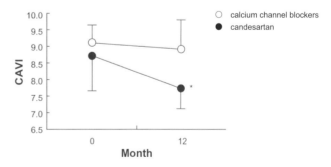

Fig. 2. Changes in the cardio-ankle vascular index during the 12-month treatment with candesartan or calcium-channel blockers. Vascular Health and Risk Management 2010; 6: 571-578; Originally published by and used with permission from Dove Medical Press Ltd[5]
*p < 0.05 vs 0 months.

Department of Endocrinology and Hypertension, Tokyo Women's Medical University, 8-1 Kawadacho, Shinjuku-ku, Tokyo 162-8666, Japan.

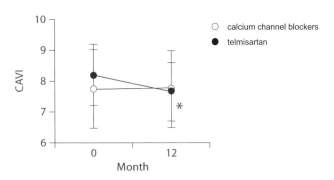

Fig. 3. Changes in the cardio-ankle vascular index during the 12-month treatment with telmisartan or calcium-channel blockers.
*p < 0.05 vs 0 months. Cited from Ref. 6. 【Copyright © 2010 Karger Publishers, Basel, Switzerland.】

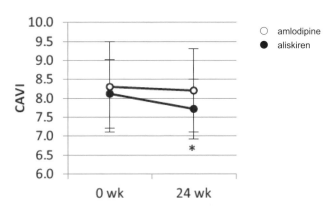

Fig. 4. Changes in the cardio-ankle vascular index during the 24-week treatment with aliskiren or amlodipine.
*p < 0.05 vs 0 weeks. Cited from Ref. 9.

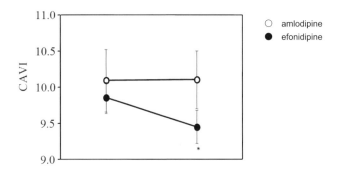

Fig. 5. Changes in the cardio-ankle vascular index during the 12-month treatment with efonidipine or amlodipine.
*p < 0.05 vs 0 months. Cited from Ref. 11.

decreased in the candesartan group (Fig. 3)[6]. In addition, in untreated hypertensive patients with concomitant type 2 diabetes mellitus, BP was significantly decreased following treatment with both olmesartan (ARB) and amlodipine (CCB), and the degree of BP reduction was similar in both groups after the 12-month treatment period[7]. Olmesartan but not amlodipine led to a significant decrease in CAVI[7].

Accordingly, ARBs are generally considered to have a CAVI-lowering effect, and a comparative study assessing these effects of ARBs has been conducted[8]. Telmisartan (40 mg/day), candesartan (8 mg/day), or losartan (50 mg/day) was administered for 12 months in patients with hypertension complicated by type 2 diabetes mellitus without RAS inhibitor treatment, and the CAVI-lowering effects of these agents were compared. BP was significantly reduced in all treatment groups with no significant difference in the degree of reduction. Although CAVI was unchanged in the telmisartan and losartan groups, it was significantly decreased in the candesartan group[8].

Direct renin inhibitor (DRI)

We investigated the effects of aliskiren, a DRI, on CAVI following 24-week administration in hypertensive patients with chronic kidney disease (CKD) without RAS inhibitor treatment. The study subjects were divided into the aliskiren group and the amlodipine group. We found that BP was significantly decreased in both groups to a similar level. Although CAVI was unchanged in the amlodipine group, it was significantly decreased in the aliskiren group (Fig. 4)[9]. Thus, aliskiren appears to have a CAVI-lowering effect similar to that of ACE inhibitors and ARBs.

Calcium-channel blockers (CCBs)

The CAVI-reducing effects of CCBs were not apparent in the studies described above[5-7, 9]. Amlodipine treatment, but not candesartan treatment, led to a significant decrease in CAVI, although both treatments showed comparable BP decreases in untreated essential hypertensive patients[10]. A previous study compared the effects of amlodipine, an L-type CCB, and efonidipine, a T-type and an L-type CCB, on type 2 diabetic patients with hypertension and nephropathy receiving ARBs. The results demonstrated that

efonidipine but not amlodipine led to a significant decrease in CAVI, while BP was significantly decreased to a similar extent in both the groups (Fig. 5)[11].

We compared the CAVI-lowering effect of olmesartan (ARB) and azelnidipine (CCB) combination therapy and olmesartan monotherapy in hypertensive patients not receiving RAS inhibitor treatment[12]. Both therapies showed similar significant reductions in BP; however, combination therapy, but not olmesartan monotherapy, led to a significant decrease in CAVI (Fig. 6)[12]. These results suggest that some CCBs have weak CAVI-lowering effects, indicating differences among CCBs regarding these effects.

Diuretics

Over a 3-month period, we compared the effects of losartan and hydrochlorothiazide (a thiazide diuretic) combination (L/HCTZ) with those of losartan alone among diabetic patients with hypertension who were not treated with RAS inhibitors[13]. The decrease in BP following L/HCTZ treatment was significantly greater than that following losartan treatment. Both treatments led to a significant decrease in CAVI to a similar extent (Fig. 7)[13]. The efficacy of a fixed-dose combination of L/HCTZ was

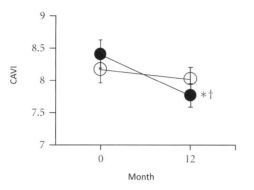

Fig. 6. Changes in the cardio-ankle vascular index during the 12-month treatment with olmesartan monotherapy or combination therapy with olmesartan and azelnidipine.
*p < 0.05 vs 0 month, †p < 0.05 vs. olmesartan monotherapy. Cited from Ref. 12.

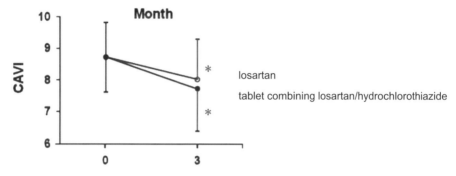

Fig. 7. Changes in the cardio-ankle vascular index during the 3-month treatment with losartan or a combination of losartan and hydrochlorothiazide.
*p < 0.05 vs 0 months. Cited from Ref. 13.

compared with that of losartan combined with controlled-release nifedipine (a CCB) for 12–16 weeks in hypertensive patients with CKD in whom medium-dose ARB monotherapy did not demonstrate sufficient antihypertensive effects[14]. The results indicated a greater reduction in BP and CAVI following treatment with losartan combined with controlled-release nifedipine[14].

Patients with hypertension who failed to achieve their target BP following treatment with the ARB olmesartan (20 mg/day) were additionally administered the CCB azelnidipine or the thiazide diuretic trichlormethiazide for 4 months. Azelnidipine and trichlormethiazide led to similar reductions in BP; moreover, although CAVI decreased following azelnidipine treatment, it remained unchanged following trichlormethiazide treatment[15].

At present, the effects of antihypertensive diuretics on CAVI have not been confirmed. However, the long-term BP-lowering effects of antihypertensive diuretics may function to suppress the increase in CAVI. Irrespective, future investigations are needed to address this concern.

Mineral corticoid receptor blocker

The mineralocorticoid receptor (MR) blocker eplerenone significantly reduces the incidenceof cardiovascular events in patients with heart failure[16]. The effects of eplerenone on CAVI in patients with hypertension was reported by Shibata et.al. They added eplerenone to the baseline medications of patients with uncontrolled hypertension and observed improvement of the degree of CAVI as early as at two

months after the beginning of treatment, independent of the blood pressure[17]. Eplerenone may directly act on the vascular wall to attenuate these processes, independent of its blood pressure-lowering actions.

Conclusion

The organ-protective effects differ among antihypertensive agents. Recent studies have revealed that different drugs have differing effects on CAVI, which might contribute to the differences in organ-protective effects among them. Moreover, a high CAVI is associated with a risk of cardiovascular events. Therefore, CAVI may be a useful surrogate marker for antihypertensive treatment, and further investigation is expected to test this presumption.

References

1) Ichihara A, Yamashita N, Takemitsu T, Kaneshiro Y, Sakoda M, Kurauchi-Mito A, et al. Cardio-ankle vascular index and ankle pulse wave velocity as a marker of arterial fibrosis in kidney failure treated by hemodialysis. *Am J Kidney Dis*, 2008; **52**: 947-55.

2) Giugliano D, Ceriello A, and Paolisso G. Oxidative stress and diabetic vascular complications. *Diabetes Care*, 1996; **19**: 257-67.

3) Watanabe Y, Takasugi E, Shitakura K, Okajima K, Hota N, Kubo Y, et al. Administration of an angiotensin-converting enzyme inhibitor improves vascular function and urinary albumin excretion in low-risk essential hypertensive patients receiving anti-hypertensive treatment with calcium channel

blockers. Organ-protecting effects independent of anti-hypertensive effect. *Clin Exp Hypertens*, 2011; **33**: 246-54. https://doi.org/10.3109/10641963.2011.583970

4) Jackson B, Cubela R, and Johnston CI. Angiotensin-converting enzyme inhibitors: measurement of relative inhibitory potency and serum drug levels by radioinhibitor binding displacement assay. *J Cardiovasc Pharmacol*, 1987; **9**: 699-704.

5) Bokuda K, Ichihara A, Sakoda M, Mito A, Kinouchi K, and Itoh H. Blood pressure-independent effect of candesartan on cardio-ankle vascular index in hypertensive patients with metabolic syndrome. *Vasc Health Risk Manag*, 2010; **6**: 571-8. https://doi.org/10.2147/vhrm.s11958

6) Kinouchi K, Ichihara A, Sakoda M, Kurauchi-Mito A, Murohashi-Bokuda K, and Itoh H. Effects of telmisartan on arterial stiffness assessed by the cardio-ankle vascular index in hypertensive patients. *Kidney Blood Press Res*, 2010; **33**: 304-12. http://dx.doi.org/10.1159%2F000316724

7) Miyashita Y, Saiki A, Endo K, Ban N, Yamaguchi T, Kawana H, et al. Effects of olmesartan, an angiotensin II receptor blocker, and amlodipine, a calcium channel blocker, on Cardio-Ankle Vascular Index (CAVI) in type 2 diabetic patients with hypertension. *J Atheroscler Thromb*, 2009; **16**: 621-6.

8) Uehara G and Takeda H. Relative effects of telmisartan, candesartan and losartan on alleviating arterial stiffness in patients with hypertension complicated by diabetes mellitus: an evaluation using the cardio-ankle vascular index (CAVI). *J Int Med Res*, 2008; **36**: 1094-102.

9) Bokuda K, Morimoto S, Seki Y, Yatabe M, Watanabe D, Yatabe J, et al. Greater reductions in plasma aldosterone with aliskiren in hypertensive patients with higher soluble (Pro)renin receptor level. *Hypertens Res*, 2018; **41**: 435-443. https://doi.org/10.1038/s41440-018-0037-1

10) Kurata M, Okura T, Watanabe S, Irita J, Enomoto D, Johtoku M, et al. Effects of amlodipine and candesartan on arterial stiffness estimated by cardio-ankle vascular index in patients with essential hypertension: A 24-week study. *Curr Ther Res*

Clin Exp, 2008; **69**: 412-22.

11) Sasaki H, Saiki A, Endo K, Ban N, Yamaguchi T, Kawana H, et al. Protective effects of efonidipine, a T- and L-type calcium channel blocker, on renal function and arterial stiffness in type 2 diabetic patients with hypertension and nephropathy. *J Atheroscler Thromb*, 2009; **16**: 568-75. https://doi.org/10.5551/jat.1628

12) Kinouchi K, Ichihara A, Bokuda K, Kurosawa H, and Itoh H. Differential Effects in Cardiovascular Markers between High-Dose Angiotensin II Receptor Blocker Monotherapy and Combination Therapy of ARB with Calcium Channel Blocker in Hypertension (DEAR Trial). *Int J Hypertens*, 2011; **2011**: 284823. https://doi.org/10.4061/2011/284823

13) Kinouchi K, Ichihara A, Sakoda M, Kurauchi-Mito A, and Itoh H. Safety and benefits of a tablet combining losartan and hydrochlorothiazide in Japanese diabetic patients with hypertension. *Hypertens Res*, 2009; **32**: 1143-7. https://doi.org/10.1038/hr.2009.162

14) Ishimitsu T, Ohno E, Nakano N, Furukata S, Akashiba A, Minami J, et al. Combination of angiotensin II receptor antagonist with calcium channel blocker or diuretic as antihypertensive therapy for patients with chronic kidney disease. *Clin Exp Hypertens*, 2011; **33**: 366-72.

15) Ishimitsu T, Numabe A, Masuda T, Akabane T, Okamura A, Minami J, et al. Angiotensin-II receptor antagonist combined with calcium channel blocker or diuretic for essential hypertension. *Hypertens Res*, 2009; **32**: 962-8.

16) Zannad F, McMurray JJ, Krum H, et al. Eplerenone in patients with systolic heart failure and mild symptoms. N Engl J Med 364:11-21, 2011.

17) Takahiro Shibata, Joshi Tsutsumi, Jun Hasegawa, Nobutaka Sato, Eitatsu Murashima, Chikara Mori, Kenichi Hongo, Michihiro Yoshimura. Effects of Add-on Therapy Consisting of a Selective Mineralocorticoid Receptor Blocker on Arterial Stiffness in Patients with Uncontrolled Hypertension. Intern Med 54: 1583-1589, 2015. DOI: 10.2169/internalmedicine.54.3427

CAVI in Diabetic Patients

Hideyuki Sasaki

Summary

1. The CAVI increases in the early stages of diabetes and partially improves with glycemic control.
2. Elevated CAVI is significantly associated with both macro-and microangiopathies (retinopathy, nephropathy, and neuropathy).

The cardio ankle vascular index (CAVI) is used worldwide as an indicator of arterial stiffness and is not depend on blood pressure at the time of measurement[1]. The author measured and compared the CAVI and brachial-ankle pulse wave velocity (baPWV) in 33 patients with diabetes mellitus (DM) and 35 participants without diabetes but with increased blood pressure induced by exercise (stair climbing) followed by stabilized blood pressure after 10 minutes of resting supine. The findings confirmed that the effect of blood pressure fluctuation was significantly less on the CAVI than on baPWV[2] (Fig. 1). This article outlines the relationship between the CAVI and DM and chronic complications of diabetes.

CAVI in DM patients is high

The CAVI in patients with type 1 and type 2 DM is higher than in participants without diabetes in the early stages of DM. Glycation, hyperinsulinemia, and autonomic dysfunction are considered possible mechanisms by which the CAVI is elevated in patients with hyperglycemia. The author investigated the effect of glycemic control on CAVI in 36 patients who had diabetes for less than 5 years and no microangiopathies. The patients were admitted to the hospital for 2 weeks for glycemic control. The association between changes in HbA1c and CAVI was observed at admission and after 8 weeks. It was found that the CAVI decreased significantly in the group with a significant improvement in HbA1c ($> 1.0\%$), but no significant change was observed in the group that showed a small improvement in HbA1c ($< 1.0\%$) (Fig. 2)[3]. This suggests that the elevated CAVI caused by chronic hyperglycemia (DM) is not only due to the organic changes but also due to functional stiffness of the arteries.

CAVI is associated with diabetic macroangiopathy

Several researchers, including the author, have reported that carotid plaque lesions and intima-media thickness (IMT) are associated with an increased CAVI in patients with diabetes[2]. A Korean retrospective study reported that

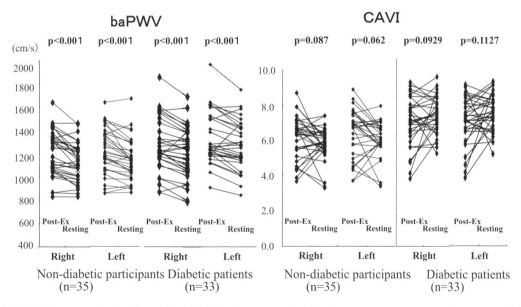

Fig. 1. The baPWV decreased significantly with the decrease in blood pressure post-exercise (post-EX) to after 10 minutes of resting in the supine position (Resting); however, the CAVI did not change significantly.

Faculty of Health Care, Kansai University of Health Science, 2-11-1, Wakaba, Kumatori-cho, Sennan-Gun, Osaka 590-0480, Japan.

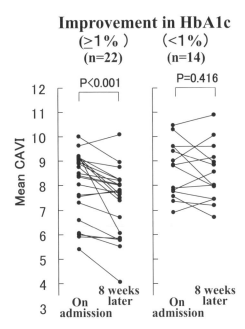

Improvement in HbA1c

Fig. 2. The CAVI decreased significantly in the group with a considerable improvement in HbA1c (>1.0%), but no significant change was observed in the group with a small improvement (<1.0%).
Adapted from ref.3

a high CAVI was a significant risk factor for cardiovascular diseases and IMT thickening (>1.1 mm) and was the most sensitive surrogate marker to detect subclinical arteriosclerosis in patients with diabetes[4]. Recently, Niwa et al. showed that the CAVI was significantly correlated with macroangiopathies, including coronary artery disease, arteriosclerosis obliterans, and stroke, in Japanese patients with diabetes[5].

CAVI may be associated with diabetic microangiopathies

① Retinopathy: Although a significant association between diabetic retinopathy and arterial stiffness has been reported, the relationship between retinopathy and CAVI has not been fully evaluated. Recently, it has been reported that abnormalities in the retinal and choroidal microvessels of patients with diabetes, quantitatively evaluated by optical coherence tomography (OCT) and OCT angiography, were significantly associated with elevated CAVI and autonomic neuropathy[6].

② Nephropathy: Patients with renal insufficiency often have hypertension and dyslipidemia, and the CAVI is expected to be high. In fact, the CAVI and eGFR showed a significant negative correlation in 881 participants in the general population, and multivariate analyses showed that the CAVI was an independent determinant of renal dysfunction[7]. High CAVI levels have also been reported to be significantly associated with microalbuminuria in patients with type 2 diabetes.

③ Neuropathy: An association between the CAVI and diabetic polyneuropathy (DPN) has been reported. Kim et al. found that the CAVI was significantly associated with DPN (diagnosed by two or more neuropathic symptoms,

10-g monofilament insensitivity, and abnormal current perception threshold) in 731 patients with diabetes[8]. Ando et al. also reported a negative correlation between the CAVI and sural nerve conduction velocity and median nerve F-wave conduction velocity in 166 patients with diabetes[9]. Elevated CAVI represents a decrease in the elasticity of the arterial wall and does not reflect a narrowing of the lumen; however, it leads to a decrease in the peripheral blood flow. An increase in the CAVI reflects decreased blood flow in the lower extremity; thus, the possibility that the decreased blood flow induces DPNs, especially the sensory and nerve conduction impairment, is contemplated. In addition, a significant relationship between a fall in the systolic blood pressure during postural change (sit-to-stand) and an increase in the CAVI has been reported in 159 patients with diabetes[10]. Therefore, CAVI may also be associated with autonomic neuropathy.

The CAVI indicates the vascular elasticity between the aorta and the arteries at the ankle, and its usefulness in the diagnosis and follow-up of diabetic macroangiopathy has been established. The associations between diabetic microangiopathies and the CAVI have also been reported; however, its pathophysiology and clinical significance are yet to be elucidated. Since renal failure is a risk factor for arteriosclerosis, the CAVI is high in patients with advanced diabetic nephropathy. In addition, the association between DPN and CAVI suggests that decreased blood flow in the lower extremities is related to the development of DPN. Further research is necessary to understand the significance of the CAVI in the clinical treatment of diabetes.

Dr. Hideaki Sasaki passed away in July, 2021. We would like to express our thanks for his contribution to the study on CAVI, and to express our sincere condolences.

References

1) Asmar R. Principles and usefulness of the cardio-ankle vascular index (CAVI): a new global arterial stiffness index. European Heart J. 2017; 19: B4–B1.
2) Ibata J, Sasaki H, Kakimoto T, et al. Cardio-ankle vascular index measures arterial wall stiffness independent of blood pressure. Diabetes Res Clin Pract. 2008; 80: 265-270.
3) Ibata J, Sasaki H, Hanabusa T, et al. Increased arterial stiffness is closely associated with hyperglycemia and improved by glycemic control in diabetic patients. J Diabetes Invest. 2013; 4: 82-87. https://doi.org/10.1111/j.2040-1124.2012.00229.x
4) Park SY, Chin SO, Rhee SY, et al. Cardio-ankle vascular index as a surrogate marker of early atherosclerotic cardiovascular disease in Koreans with type 2 diabetes mellitus. Diabetes Metab J. 2018; 42: 285-295.
5) Niwa H, Takahashi K, Dannoura M, et al. The association of cardio-ankle vascular index and ankle-brachial index with macroangiopathy in patients with type 2diabtes. J Atheroscler Thromb. 2018; 26: 616-623.
6) Kim M, Kim RY, Kim JY, et al. Correlation of systemic arterial stiffness with changes in retinal and choroidal microvasculature in type 2 diabetes. Sci Rep. 2019; 9: 1401. https://doi.org/10.1038/s41598-018-37969-7
7) Kubozono T, Miyata M, Ueyama K, et al. Association between arterial stiffness and estimated glomerular filtration rate in the Japanese general population. J Atheroscler

Thromb. 2009; 16: 840-845.

8) Kim ES, Ahn CW, Moon S, et al. Diabetic peripheral neuropathy is associated with increased arterial stiffness without changes in carotid intima–media thickness in type 2 diabetes. Diabetes Care. 2011; 34: 1403-1405.

9) Ando A, Miyamto M, Kotani K, et al. Cardio-ankle vascular index and indices of diabetic polyneuropathy in patients with type 2 diabetes. J Diabet Res. 2017; 2017. https://doi.org/10.1155/2017/2810914

10) Kobayashi Y, Fujikawa T, Kobayashi H, et al. Relationships between arterial stiffness and blood pressure drop during the sit-to-stand test in patients with diabetes mellitus. J Atheroscler Thromb. 2017; 24: 147-156.

CAVI Epidemiology: Diabetes Mellitus

Tsukasa Namekata

Purpose

This section describes a method for examining the association of the cardio-ankle vascular index (CAVI) with established cardiovascular disease (CVD) risk factors, including diabetes mellitus.

Method

Subjects were 9,881 male and 12,033 female company employees and their families, aged 20 years and over who participated in CVD screening in Japan. For the sake of brevity, I focus on the procedure of converting CAVI scores (a continuous variable) to a binary variable for logistic regression analysis. Details are described in reference 1. To examine the association of CAVI with CVD risk factors, CAVI scores of screening participants were stratified as shown in Table 1, according to the means and standard deviations (SDs) of CAVI scores of 2,239 men and 3,730 women without clinical CVD-related abnormalities. All CAVI scores were converted to 1 for scores less than (mean − 1 SD), 2 for scores between (mean − 1 SD) and (mean − ½ SD), 3 for scores between (mean − ½S D) and mean, 4 for scores between mean and (mean + ½ SD), 5 for scores between (mean + ½ SD) and (mean + 1 SD), and 6 for scores greater than (mean + 1 SD). Based on the distribution of CAVI scores by coronary heart disease (CHD) status, there was a substantial increase in CHD cases for CAVI scores ≤ 5–6: the prevalence of CHD corresponding to codes 1, 2, 3, 4, 5, and 6 was 1.9%, 1.2%, 1.8%, 2.8%, 2.7%, and 4.6%, respectively, among men, and was 2.1%, 2.8%, 2.6%, 3.8%, 2.7%, and 4.7%, respectively, among women. Thus, we coded CAVI scores as a binary

variable: 1 for codes 1–5 (combined as normal) and 2 for code 6 (as an abnormally high CAVI score) to conduct logistic regression analysis.

Results

Table 2 shows odds ratios (ORs) of abnormally high CAVI scores for each CVD risk factor after adjusting for age among men. Significantly high ORs were found in persons with hypertension, 8.37 (95% confidence interval [CI]: 7.32–9.56), and in persons with diabetes mellitus, 10.02 (95%CI: 8.74–11.49). All other CVD risk factors had significant ORs ranging from 1.20 (95%CI: 1.05–1.36) in ex-smokers to 3.37 (95%CI: 2.72–4.18) for a body mass index ≥ 30 kg/m^2. Only high-density lipoprotein cholesterol (HDL-C) showed negative or protective ORs: 0.19 (95%CI: 0.17–0.23) for persons with HDL-C 40–59 mg/dL and 0.20 (95%CI: 0.17–0.24) for those with HDL-C ≥ 60 mg/dL, as compared with the reference category of HDL-C. A similar trend was found in females, as shown in Table 3, except that significantly high ORs were found in both current smokers, 2.25 (95%CI: 1.98–2.56) and ex-smokers, 2.42 (95%CI: 2.11–2.79), as compared to nonsmokers.

Discussion

The highest ORs appeared in the association between CAVI and diabetes in both sexes: 10.02 for males and 8.42 for women. This implies that, among CVD risk factors, diabetes most critically contributes to the advancement of stiffness and arteriosclerosis of the artery.

Table 1, which shows the baseline CAVI values of 2,239

Table 1. Baseline values of CAVI scores: comparison of average cardio-ankle vascular index (CAVI) scores of CVD risk-free subjects by age and sex.

Age (years)	Sex	Mean (M)	SD	M-1SD	M-0.5SD	M+0.5SD	M+1SD
20–29	Males	6.69	0.70	5.99	6.34	7.04	7.39
	Females	6.57	0.66	5.91	6.24	6.90	7.23
30–39	Males	7.12	0.68	6.44	6.78	7.46	7.80
	Females	6.79	0.63	6.16	6.48	7.11	7.42
40–49	Males	7.59	0.70	6.89	7.24	7.94	8.29
	Females	7.29	0.66	6.63	6.96	7.62	7.95
50–59	Males	8.07	0.76	7.31	7.69	8.45	8.83
	Females	7.82	0.70	7.12	7.47	8.17	8.52
60–69	Males	8.73	0.81	7.92	8.33	9.14	9.54
	Females	8.26	0.72	7.54	7.90	8.62	8.98
≥ 70	Males	9.35	1.00	8.35	8.85	9.85	10.35
	Females	8.71	0.75	7.96	8.34	9.09	9.46

Note: SD denotes standard deviation. Cited from Table 2 of reference 1.

Pacific Rim Disease Prevention Center, P.O.Box 25444, Seattle, WA 98165-2344, USA.

Table 2. Estimated risk for having abnormally high CAVI scores after adjusting for age: Males.

CVD risk factors	Reference	Covariates	persons at risk	Odds ratio		lower CI	upper CI
Hypertension	No	Yes	755	8.37	***	7.32	9.56
Diabetes Mellitus	No	Yes	548	10.02	***	8.74	11.49
Total cholesterol	<200mg/dL	200–239	2128	1.01		0.87	1.18
		≥ 240	862	1.88	***	1.56	2.26
HDL-C	<40mg/dL	40–59	4859	0.19	***	0.17	0.23
		≥ 60	4369	0.20	***	0.17	0.24
Triglycerides	<150mg/dL	150–199	1319	2.76	***	2.43	3.14
		≥ 200	1609	2.85	***	2.53	3.22
Body mass index	20-22.9	< 20	1012	2.04	***	1.72	2.41
		23–24.9	2453	0.94		0.82	1.08
		25–27.9	2205	0.90		0.78	1.04
		28–29.9	563	2.31	***	1.89	2.83
		≥ 30	429	3.37	***	2.72	4.18
Drinking	Non-drinkers	1–2 times/week	2151	1.12		0.96	1.31
		3–4 times/week	1183	1.81	***	1.53	2.14
		5–6 times/week	1216	1.87	***	1.58	2.21
		Every day	2852	1.22	**	1.06	1.40
Smoking	Non-smokers	Current smokers	4457	1.05		0.94	1.19
		Ex-smokers	2481	1.20	**	1.05	1.36

Note: *p < 0.05, **p < 0.01, ***p < 0.001, CI: Confidence Interval. Cited from Table 5 of reference 1.

Table 3. Estimated risk for having abnormally high CAVI scores after making adjustment for age: Females.

CVD risk factors	Reference	Covariates	persons at risk	Odds ratio		lower CI	upper CI
Hypertension	No	Yes	477	6.57	***	5.67	7.61
Diabetes	No	Yes	229	8.42	***	7.22	9.81
Total cholesterol	< 200 mg/dL	200–239	3793	1.13		0.99	1.29
		≥ 240	2276	1.33	***	1.15	1.54
HDL-C	< 50	50–59	1667	0.47	***	0.38	0.57
		≥ 60	9722	0.33	***	0.28	0.39
Triglycerides	< 150 mg/dL	150–199	608	2.89	***	2.46	3.40
		≥ 200	402	4.30	***	3.60	5.14
Body mass index	20–22.9	< 20	3992	1.43	***	1.28	1.60
		23–24.9	1677	1.17	*	1.01	1.35
		25–27.9	1091	0.98		0.82	1.17
		28–29.9	274	2.60	***	2.01	3.38
		≥ 30	272	2.45	***	1.87	3.20
Drinking	Non-drinkers	1–2 times/week	2473	1.05		0.93	1.19
		3–4 times/week	940	1.81	***	1.54	2.13
		5–6 times/week	654	2.50	***	2.10	2.99
		Every day	884	2.06	***	1.75	2.41
Smoking	Non-smokers	Current smokers	1430	2.25	***	1.98	2.56
		Ex-smokers	1080	2.42	***	2.11	2.79

Note: * p < 0.05, **p < 0.01, ***p < 0.001, CI: Confidence Interval. Cited from Table 6 of reference 1.

CVD risk-free men and 3,730 CVD risk-free women, can be used to stratify CAVI scores for screening participants by age and sex in studies of CVD and CAVI screening in more than 50 individuals using logistic regression analysis. Since it is difficult to find such a large number of CVD risk-free persons, and as the baseline CAVI scores can be applied to any racial population, the procedures described here can be used in logistic regression analysis to estimate risks of CVD factors associated with CAVI in different populations.

References

1) Namekata T, Suzuki K, Ishizuka N, et al. Association of Cardio-Ankle Vascular Index with cardiovascular disease risk factors and coronary heart disease among Japanese urban workers and their families. J Clin Exper Cardiol 2012; S1:003. http://dx.doi.org/10.4172/2155-9880.S1-003 SAGE as the original publissher. https://journals.sagepub.com/

2) Namekata T, Suzuki K, Ishizuka N, Shirai K. Establishing baseline criteria of cardio-ankle vascular index as a new indicator of arteriosclerosis: a cross-sectional study. BMC Cardiovasc Dis 2011; 11:51. http://www.biomedcentral.com/1471-2261/11/51

Diabetes Treatment and CAVI

Masahiro Ohira

Summary

1. Improving insulin resistance leads to improved CAVI.
2. Improvements in postprandial hyperglycemia also lead to improvements in the CAVI.

Introduction

Diabetes causes macrovascular complications, such as myocardial infarction and cerebral infarction. Therefore, diabetes is one of the factors that exacerbates Cardio-Ankle Vascular Index (CAVI), and CAVI improves with the treatment of diabetes. This article reviews the changes in CAVI caused by antidiabetic drugs.

Changes in CAVI with antidiabetic drugs.

a. Sulfonylurea (SU)

SU drugs act on pancreatic β cells to stimulate insulin secretion and exert antidiabetic effects. We reported that in a study comparing non-pharmacologically treated patients with type 2 diabetes mellitus treated with glimepiride 1.5 mg/day or glibenclamide 1.25 mg/day, CAVI improved only with glimepiride, despite a similar reduction in HbA1c with either drugs (Fig. 1)[1]. The effect of glimepiride on oxidative stress might be due to the difference in the effects of both drugs on CAVI[1]. Furthermore, glimepiride is known to increase insulin sensitivity[2], and this action may influence the CAVI. Comparisons with both drugs indicate

that the effects on improving blood glucose levels might not necessarily be the same for improving vascular toxicity in diabetes mellitus.

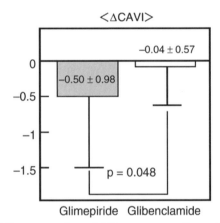

Fig. 1. Changes in CAVI upon glimepiride or glibenclamide administration. Cited from ref.1

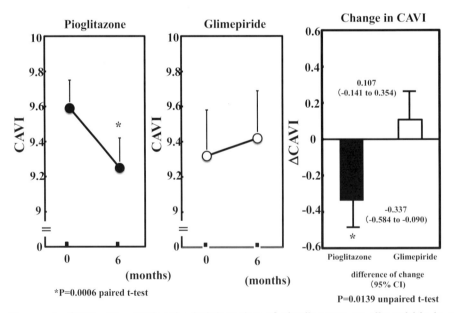

Fig. 2. Change in CAVI with additional administration of pioglitazone or glimepiride in patients with type 2 diabetes who are already treated with metformin. Diabetes, Metabolic Syndrome and Obesity : Targets and Therapy 2014:7 313-319; Originally published by and used with permission from Dove Medical Press Ltd[3]

Division of Diabetes, Metabolism and Endocrinology, Department of Internal medicine, Toho University Ohashi Medical Center, 2-17-6 Ohashi, Meguro, Tokyo, 153-8515, Japan.

b. Thiazolidines

Thiazolidinediones enhance insulin-induced uptake of glucose into skeletal muscle, inhibit hepatic gluconeogenesis, and decrease insulin levels with blood glucose. In addition, insulin sensitivity is strengthened in adipocytes through differentiation into the maturation adipocyte, the expression lowering action of the inflammatory cytokine, and the adiponectin expression enhancement action. It is a drug that exerts a hypoglycemic effect through these actions.

Administration of pioglitazone 15 mg daily, not glimepiride 1 mg daily, improved CAVI in type 2 diabetes patients already receiving metformin 500 mg daily (Fig. 2)[3]. When administered alone, glimepiride improved CAVI in relation to its insulin-resistant ameliorating effect[1]. However, in this study, the ameliorating effect of glimepiride on insulin resistance has not been recognized[3]. Because glimepiride may be incapable of reducing insulin resistance in patients with type 2 diabetes who are already treated with metformin, there may have been no improvements in CAVI with glimepiride.

c. DPP-4(Dipeptidyl Peptidase-4) inhibitor

When orally ingested glucose reaches the intestinal tract, glucose-dependent insulinotropic polypeptide (GIP) and glucagon-like peptide-l (GLP-l) are secreted from the gastrointestinal tract. GIP and GLP-1 act on pancreatic β cells to promote insulin secretion, but they are rapidly degraded and lose their bioactivity by DPP-4 (dipeptidyl peptidase-4). DPP-4 inhibitors inhibit the activity of DPP-4 and exert hypoglycemic effects by inhibiting the inactivation of GIP and GLP-1. The DPP-4 inhibitor, anagliptin (200 mg/day or 400 mg/day), significantly improved CAVl (Fig. 3)[4]. In this study, anagliptin also improved lipids such as low-density lipoprotein cholesterol (LDL-C), malondialdehyde-modified LDL (MDA-LDL), and remnant-like particle cholesterol (RLP-C)[3]. Changes in CAVI were correlated with improvements in the RLP-C[4]. In addition to improving glucose metabolism, anagliptin has a lipid-improving effect[5], and this characteristic seems to contribute to the improvement of vascular function.

d. Sodium-glucose cotransporter-2 (SGLT-2) Inhibitors

SGLT-2 inhibitors exert hypoglycemic effects by inhibiting the reabsorption of glucose in the renal tubules. In patients with type 2 diabetes treated with DPP-4 inhibitors, switching the DPP-4 inhibitor to the SGLT-2 inhibitor tofogliflozin 20 mg/day significantly improves CAVI (Fig. 4)[6], and improvement of uric acid correlates with changes in CAVI. Although there are factors beyond uric acid that improve CAVI, uric acid levels are known to be associated with CAVI[7]. However, luseogliflozin does not change CAVI in patients with type 2 diabetes patients[8]. Further studies are needed to clarify the relationship between SGLT-2 inhibitors and CAVI.

e. Insulin

Although human insulin was used in the past, analog preparations have been used frequently in recent years. Improvement of postprandial blood glucose is expected by

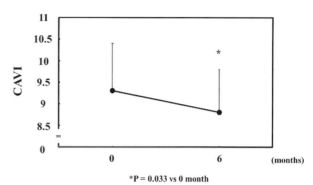

*P = 0.033 vs 0 month

Fig. 3.   Change in CAVI after administration of anagliptin.

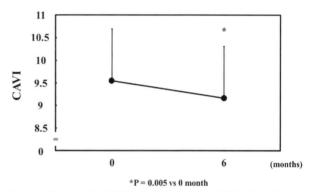

*P = 0.005 vs 0 month

Fig. 4.   Change in CAVI after switching DPP-4 inhibitor to tofogliflozin.

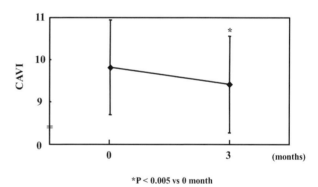

*P < 0.005 vs 0 month

Fig. 5.   Change in CAVI after switching from premixed human insulin 30/70 to biphasic insulin aspart 30/70. [with permission of Elsevier][9]

switching the rapid-acting human insulin, which is the human insulin, to the rapid-acting insulin, which is the analog preparation. In patients with type 2 diabetes, switching premixed human insulin 30/70 to biphasic insulin aspart 30/70 significantly reduces CAVI (Fig. 5)[9]. Improvement of 1,5-AG (anhydroglucitol) is correlated with the improvement of CAVI, and it is considered that the improvement of postprandial blood glucose improves vascular function[9].

Conclusions

The effects of various antidiabetic drugs on CAVI are outlined. The degree of glycemic control and degree of improvement in CAVI were not identical among the various drugs. Diabetes treatment indiscriminately has as primary objective to lower blood glucose levels, as well as to prevent vasculopathy. However, given the lack of a sensitive and simple test required to assess vasculopathy prevention, large prospective studies have been conducted over several years, and each reported different efficacies in preventing vasculopathy. If there are differences in CAVI improvements and their relationships with large prospective studies, internists might be able to measure the CAVI to determine the likelihood of future complications. We expect future investigations in this area.

Future issues: Some drugs, such as GLP-1 receptor agonists, have not yet been shown to be effective against CAVI and should be investigated.

References

1) Nagayama D, Saiki A, Endo K, et al. Improvement of cardio-ankle vascular index by glimepiride in type 2 diabetic patients. Int J Clin Pract. 2010;64:1796-1801. https://doi.org/10.1111/j.1742-1241.2010.02399.x

2) Mori, S M Hirabara, A E Hirata, M M Okamoto, U F Machado. Glimepiride as insulin sensitizer: increased liver and muscle responses to insulin, Diabetes Obes Metab. 2008;10:596-600.

3) Ohira M, Yamaguchi T, Saiki A, et al. Pioglitazone improves the cardio-ankle vascular index in patients with type 2 diabetes mellitus treated with metformin. Diabetes Metab Syndr Obes. 2014;7:313-319. https://doi.org/10.2147/dmso.s65275

4) Tahara N, Yamagishi SI, Bekki M, et al. Anagliptin, A Dipeptidyl Peptidase-4 Inhibitor Ameliorates Arterial Stiffness in Association with Reduction of Remnant-Like Particle Cholesterol and Alanine Transaminase Levels in Type 2 Diabetic Patients. Curr Vasc Pharmacol. 2016;14:552-562.

5) Nishio S, Abe M, Ito H. Anagliptin in the treatment of type 2 diabetes: safety, efficacy, and patient acceptability. Diabetes Metab Syndr Obes. 2015;8:163-171.

6) Bekki M, Tahara N, Tahara A, et al. Switching dipeptidyl peptidase-4 inhibitors to tofogliflozin, a selective inhibitor of sodium-glucose cotransporter 2 improves arterial stiffness evaluated by cardio-ankle vascular index in patients with type 2 diabetes: a pilot study. Curr Vasc Pharmacol. 2019;17:411-420.

7) Nagayama D, Yamaguchi T, Saiki A, et al. High serum uric acid is associated with increased cardio-ankle vascular index (CAVI) in healthy Japanese subjects: a cross-sectional study. Atherosclerosis. 2015;239:163-168.

8) Kario K, Okada K, Murata M, et al. Effects of luseogliflozin on arterial properties in patients with type 2 diabetes mellitus: The multicenter, exploratory LUSCAR study. J Clin Hypertens. 2020;22:1585-1593. doi: 10.1111/jch.13988.

9) Ohira M, Endo K, Oyama T, et al. Improvement of postprandial hyperglycemia and arterial stiffness upon switching from premixed human insulin 30/70 to biphasic insulin aspart 30/70. Metabolism. 2011;60:78-85. https://doi.org/10.1016/j.metabol.2010.06.001

Dyslipidemia and its Treatments

Daiji Nagayama

Summary

1. CAVI was positively correlated with LDL cholesterol, non-HDL cholesterol, total cholesterol, and triglycerides and negatively correlated with HDL cholesterol.
2. Young patients with heterozygous familial hypercholesterolemia did not necessarily show high CAVI values, but those with high CAVI (> 9) often showed severe coronary atherosclerosis.
3. The administration of eicosapentaenoic acid, bezafibrate, pitavastatin, and ezetimibe improved the CAVI.
4. It has been reported that the decrease in the CAVI with pitavastatin therapy was associated with the prevention of cardiovascular events. Further studies on the pleiotropic effects of statins using the CAVI might be required.

Introduction

Dyslipidemia, including hyper-LDL cholesterolemia, hypertriglyceridemia, or hypo-HDL cholesterolemia, are known to be risk factors for the progression of atherosclerosis. In particular, familial hypercholesterolemia (FH) causes a significant progression of atherosclerosis. However, comparisons between the atherogenicity of various lipids and/or lipoprotein cholesterols are not easy because the evaluation of the degree of atherosclerosis in each person cannot be detected by conventional indices or markers in routine clinical practice. CAVI could indicate the degree of arteriosclerosis quantitatively. We studied the relationship of various lipids and/or lipoprotein cholesterols with the CAVI

in Japanese workers and their families and tried to define the cut-off values of lipids and/or lipoprotein cholesterols in terms of the CAVI.

In the last twenty years, various lipid-lowering agents with different mechanisms of action have been developed and used worldwide. The purpose of treatment for dyslipidemia is to prevent or improve the atherosclerosis. To prove it, many large-scale clinical trials had been performed by evaluating the incidences of mortality and morbidity. To compensate or support the results of those studies, studies using the CAVI might be helpful. In this chapter, we summarize the effects of various lipid-lowering agents on the CAVI. In addition, the prospective role of decreasing the

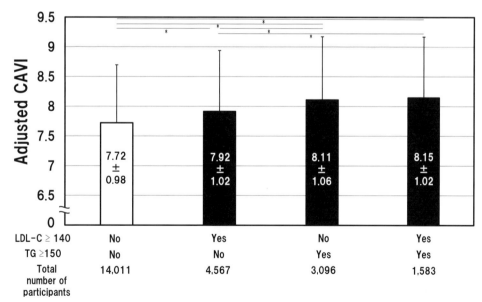

Fig. 1. Comparison of adjusted CAVI between the three types of dyslipidemia.

23,257 healthy Japanese subjects; 54.7% men, 47 ± 13 years, TG: 113 ± 95 mg/dl, LDL-C: 121 ± 34 mg/dl.
The CAVI was adjusted by gender, age, sBP, and BMI. Data are presented as mean ± SD.
*P <0.01: one-way ANOVA followed by Bonferroni multiple comparison test.
Adapted from Ref. (1).

Nagayama Clinic, 2-12-22, Tenjin-Cho, Oyama-City, Tochigi 323-0032, Japan

CAVI by pitavastatin, one of the strong statins, is discussed.

1. The relationship between serum lipids and/ or lipoprotein cholesterols with the CAVI in Japanese workers and their families

We reported the relationships of each lipid parameter with the CAVI in 23,257 Japanese workers and their families (12,729 males and 10,528 females, mean age 47.1 years) with no history of heart disease or therapeutic interventions for metabolic disorders[1]. In the total sample, 5.0% had hypo-HDL cholesterolemia [HDL cholesterol (HDL-C) < 40 mg/dl], 24.8% had hypertriglyceridemia [fasting triglyceride (TG) ≥ 150 mg/dl], and 20.1% had hyper-LDL cholesterolemia [LDL cholesterol (LDL-C) ≥

140 mg/dl]. After adjusting for confounders, including gender, age, systolic blood pressure, and body mass index (BMI), the multiple regression analysis showed that the adjusted CAVI was lower in normolipidemic participants than in dyslipidemic patients (**Fig. 1**). The combination of hyper-LDL cholesterolemia and hypertriglyceridemia was the type of dyslipidemia with the highest risk.

A trend test detected linear relationships between the adjusted CAVI and TC, LDL-C, non-HDL-C, TG, and HDL-C. It was seen that the adjusted CAVI was correlated positively with LDL-C, non-HDL-C, and TG and negatively with HDL-C (Fig. 2-5). The adjusted CAVI was rising up to LDL-C = 160 mg/dl, to non-HDL-C = 190 mg/dl, and to TG = 140 mg/dl, and is declining to HDL-C ≥ 90 mg/dl.

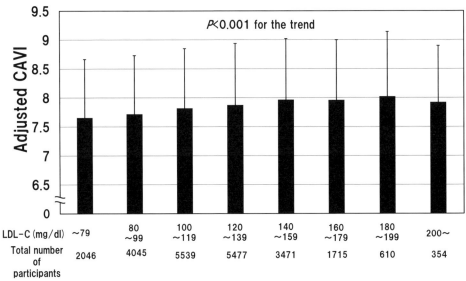

Fig. 2. Relationship between adjusted CAVI and LDL-C.
The CAVI was adjusted by gender, age, sBP, and BMI. Data are presented as mean ± SD. P value for trend by one-way ANOVA. Adapted from Ref. (1).

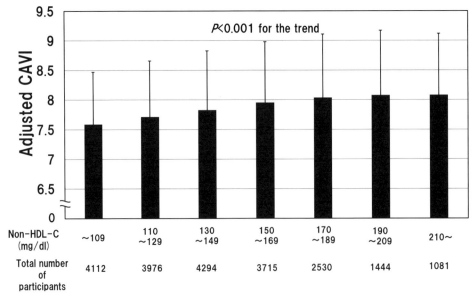

Fig. 3. Relationship between adjusted CAVI and Non-HDL-C.
The CAVI was adjusted by gender, age, sBP and BMI. Data are presented as mean ± SD. P value for trend by one-way ANOVA. Adapted from Ref. (1).

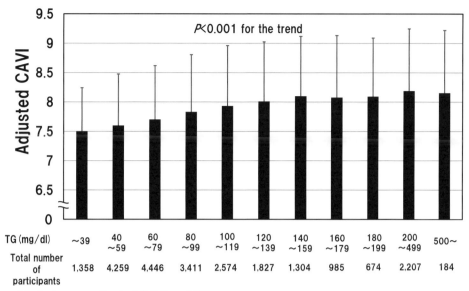

Fig. 4. Relationship between adjusted CAVI and TG.
The CAVI was adjusted by gender, age, sBP and BMI. Data are presented as mean ± SD. P value for trend by one-way ANOVA. Adapted from Ref. (1).

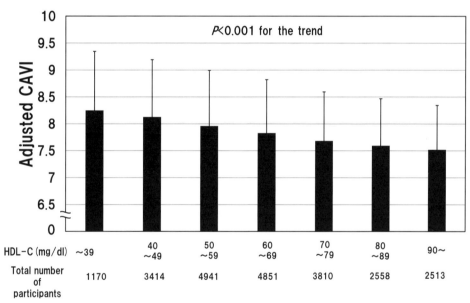

Fig. 5. Relationship between adjusted CAVI and HDL-C.
The CAVI was adjusted by gender, age, sBP and BMI. Data are presented as mean ± SD. P value for trend by one-way ANOVA. Adapted from Ref. (1)

Then, CAVI reached its peaks over those levels. In other words, the positive correlations disappeared over those ranges, and CAVI did not increase much more. In the pathophysiology of atheroma formation, the initial stage is lipidosis, and a complicated lesion is formed later. At the stage of lipidosis, the CAVI might not be elevated. This point will be discussed in a subsequent chapter.

We also analyzed the relationship between various types of lipids and CAVI. After adjusting for confounders, the logistic regression models showed that all lipid parameters contributed independently to a high CAVI (≥ 90th percentile), which was approximately equivalent to the cut-off value for coronary artery disease (CAD). The ROC analysis determined reliable cut-off values of 93 mg/dl for

TG [area under the curve (AUC) = 0.735], 114 mg/dl for LDL-C (AUC = 0.614), and 63 mg/dl for HDL-C (AUC = 0.728) in predicting a high CAVI. These cut-off values of lipid parameters were confirmed to independently predict a high CAVI in a bivariate logistic regression model, indicating a possible association between lipid parameters and early vascular damage.

2. FH and CAVI

As previously mentioned, each lipid parameter is independently associated with the CAVI. However, several studies have reported that the CAVI was not necessarily high in heterozygous patients with FH[2)].

With respect to the pulse wave velocity (PWV), an index

of arterial stiffness, Reiner et al.[3] performed 8 meta-analyses and reported that patients with FH did not have a significantly altered PWV compared with normo-cholesterolemic individuals. However, this meta-analysis indicated that carotid intima-media thickness increased in patients with FH. From these reports, it can be inferred that the arterial tree from the origin of the aorta to the ankle did not become rigid in the initial stage in patients with FH. However, Suzuki reported that the CAVI in patients with FH who took interventional treatment for CAD was extremely high. One of the interpretations is that the initial stage of an atheromatous lesion is the deposition of cholesterol in the intima, forming a fatty streak. In this stage, the arterial stiffness might decrease due to the infiltration of the lipids into the arterial wall. This is followed by an inflammatory reaction leading to vascular smooth muscle cell proliferation and foam cell formation. A fibromuscular lesion is formed as a result, in which macrophages congregate to form a complicated lesion. The increase in the CAVI in patients with dyslipidemia may be attributed primarily to these pathological changes inherent in the vascular wall.

3. Treatment with lipid-lowering agents and CAVI

As stated at the beginning of this chapter, our data demonstrated that TG, HDL-C, and LDL-C each affect CAVI independently.

Moreover, it has been reported that some drugs used in the treatment of dyslipidemia can improve the CAVI.

3-1. Eicosapentaenoic acid (EPA, n-3 polyunsaturated fatty acids)

Satoh et al. reported that EPA might reduce CAVI in Japanese subjects with obesity[4]. Three months of treatment with EPA significantly reduced the levels of immunoreactive insulin, TG, serum amyloid A-low-density lipoprotein (SAA-LDL) as a marker of oxidized LDL, C-reactive protein (CRP), and CAVI (7.87 to 7.59) and increased the serum levels of adiponectin compared to those in the control group. Stepwise multivariate linear regression analysis revealed that the only significant determinant for a decrease in the CAVI by EPA is the reduction in SAA-LDL (P < 0.05), suggesting that the decrease in oxidized LDL modification is a part of the mechanism of the anti-atherogenic effect of EPA.

3-2. Bezafibrate

It has been reported that fibrates that are typical TG-lowering agents also decreased the CAVI[5]. We conducted a multicenter, open-label, randomized controlled trial that involved a head-to-head comparison between bezafibrate 400 mg/day and EPA 1.8 g/day. This trial enrolled 66 patients with hypertriglyceridemia and type 2 diabetes, who were assigned to the respective treatment groups for 12 weeks. The levels of serum TG, remnant-like particle cholesterol (RLP-C), fasting plasma glucose, HbA1c, and diacron-reactive oxygen metabolites (d-ROMs), a marker of oxidative stress, decreased, while the levels of HDL-C increased significantly in the bezafibrate group but did not change in the EPA group. The decrease in the levels of TG, RLP-C, HbA1c, and d-ROMs was significantly greater in the bezafibrate group than in the EPA group. The

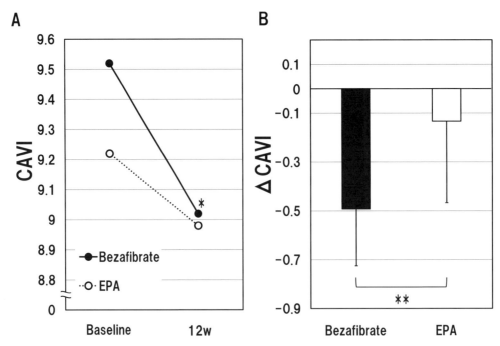

Fig. 6. Changes in the CAVI during 12-week treatment by bezafibrate and EPA.
(A) Relationship between baseline CAVI and CAVI after 12-week treatment in bezafibrate and EPA groups. *P < 0.05, Paired *t*-test. (B) Comparison of changes in CAVI after 12-week treatment between bezafibrate and EPA groups. **P < 0.05, Student's t –test. Adapted from Ref. (5).

CAVI decreased significantly only in the bezafibrate group (9.52 to 9.02, P < 0.05), and the decrease in the CAVI was significantly greater in the bezafibrate group than in the EPA group (-0.492 vs. -0.133, P < 0.05) (**Fig. 6**). Multivariate logistic regression analysis revealed that high baseline CAVI, low HDL-C level, and bezafibrate administration were significant independent predictors for a decrease in the CAVI. Notably, bezafibrate treatment reduces arterial stiffening accompanied by an improvement in glycolipid metabolism and oxidative stress.

3-3. Statins

Mere LDL-C lowering therapy does not necessarily contribute to a decrease in the CAVI; however, certain types of LDL-C lowering agents have been reported to contribute to a decrease in the CAVI. For example, Miyashita et al. reported that the administration of pitavastatin decreased the CAVI[6]. Forty-five patients with type 2 diabetes and hypercholesterolemia were enrolled and treated with pitavastatin 2 mg/day for 12 months. A significant decrease in the oxidative stress marker (urinary 8-OHdG; 11.3 to 8.4 ng/mg/Cr), oxidized LDL (malondialdehyde-LDL; 170 to 114 U/L), and CAVI (9.54 to 8.91) were observed, and the change in the CAVI significantly correlated with the change in malondialdehyde-LDL (R = 0.549, P = 0.02). To summarize, pitavastatin may be effective in improving the arterial stiffness in patients with high oxidative stress.

3-4. Ezetimibe

Miyashita et al. reported that ezetimibe, a cholesterol absorption inhibitor, improved the CAVI[7]. The administration of ezetimibe (10 mg/day) for 6 months in 40 patients with hypercholesterolemia and diabetes decreased RLP-C (9.44 to 7.41 mg/dl) and CAVI (9.17 to 9.00). Recently, it has been reported that high absorption of cholesterol in the small intestine may be one of the risk factors for atherosclerosis. In this study, the LDL-C-lowering response to ezetimibe treatment was higher in patients who achieved the LDL-C goal than in patients who did not achieve the goal. From these findings, it was hypothesized that patients who achieved the LDL-C goal may have a high absorption of cholesterol, which might be the reason for the high CAVI; however, the change in RLP-C, which is atherogenic, was not significant between the two groups.

4. TOHO Lipid Intervention Trial Using Pitavastatin (TOHO-LIP)

We conducted a multicenter randomized trial named the TOHO-LIP, and the outcomes showed that the administration of pitavastatin (2 mg/day) was superior to that of atorvastatin (10 mg/day) in reducing the incidence of

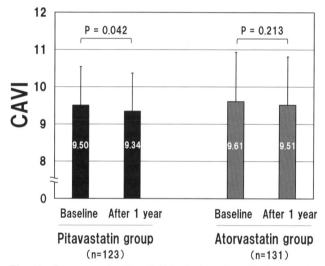

Fig. 7. Changes in the CAVI during the first year in pitavastatin and atorvastatin groups.

P values were calculated by paired *t*-test. Adapted from Ref. (10).

Table 1. Cox proportional-hazards regression analysis of the association between 3P-MACE and clinical variables.

3P-MACE, 3-point major cardiac adverse events. Adapted from Ref. (10).

(a) Model 1

Variables	Hazard Ratio	95% Confidence Interval		P-value
ΔLDL-C (Δmg/dl)	1.007	0.994 –	1.021	0.280
ΔCAVI	1.758	0.926 –	3.338	0.084
Group (Atorvastatin; 0, Pitavastatin; 1)	0.493	0.171 –	1.420	0.190

(b) Model 2

Variables	Hazard Ratio	95% Confidence Interval		P-value
Gender (male; 0, female; 1)	0.666	0.245 –	1.813	0.426
Age (years)	1.039	0.978 –	1.104	0.215
ΔLDL-C (Δmg/dl)	1.006	0.993 –	1.020	0.363
ΔCAVI	1.736	0.938 –	3.213	0.079
Group (Atorvastatin; 0, Pitavastatin; 1)	0.501	0.172 –	1.461	0.206

cardiovascular (CV) events despite a similar LDL-C-lowering effect[8]. In this study, only pitavastatin reduced the levels of high-sensitive CRP, indicating the pleiotropic effects of pitavastatin, including anti-oxidant and anti-inflammatory effects. In addition, increased serum lipoprotein lipase (LPL) mass during the first year of pitavastatin treatment might be associated with the decrease in CV events[9]. Considering that LPL, produced mainly in the adipose tissue, is an indicator of insulin sensitivity and vascular endothelial function, pitavastatin may have a unique class effect on the adipose tissue. Saiki et al. examined whether the decrease in the incidence of CV events was associated with the CAVI-lowering effect of pitavastatin in the subgroup analysis of the TOHO-LIP study[10]. The CAVI decreased significantly only in the pitavastatin group during the first year (9.50 to 9.34, P = 0.042), while the change in LDL-C did not differ between the two groups (**Fig. 7**). In this study, the change in the CAVI during the first year correlated positively with 3-point major adverse cardiovascular events (3P-MACE: CV death, nonfatal myocardial infarction, and nonfatal stroke) and was an independent predictor for 3P-MACE in the Cox proportional-hazards model (hazard ratio: 1.736, P = 0.079) (**Table 1**). Annual changes in the CAVI throughout the observation period were significantly higher in subjects who had CV events than in those who did not. These findings revealed that the CAVI-lowering effect of pitavastatin might be associated with a reduction in CV events. The extent to which the decreased CAVI reflects the improvements in oxidative stress, inflammation, and TG metabolism needs further investigation.

5. Challenges and prospects for the treatment of dyslipidemia today

The latest guideline establishes a target value for the management of LDL-C in the primary prevention group of middle-aged and elderly dyslipidemic patients, considering the multiple coronary risks[11], while there is a single target value for the management of TG and HDL-C. Essentially, the control targets for TG and HDL-C may need to be determined in the same way as for LDL-C, taking into account multiple risks. Furthermore, it may be worthwhile to focus on the vascular pleiotropic effect of each statin independent of its lipid-lowering effect. Routine CAVI assessment of arterial stiffness in dyslipidemic patients would allow appropriate customization of the treatment for every individual patient.

References

1) Nagayama D, Watanabe Y, Saiki A, Shirai K, Tatsuno I. Lipid parameters are independently associated with cardio-ankle vascular index (CAVI) in healthy Japanese subjects. J Atheroscler Thromb. 2018;25:621-633. https://doi.org/10.5551/jat.42291

2) Soska V, Dobsak P, Dusek L, Shirai K, Jarkovsky J, Novakova M, Brhel P, Stastna J, Fajkusova L, Freiberger T, Yambe T. Cardio-ankle vascular index in heterozygous familial hypercholesterolemia. J Atheroscler Thromb. 2012;19:453-461.

3) Reiner Ž, Simental-Mendía LE, Ruscica M, Katsiki N, Banach M, Al Rasadi K, Jamialahmadi T, Sahebkar A. Pulse wave velocity as a measure of arterial stiffness in patients with familial hypercholesterolemia: a systematic review and meta-analysis. Arch Med Sci. 2019;15:1365-1374.

4) Satoh N, Shimatsu A, Kotani K, Himeno A, Majima T, Yamada K, Suganami T, Ogawa Y. Highly purified eicosapentaenoic acid reduces cardio-ankle vascular index in association with decreased serum amyloid A-LDL in metabolic syndrome. Hypertens Res. 2009;32:1004-1008.

5) Yamaguchi T, Shirai K, Nagayama D, Nakamura S, Oka R, Tanaka S, Watanabe Y, Imamura H, Sato Y, Kawana H, Ohira M, Saiki A, Shimizu N, Tatsuno I. Bezafibrate ameliorates arterial stiffness assessed by cardio-ankle vascular index in hypertriglyceridemic patients with type 2 diabetes mellitus. J Atheroscler Thromb. 2019;26:659-669. http://doi.org/10.5551/jat.45799

6) Miyashita Y, Endo K, Saiki A, Ban N, Yamaguchi T, Kawana H, Nagayama D, Ohira M, Oyama T, Shirai K. Effects of pitavastatin, a 3-hydroxy-3-methylglutaryl coenzyme a reductase inhibitor, on cardio-ankle vascular index in type 2 diabetic patients. J Atheroscler Thromb. 2009;16:539-545.

7) Miyashita Y, Endo K, Saiki A, Ban N, Nagumo A, Yamaguchi T, Kawana H, Nagayama D, Ohira M, Oyama T, Shirai K. Effect of ezetimibe monotherapy on lipid metabolism and arterial stiffness assessed by cardio-ankle vascular index in type 2 diabetic patients. J Atheroscler Thromb. 2010;17:1070-1076.

8) Moroi M, Nagayama D, Hara F, Saiki A, Shimizu K, Takahashi M, Sato N, Shiba T, Sugimoto H, Fujioka T, Chiba T, Nishizawa K, Usui S, Iwasaki Y, Tatsuno I, Sugi K, Yamasaki J, Yamamura S, Shirai K. Outcome of pitavastatin versus atorvastatin therapy in patients with hypercholesterolemia at high risk for atherosclerotic cardiovascular disease. Int J Cardiol. 2020;305:139-146.

9) Nagayama D, Saiki A, Watanabe Y, Yamaguchi T, Ohira M, Sato N, Kanayama M, Moroi M, Miyashita Y, Shirai K, Tatsuno I. Prevention of cardiovascular events with pitavastatin is associated with increased serum lipoprotein lipase mass level: subgroup analysis of the TOHO-LIP. J Atheroscler Thromb. 2020. Online ahead of print.

10) Saiki A, Watanabe Y, Yamaguchi T, Ohira M, Nagayama D, Sato N, Kanayama M, Takahashi M, Shimizu K, Moroi M, Miyashita Y, Shirai K, Tatsuno I. CAVI-lowering Effect of Pitavastatin may be Involved in Prevention of Cardiovascular Disease: Subgroup Analysis of the TOHO-LIP. J Atheroscler Thromb. 2020. Online ahead of print. https://doi.org/10.5551/jat.60343

11) Kinoshita M, Yokote K, Arai H, Iida M, Ishigaki Y, Ishibashi S, Umemoto S, Egusa G, Ohmura H, Okamura T, Kihara S, Koba S, Saito I, Shoji T, Daida H, Tsukamoto K, Deguchi J, Dohi S, Dobashi K, Hamaguchi H, Hara M, Hiro T, Biro S, Fujioka Y, Maruyama C, Miyamoto Y, Murakami Y, Yokode M, Yoshida H, Rakugi H, Wakatsuki A, Yamashita S. Committee for Epidemiology and Clinical Management of Atherosclerosis. Japan Atherosclerosis Society (JAS) Guidelines for Prevention of Atherosclerotic Cardiovascular Diseases 2017. J Atheroscler Thromb. 2018;25:846-984.

Obesity: Body Mass Index, Waist Circumstance and A Body Shape Index (ABSI)

Daiji Nagayama

Summary

1. Inverse relationship between CAVI and body mass index (BMI) is observed in healthy Japanese population.
2. CAVI is correlated positively with visceral fat accumulation, and negatively with subcutaneous fat accumulation. This is the so-called "obesity paradox of CAVI."
3. Recently, a body shape index (ABSI) has been proposed to reflect visceral fat accumulation, and is related positively with CAVI.
4. Metabolic syndrome (MS) is known to be caused by visceral fat accumulation. CAVI reflects the severity of obesity-related metabolic disorders; but, CAVI was not necessarily high in subjects with MS defined by several classical criteria using waist circumference (WC). However, when newly proposed ABSI was used to define MS instead of WC, the subjects with high CAVI were accurately identified.

Introduction

In the healthy population, an inverted relationship of CAVI with body mass index (BMI) has been reported. However, obesity is not simple, and is classified into intra-abdominal fat (visceral type) obesity and extra-abdominal fat (subcutaneous type) obesity. The former is related to multiple metabolic disorders, such as the so-called metabolic syndrome (MS). CAVI is reported to be high in subjects with intra-abdominal obesity, and may decrease after body weight reduction in patients with obesity-related metabolic disorders, whereas CAVI is low in extra-abdominal obesity. Therefore, there seems to exist an "obesity paradox of CAVI". In this chapter, the meaning of this paradox will be discussed.

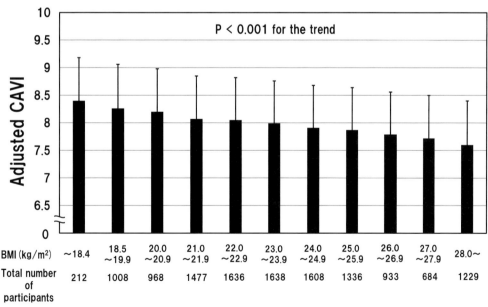

Fig. 1. Relationship between adjusted CAVI and BMI in Japanese male subjects. Vascular Health and Risk Management 2016; 13:1-9; Originally published by and used with permission from Dove Medical Press Ltd[1]

Japanese male subjects without a past history of cardiovascular disease, stroke, hypertension, diabetes, or dyslipidemia (N = 12,729, Age: 47 ± 13 years, BMI: 23.9 ± 3.2 kg/m²).
F = 53.732, P < 0.001. CAVI was adjusted by age, sBP, and HDL-C. Data are presented as mean ± SD.

Nagayama Clinic, 2-12-22, Tenjin-Cho, Oyama-City, Tochigi 323-0032, Japan

1. Inverse relationship of CAVI with BMI in healthy Japanese subjects

We reported the relationship of CAVI with BMI in a cross-sectional study in 23,257 healthy Japanese subjects (12,729 men and 10,528 women, aged 47.1 years)[1]. Male subjects showed a significantly higher BMI (23.9 vs. 21.7 kg/m^2), CAVI (7.96 vs. 7.69) and level of triglycerides (TG), and lower high-density lipoprotein cholesterol (HDL-C) compared to female subjects. After adjusting for confounders including age, systolic blood pressure (sBP) and HDL-C identified by multiple regression analysis, the mean CAVI decreased progressively as the BMI tertile increased in both genders. Furthermore, an inverse relationship between BMI and adjusted CAVI was observed throughout the BMI distribution of less than 18 to over 28 kg/m^2 (**Fig. 1**). The multivariate logistic regression model for contributors of high CAVI ($\geq 90^{th}$ percentile,

equal to 9.20 in all participants), which was roughly equivalent to the cut-off value for coronary artery disease (CAD), identified obesity [odds ratios (95% confidence interval): 0.804 (0.720-0.899)], elderly (Age $\geq$ 65 years) [15.6 (14.0-17.4)], male gender [2.26 (2.03-2.51)], hypertension [2.28 (2.06-2.54)] and impaired fasting glucose [1.17 (1.01-1.37)] to be independent factors.

The inverse relationship of CAVI with BMI in healthy Japanese subjects suggests that systemic accumulation of adipose tissue per se may lead to a linear decrease of arterial stiffness at least in non-obese and obese subjects without metabolic disorders. The reason for this has been discussed in the next session.

2. Various types of regional fat accumulation and CAVI

Currently, it is generally accepted that obesity is classified

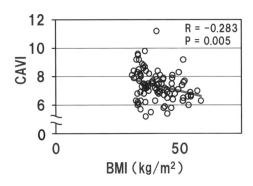

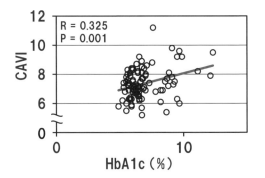

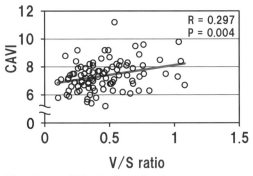

Fig. 2. Relationship of CAVI with body adiposity composition in morbid obese patients.
Simple linear regression analysis. N = 95, Mean BMI: 41.2 kg/m^2.
V/S ratio, visceral fat area/subcutaneous fat area ratio calculated using CT.
(unpublished)

Table 1. Correlation between BMI and body adiposity indices according to gender and obesity status.
*p < 0.001, ρ, Spearman's correlation coefficient. Adapted from Ref. (6).

BMI vs.	ρ				
	All (n = 62,514)	Male (n = 26,037)	Female (n = 36,477)	Subjects with BMI ≥ 25 (n = 11,251)	Subjects with BMI < 25 (n = 51,263)
WC	0.885*	0.881*	0.823*	0.675*	0.796*
WC/Height ratio	0.832*	0.880*	0.832*	0.621*	0.716*
WC/BMI ratio	−0.583*	−0.592*	−0.544*	−0.425*	−0.414*
ABSI	0.043*	0.160*	0.100*	−0.001	0.055*

into intra-abdominal fat (visceral type) obesity and extra-abdominal fat (subcutaneous type) obesity. The former is related to many metabolic disorders such so-called metabolic syndrome[2]. Thus, it can be called "malignant obesity." On the other hand, the latter subcutaneous type obesity can be called "benign obesity." Interestingly, CAVI is reported to be correlated with visceral fat area measured with CT[3]. Furthermore, Park HE et al. demonstrated that CAVI was correlated with pericardial fat mass[4]. Therefore, malignant obesity is also involved in ectopic adipose tissue such as pericardial fat in addition to mesenteric fat tissue. In addition, we examined the relationship of CAVI with

Table 2. Discriminatory powers of body adiposity indices for high CAVI (≥ 90th percentile). ROC analyses for discriminating the probability of high CAVI. Adapted from Ref. (6).

Indices	AUC	95% CIs	P value
ABSI	0.709	0.703–0.716	< 0.001
WC/Height ratio	0.642	0.635–0.649	< 0.001
WC/BMI ratio	0.624	0.617–0.631	< 0.001
WC	0.594	0.587–0.601	< 0.001
BMI	0.520	0.513–0.528	< 0.001

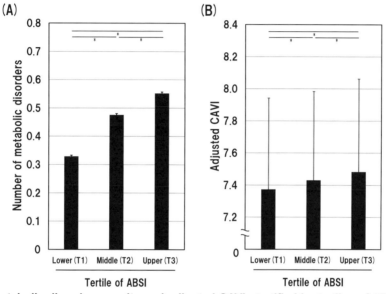

Fig. 3.   Comparison of metabolic disorder severity and adjusted CAVI stratified by tertiles of ABSI.

(A) Relationship of a number of metabolic disorders with tertiles of ABSI. Metabolic disorders comprise untreated hypertension (sBP ≥ 130 and/or dBP ≥ 85 mmHg), dyslipidemia (TG ≥ 150 mg/dL and/or HDL-C < 40 mg/dL), and IFG (FPG ≥ 110 mg/dL). (B) Relationship of adjusted CAVI with tertiles of ABSI. CAVI was adjusted by gender, age, and sBP.
Data are presented as mean ± SE in (A), or mean ± SD in (B). *p < 0.001, ANOVA followed by post-hoc Bonferroni method.
Adapted from Ref. (6).

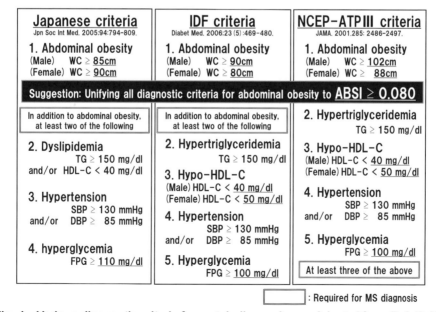

Fig. 4.   Various diagnostic criteria for metabolic syndrome. Adapted from Ref. (8-10).

body adiposity composition in morbid obese patients whose BMI ≥ 35 kg/m^2 requiring bariatric surgery shown in **Fig. 2**. CAVI was correlated positively with HbA1c and visceral fat area/subcutaneous fat area (V/S ratio), and negatively with BMI, indicating that visceral fat accumulation contributed to arterial stiffening even in morbid obesity. These results suggested that visceral fat tissue might secrete some direct/indirect vascular toxic factors, resulting in the occurrence of chronic inflammation, oxidative stress, and insulin resistance. On the other hand, the negative correlation between CAVI and subcutaneous adipose tissue might suggest that subcutaneous adipose tissue might work to improve vascular function. However, the precise mechanism was not clear. Factors that influence the accumulation of subcutaneous adipose tissue through adjustments to insulin sensitivity or angiogenesis may be

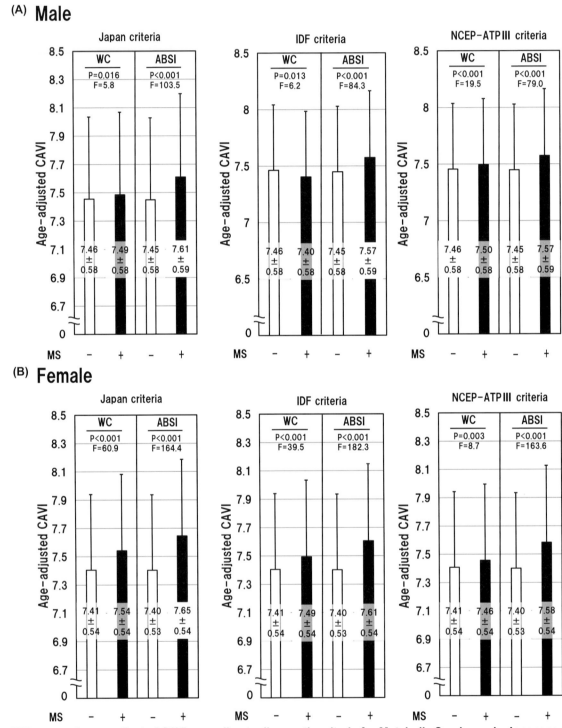

Fig. 5. Differences in age-adjusted CAVI according to diagnostic criteria for Metabolic Syndrome in Japanese subjects.
(A) Male and (B) Female. Data are presented as mean ± SD, Bonferroni method.
"WC" was diagnosed using the WC cut-off value for each MS criterion, and "ABSI" was diagnosed using ABSI ≥ 0.080 instead of WC cut-off value. Non-publication data.

involved.

Further studies are needed to clarify the role of factors from subcutaneous adipose tissue in the decrease of CAVI, as they may be factors that promote vascular health.

3. Estimation of visceral fat mass using a body shape index (ABSI)

Although it is not easy to accurately assess visceral fat volume, evaluation of visceral adiposity using computed tomography (CT) from an umbilical slice is currently believed to be the golden standard. However, it is difficult to use CT in routine clinical practice or mass examination of health check. Then, waist circumference (WC) is used as the evaluation of visceral adiposity. Furthermore, Krakauer NY et al. proposed a body shape index (ABSI), which is calculated using the height, body weight and WC by the following formula: $ABSI = WC/BMI^{2/3} \times height^{1/2}$ [5]. We studied the relationship of CAVI with WC and ABSI during the mass examination of health check in 62,514 Japanese subjects (mean age 44.4 years, mean BMI 22.2 kg/m^2) without a past history of cardiovascular disease, stroke or treatment for obesity-related metabolic disorders[6]. Resultantly, the WC, WC/height ratio, and WC/BMI ratio correlated with BMI regardless of gender or obesity, whereas a body shape index (ABSI) hardly correlated with BMI (**Table 1**). Additionally, ROC analyses demonstrated that ABSI had the highest discriminatory power compared to other body adiposity indices, and the cut-off value for high CAVI ($\geq 90^{th}$ percentile, equal to 9.0 in all participants) was 0.080 (**Table 2**) in both genders. The number of metabolic disorders and confounders-adjusted CAVI increased with increasing tertiles of ABSI (**Fig. 3**). Additionally, the contribution of high ABSI (≥ 0.080) for high CAVI was independent of gender, elderly, obesity, and obesity-related metabolic disorders in the multivariate logistic regression model. These results indicated that ABSI could be an index reflecting visceral fat obesity. In other words, the utility of ABSI was shown by its association with CAVI.

4. The usefulness of ABSI for the diagnosis of metabolic syndrome in term of CAVI

MS is known to be caused by visceral fat accumulation. CAVI increased as the number of the obesity-related metabolic disorders such as hypertension, diabetes mellitus and dyslipidemia increased. However, in some cases, CAVI was not necessarily high in patients with MS defined by several classical criteria using WC[7].

The Japanese original definition of MS was established by the Japanese Committee for the Diagnostic Criteria of MetS in April 2005[8], which defined MS as two or more metabolic disorders based on abdominal obesity defined as large WC. On the other hand, other well-known MS diagnostic criteria include International Diabetes Federation (IDF) criteria[9] and National Cholesterol Education Program-Third Adult Treatment Panel (NCEP-ATP III) criteria[10]. In the diagnostic criteria for MS, the Japanese and IDF criteria assume abdominal obesity, while the NCEP-ATP III criteria treat abdominal obesity as being of

the same magnitude as other metabolic disorders (**Fig. 4**).

We proposed the adoption of ABSI ≥ 0.080 instead of the conventionally used "large WC," and compared how age-adjusted CAVI differs with and without MS when diagnosed using WC or ABSI in 62,514 Japanese subjects without a past history of cardiovascular disease, stroke, or treatment for obesity-related metabolic disorders (Male in **Fig. 5A**, and female in **Fig. 5B**). The results showed that age-adjusted CAVI in MS patients was significantly higher when ABSI was used instead of WC to diagnose MS based on the Japanese, IDF, or NCEP-ATP III criteria. This finding suggests that ABSI can identify patients with vascular toxicity more efficiently than WC.

Since WC is strongly correlated with BMI, subjects with a large WC are more likely to have benign obesity. It is therefore useful to diagnose abdominal obesity using ABSI instead of WC, and to evaluate vascular toxicity caused by abdominal obesity using CAVI.

References

1) Nagayama D, Imamura H, Sato Y, et al. Inverse relationship of cardio-ankle vascular index with BMI in healthy Japanese subjects: a cross-sectional study. Vasc Health Risk Manag. 2016; 13:1-9. http://dx.doi.org/10.2147/VHRM.S119646

2) Mottillo S, Filion KB, Genest J, Joseph L, Pilote L, Poirier P, Rinfret S, Schiffrin EL, Eisenberg MJ. The metabolic syndrome and cardiovascular risk a systematic review and meta-analysis. J Am Coll Cardiol. 2010; 56: 1113-1132.

3) Nagayama D, Endo K, Ohira M, Yamaguchi T, Ban N, Kawana H, Nagumo A, Saiki A, Oyama T, Miyashita Y, Shirai K. Effects of body weight reduction on cardio-ankle vascular index (CAVI). Obes Res Clin Pract. 2013; 7: e139-e145.

4) Park HE, Choi SY, Kim HS, Kim MK, Cho SH, Oh BH. Epicardial fat reflects arterial stiffness: assessment using 256-slice multidetector coronary computed tomography and cardio-ankle vascular index. J Atheroscler Thromb. 2012;19:570-576.

5) Krakauer NY and Krakauer JC. A new body shape index predicts mortality hazard independently of body mass index. PLoS ONE. 2012. 7: e39504.

6) Nagayama D, Watanabe Y, Yamaguchi T, Maruyama M, Saiki A, Shirai K, Tatsuno I. New index of abdominal obesity, a body shape index, is BMI-independently associated with systemic arterial stiffness in real-world Japanese population. Int J Clin Pharmacol Ther. Int J Clin Pharmacol Ther. 2020;58:709-717. https://doi.org/10.5414/cp203778

7) Topouchian J, Labat C, Gautier S, et al. Effects of metabolic syndrome on arterial function in different age groups: the Advanced Approach to Arterial Stiffness study. J Hypertens. 2018;36:824-833.

8) Matsuzawa Y. Metabolic syndrome – definition and diagnostic criteria in Japan. J Atheroscler Thromb. 2005; 12: 301.

9) Alberti KGMM, Zimmet P, Shaw J, Metabolic syndrome--a new world-wide definition. A Consensus Statement from the International Diabetes Federation. Diabet Med. 2006;23:469-480.

10) Expert Panel on Detection, Evaluation, and Treatment of High Blood Cholesterol in Adults. Executive Summary of The Third Report of The National Cholesterol Education Program (NCEP) Expert Panel on Detection, Evaluation, And Treatment of High Blood Cholesterol In Adults (Adult Treatment Panel III). JAMA. 2001;285:2486-97.

Effects of metabolic syndrome on arterial function
The Advanced Approach to Arterial Stiffness (AAA) Study

Jirar Topouchian

Introduction

The prevalence of cardiovascular risk factors and metabolic syndrome (MetS) dramatically increases with age at least until the age of 60 years[1]. MetS is becoming a pandemic disease with major consequences on public health.

The influence of the different metabolic and hemodynamic components of MetS on the arterial system has been assessed in different clinical studies. A relationship has been demonstrated between the presence of MetS and progression of arterial stiffness of the aorta and other large arteries[2,3].

It was described that the interaction of MetS components could have synergistic impact on arterial parameters like carotid Intima Media Thickness (IMT), Pulse Wave Velocity (PWV), Ankle Brachial Index (ABI), Cardio-Ankle Vascular Index (CAVI), etc. At the same time, a considerable heterogeneity was observed in the relationship between MetS components and arterial stiffness[4-7].

Therefore, several aspects of the impact of MetS and its components have been described but some others not, mainly age.

The AAA study was designed to contribute to bringing some answers and clarification about the role of age in the impact of MetS and its components on arterial stiffness.

The AAA study is an international multicenter prospective longitudinal study with three scheduled visits at baseline and after 2 and 5 years of follow-up.

Patients aged 40 years and older were recruited at 32 outpatient centers participating in the AAA study network from 18 countries. To assess the influence of age on the effects of MetS on arterial stiffness, four age groups were prespecified: Group 1: 40–49 years, Group 2: 50–59 years, Group 3: 60–74 years and Group 4: at least 75 years.

The arterial evaluation was performed using two methods:

1 – *The carotid–femoral pulse wave velocity (CF-PWV)*[8-11] which is considered to be the "gold standard" measurement of arterial stiffness. However, it presents a number of limitations and sources of inaccuracy, like the transit distance measurements of the arterial segment. Also, some physiological factors could affect

PWV, such as blood pressure (BP) and heart rate[9-11]. PWV was measured using a validated automatic device [Complior (ALAM Medical, Pantin, France), Sphygmocor (AtCor Medical, Sydney, Australia) and PulsePen (Diatecne, Milan, Italy)]. Because of the use of several devices, normalization of the measurement values was performed according to the European Experts recommendations[11].

2- *The cardio-ankle vascular index (CAVI)*[12] assesses arterial mechanical and elastic properties by means of the beta stiffness index, which is relatively independent of BP levels at the time of the measurement. *CAVI* was measured and automatically calculated using the VaSera system (Fukuda Denshi Co, Japan)[12].

Non-inclusion criteria were factors potentially impairing the quality of the CAVI or PWV measurements or rending PWV recording unreliable, namely: known significant peripheral arterial disease, ankle brachial index < 0.9 (even unilateral), limb amputation; history of vascular surgery at the level of the carotid artery, femoral artery or aorta; body mass index > 40 kg/m^2; atrial fibrillation and/or other major arrhythmia; and pregnancy.

Metabolic syndrome was defined using the National Cholesterol Education Program – Adult treatment Panel revised version (NCEP-R) definition[17,18]. *Blood pressure* was measured in clinic according to the European Society of Hypertension guidelines using validated equipment that meets certification criteria[19]. *Ankle-brachial index (ABI)* was automatically obtained from the CAVI measurements performed with the VaSera device (Fukuda Denshi Co)[12].

Plasma measurement: Glycaemia, total cholesterol, triglycerides, LDL cholesterol, HDL cholesterol, serum creatinine, creatinine clearance (modification of diet in renal disease) and hemoglobin A1c were measured ± 12 weeks of the study visit.

The results of the AAA-Study baseline values were published previously in detail[20]. In this chapter we will focus on some of them.

Characteristics of the population: 2348 patients were enrolled at 32 centers from 18 countries. 124 patients were excluded from the analysis due to either missing information on elements for the NCEP-2005 MetS classification or

Diagnostic Center, Hôtel-Dieu de Paris, France.

lacking CAVI measurements. 1664 patients (74.8%) were classified with MetS and 560 without.

Patients with MetS were older, had more often a family history of cardiovascular disease (CVD) and presented a higher prevalence of cardiovascular risk factors, stroke, myocardial infarction, angina, heart failure and renal failure. Patients with MetS had higher PWV and CAVI values, this difference was maintained after adjustment for age and sex for PWV (P < 0.0001) but not for CAVI (P = 0.40).

Age and arterial stiffness: Both CAVI and CF-PWV increased with age, stronger correlation coefficient was observed with CAVI (r^2 = 0.37; P < 0.0001), y = 0.07 + 3.87 than with PWV (r^2 = 0.14; P < 0.0001), y = 0.09 + 4.39. Comparison of the correlation coefficients using the Hotelling–Williams test showed that the age/CAVI relationship was statistically stronger (P < 0.001) than the

age/PWV relationship. Effects of age on arterial stiffness did not differ between men and women (Fig. 1).

Metabolic syndrome and arterial stiffness: In the presence of MetS, age-adjusted and sex-adjusted values of CF-PWV but not CAVI were higher (Fig. 2, 3). The effects of MetS on sex-adjusted CAVI and PWV values in the four predefined age-groups are shown in Fig. 3. While analysing the effects of each of the five MetS components, higher CAVI values were associated with Glycemia (p < 0.0001) and BP (p < 0.02) components, whereas the HDL and triglyceride components did not influence CAVI. Finally, high waist circumference was associated with lower age-adjusted and sex-adjusted CAVI values. In contrast, all five MetS components showed positive correlations with CF-PWV (Fig. 4). The multiple regression analysis testing the arterial effect of the five MetS components showed that

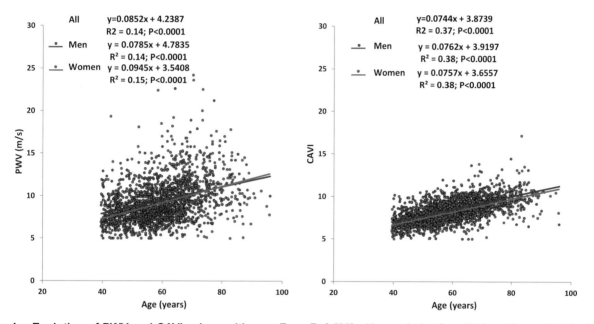

Fig. 1. Evolution of PWV and CAVI values with age. From Ref. [20] with permission from Wolters Kluwer Health, Inc.

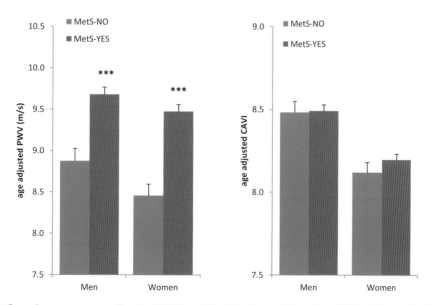

Fig. 2. Effects of MetS and sex on age-adjusted PWV and CAVI values. From Ref. [20] with permission from Wolters Kluwer Health, Inc.

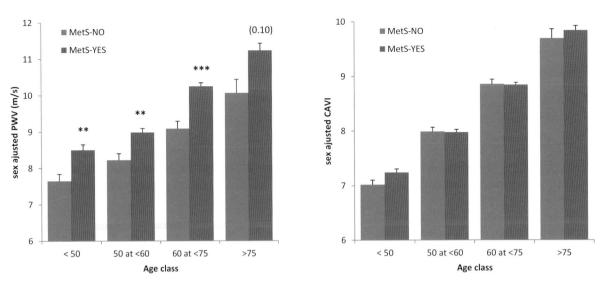

Fig. 3. **Effects of MetS on sex-adjusted PWV and CAVI values according to age groups.** From Ref. [20] with permission from Wolters Kluwer Health, Inc.

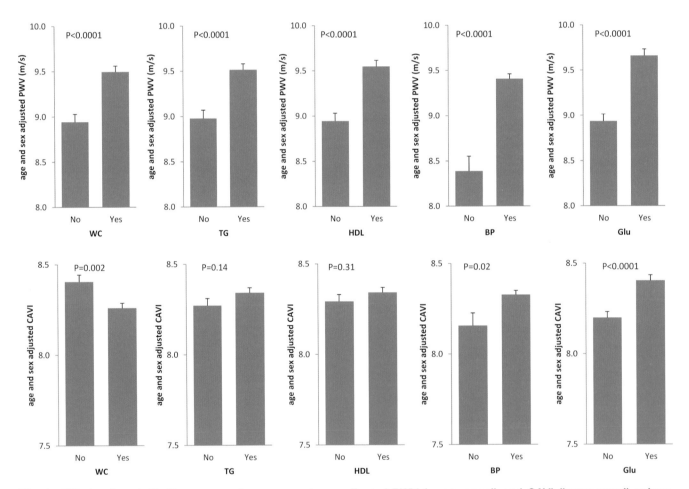

Fig. 4. **Effects of each MetS component on sex- and age-adjusted PWV (upper panel) and CAVI (lower panel) values.** From Ref. [20] with permission from Wolters Kluwer Health, Inc.

older age, male sex, presence of the BP and glycaemia components and absence of the overweight component were all independent determinants of higher CAVI values.

Discussion

Although CF-PWV and CAVI both represent

measurements of arterial stiffness, their fundamental principles differ, for mainly two reasons:

a- PWV is based on the Moens–Korteweg/Bramwell–Hill Eqs.[21] and measures the velocity of the pulse waves between two arterial sites. It is well known that this velocity is dependent on both arterial structure/function but also on distension pressure at the time of the measurement[22–24], thereby explaining a more pronounced influence of BP variations during PWV assessment. On the other hand, CAVI corresponds to the β index, which reflects the slope of the relationship between changes in pressure and changes in volume[12–15,25], thus explaining why this index is much less dependent on acute pressure variations at the time of the measurements.

b- CF-PWV measures arterial stiffness primarily of the descending aorta, whereas CAVI estimates stiffness of a more general territory including ascending aorta, aortic arch, descending aorta and lower limb arteries[26].

The AAA study showed that in this specific population both CAVI and CF-PWV were correlated with age although with a stronger correlation coefficient with CAVI ($r^2 = 0.37$) than with CF-PWV ($r^2 = 0.14$). Furthermore, effects of sex (higher arterial stiffness in men than in women) were detected with CAVI but not with CF-PWV. The fact that CAVI explores a larger vascular territory as stated above could explain such differences between the two methods.

The AAA-study results indicate differential effects according to the different MetS components as well as according to the different methods for evaluating vascular stiffness. Patients with MetS exhibited significantly higher CF-PWV in all age groups. In contrast, CAVI was less affected in the presence of MetS, thereby further reinforcing that these two methods reflect different aspects of arterial stiffness. CAVI was positively associated with high glycemia and high BP components whereas it lacked significant associations with the HDL cholesterol and triglycerides components while exhibiting a negative association with the overweight component.

Interest in cardio-ankle vascular index for the evaluation of arterial stiffness: In Europe, CF-PWV is used in several specialized centers and recommended by scientific societies as the gold standard to assess arterial stiffness[8–11]. The results of this study show that CAVI, as an alternative approach to measure arterial stiffness, provides complementary information to that obtained by PWV. Clinical studies now show that CAVI could represent a useful tool for the assessment of arterial health in large multicenter studies, owing to several advantages related to feasibility, reproducibility and facility of use, with little or no observer bias[12,16,27].

Beyond these practical aspects, the interest in CAVI is also related to the minimal impact of BP values at the time of the measurements, which allows a better assessment of the intrinsic elastic properties of the vascular system. This may be of major interest in some subgroups of patients especially in very old patients in whom BP levels are very often influenced by comorbidities and poor general condition[28].

In conclusion, the current large European multicenter study shows the differential impact of MetS and age on CAVI and CF-PWV. Age had a more pronounced effect on CAVI, whereas MetS increased CF-PWV but not CAVI. This important finding is probably due to the heterogeneous effects of the MetS components on CAVI.

Prospects: The ongoing longitudinal component of the current study that has already registered more than 1000 patients' follow-up visits and around 100 morbi-mortality events, should provide answers to several questions not yet clarified at this stage of the study by assessing the long-term evolution of CAVI values.

References

1) Akbulut G, Koksal E, Bilici S, Acar Tek N, Yildiran H, Karadag MG, Sanlier N. Metabolic syndrome (MS) in elderly: a cross sectional survey. Arch Gerontol Geriatr 2011; 53:e263–e266.

2) Henry RM, Kostense PJ, Spijkerman AM, Dekker JM, Nijpels G, Heine RJ, et al. Arterial stiffness increases with deteriorating glucose tolerance status: the Hoorn Study. Circulation 2003; 107:2089–2095.

3) Scuteri A, Najjar SS, Orru M, Usala G, Piras MG, Ferrucci L, et al. The central arterial burden of the metabolic syndrome is similar in men and women: the SardiNIA Study. Eur Heart J 2010; 31:602–613.

4) Sri-Amad, R., Huipao, N., Prasertsri, P., & Roengrit, T. (2020). Aortic Pulse Wave Velocity, Ankle-Brachial Index, and Malondialdehyde in Older Adults with or without Metabolic Syndrome. Pulse (Basel, Switzerland), 8(1-2), 31–39.

5) Ryliškytė L, Navickas R, Šerpytis P, Puronaitė R, Zupkauskienė J, Jucevičienė A, Badarienė J, Rimkienė MA, Ryliškienė K, Skiauterytė E, Laucevičius A. Association of aortic stiffness, carotid intima-media thickness and endothelial function with cardiovascular events in metabolic syndrome subjects. Blood Press. 2019;28:131-138. doi: 10.1080/08037051.2019.1569461

6) Nam S. H., Kang, S. G., Lee, Y. A., Song, S. W., & Rho, J. S. (2015). Association of Metabolic Syndrome with the Cardioankle Vascular Index in Asymptomatic Korean Population. Journal of diabetes research, 2015, 328585.

7) Scuteri A, Cunha PG, Agabiti Rosei E, Badariere J, et al. MARE Consortium. Arterial stiffness and influences of the metabolic syndrome: a cross-countries study. Atherosclerosis. 2014 Apr;233(2):654-660.

8) Asmar R. Factors influencing pulse wave velocity.Arterial stiffness and pulse wave velocity. Clinical applications, Editions scientifiques et me´dicales Paris: Elsevier SAS; 1999. pp. 57–86; Chap. IV.

9) Laurent S, Cockcroft J, Van Bortel L, Boutouyrie P, Giannattasio C, Hayoz D, et al. Expert Consensus document on arterial stiffness: methodological issues and clinical applications. Eur Heart J 2006; 27:2588–2605.

10) Townsend RR, Wilkinson IB, Schiffrin EL, Avolio AP, Chirinos JA, Cockcroft JR, et al. Recommendations for improving and standardizing vascular research on arterial stiffness: a scientific statement from the American Heart Association. Hypertension 2015; 66:698–722.

11) Reference Values for Arterial Stiffness' Collaboration. Determinants of pulse wave velocity in healthy people and in the presence of cardiovascular risk factors: 'establishing normal and reference values'. Eur Heart J. 2010;31:2338–2350. doi: 10.1093/eurheartj/ehq165

12) Shirai K, Utino J, Otsuka K, Takata M. A novel blood pressure-independent arterial wall stiffness parameter: cardio-ankle vascular index (CAVI). J Atheroscler Thromb 2006; 13:101–107.

13) Shirai K, Song M, Suzuki J, Kurosu T, Oyama T, Nagayama D, et al. Contradictory effects of b1- and a1-aderenergic receptor blockers on cardio-ankle vascular stiffness index (CAVI)-the independency of CAVI from blood pressure. J Atheroscler Thromb 2011; 18:49–55.

14) Ogawa T, Shimada M, Ishida H, Matsuda N, Fujiu A, Ando Y, Nitta K. Relation of stiffness parameter beta to carotid arteriosclerosis and silent cerebral infarction in patients on chronic hemodialysis. Int Urol Nephrol 2009; 41:739–745.

15) Hayashi k, Yamamoto T, Takahara A, Shirai K. Clinical assessment of arterial stiffness with cardio-ankle vascular index: theory and applications. J Hypertens 2015; 33:1742–1757.

16) Gomez-Sanchez L, Garcia-Ortiz L, Patino-Alonso M, Recio-Rodriguez J, Frontera G, Ramos R, et al., MARK group. The association between the cardio ankle vascular index and other parameters of vascular structure and function in Caucasian adults: the MARK study. J Atheroscler Thromb 2015; 22:901–911.

17) Grundy SM, Cleeman JI, Daniels SR, Donato KA, Eckel RH, Franklin BA, et al., AHA/NHLBI Scientific Statement. Diagnosis and management of the metabolic syndrome. An American Heart Association/National Heart, Lung, and Blood Institute scientific statement. Circulation 2005; 112:2735–2752.

18) Alberti KG, Eckel RH, Grundy SM, Zimmet PZ, Cleeman JI, Donato KA, et al. Harmonizing the metabolic syndrome: a joint interim statement of the International Diabetes Federation Task Force on Epidemiology and Prevention; National Heart, Lung, and Blood Institute; American Heart Association; World Heart Federation; International Atherosclerosis Society; and International Association for the Study of Obesity. Circulation 2009; 120:1640–1645.

19) Williams B, Mancia G, Spiering W, Agabiti Rosei E, et al. 2018 Practice Guidelines for the management of arterial hypertension of the European Society of Cardiology and the European Society of Hypertension. Blood Press. 2018; 27:314-340. doi: 10.1080/08037051.2018.1527177 Erratum in: Blood Press. 2019;28:74.

20) Topouchian J, Labat C, Gautier S, Bäck M, Achimastos A, Blacher J, et al. Effects of metabolic syndrome on arterial function in different age groups: the Advanced Approach to Arterial Stiffness study. J Hypertens. 2018;36:824-833.

21) Bramwell JC, Hill AV. The velocity of the pulse wave in man. Proc R Soc London Series B 1926; 93:298–306.

22) Nichols WW, O'Rourke MF, Vlachopoulos C. McDonald's blood flow in arteries. Theoretical, experimental and clinical principles, 6th ed. London: Hodder Arnold; 2011.

23) Salvi P, Palombo C, Salvi GM, Labat C, Parati G, Benetos A. Leftventricular ejection time, not heart rate, is an independent correlate of aortic pulse wave velocity. J Appl Physiol 2013; 115:1610–1617.

24) Spronck B, Heusinkveld MHG, Vanmolkot FH, Op't Roodt J, Hermeling E, Delhass T, et al. Pressure-dependence of arterial stiffness: potential clinical implications. J Hypertens 2015; 33:330–338.

25) Benetos A. Assessment of arterial stiffness in an older population: theinterest of the cardio-ankle vascular index (CAVI). Eur Heart J Suppl. 2017; 19:B11–B16.

26) Asmar R. Principles & usefulness of the cardio ankle vascular index (CAVI). A new global arterial stiffness index. Eur Heart J Suppl 2017; 19:B4–B10.

27) Li Y, Cordes M, Recio-Rodriguez JI, Garcı´a-Ortiz L, Hanssen H, Schmidt-Trucksa¨ss A. Diurnal variation of arterial stiffness in healthy individuals of different ages and patients with heart disease. Scand J Clin Lab Invest 2014; 74:155–162.

28) Benetos A, Gautier S, Labat C, Salvi P, Valbusa F, Marino F, et al. Mortality and cardiovascular events are best predicted by low central/peripheral pulse pressure amplification but not by high blood pressure levels in elderly nursing home subjects: the PARTAGE (Predictive Values of Blood Pressure and Arterial Stiffness in Institutionalized Very Aged Population) study. J Am Coll Cardiol. 2012;60:1503-1511. doi: 10.1016/j.jacc.2012.04.055

The role of CAVI in cardiovascular risk assessments in Spain

Rafel Ramos

Introduction

Cardiovascular diseases (CVDs) are a major cause of mortality and morbidity, despite improvements in tackling their complications. Indeed, a high proportion of deaths occurring in persons under 60 years old could have been prevented[1,2]. Moreover, estimates indicate that 80% of CVDs are preventable by modifying health-risk behaviour[3-6]. Thus, greater focus on preventive strategies is certainly required to reduce the burden of CVD.

CVD prevention is defined as a coordinated set of actions at a population or individual level, to minimize the impact of CVD[7]. It remains a challenge for the general population, healthcare professionals and managers. In this regard, the European guidelines on cardiovascular disease prevention[8] concur with Rose's[3,9] in recommending to consider two main prevention strategies. First, a strategy at a population level that would promote lifestyle and environmental changes to reduce CVD incidence. Second, a strategy for high-risk individuals that would include measures on primary and secondary prevention to reduce risk factors in individuals with no established or with established CVD, respectively. These measures target unhealthy lifestyles such as poor-quality diets, physical inactivity, smoking, and alcohol consumption. Both strategies provide the same estimated benefits[10], and are complementary and important for reducing the CVD burden[3,9].

In the second strategy, identifying high risk individuals -with risk functions- is key. Nevertheless, there are certain limitations, as most events occur in non-high-risk categories[3,11]. This is the case for the Mediterranean region, the inhabitants of which have low incidence of CVDs[12,13]. However, more than 50% of cardiovascular (CV) events occur in the population at intermediate CV risk, which is approximately 30% of the total population. This represents the most numerous group, and thus relevant regarding the efforts aimed at reducing CV events. Indeed, measures to improve CV risk classification of the intermediate risk population are needed, to be able to recommend lifestyle changes or monitor arterial stiffness.

A promising approach in the high-risk strategy is the early detection of asymptomatic atherosclerosis, which usually develops silently over decades. Increased arterial stiffness, which reflects loss of elasticity and collagen, is a measure of subclinical atherosclerosis and a predictor of CV events[15]. Its detection has been proposed in persons at high risk[16]. Even more, it has also been associated with age, sex, lifestyles, and classical CV risk determinants in general population[17]. Thus, it may play a major role in primary prevention of CVD.

Amid a vast array of non-invasive methods to assess arterial stiffness, the most commonly used are the augmentation index (Aix), the stiffness parameter β, the pulse wave velocity (PWV), and the cardio-ankle vascular index (CAVI). This last one -CAVI- presents an advantage: it is independent from blood pressure levels during measurement[14].

Characteristics and methods of the main studies with CAVI in Spain

The MARK study[18] is a cross-sectional analysis of persons from three Spanish regions (Catalonia, Castile and Leon and Balearic Community). Selection of participants was random and included 2495 individuals (participation rate 70%) aged 35-74 at intermediate CV risk. The study includes demographic and social baseline information, received medications related to cardiovascular diseases, clinical history of cardiovascular risk factors, lifestyles, arterial stiffness, and laboratory data. CAVI was selected as the measure of arterial stiffness.

The REGICOR study is a descriptive, population-based, cross-sectional study developed by the *Registre Gironídel Cor* (REGICOR) research group. From 2003 to 2006, a population-based cohort was recruited in Girona (Catalonia) in the context of the REGICOR study, and 6556 individuals aged 35 to 79 years were included[19]. Between September 2007 and November 2013, all participants were invited to participate in a follow-up visit and 4280 attended (participation rate > 70%). The population in this analysis is a random subsample of the participants with VaSera measurements, recorded in the follow-up visit. Eligible participants were aged 40 to 90 years. Nurses received training to perform the examinations following a standardized protocol. CAVI measurement was performed using the VaSera VS-1500 device (FukudaDenshi Co Ltd), following the manufacturer's instructions for the best accuracy of the measurement.

The early vascular aging (EVA) study[20] is an observational, descriptive, cross-sectional study that used a cluster random sampling stratified by age and gender to obtain 500 participants aged between 35 and 75. The two main dependent variables were the carotid-femoral pulse wave velocity (cf-PWV), determined using the SphygmoCor

Institut Universitari per a la recerca a l'Atenció Primària Jordi Gol i Gurina (IDIAPJGol), Institut d'Investigació Biomèdica de Girona (IdIBGi), Department of Medical Sciences, University of Girona, Spain.

System, and CAVI, measured with VaSera. Other registered variables were carotid intima-media thickness, central and peripheral augmentation index, ankle-brachial pulse wave velocity, ankle-brachial index, retinal arteriovenous index, renal and cardiac organ damage, lifestyles (physical activity, adherence to the Mediterranean diet, alcohol and tobacco consumption), psychological factors (depression, anxiety, and chronic stress), inflammatory factors and oxidative stress.

The LOD-DIABETES study[21] is an observational prospective study with 5 years of follow-up. A consecutive sampling was carried out to include 110 patients aged between 20-80 years with type 2 diabetes. Registered variables were: patient's age and sex, family and personal history of cardiovascular disease, and cardiovascular risk factors; height, weight, heart rate and abdominal circumference; laboratory tests: hemoglobin, lipid profile, creatinine, microalbuminuria, glomerular filtration rate, blood glucose, glycosylated hemoglobin, blood insulin, fibrinogen, and high sensitivity C-reactive protein; clinical and 24-hour ambulatory (home) blood pressure monitoring and self-measured blood pressure; common carotid artery ultrasound, to measure mean carotid intima-media thickness; electrocardiogram, to assess left ventricular hypertrophy; ankle-brachial index; retinal vascular study based on funduscopy with non-mydriatic retinography, and evaluation of pulse wave morphology and pulse wave velocity using the SphygmoCor system; medications used for diabetes, arterial hypertension and hyperlipidemia were also registered, together with antiplatelet drugs.

Results

Epidemiology of CAVI in Spain

The REGICOR study provided population reference values for CAVI assessment in men and women and across age groups[19]. Mean (standard deviation –SD-) CAVI was 8.76 (1.35), it increased with age and was significantly higher in men than in women in all age-groups. The prevalence of CAVI>9 among the 2,613 participants recruited in the REGICOR study was 41.1% (95% CI: 39.2-43.0). The prevalence of CAVI>9 was particularly high among participants aged 70-90 years. Fig. 1 shows original data from the REGICOR study analysed for the present publication that illustrate mean of CAVI values by age groups and sex in the Spanish population. Similarly, the mean (SD) CAVI value was 8.01 (1.44) in the EVA study, and arterial stiffness measured with CAVI also increased with age and was higher in men[22].

Association of CAVI with CV risk factors

All studies that included CAVI measurements in Spain assessed their association with cardiovascular risk factors. The REGICOR study established the association of classical cardiovascular risk factors -with the exception of BMI- and lack of physical activity with a CAVI ≥ 9[19].

The MARK study showed a positive association of fasting plasma glucose and HbA1c with CAVI in adults at intermediate cardiovascular risk, predominantly in those with type 2 diabetes mellitus[23]. In fact, all the components of the metabolic syndrome (except HDL-cholesterol) were associated with CAVI[24]. These findings were confirmed in the LOD-DIABETES study, where an association of CAVI

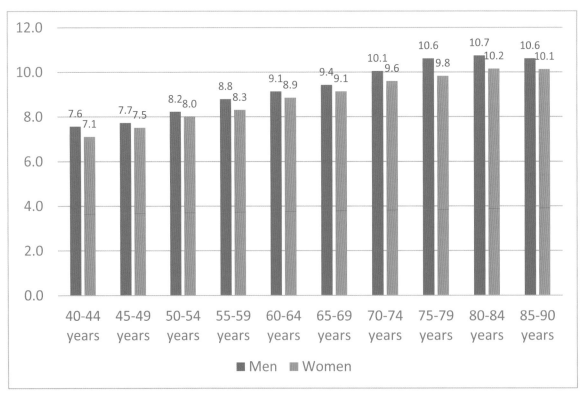

Fig. 1. Mean of CAVI values by age groups and sex in the Spanish population.
Source of data: the REGICOR study, original data analyzed for this publication.

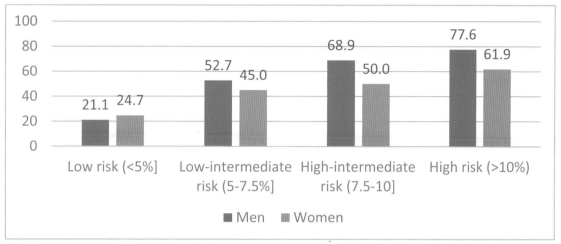

**Fig. 2. Proportion of individuals with CAVI ≥ 9 by sex and cardiovascular risk in the population of Spain.
Source of data: the REGICOR study, original data analyzed for this publication.**

with metabolic syndrome was also evidenced in patients with diabetes[25].

The EVA study showed an association of vascular aging as measured with VaSera with tobacco consumption, blood pressure, waist circumference, and altered baseline glycemia[26].

Role of CAVI in risk assessment in Spain

Results from the REGICOR study showed that the higher the coronary risk, the greater the prevalence of CAVI ≥ 9. Furthermore, the prevalence of CAVI ≥ 9 in groups not classified as high-risk reached 50%. Fig. 2 shows original data from the REGICOR study analysed for the present publication that illustrate the proportion of individuals with CAVI ≥ 9 by sex and cardiovascular risk in the population of Spain. CAVI ≥ 9 was frequent in individuals with low, low-intermediate, and high-intermediate coronary risk in both groups. A remarkable proportion of these participants could be reclassified to the high-risk group as previously published[19]. In both sexes, cardiovascular healthy individuals had a lower prevalence of CAVI ≥ 9 as well as lower mean CAVI scores than individuals with cardiovascular risk factors, across all 10 year-age categories from 40 to 69 years. These results suggest that CAVI assessment could be a useful tool to detect asymptomatic arteriosclerosis, and thus improve cardiovascular risk stratification[27].

The usefulness of CAVI to identify persons at high CV was also supported by the results of the MARK study. This study showed a positive association of CAVI with vascular structure and function parameters and this association was independent of cardiovascular risk and of any medications received[28]. Finally, the LOD-DIABETES study showed association of CAVI with cardiovascular target organ damage and vascular structure and function in patients with diabetes[25].

Future of CAVI in Spanish research

Three new studies including CAVI measurement have been recently funded in Spain. The EIRA study aims to evaluate the effectiveness and costs of a complex multiple risk behaviour intervention to promote healthy attitudes in people aged between 45 and 75 years attended in Primary Health Care services[29]. The Aging Imagenomics Study[30] aims to identify biomarkers of human aging by analysing imaging, biopsychosocial, cardiovascular, metabolomic, lipidomic, and microbiome variables. Finally, the DESVELA study proposes to analyse whether personal determinants related to certain behaviours, social and family support, and social capital are independently associated with results in physical health, mental health, quality of life, lifestyles, and use of health services.

Conclusions

Almost 31% of persons aged 35-74 years, with CAVI > 9 and no CHD were at ≥ 10% 10-year CHD risk. Including CAVI > 9 in the screening process results in a considerable increase in the proportion of possible high-risk population when combined with 10-year CHD risk ≥ 10% using risk functions. All these results support the idea that CV risk screening strategies could be improved by adding CAVI measurement to CV risk assessment, particularly for older people. The analysed studies suggest this hypothesis considering a Mediterranean population with a known low risk of CHD. Primary prevention of CVDs is a priority in public health policies in developed and developing countries. The current main strategies include identification of people in a high-risk situation in whom preventive measures are effective and efficient. Improvement of this identification in our country would have an immediate impact, clinical and on well-being, and a short-term effect on public health. Information provided by CAVI measurement could be combined with the 10-year CHD risk estimation by risk functions, or incorporated in future cardiovascular prediction functions.

References

1) O'Flaherty M, Sans-Menendez S, Capewell S, Jørgensen T. Epidemiology of atherosclerotic cardiovascular disease:

scope of the problem and its determinants. In: The ESC Textbook of Preventive Cardiology. 2017. p. on line.

2) Mendis S, Puska P, Norrving B, editors. Global Atlas on cardiovascular disease prevention and control. Geneva: World Health Organization; 2011.

3) Cooney MT, Dudina A, Whincup P, Capewell S, Menotti A, Jousilahti P, et al. Re-evaluating the Rose approach: Comparative benefits of the population and high-risk preventive strategies. Eur J Cardiovasc Prev Rehabil. 2009;16(5):541–9.

4) Peters RJG. Health literacy skills and the benefits of cardiovascular disease prevention. Netherlands Hear J. 2017;25:407–8.

5) McGill HC, McMahan CA, Gidding SS. Preventing heart disease in the 21st century: Implications of the pathobiological determinants of atherosclerosis in youth (PDAY) study. Circulation. 2008;117(9):1216–27.

6) Liu K, Daviglus ML, Loria CM, Colangelo LA, Spring B, Moller AC, et al. Healthy lifestyle through young adulthood and the presence of low cardiovascular disease risk profile in middle age: The Coronary Artery Risk Development in (Young) Adults (CARDIA) study. Circulation. 2012;125(8):996–1004.

7) Last JM, editor. A Dictionary of Epidemiology. 4th ed. New York: Oxford University Press; 2001.

8) Perk J, De Backer G, Gohlke H, Graham I, Reiner Ž, Verschuren M, et al. European Guidelines on cardiovascular disease prevention in clinical practice (version 2012). Eur Heart J. 2012;33(13):1635–701.

9) Rose G. Sick individuals and sick populations. Int J Epidemiol. 1985 Mar 1;14(1):32–8.

10) Manuel DG. Revisiting Rose: strategies for reducing coronary heart disease. BMJ. 2006;332(7542):659–62.

11) Amor AJ, Serra-Mir M, Martínez-González MA, Corella D, Salas-Salvadó J, Fitó M, et al. Prediction of Cardiovascular Disease by the Framingham-REGICOR Equation in the High-Risk PREDIMED Cohort: Impact of the Mediterranean Diet Across Different Risk Strata. J Am Heart Assoc. 2017;6(3):e004803.

12) Marrugat J, Vila J, Baena-Díez JM, Grau M, Sala J, Ramos R, Subirana I, Fitó M, Elosua R. Relative validity of the 10-year cardiovascular risk estimate in a population cohort of the REGICOR study. Rev Esp Cardiol. 2011;64:385–394. doi:10.1016/j.rec.2010.12.017

13) Masiá R, Pena A, Marrugat J, Sala J, Vila J, Pavesi M, Covas M, Aubó C, Elosua R. High prevalence of cardiovascular risk factors in Gerona, Spain, a province with low myocardial infarction incidence. REGICOR Investigators. J Epidemiol Community Health. 1998;52:707–715. doi:10.1136/jech.52. 11.707

14) Shirai K, Hiruta N, Song M, Kurosu T, Suzuki J, Tomaru T, Miyashita Y, Saiki A, Takahashi M, Suzuki K, Takata M. Cardio-ankle vascular index (CAVI) as a novel indicator of arterial stiffness: theory, evidence and perspectives. J Atheroscler Thromb. 2011;18:924–938.

15) Sakuragi S, Abhayaratna WP. Arterial stiffness: methods of measurement, physiologic determinants and prediction of cardiovascular outcomes. Int J Cardiol. 2010;138:112–118.

16) Shah PK. Screening Asymptomatic Subjects for Subclinical Atherosclerosis. Can We, Does It Matter, and Should We? J Am Coll Cardiol. 2010;56:98–105. doi:10.1016/j. jacc.2009.09.081

17) Namekata, T., Suzuki, K., Ishizuka, N., & Shirai, K. Establishing baseline criteria of cardio-ankle vascular index as a new indicator of arteriosclerosis: a cross-sectional study. BMC Cardiovasc Disord. 2011;11: 51. doi:10.1186/1471-2261-11-51

18) Martí R, Parramon D, García-Ortiz L, Rigo F, Gómez-Marcos MA, Sempere I,García-Regalado N, Recio-Rodriguez JI,

Agudo-Conde C, Feuerbach N, Garcia-Gil M, Ponjoan A, Quesada M, Ramos R. Improving interMediAte risk management. MARK study. BMC Cardiovasc Disord. 2011 Oct 13;11:61.

19) Elosua-Bayés M, Martí-Lluch R, García-Gil MDM, Camós L, Comas-Cufí M, Blanch J, Ponjoan A, Alves-Cabratosa L, Elosua R, Grau M, Marrugat J, Ramos R. Association of Classic Cardiovascular Risk Factors and Lifestyles With the Cardio-ankle Vascular Index in a General Mediterranean Population. Rev Esp Cardiol (Engl Ed). 2018 Jun;71(6):458-465.

20) Gomez-Marcos MA, Martinez-Salgado C, Gonzalez-Sarmiento R,Hernandez-Rivas JM, Sanchez-Fernandez PL, Recio-Rodriguez JI, Rodriguez-Sanchez E, García-Ortiz L. Association between different risk factors and vascular accelerated ageing (EVA study): study protocol for a cross-sectional, descriptive observational study. BMJ Open. 2016 Jun 7;6(6):e011031. doi: 10.1136/bmjopen-2016-011031

21) Gómez-Marcos MA, Recio-Rodríguez JI, Rodríguez-Sánchez E, Castaño-Sánchez Y, de Cabo-Laso A, Sánchez-Salgado B, Rodríguez-Martín C, Castaño-Sánchez C, Gómez-Sánchez L, García-Ortiz L. Central blood pressure and pulse wave velocity: relationship to target organ damage and cardiovascular morbidity-mortality in diabetic patients or metabolic syndrome. An observational prospective study. LOD-DIABETES study protocol. BMC Public Health. 2010 Mar 18;10:143. doi: 10.1186/1471-2458-10-143

22) Gómez-Sánchez M, Patino-Alonso MC, Gómez-Sánchez L, Recio-Rodríguez JI, Rodríguez-Sánchez E, Maderuelo-Fernández JA, García-Ortiz L, Gómez-Marcos MA; EVA Group. Reference values of arterial stiffness parameters and their association with cardiovascular risk factors in the Spanish population. The EVA Study. Rev Esp Cardiol (Engl Ed). 2020 Jan;73(1):43-52.

23) Gomez-Sanchez L, Garcia-Ortiz L, Patino-Alonso MC, Recio-Rodriguez JI, Feuerbach N, Marti R, Agudo-Conde C, Rodriguez-Sanchez E, Maderuelo-Fernandez JA, Ramos R, Gomez-Marcos MA; MARK Group. Glycemic markers and relation with arterial stiffness in Caucasian subjects of the MARK study. PLoS One. 2017 Apr 17;12(4):e0175982.

24) Gomez-Sanchez L, Garcia-Ortiz L, Patino-Alonso MC, Recio-Rodriguez JI, Fernando R, Marti R, Agudo-Conde C, Rodriguez-Sanchez E, Maderuelo-Fernandez JA, Ramos R, Gomez-Marcos MA; MARK Group. Association of metabolic syndrome and its components with arterial stiffness in Caucasian subjects of the MARK study: a cross-sectional trial. Cardiovasc Diabetol. 2016 Oct 24;15(1):148.

25) Gómez-Marcos MÁ, Recio-Rodríguez JI, Patino-Alonso MC, Agudo-Conde C, Gómez- Sánchez L, Gomez-Sanchez M, Rodríguez-Sanchez E, Maderuelo-Fernandez JA, García-Ortiz L; LOD-DIABETES Group. Cardio-ankle vascular index is associated with cardiovascular target organ damage and vascular structure and function in patients with diabetes or metabolic syndrome, LOD-DIABETES study: a case series report. Cardiovasc Diabetol. 2015 Jan 16;14:7.

26) Gómez-Sánchez M, Gómez-Sánchez L, Patino-Alonso MC, Alonso-Domínguez R, Sánchez-Aguadero N, Recio-Rodríguez JI, González-Sánchez J, García-Ortiz L, Gómez-Marcos MA; EVA group. Relationship of healthy vascular aging with lifestyle and metabolic syndrome in the general Spanish population. The EVA study. Rev Esp Cardiol (Engl Ed). 2020 Oct 29;S1885-5857(20)30423-0.

27) Martí-Lluch R, Garcia-Gil MDM, Camós L, Comas-Cufí M, Elosua-Bayés M, Blanch J, Ponjoan A, Alves-Cabratosa L, Elosua R, Grau M, Marrugat J, Ramos R. Differences in cardio-ankle vascular index in a general Mediterranean population depending on the presence or absence of metabolic cardiovascular risk factors. Atherosclerosis. 2017 Sep;264:29-35.

28) Gomez-Sanchez L, Garcia-Ortiz L, Patino-Alonso MC, Recio-Rodriguez JI, Frontera G, Ramos R, Martí R, Agudo-Conde C, Rodriguez-Sanchez E, Maderuelo-Fernández JA, Gomez-Marcos MA; MARK Group. The Association Between the Cardio-ankle Vascular Index and Other Parameters of Vascular Structure and Function in Caucasian Adults: MARK Study. J Atheroscler Thromb. 2015;22(9):901-11.

29) Zabaleta-Del-Olmo E, Pombo H, Pons-Vigués M, Casajuana-Closas M, Pujol-Ribera E, López-Jiménez T, Cabezas-Peña C, Martín-Borràs C, Serrano-Blanco A, Rubio-Valera M, Llobera J, Leiva A, Vicens C, Vidal C, Campiñez M, Martín-Álvarez R, Maderuelo JÁ, Recio JI, García-Ortiz L, Motrico E, Bellón JÁ, Moreno-Peral P, Martín-Cantera C, Clavería A, Aldecoa-Landesa S, Magallón-Botaya R, Bolíbar B. Complex multiple risk intervention to promote healthy behaviours in people between 45 to 75 years attended in primary health care (EIRA study): study protocol for a hybrid trial. BMC Public Health. 2018 Jul 13;18(1):874.

doi: 10.1186/s12889-018-5805-y. Erratum in: BMC Public Health. 2018 Aug 13;18(1):1004.

30) Puig J, Biarnes C, Pedraza S, Vilanova JC, Pamplona R, Fernández-Real JM, Brugada R, Ramos R, Coll-de-Tuero G, Calvo-Perxas L, Serena J, Ramió-Torrentà L, Gich J, Gallart L, Portero-Otin M, Alberich-Bayarri A, Jimenez-Pastor A, Camacho-Ramos E, Mayneris-Perxachs J, Pineda V, Font R, Prats-Puig A, Gacto ML, Deco G, Escrichs A, Clotet B, Paredes R, Negredo E, Triaire B, Rodríguez M, Heredia-Escámez A, Coronado R, de Graaf W, Prevost V, Mitulescu A, Daunis-I- Estadella P, Thió-Henestrosa S, Miralles F, Ribas-Ripoll V, Puig-Domingo M, Essig M, Figley CR, Figley TD, Albensi B, Ashraf A, Reiber JHC, Schifitto G, Md Nasir U, Leiva-Salinas C, Wintermark M, Nael K, Vilalta-Franch J, Barretina J, Garre-Olmo J. The Aging Imageomics Study: rationale, design and baseline characteristics of the study population. Mech Ageing Dev. 2020 Jul;189:111257.

Association of CAVI with Cardiovascular Risk Factors and Cardiovascular Events in Metabolic Syndrome in Lithuania

Ligita Ryliškytė[1,2] and Agnė Jucevičienė[1,2]

1. Introduction

The term "metabolic syndrome" (MetS) describes a cluster of proatherogenic risk factors for cardiovascular (CV) disease[1] and type 2 diabetes mellitus[2]. Metabolic syndrome subjects have a 5-fold increased risk of diabetes[2,3] and 3-fold increase of cardiovascular disease mortality, as compared to the individuals without metabolic syndrome[3]. The prominent pathophysiological mechanisms of the increased risk involve insulin resistance, oxidative stress, and chronic inflammatory condition, which manifest itself in early arterial aging, and proinflammatory and prothrombotic states[4]. The main components of metabolic syndrome are increased blood pressure, dyslipidemia (increased level of triglycerides and decreased level of high-density lipoprotein cholesterol), increased fasting glucose level and visceral obesity measured by waist circumference[5].

It has been shown that metabolic syndrome and its various components are associated with an increase in arterial stiffness[6,7,8,9,10]. Multiple studies performed in various populations have demonstrated that elevated arterial stiffness, in turn, predicts higher cardiovascular and all-cause mortality[11]. Though longitudinal CV outcome studies in MetS subjects are lacking, this data suggests that the increase in CV risk in MetS might be mediated by early vascular aging, especially, by the increase in arterial stiffness[12]. Correspondingly, this provides a rationale for evaluating the association between arterial stiffness and cardiovascular outcomes in MetS subjects. But what methods should be used?

There is a number of methods that help to evaluate arterial stiffness[13]. CAVI index stands out for its wide applicability, as it does not require sophisticated technical skills. Moreover, as a potential prognostic marker of CV risk, the CAVI index is especially promising because it does not depend on the variation of blood pressure, as it is calculated by the stiffness parameter beta and Bramwell-Hill equation, correcting for blood pressure parameters during the measurement[14,15,16]. Because of this advantage, CAVI has been used in the evaluation of the real effect of blood pressure control on the arteries during antihypertensive

therapy[17,18]. Accumulating evidence suggests that CAVI might be equal or superior to PWV as a long-term cardiovascular (CV) risk predictor[19,20,21]. To further evaluate this, more large longitudinal studies are needed.

At the Vilnius University Hospital Santaros Klinikos, we performed several studies to assess the relation of CAVI to traditional cardiovascular and cardiometabolic risk factors and to evaluate its association with cardiovascular events among middle-aged subjects with metabolic syndrome[22,23,24]. This paper summarizes our experience gathered since the year 2009. The main objective was to evaluate the relation between CAVI and cardiovascular outcomes.

2. Study Subjects and Design

To achieve this objective, we carried out the follow-up study of 3.9 ± 1.7 years. The study included 2728 middle-aged (53.95 ± 6.18 years old, 63% women) MetS subjects. All study subjects were participants of the Lithuanian High Cardiovascular Risk (LitHiR) primary prevention program. All participants were recruited at a single specialized health care centre, Vilnius University Hospital Santaros Klinikos during the years 2009-2011.

As described in more detail earlier, the LitHir program focuses on women (aged 50–65) and men (aged 40–55) without a history of cardiovascular disease[25,26]. Out of a total of 413 155 subjects screened in the Lithuanian primary health care centers according to the LitHir protocol in 2009-2011, 2941 subjects with the initial diagnosis of MetS were referred to Santaros Klinikos for further evaluation. After a detailed assessment, MetS was confirmed in 2728 subjects. As previously reported[19], the subjects with available CAVI data comprised n = 2106 of the follow-up cohort, and the data of these subjects is analyzed below.

MetS was defined in accordance to the revised National Cholesterol Education Program Adult Treatment Panel III (NCEP ATPIII) criteria[27], when at least 3 out of 5 of the following criteria were present:

- Waist circumference $\geq$ 102 cm in men, $\geq$ 88 cm in women;
- Triglycerides $\geq$ 1.7 mmol/l;

[1]Vilnius University Hospital Santaros Klinikos, Santariškių str. 2, Vilnius, Lithuania.
[2]Clinic of Cardiac and Vascular Diseases Institute of Clinical Medicine of the Faculty of Medicine of Vilnius University, M. K. Čiurlionio str. 21, Vilnius, Lithuania.

– High-density lipoprotein cholesterol < 1.03 mmol/l in men, < 1.29 mmol/l in women;
– Blood pressure (BP) ≥ 130/85 mmHg (or on antihypertensive drug treatment in a patient with a history of hypertension);
– Fasting plasma glucose ≥ 5.6 mmol/l.

The outcome data for these subjects was retrieved from Lithuanian National Death Registry and National Healthcare Fund Disease and Services Database. The outcome included the following CV events: fatal and non-fatal myocardial infarction, cerebrovascular events (stroke or transient ischemic attack), and sudden cardiac death.

The study was approved by the Regional Ethics Committee (Permission No. 158200-13-641-205).

3. Methods

All patients underwent detailed assessment of the anthropometric data and CV risk profile, as well as detailed physical examination and clinical evaluation. The clinical evaluation included blood sampling, ECG, stress and cardiac ultrasound tests, and the non-invasive measurements of the vascular structure and function, as described earlier[22]. The fasting venous blood sample was collected for each

patient at baseline to assess renal function, serum lipid profile, high sensitivity C-reactive protein (hsCRP), and glucose metabolism (fasting and oral glucose tolerance test [OGTT] glucose and insulin).

A comprehensive noninvasive assessment of arterial markers of vascular aging and subclinical atherosclerosis was carried out in all patients. VaSera-1000 device (Fukuda Denshi Co. Ltd., Tokyo, Japan) was used to measure CAVI arterial stiffness index. Right CAVI and left CAVI measurements were obtained on the right and left side of the body in accordance to the specification of the device, as described earlier[28]. Mean CAVI was then calculated and used for the CV outcome statistical analysis.

Statistical analysis was performed using STATISTICA (StatSoft, version 10). Kaplan-Meier survival curves were constructed for comparison of the cumulative proportion of the event-free survival in subjects with CAVI above and below the median. In all comparisons, values of p < 0.05 were considered statistically significant.

4. Results

4.1. The Baseline Characteristics

All 2106 MetS subjects included into the CV outcome

Table 1. The Baseline Characteristics of the Participants.

Characteristic variable	All subjects Mean ± SD	Women Mean ± SD	Men Mean ± SD	P value*
Age, years	53.83 ± 6.17	57.39 ± 4.08	48.02 ± 4.31	<0.001
Height, m	1.68 ± 0.10	1.61 ± 0.06	1.78 ± 0.07	<0.001
Weight, kg	90.66 ± 17.07	84.19 ± 14.23	101.25 ± 16.01	<0.001
BMI, kg/m^2	32.20 ± 4.89	32.29 ± 5.19	32.06 ± 4.34	0.283
Waist circumference, cm	107.08 ± 10.80	104.77 ± 10.58	110.87 ± 10.08	<0.001
TC, mmol/L	6.98 ± 1.54	7.12 ± 1.40	6.75 ± 1.71	<0.001
LDL-C, mmol/L	4.51 ± 1.29	4.74 ± 1.25	4.14 ± 1.26	<0.001
HDL-C, mmol/L	1.26 ± 0.34	1.35 ± 0.30	1.11 ± 0.34	<0.001
TG, mmol/L	2.66 ± 2.69	2.22 ± 1.29	3.37 ± 3.94	<0.001
Fasting glucose, mmol/L	6.26 ± 1.31	6.16 ± 1.16	6.44 ± 1.50	<0.001
Plasma glucose after OGTT, mmol/L	6.66 ± 2.45	7.12 ± 2.56	5.94 ± 2.06	<0.001
Plasma fasting insulin, pmol/L	100.40 ± 61.75	93.66 ± 60.37	111.14 ± 62.44	<0.001
Plasma insulin after OGTT, pmol/L	385.39 ± 329.04	421.57 ± 324.89	330.32 ± 328.01	<0.001
HbA1c (%)	5.98 ± 0.69	5.97 ± 0.59	5.99 ± 0.82	0.337
Right CAVI	7.98 ± 1.51	8.00 ± 1.41	7.95 ± 1.66	0.430
Left CAVI	7.86 ± 1.53	7.91 ± 1.39	7.76 ± 1.72	0.030
Mean CAVI	7.92 ± 1.43	7.96 ± 1.35	7.85 ± 1.54	0.098
hsCRP, mg/dL	3.50 ± 4.76	3.51 ± 4.84	3.49 ± 4.62	0.926
Heart rate (bpm)	65.87 ± 9.31	65.34 ± 9.16	66.73 ± 9.51	0.009
MAP, mmHg	108.31 ± 13.17	107.85 ± 13.22	109.07 ± 13.06	0.047
ISI-Matsuda	5.61 ± 6.07	5.37 ± 6.81	5.99 ± 4.71	0.095
HOMA-IR	4.20 ± 3.44	3.87 ± 3.23	4.71 ± 3.68	<0.001
Smoking	513 (24%)	188 (14%)	325 (41%)	<0.001
Family history of CVD	723 (34%)	448 (34%)	275 (35%)	0.920
Diabetes	394 (19%)	245 (19%)	149 (19%)	0.960

*P value is provided for comparison between men and women; Abbreviations: BMI – body mass index; TC – total cholesterol; LDL-C – low density lipoprotein cholesterol; HDL-C – high density lipoprotein cholesterol; TG – triglycerides; OGTT - oral glucose tolerance test; HbA$_{1c}$ - glycated hemoglobin; CAVI - cardio-ankle vascular index; hsCRP – high sensitivity C-reactive protein; MAP - mean arterial pressure; HOMA-IR – Homeostasis Model Assessment of Insulin Resistance Index; ISI-Matsuda – Matsuda Insulin Sensitivity Index; CVD - cardiovascular disease.
[Cited from: Laucevičius A, Ryliškytė L, Balsytė J, et al. Association of cardio-ankle vascular index with cardiovascular risk factors and cardiovascular events in metabolic syndrome patients. Medicina. 2015;51:155][22].

analysis were middle-aged individuals (53.83 ± 6.17 years old) without overt CV disease. Women comprised more than a half of our study group (n = 1307, 62%). The baseline characteristics of the entire study population are presented in **Table 1**.

4.2. Relation between CAVI Values and CV Risk Factors

To estimate the relationship between CAVI index and cardiometabolic risk factors, we divided the follow-up cohort into two subgroups according to the median of CAVI (7.95). CAVI above the median was more frequent among the women as compared to men (n = 691 vs. 346, 54% vs. 44%, p < 0.0001). The comparison of the subgroups above and below CAVI median is presented in **Table 2**.

We found that subjects with higher CAVI were older (p < 0.001), had higher heart rate (p = 0.016) and mean arterial pressure (p < 0.001), as well as worse lipid and glucose metabolism profile. In particular, CAVI above the median was associated with elevated total and low-density lipoprotein (LDL) cholesterol and decreased high-density lipoprotein (HDL) cholesterol (all p < 0.01). Subjects above the CAVI median also had higher fasting and OGTT glucose levels (p < 0.05). However, serum triglyceride (TG) levels and insulin resistance and sensitivity indices did not differ significantly between low and high CAVI groups. Neither did the frequency of smoking (p = 0.74), diabetes (p = 0.25), family CV disease history (p = 0.72), or the presence of central obesity (p = 0.23).

4.3. Association between CAVI and Cardiovascular Outcome

During the follow-up, 93 (4.4%) subjects developed a cardiovascular event: myocardial infarction occurred in 55 (2.6%) subjects, while cerebrovascular event in 38 (1.8%) subjects. There were 6.5% (n = 6) fatal CV events and 2 deaths due to cancer.

Kaplan-Meier analysis revealed that CAVI above median was statistically significantly (Z = 2.079, p = 0.038) associated with better CV event-free survival (**Fig. 1**).

The Cox proportional hazard regression analysis showed that, in the univariate analysis, an increase in CAVI is associated with the higher risk of fatal or non-fatal CV event (HR 1.26 [1.03 – 1.55], p = 0.026). The multivariate analysis revealed that this association was mediated by the CV risk factors. After entering all variables into the model, only the hazard ratios for gender (HR 2.77 [1.49 – 5.14], p = 0.001) and age (HR 1.74 [1.27 – 2.38], p < 0.001) remained significantly associated with the occurrence of the cardiovascular event. Meanwhile, CAVI (HR 1.12 [0.9 – 1.4], p = 0.302) and fasting glucose (HR 1.16 [0.98 – 1.39], p = 0.085) did not retain independent association with the CV outcome.

When comparing the event and event-free groups, higher CAVI index was statistically significantly associated with the occurrence of all cardiovascular events (p = 0.045) and myocardial infarction (p = 0.027) but not with the occurrence of cerebrovascular events (p = 0.651). As compared to the event-free group, subjects who had a CV event were older (55.3 ± 5.9 vs. 53.8 ± 6.2, p = 0.017) and had slightly higher fasting glucose levels (6.54 ± 1.51 vs. 6.25 ± 1.30, p = 0.049)

Table 2. The Comparison between CV Risk Factors and CAVI Values (Student T-test, age and gender unadjusted).

Characteristic variable	CAVI value below the median Mean ± SD	CAVI value above the median Mean ± SD	P value
Age, years	52.23 ± 6.07	55.36 ± 5.92	<0.001
TC, mmol/L	6.88 ± 1.56	7.07 ± 1.51	0.004
LDL-C, mmol/L	4.42 ± 1.29	4.59 ± 1.28	0.004
HDL-C, mmol/L	1.28 ± 0.33	1.23 ± 0.34	0.004
TG, mmol/L	2.66 ± 2.55	2.68 ± 2.86	0.860
Fasting glucose, mmol/L	6.20 ± 1.18	6.34 ± 1.44	0.023
Plasma glucose after OGTT, mmol/L	6.51 ± 2.30	6.81 ± 2.58	0.031
Plasma fasting insulin, pmol/L	104.22 ± 69.08	97.07 ± 54.15	0.021
Plasma insulin after OGTT, pmol/L	371.72 ± 307.32	396.41 ± 345.19	0.198
HbA1c (%)	5.96 ± 0.67	6.00 ± 0.71	0.201
hsCRP, mg/dL	3.69 ± 4.95	3.32 ± 4.60	0.083
Heart rate (bpm)	65.40 ± 9.05	66.48 ± 9.57	0.040
MAP, mmHg	107.00 ± 12.91	109.30 ± 13.21	<0.001
ISI Matsuda	5.72 ± 6.34	5.53 ± 5.90	0.592
HOMA-IR	4.28 ± 3.44	4.14 ± 3.48	0.408

BMI – body mass index; TC – total cholesterol; LDL-C – low density lipoprotein cholesterol; HDL-C – high density lipoprotein cholesterol; TG – triglycerides; OGTT - oral glucose tolerance test; HbA1c - glycated hemoglobin; CAVI - cardio-ankle vascular index; hsCRP – high sensitivity C-reactive protein; MAP - mean arterial pressure; ISI-Matsuda – Matsuda Insulin Sensitivity Index; HOMA-IR – Homeostasis Model Assessment of Insulin Resistance Index.
[Cited from: Laucevičius A, Ryliškytė L, Balsytė J, et al. Association of cardio-ankle vascular index with cardiovascular risk factors and cardiovascular events in metabolic syndrome patients. Medicina. 2015;51:155][22].

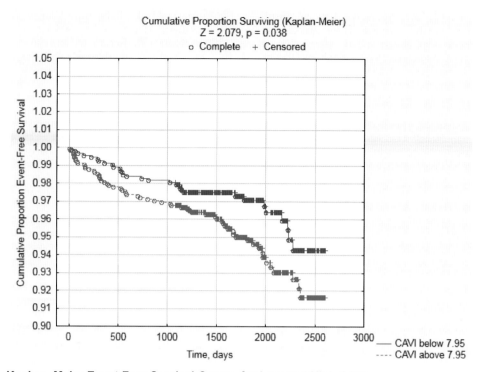

Fig. 1. Kaplan–Meier Event-Free Survival Curves for Low and High CAVI.

[Cited from: Laucevičius A, Ryliškytė L, Balsytė J, et al. Association of cardio-ankle vascular index with cardiovascular risk factors and cardiovascular events in metabolic syndrome patients. Medicina. 2015;51:156][22].

but did not differ by other variables.

5. Discussion

This study evaluated the relation between cardiometabolic risk factors and CAVI in the middle-aged Lithuanian subjects with metabolic syndrome. In concurrence with previously published data, we found that higher CAVI values were associated with older age, dyslipidemia, and dysglycemia[17,21,29,30].

The follow-up analysis revealed that higher CAVI values are associated with the total number of cardiovascular events and with the incidence of myocardial infarction. While cerebrovascular events showed a similar tendency, this tendency did not reach statistical significance. This might be explained by the relatively low number of strokes in our cohort. In a larger cohort, the association between cerebrovascular events and increased arterial stiffness still can be expected, as a recent cross-sectional study demonstrated that stroke patients with metabolic syndrome, compared control subjects without stroke, showed higher PWV[31]. The fact that the association between CAVI and CV outcome in our Cox proportional hazard regression model was mitigated by the inclusion of other cardiometabolic risk factors suggests that CAVI might be considered as a surrogate marker for CV risk and reflects the total burden of MetS and traditional CV risk factors on the arteries.

Though data on the predictive value of CAVI in MS patients was not previously available, CAVI has been shown to be associated with CV outcomes in patients with coronary heart disease (p < 0.01)[17,32]. However, to the best of our knowledge, we were first to demonstrate the relation between CV outcome and CAVI in MetS subjects.

Conclusion

To conclude, the data analysis in subjects with MetS, recruited according to LitHir program at the Vilnius University Hospital Santaros Klinikos, demonstrated that higher CAVI values are associated with an elevated total and low-density lipoprotein cholesterol, decreased high-density lipoprotein cholesterol, higher fasting and OGTT glucose levels, and lower fasting insulin level, as well as with greater age, heart rate, and mean arterial pressure. Most importantly, according to Kaplan-Meier event-free survival analysis, CAVI above the median was predictive of cardiovascular outcome.

References

1) Sookoian S, Pirola CJ. Metabolic syndrome: from the genetics to the pathophysiology. Curr Hypertens Rep. 2011 Apr;13:149–57.
2) Ford ES, Li C, Sattar N. Metabolic syndrome and incident diabetes: current state of the evidence. Diabetes Care. 2008;31:1898-1904.
3) Malik S, Wong ND, Franklin SS, Kamath TV, L'Italien GJ, Pio JR, et al. Impact of the metabolic syndrome on mortality from coronary heart disease, cardiovascular disease, and all causes in United States adults. Circulation 2004;110:1245–50.
4) Kim M, Kim M, Yoo HJ, Lee SY, Lee S, Lee JH. Age-specific determinants of pulse wave velocity among metabolic syndrome components, inflammatory markers, and oxidative stress. J Atheroscler Thromb. 2018;25:178-185.
5) Alberti KG, Eckel RH, Grundy SM, Zimmet PZ, Cleeman JI, Donato KA, Fruchart JC, James WP, Loria CM, Smith SC Jr. International Diabetes Federation Task

Force on Epidemiology and Prevention; Hational Heart, Lung, and Blood Institute; American Heart Association; World Heart Federation; International Atherosclerosis Society; International Association for the Study of Obesity. Harmonizing the metabolic syndrome: a joint interim statement of the International Diabetes Federation Task Force on Epidemiology and Prevention; National Heart, Lung, and Blood Institute; American Heart Association; World Heart Federation; International Atherosclerosis Society; and International Association for the Study of Obesity. Circulation 2009; 120:1640–1645.

6) Scuteri A, Najjar SS, Muller DC, et al. Metabolic syndrome amplifies the age-associated increases in vascular thickness and stiffness. J Am Coll Cardiol. 2004;43:1388-1395.

7) Scuteri A, Cunha PG, Rosei EA, et al. Arterial stiffness and influences of the metabolic syndrome: A cross-countries study. Atherosclerosis. 2014;233:654.

8) Chen L, Zhu W, Mai L, Fang L, Ying K. The association of metabolic syndrome and its components with brachial-ankle pulse wave velocity in South China. Atherosclerosis. 2015;240:345-350.

9) Topouchian J., Labat C., Gautier S., et al. Effects of metabolic syndrome on arterial function in different age groups: the Advanced Approach to Arterial Stiffness study. Journal of Hypertension 2018;36:824-833.

10) Lopes-Vicente W, Rodrigues S, Cepeda FX, et al. Arterial stiffness and its association with clustering of metabolic syndrome risk factors. Diabetology & metabolic syndrome. 2017;9:87.

11) Vlachopoulos C, Aznaouridis K, Stefanadis C. Prediction of cardiovascular events and all-cause mortality with arterial stiffness: a systematic review and meta-analysis. J Am Coll Cardiol 2010; 55:1318–1327.

12) Nilsson PM. Arterial stiffness, the metabolic syndrome, and the brain. Am J Hypertens. 2018;31:24-26. doi: 10.1093/ajh/hpx152

13) Laurent S, Marais L, Boutouyrie P. The noninvasive assessment of vascular aging. Can J Cardiol. 2016;32:669-679. doi: 10.1016/j.cjca.2016.01.039

14) Ibata J, Sasaki H, Kakimoto T, et al. Cardio-ankle vascular index measures arterial wall stiffness independent of blood pressure. Diabetes Res Clin Pract 2008;80:265–70.

15) Wang H, Liu J, Zhao H, Fu X, Shang G, Zhou Y, et al. Arterial stiffness evaluation by cardio-ankle vascular index in hypertension and diabetes mellitus subjects. J Am Soc Hypertens 2013;7:426–31.

16) Gómez-Marcos MÁ, Recio-Rodríguez JI, Patino-Alonso MC, et al. Cardio-ankle vascular index is associated with cardiovascular target organ damage and vascular structure and function in patients with diabetes or metabolic syndrome, LOD-DIABETES study: a case series report. Cardiovasc Diabetol 2015;14:7.

17) Shirai K, Utino J, Otsuka K, Takata M. A novel blood pressure-independent arterial wall stiffness parameter; cardio-ankle vascular index (CAVI). J Atheroscler Thromb 2006;13:101–7.

18) Shirai K, Utino J, Saiki A, Endo K, Ohira M, Nagayama D, et al. Evaluation of Blood Pressure Control using a New Arterial Stiffness Parameter, Cardio-ankle Vascular Index (CAVI). Curr Hypertens Rev 2013;9:66–75.

19) Takaki A, Ogawa H, Wakeyama T, Iwami T, Kimura M, Hadano Y, et al. Cardio-Ankle Vascular Index Is Superior to Brachial-Ankle Pulse Wave Velocity as an Index of Arterial Stiffness. Hypertens Res 2008;31:1347–55.

20) Nakamura K, Tomaru T, Yamamura S, Miyashita Y, Shirai K, Noike H. Cardio-ankle vascular index is a candidate predictor of coronary atherosclerosis. Circ J 2008;72:598–604.

21) Tian G, Wei W, Zhang W, Zhang L, You H, Liu W, et al. Increasing age associated with elevated cardio-ankle vascular index scores in patients with type 2 diabetes mellitus. J Int Med Res 2013;41:435–44.

22) Laucevicius A, Ryliškytė L, Balsytė J, et al. Association of cardio-ankle vascular index with cardiovascular risk factors and cardiovascular events in metabolic syndrome patients. Medicina. 2015;51:152-158. doi: 10.1016/j.medici. 2015.05.001

23) Solovjova S., Ryliškytė L., Čelutkienė J., et al. Aortic stiffness is an independent determinant of left ventricular diastolic dysfunction in metabolic syndrome patients. Blood Pressure 2016;25:11-20.

24) Ryliškytė L., Navickas R., Šerpytis P., Puronaitė R., Zupkauskienė J., Jucevičienė A., Badarienė J., Rimkienė M.A., Ryliškienė K., Skiauterytė E., Laucevičius A. Association of aortic stiffness, carotid intima-media thickness and endothelial function with cardiovascular events in metabolic syndrome subjects. Blood Pressure 2019;28:131-138.

25) Laucevicius A, Kasiulevičius V, Jatužis D, et al. Lithuanian High Cardiovascular Risk (LitHiR) primary prevention programme – rationale and design. Semin Cardiovasc Med 2012;18:1–6.

26) Laucevičius A, Rinkūnienė E, Petrulionienė Ž, et al. Trends in cardiovascular risk factor prevalence among Lithuanian middle-aged adults between 2009 and 2018. Atherosclerosis. 2020;299:9-14.

27) National Cholesterol Education Program (NCEP) Expert Panel on Detection, Evaluation, and Treatment of High Blood Cholesterol in Adults (Adult Treatment Panel III). Third report of the National Cholesterol Education Program (NCEP) Expert Panel on detection, evaluation, and treatment of high blood cholesterol in adults (adult treatment panel III) final report. Circulation 2002;106:3143–421.

28) Slivovskaja I, Ryliskyte L, Serpytis P, et al. Aerobic Training Effect on Arterial Stiffness in Metabolic Syndrome. Am J Med. 2018;131:148-5.

29) Gomez-Sanchez L, Garcia-Ortiz L, Patino-Alonso M, et al. Association of metabolic syndrome and its components with arterial stiffness in caucasian subjects of the MARK study: A cross-sectional trial. Cardiovascular diabetology. 2016;15:148.

30) Kim KJ, Lee B-W, Kim H-M, Shin JY, Kang ES, Cha BS, et al. Associations between cardio-ankle vascular index and microvascular complications in type 2 diabetes mellitus patients. J Atheroscler Thromb 2011;18:328–36.

31) Tuttolomondo A, Di Raimondo D, Di Sciacca R, et al. Arterial stiffness and ischemic stroke in subjects with and without metabolic syndrome. Atherosclerosis. 2012;225:216-219. doi: 10.1016/j.atherosclerosis.2012.08.027

32) Otsuka K, Fukuda S, Shimada K, Suzuki K, Nakanishi K, Yoshiyama M, et al. Serial assessment of arterial stiffness by cardio-ankle vascular index for prediction of future cardiovascular events in patients with coronary artery disease. Hypertens Res 2014;37:1014–20.

The role of cardio-ankle vascular index and fat deposition in coronary arterial disease in an asymptomatic general population

Su-Yeon Choi[1,2] and Byung-Hee Oh[1,3]

Introduction

Arterial stiffness is an early marker of systemic atherosclerosis and an independent predictor of the progression of atherosclerosis, cardiovascular events, and all-cause mortality independent of traditional risk factors[1-3]. Pulse wave velocity (PWV) has been widely used to estimate arterial stiffness using non-invasive methods; however, it may be influenced by blood pressure (BP) at the time of measurement[4]. Cardio-ankle vascular index (CAVI) representing the stiffness of the whole artery, including the aorta, femoral, and tibial arteries, is easy to measure, not affected by BP during measurement, and has better reproducibility than PWV[4, 5].

Inflammation plays an important role in the pathogenesis of atherosclerosis, which underlies the development of all cardiovascular diseases (CVDs)[6]. Visceral fat as "sick fat" secretes large quantities of inflammatory cytokines and is the primary mediator of adverse effects, particularly increased cardiovascular (CV) risk, associated with obesity[7-9].

We addressed the clinical validity and application of the arterial stiffness measured using CAVI associated with different fat compartments (according to distribution or extent of the fat compartment) and with coronary artery disease in an asymptomatic general population.

The Association of Arterial Stiffness with Different Fat Compartments

Epicardial fat is correlated with CVD risk factors and is associated with vascular calcification with adjustment for metabolic risk factors and visceral adipose tissue, body mass index, and waist circumference, suggesting that these fat depots may exert local toxic effects on the vasculature[10]. Moreover, epicardial fat independently predicts the development of non-calcified coronary plaque[11] and is associated with fatal and nonfatal coronary events in the general population independent of traditional CV risk factors[12].

We investigated the association of fat burden with CAVI in the asymptomatic general population[13]. On the assessment of quartiles of CAVI, epicardial adipose tissue (EAT) showed serial increment, whereas abdominal subcutaneous to visceral adipose tissue ratio demonstrated a stepwise decrease from the first to the fourth quartile of CAVI. Abdominal visceral adipose tissue, EAT, and the abdominal subcutaneous to visceral adipose tissue ratio have shown significant correlations with arterial stiffness measured using CAVI, whereas the amount of total abdominal fat and subcutaneous adipose tissue did not. EAT showed the strongest correlation with CAVI and an independent association with arterial stiffness using multivariate correlation analysis.

Epicardial adipocytes have intrinsic pro-inflammatory and atherogenic secretion profiles through macrophage activation, oxidative stress, and the production of proinflammatory adipokines. The secretion of epicardial inflammatory molecules into the coronary bloodstream promotes atherogenesis[14]. Epicardial fat has been associated with fat accumulation in the liver, and increased release of free fatty acid and a state of intrinsic insulin resistance are the most likely mechanisms that link epicardial fat with infiltration of intrahepatic fat[15].

Nonalcoholic fatty liver disease (NAFLD) is associated with the risk factors for CVD, coronary artery calcification (CAC), and the development of CAC[16, 17]. We investigated whether NAFLD is associated with arterial stiffness in apparently healthy participants without any known liver or CV diseases[18]. On adjusting age, sex, body mass index, waist circumference, smoking status, diabetes, and hypertension, NAFLD was associated with a 32% increased risk of arterial stiffness (age- and sex-specific highest quartile of the CAVI). The risk of arterial stiffness increased according to the severity of NAFLD (adjusted odds ratio [OR], 95% confidence interval [CI] 1.20 [0.96–1.50] vs. 1.59 [1.21–2.08], for mild vs. moderate-to-severe with the reference of no NAFLD). The association between NAFLD and arterial stiffness was significant even in the non-obese groups. In subgroup analysis, the association between NAFLD and arterial stiffness was significant in the younger and non-obese group. The presence of cardiometabolic risk

[1]Department of Internal Medicine, Seoul National University College of Medicine, Seoul, Korea.
[2]Division of Cardiology, Healthcare System Gangnam Center, Seoul National University Hospital, Seoul, Korea.
[3]Division of Cardiology, Cardiovascular Center, Incheon Sejong Hospital, Incheon, Korea.

Table 1. Multivariate analysis of the association between nonalcoholic fatty liver disease and increased arterial stiffness (age-and sex-specific highest quartile of the CAVI) according to age and obesity.

Table 1. Multivariate analysis of the association between nonalcoholic fatty liver disease and increased arterial stiffness (age-and sex-specific highest quartile of the CAVI) according to age and obesity.

(Total N = 2954)	OR (95% CI)	*p*-value
No NAFLD	1 (reference)	
NAFLD	1.32 (1.08–1.61)	0.007
NAFLD grade		0.001*
Mild NAFLD	1.20 (0.96–1.50)	0.104
Moderate–severe NAFLD	1.59 (1.21–2.08)	0.001
Age <55 (n = 1343)		
NAFLD	1.54 (1.11–2.12)	0.009
NAFLD grade		0.002*
Mild NAFLD	1.34 (0.92–1.93)	0.122
Moderate–severe NAFLD	1.97 (1.28–3.01)	0.002
Age ≥ 55 (n = 1611)		
NAFLD	1.16 (0.90–1.49)	0.257
NAFLD grade		0.104*
Mild NAFLD	1.07 (0.81–1.42)	0.623
Moderate–severe NAFLD	1.37 (0.96–1.96)	0.081
BMI < 25 (n = 1875)		
NAFLD	1.35 (1.05–1.73)	0.018
NAFLD grade		0.004*
Mild NAFLD	1.23 (0.94–1.62)	0.134
Moderate–severe NAFLD	1.80 (1.19–2.71)	0.005
BMI ≥ 25 (n = 1079)		
NAFLD	1.24 (0.89–1.74)	0.205
NAFLD grade		0.128*
Mild NAFLD	1.15 (0.78–1.69)	0.490
Moderate–severe NAFLD	1.35 (0.92–1.98)	0.128

No NAFLD as the reference of OR. The multivariate model was adjusted for age, sex, BMI, WC, smoking status, diabetes, and hypertension. BMI = body mass index, CI = confidence interval, NAFLD = nonalcoholic fatty liver disease, OR = odds ratio, WC = waist circumference. *P value for the test of trend of odds.

factors in the older and obese group may attenuate the prediction (Table 1).

Liver fibroscan has recently been suggested as an alternative method to non-invasively diagnosed liver steatosis, while measurement of the controlled attenuation parameter (CAP) during transient elastography has shown high sensitivity for detecting low-grade steatosis, and a good correlation with the level of steatosis[19]. In asymptomatic patients without potential cause of liver disease, fatty liver defined as CAP ≥ 222 dB/m demonstrated a significant association with increased arterial stiffness (CAVI ≥ 8) (OR 2.309, 95% CI 1.419–3.756, p = .001) using adjusted regression analyses[20].

In these studies, fat compartments of visceral obesity have shown correlations with CAVI and is a possible risk factor for increased arterial stiffness. Excess visceral fat is accompanied by metabolic disease, and additionally, secretes large quantities of proinflammatory adipocytokines, including tumor necrosis factor α, interleukin 1 (IL-1), and IL-6, which are associated with CVDs[9, 21].

The Relation between Arterial Stiffness and Coronary Artery Calcification or Stenosis

Previous studies demonstrate that CAVI was related to CV risk factors and independently associated with the intima-media thickness of carotid artery and the presence and severity of coronary artery multivessel disease for assessment in patients with suspected coronary artery diseases[22].

We investigated the association of CAVI with the severity of CAC and coronary stenosis using coronary computed tomography angiography in an asymptomatic population without coronary artery disease[23]. After adjustment for age, sex, hypertension, diabetes, and dyslipidemia, a predefined cutoff value of CAVI ≥ 8 was associated with advanced CAC (CAC ≥ 300) and significant coronary stenosis

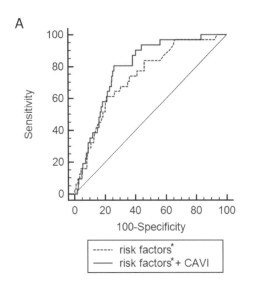

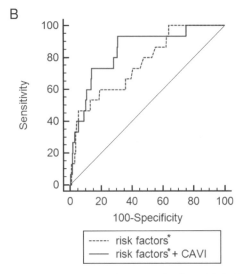

Fig. 1. Comparison of the area under curves for predicting coronary artery calcification (CAC ≥ 300) [A] and coronary stenosis ≥50% [B] for cardio-ankle vascular index (CAVI) additional to traditional risk factors. The area under curves shows increase from 0.739 to 0.791 (*p* = 0.023) [A] and from 0.761 to 0.842 (*p* = 0.032) [B].

*Risk factors include age ≥50 years, sex, hypertension, diabetes mellitus, dyslipidemia, and high sensitive C-reactive protein (cited from Park et al. J Atheroscler Thromb 2013;20:557-67.)

(stenosis $\geq$ 50%). Specifically, the adjusted OR (95% CI) of CAC $\geq$ 300 and coronary stenosis $\geq$ 50% was 3.57 (1.92–6.66) and 2.81 (1.13–7.00), respectively. Additional inclusion of CAVI improved the predictive power of the receiver operating characteristic curves for predicting coronary atherosclerosis based on traditional risk factors (Fig. 1).

These results suggest that CAVI reflects coronary atherosclerosis and may be used as a screening tool for assessing subclinical atherosclerotic burden in an asymptomatic population.

Conclusions

Increased epicardial fat and the presence of NAFLD are significantly associated with increased arterial stiffness independent of traditional CV risk factors in an asymptomatic general population. Moreover, the increased arterial stiffness is a surrogate and prognostic factor for coronary atherosclerosis with advanced CAC or significant coronary stenosis in an asymptomatic population.

CAVI is a non-invasive, readily available, and non-harmful clinical test to evaluate for subclinical atherosclerosis. Increased arterial stiffness particularly in individuals with high-visceral fat compartments is an indicator of increased risk for CVD. Assessment of arterial stiffness using CAVI may provide further risk discrimination in participants with increase epicardial fat or NAFLD. Therefore, active surveillance using CAVI may help screen and further stratify risk for CVD, particularly in individuals with high-fat compartments, and arterial stiffness measurement could guide more intensive therapeutic strategies for early primary CVD prevention. In those with increased epicardial fat or NAFLD and increased arterial stiffness, the development and progression of atherosclerosis and comorbidities should be actively screened and managed.

References

1) Vlachopoulos C, Aznaouridis K, Stefanadis C. Prediction of cardiovascular events and all-cause mortality with arterial stiffness: a systematic review and meta-analysis. J Am Coll Cardiol. 2010;55:1318-27.

2) Shirai K, Hiruta N, Song M, Kurosu T, Suzuki J, Tomaru T, et al. Cardio-ankle vascular index (CAVI) as a novel indicator of arterial stiffness: theory, evidence and perspectives. J Atheroscler Thromb. 2011;18:924-38.

3) Laurent S, Cockcroft J, Van Bortel L, Boutouyrie P, Giannattasio C, Hayoz D, et al. Expert consensus document on arterial stiffness: methodological issues and clinical applications. Eur Heart J. 2006;27:2588-605.

4) Shirai K, Utino J, Otsuka K, Takata M. A novel blood pressure-independent arterial wall stiffness parameter; cardio-ankle vascular index (CAVI). J Atheroscler Thromb. 2006;13:101-7.

5) Kubozono T, Miyata M, Ueyama K, Nagaki A, Otsuji Y, Kusano K, et al. Clinical significance and reproducibility of new arterial distensibility index. Circ J. 2007;71(1):89-94.

6) Ross R. Atherosclerosis--an inflammatory disease. N Engl J Med. 1999;340:115-26.

7) Bays HE. Adiposopathy is "sick fat" a cardiovascular disease? J Am Coll Cardiol. 2011;57:2461-73.

8) Despres JP. Body fat distribution and risk of cardiovascular disease: an update. Circulation. 2012;126(10):1301-13.

9) Van Gaal LF, Mertens IL, De Block CE. Mechanisms linking obesity with cardiovascular disease. Nature. 2006;444(7121):875-80.

10) Rosito GA, Massaro JM, Hoffmann U, Ruberg FL, Mahabadi AA, Vasan RS, et al. Pericardial fat, visceral abdominal fat, cardiovascular disease risk factors, and vascular calcification in a community-based sample: the Framingham Heart Study. Circulation. 2008;117:605-13.

11) Hwang IC, Park HE, Choi SY. Epicardial Adipose Tissue Contributes to the Development of Non-Calcified Coronary Plaque: A 5-Year Computed Tomography Follow-up Study. J Atheroscler Thromb. 2017;24:262-74.

12) Mahabadi AA, Berg MH, Lehmann N, Kalsch H, Bauer M, Kara K, et al. Association of epicardial fat with cardiovascular risk factors and incident myocardial infarction in the general population: the Heinz Nixdorf Recall Study. J Am Coll Cardiol. 2013;61:1388-95.

13) Park HE, Choi SY, Kim HS, Kim MK, Cho SH, Oh BH. Epicardial fat reflects arterial stiffness: assessment using 256-slice multidetector coronary computed tomography and cardio-ankle vascular index. J Atheroscler Thromb. 2012;19:570-6.

14) Iacobellis G. Local and systemic effects of the multifaceted epicardial adipose tissue depot. Nat Rev Endocrinol. 2015;11:363-71.

15) Kankaanpaa M, Lehto HR, Parkka JP, Komu M, Viljanen A, Ferrannini E, et al. Myocardial triglyceride content and epicardial fat mass in human obesity: relationship to left ventricular function and serum free fatty acid levels. J Clin Endocrinol Metab. 2006;91:4689-95.

16) Park HE, Kwak MS, Kim D, Kim MK, Cha MJ, Choi SY. Nonalcoholic Fatty Liver Disease Is Associated With Coronary Artery Calcification Development: A Longitudinal Study. J Clin Endocrinol Metab. 2016;101:3134-43.

17) Kim D, Choi SY, Park EH, Lee W, Kang JH, Kim W, et al. Nonalcoholic fatty liver disease is associated with coronary artery calcification. Hepatology. 2012;56:605-13.

18) Chung GE, Choi SY, Kim D, Kwak MS, Park HE, Kim MK, et al. Nonalcoholic fatty liver disease as a risk factor of arterial stiffness measured by the cardioankle vascular index. Medicine (Baltimore). 2015;94:e654.

19) Myers RP, Pollett A, Kirsch R, Pomier-Layrargues G, Beaton M, Levstik M, et al. Controlled Attenuation Parameter (CAP): a noninvasive method for the detection of hepatic steatosis based on transient elastography. Liver Int. 2012;32:902-10.

20) Park HE, Lee H, Choi SY, Kwak MS, Yang JI, Yim JY, et al. Usefulness of controlled attenuation parameter for detecting increased arterial stiffness in general population. Dig Liver Dis. 2018;50:1062-7.

21) Alexopoulos N, Katritsis D, Raggi P. Visceral adipose tissue as a source of inflammation and promoter of atherosclerosis. Atherosclerosis. 2014;233:104-12.

22) Izuhara M, Shioji K, Kadota S, Baba O, Takeuchi Y, Uegaito T, et al. Relationship of cardio-ankle vascular index (CAVI) to carotid and coronary arteriosclerosis. Circ J. 2008;72:1762-7.

23) Park JB, Park HE, Choi SY, Kim MK, Oh BH. Relation between cardio-ankle vascular index and coronary artery calcification or stenosis in asymptomatic subjects. J Atheroscler Thromb. 2013;20:557-67.

Metabolic Syndromes and CAVI

Noriko Satoh-Asahara

Summary

1. Cardio-ankle vascular index (CAVI) is associated with metabolic syndrome severity (MetS) [i.e., increased numbers of risk factors for MetS] and hypoadiponectinemia.

2. CAVI is a useful therapeutic assessment indicator in weight reduction therapy and relevant pharmacotherapy.

Aortic stiffness is predictive of cardiovascular diseases (CVD) and mortality from lifestyle-related diseases. Metabolic syndrome (MetS) includes a high-risk group of fatal atherosclerotic CVDs, such as myocardial infarction and stroke. Therefore, the establishment of early prediction and diagnostic indicator of arteriosclerosis progress is essential. The cardio-ankle vascular index (CAVI) has been established as an atherosclerosis index independent of blood pressure (BP) based on the β method, which is an index of vascular intrinsic stiffness. In our National Hospital Organization Obesity Multicenter Study, CAVI was associated with the severity of risk factors for MetS and hypoadiponectinemia. In addition, CAVI was useful as a sensitive indicator for evaluation of weight reduction therapy and pharmacotherapy. Thus, regular monitoring with CAVI in MetS may be crucial for the comprehensive management toward prevention of CVD and CKD.

Introduction

Metabolic syndrome (MetS) is a disease state combining hypertension, diabetes mellitus, and dyslipidemia in individuals with a visceral obesity status. MetS refers to a high-risk group of fatal atherosclerotic CVD diseases such as myocardial infarction and stroke. For the prevention of CVD events, it is urgent to establish and standardize the use of an accurate and simple indicator that can comprehensively diagnose atherosclerosis progression at early stages and not just manage blood sugar, blood pressure (BP), and lipid profiles.

Atherosclerosis in MetS

In MetS, the abnormal secretion of adipocytokines (e.g., hypoadiponectinemia and increased TNF-α and PAI-1) (which is associated with visceral adiposity) leads to insulin-resistance and increased inflammatory cytokine levels, which may promote vascular endothelial dysfunction, foam-cell formation, decreased vasorelaxant capacity, and vasospasm, which in turn lead to atherosclerosis progression[1].

Issues with measuring brachial-ankle pulse wave velocity (baPWV) in MetS

baPWV, a simple and non-invasive examination method of atherosclerosis, is challenged by BP's influence in the measurement[2]. Since hypertension is a risk factor for MetS, BP dependency is a key issue in baPWV measurements in MetS. To overcome this issue, cardio-ankle vascular index (CAVI) was developed as an arteriosclerotic indicator, independent of BP, based on the β method, a specific index for blood vessel sclerosis[3]. Recently, CAVI which is measuring PWV and BP is often used as a new index of arterial stiffness independent of BP[3].

MetS and CAVI

When CAVI was first released, there were no reports on the usefulness of CAVI as an atherogenic index in obesity. Therefore, we investigated its usefulness in obese patients, including MetS, in a multicenter study (Japan Obesity and Metabolic Syndrome Study [JOMS]) involving the National Hospital Organization Hospitals (NHO), since 2006. Among 325 obese Japanese outpatients in JOMS, CAVI was significantly higher in the 216 (67%) MetS patients meeting the criteria of the modified NCEP-ATPIII than in non-MetS patients, whereas no significant difference was observed in body mass index (BMI), total cholesterol (TC) BMI, TC, and LDL-C between both the groups.

In this study, baPWV values were highly positively correlated with systolic BP (SBP); CAVI values were also correlated with SBP, although the correlation was weaker (Fig. 1)[4]. Accordingly, these results suggested its superiority over baPWV in patients with obesity and MetS. In addition, CAVI values were significantly correlated with the severity of MetS and MetS-related parameters, such as hypoadiponectinemia, compared to that with baPWV severity (Fig. 2)[4].

Furthermore, we reported that CAVI was independently correlated with salivary cortisol levels, a typical stress marker, among obese patients, suggesting the significant association between stress status and CAVI in obese and MetS patients[5].

Based on these results, we suggest that CAVI may be a

Clinical Research Institute for Endocrine Metabolic Diseases, Kyoto Medical Center, 1-1 Fukakusa Mukaihata-cho, Fushimi-ku, Kyoto-shi, Kyoto 612-8555, Japan.

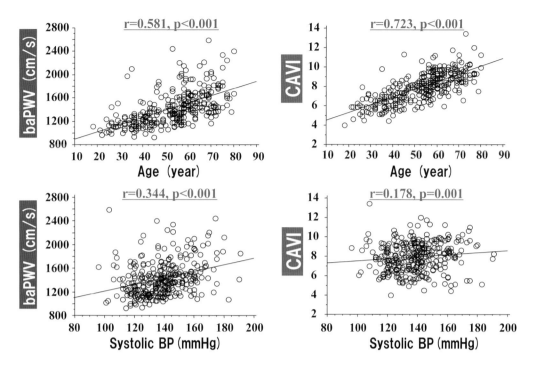

Adapted from ref.3

Fig. 1. Baseline correlations of baPWV and CAVI with age and systolic BP in obese patients.
baPWV: brachial-ankle Pulse Wave Velocity
CAVI: Cardio Ankle Vasucular Index
BP: Blood Pressure

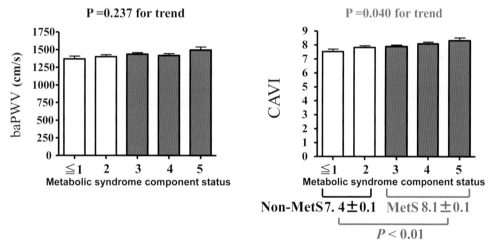

Metabolic syndrome components: abdominal obesity, high blood glucose, high blood
pressure (BP), low HDL, and high TG according to the criteria proposed by the NCEP-ATPIII

☐ Non-Mets:without metabolic syndrome

▨ Mets:with metabolic

In the analysis after correcting for age and BP, only CAVI increased
significantly with increasing numbers of MetS components.   Adapted from ref.4

**Fig. 2. Comparison of baPWV and CAVI means in obese patients stratified by number of components for metabolic
syndrome (MetS) (age- and BP-adjusted ANCOVA).**
baPWV: brachial-ankle Pulse Wave Velocity
CAVI: Cardio Ankle Vasucular Index
BP: Blood Pressure
HDL: High-Density Lipoprotein cholesterol
TG: Triglyceride
MetS: Metabolic Syndrome

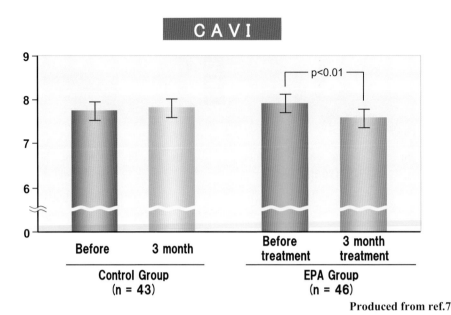

Produced from ref.7

Fig. 3. Highly purified eicosapentaenoic acid (EPA) significantly reduces CAVI values in patients with metabolic syndrome (MetS).

CAVI: Cardio Ankle Vasucular Index
EPA: Eicosapentaenoic Acid
MetS: Metabolic Syndrome

useful atherosclerotic indicator (independent of BP) that reflects atherosclerotic status influenced by lifestyle-related diseases and psychological status in patients with obesity and MetS.

CAVI as a therapeutic efficacy indicator for MetS

In the JOMS, a multicenter study by NHO revealed a significant reduction in CAVI values only in patients who successfully lost $\geq 3\%$ of their initial body weight after 3 months of weight reduction therapy through diet and exercise therapy[4].

In addition, in patients with obstructive sleep apnea syndromes in our obesity clinic, we found that CAVI was significantly correlated with the apnea-hypopnea index (AHI) and that an improvement in CAVI was significantly associated with AHI reduction through weight reduction therapy[6]. Furthermore, after a 3-month treatment with eicosapentaenoic acid (EPA), a lipid-lowering agent, CAVI was significantly decreased while there was an increase in adiponectin, oxidative LDL, and inflammatory index Furthermore, we examined the effect of eicosapentaenoic acid (EPA), on CAVI values in the patients with metabolic syndrome. A 3-month treatment with EPA significantly reduced the levels of CAVI in accordance with an increase in adiponectin, and decreases in oxidative LDL, and inflammatory markers in the patients with metabolic syndrome (Fig. 3)[7-10].

Based on the above, it seems that the CAVI value reflects the severity of MetS and hypoadiponectin, an abnormal adipocytokine status, and that CAVI can act as a useful atherosclerotic index not only for the detection of early atherosclerosis but also for evaluation of interventions against obesity, including weight reduction therapy and pharmacotherapy.

CAVI as a predictive indicator of CVD events in MetS

In recent years, international studies have suggested that high CAVI values are associated with the onset of CVD events in MetS[11,12].

In the longitudinal analysis of our NHO-JOMS study, we also reported that a high CAVI was a significant factor for the incidence of CVD events in 5-years in obese patients. In this study, we found that the CAVI threshold for CVD events was 7.8 in obese patients, indicating that careful monitoring is important, and especial caution is necessary in obese patients with CAVI values ≥ 7.8[13].

Conclusions

Based on national and international reports, CAVI is expected to serve as an early atherosclerotic indicator reflecting BP-independent vascular function in MetS and as a sensitive useful index for therapeutic evaluation of weight reduction therapy and drug treatments. Therefore, monitoring CAVI as an index of arterial stiffness may lead to the prevention of CVD events and vascular complications in MetS and an extension of healthy life span.

For early diagnosis and comprehensive management of atherosclerotic CVD diseases in MetS, regular CAVI monitoring is crucial, and the correction of lifestyle habit and the selection of relevant pharmacotherapy by monitoring CAVI as an index of arterial stiffness may lead to the prevention of vascular complications in MetS and an extension of healthy life span.

Future challenges

1. Whether CAVI may act as an early diagnostic indicator

for the development of cardiovascular events in the general population as well as in MetS needs to be validated in large-scale studies.

2. Prospective studies are warranted to determine whether CAVI may act as a long-term care indicator for MetS.

References

1) Fantuzzi G, Mazzone T. Adipose tissue and atherosclerosis: exploring the connection. *Arterioscler Thromb Vasc Biol* 2007; **27**: 996-1003.

2) Ibata J, Sasaki H, K Nanjo et al. Cardio-ankle vascular index measures arterial wall stiffness independent of blood pressure. *Diabetes Res Clin Pract* 2008; **80**: 265-270.

3) Shirai K, Utino J, Otsuka K et al. A novel blood pressure-independent arterial wall stiffness parameter; cardio-ankle vascular index (CAVI). *J Atheroscler Thromb* 2006; **13**:101-107. https://doi.org/10.5551/jat.13.101

4) Satoh N, Shimatsu A, Ogawa Y et al, For the Japan Obesity and Metabolic Syndrome Study (JOMS) Group. Evaluation of cardio-ankle vascular index, a new indicator of arterial stiffness independent of blood pressure, in obesity and metabolic syndrome. *Hypertens Res* 2008; **31**: 1921-1930. https://doi.org/10.1016/j.atherosclerosis.2015.08.003

5) Himeno A, Satoh-Asahara N, Shimatsu A et al. Salivary cortisol levels are associated with outcomes of weight reduction therapy in obese Japanese patients. *Metabolism* 2012; **61**: 255-261.

6) Iguchi A, Yamakage H, Satoh-Asahara N et al. Effect of weight reduction therapy on obstructive sleep apnea syndrome and arterial stiffness in the patients with obesity and metabolic syndrome. *J Atheroscler Thromb* 2013; **20**: 807-820.

7) Satoh N, Shimatsu A, Ogawa Y et al. Highly purified eicosapentaenoic acid reduces cardio-ankle vascular index in association with decrease in serum amyloid A-LDL in metabolic syndrome. *Hypertens Res* 2009; **32**: 1004-1008.

8) Satoh N, Shimatsu A, Kotani K, et al. Purified eicosapentaenoic acid reduces small dense LDL, remnant lipoprotein particles, and CRP in metabolic syndrome. *Diabetes Care* 2007; **30**: 144-146.

9) Itoh M, Suganami T, Satoh N, et al. Increased Adiponectin Secretion by Highly Purified Eicosapentaenoic Acid in Rodent Models of Obesity and Human Obese Subjects. *Arterioscler Thromb Vasc Biol* 2007; **27**: 1918-1925.

10) Yamada H, Satoh N, Ogawa Y et al. *In vivo* and *In vitro* Inhibition of Monocyte Adhesion to Endothelial Cells and Endothelial Adhesion Molecules by Eicosapentaenoic Acid. *Arterioscler Thromb Vasc Biol* 2008; **28**: 2173-2179.

11) Laucevičius A, Ryliškytė L, Solovjova S et al. Association of cardio-ankle vascular index with cardiovascular risk factors and cardiovascular events in metabolic syndrome patients. *Medicina* 2015; **51**: 152-158.

12) Sato Y, Nagayama D, Saiki A, et al. Cardio-Ankle Vascular Index is Independently Associated with Future Cardiovascular Events in Outpatients with Metabolic Disorders. *J Atheroscler Thromb* 2016; **23**: 596-605.

13) Satoh-Asahara N, Kotani K, Shimatsu A et al, Japan Obesity and Metabolic Syndrome Study (JOMS) Group. Cardio-Ankle Vascular Index Predicts for the Incidence of Cardiovascular Events in Obese Patients: A multicenter prospective cohort study (Japan Obesity and Metabolic Syndrome Study: JOMS). *Atherosclerosis* 2015; **242**: 461-468.

Commentary: Why was CAVI not necessarily high in metabolic syndrome?

Daiji Nagayama[1] and Kohji Shirai[2,3]

Metabolic syndrome (MetS) is the result of the complex interplay of cardiovascular risk factors such as impaired glucose tolerance, high blood pressure, dyslipidemia and abdominal obesity[1]. Patients with MetS frequently manifest cardiovascular disease, with high morbidity and mortality[2]. Progression of arteriosclerosis is remarkable. Therefore, CAVI would be expected to be high in patients with MS. However, high CAVI values in MetS were not uniformly reported[3-7] as described in this section. We considered those contradictory results as the "obesity paradox about CAVI".

Metabolic syndrome is essentially derived from visceral fat accumulation, and the criterion for obesity should adopt an index reflecting visceral adipose accumulation[8]. However, it is not easy to measure visceral adipose tissue mass, then, waist circumference (WC) was used in National Cholesterol Education Program-Adult Treatment Panel III (NCEP-ATP III)[9] and international diabetic federation (IDF) criteria[10]. In Japan, visceral fat area $= 100$ cm^2 obtained by computed tomography (CT) was originally proposed, but WC was adopted finally for convenience. WC threshold value (man $= 85$ cm, woman $= 90$ cm) was corresponding to visceral fat area $= 100$ cm^2 [11]. However, the "obesity paradox about CAVI" was found. Nagayama reported that CAVI was negatively related with body mass index (BMI)[12]. Park et al. reported that CAVI was positively related with visceral and pericardial fat, and negatively related with subcutaneous adipose tissue[13]. Sugiura[14] also reported that CAVI was positively related with visceral fat area and negatively with other adiposity indices, BMI, WC and percent body fat, as measured by CT. Therefore, CAVI might properly discriminate obesity type between so-called benign obesity (subcutaneous) and malignant obesity (visceral). Moreover, CAVI in MetS as defined by criteria using WC, could be low especially among people whose CAVI was negatively related with WC.

We studied the relationship between CAVI and BMI, WC and a body shape index (ABSI) among 62,514 Japanese people. ABSI was proposed by Krakauer as a new body shape index predicting mortality and was independent of BMI[15],

Table 1. Association between CAVI and each obesity index.

CAVI vs.	R	P value
BMI	-0.011	0.006
WC	0.116	<0.001
ABSI	0.347	<0.001

Pearson's correlation analysis.

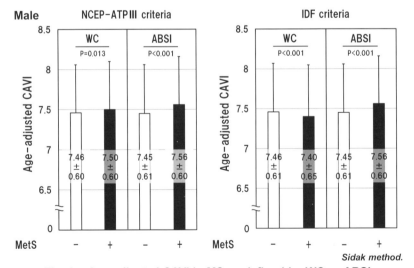

Fig. 1. Age-adjusted CAVI in MS as defined by WC or ABSI.

[1]Emeritus professor, Medical School, Toho university.
[2]Director, Seijinkai Mihama Hospital, 1-1-5 Utase, Mihama-ku, Chiba-shi, Chiba 261-0013, Japan.

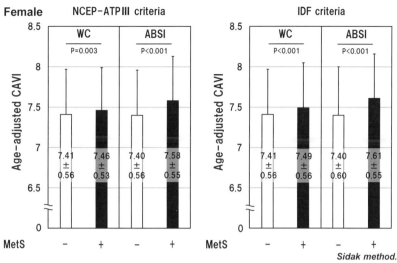

Fig. 2. Age-adjusted CAVI in MS defined by WC or ABSI.

and we found that ABSI, unlike WC is strongly associated with CAVI, and the results are shown in table 1: CAVI correlated negatively with BMI and positively with ABSI, but weakly with WC. Anoop et.al reported that ABSI was correlated with visceral fat volume as measured by MRI[16]. These results suggest that CAVI could be low in people with MetS defined using WC according to NCEP-PIII and IDF criteria. Therefore, we studied CAVI values in Japanese people with MetS defined using ABSI ($\geq$ 0.080: visceral obesity) instead of WC. The results are shown in Fig. 1 (men) and Fig. 2 (women). CAVI was higher under both NCEP-PIII and IDF criteria using ABSI than using WC. And the difference between MS – and MS + was more remarkable both in men and women. Further studies on the replacement of WC by ABSI in MetS definition, including follow-up studies on morbidities and mortality, were required.

Now, we recommend ABSI instead of WC for MetS definition.

References

1) Eckel RH, Grundy SM, Zimmet PZ. The metabolic syndrome. *The Lancet.* 2005; **365**(9468): 1415-1428.
2) Galassi A, Reynolds K, He J. Metabolic syndrome and risk of cardiovascular disease: a meta-analysis. *Am J Med* 2006; 119: 812-9.
3) Liu H, Zhang X, Feng X, Li J, Hu M, Yambe T. Effects of metabolic syndrome on cardio-ankle vascular index in middle-aged and elderly Chinese. *Metab Syndr Relat Disord* 2011; **9**: 105-10.
4) Topouchian J, Labat C, Gautier S, Bäck M, Achimastos A, Blacher J, et al. Effects of metabolic syndrome on arterial function in different age groups: the Advanced Approach to Arterial Stiffness study. *J Hypertens* 2018; **36**: 824-833.
5) Gomez-Sanchez L, Garcia-Ortiz L, Patino-Alonso MC, Recio-Rodriguez JI, Fernando R, Marti R, et al. Association of metabolic syndrome and its components with arterial stiffness in Caucasian subjects of the MARK study: a cross-sectional trial. *Cardiovasc Diabetol* 2016; **15**: 148.
6) Nam SH, Kang SG, Lee YA, Song SW, Rho JS. Association

of Metabolic Syndrome with the Cardioankle Vascular Index in Asymptomatic Korean Population. *J Diabetes Res* 2015; **2015**: 328585.
7) Satoh N, Shimatsu A, Kato Y, Araki R, Koyama K, Okajima T, Tanabe M, Ooishi M, Kotani K, Ogawa Y. Evaluation of the cardio-ankle vascular index, a new indicator of arterial stiffness independent of blood pressure, in obesity and metabolic syndrome. *Hypertens Res* 2008; **31**: 1921-30.
8) Kishida K, Funahashi T, Matsuzawa Y, Shimomura I. Visceral adiposity as a target for the management of the metabolic syndrome. *Ann Med* 2012; **44**: 233-41.
9) Executive Summary of The Third Report of The National Cholesterol Education Program (NCEP) Expert Panel on Detection, Evaluation, And Treatment of High Blood Cholesterol In Adults (Adult Treatment Panel III). *JAMA* 2001; **285**: 2486-97.
10) Alberti KG, Zimmet P, Shaw J. Metabolic syndrome--a new world-wide definition. A Consensus Statement from the International Diabetes Federation. Diabet Med 2006; **23**: 469-80.
11) [Definition and the diagnostic standard for metabolic syndrome--Committee to Evaluate Diagnostic Standards for Metabolic Syndrome]. *Nihon Naika Gakkai Zasshi* 2005; **94**: 794-809. in Japanese.
12) Nagayama D, Imamura H, Sato Y, Yamaguchi T, Ban N, Kawana H, et al. Inverse relationship of cardio-ankle vascular index with BMI in healthy Japanese subjects: a cross-sectional study. *Vasc Health Risk Manag* 2016; **13**: 1-9.
13) Park HE, Choi SY, Kim HS, Kim MK, Cho SH, Oh BH. Epicardial fat reflects arterial stiffness: assessment using 256-slice multidetector coronary computed tomography and cardio-ankle vascular index. *J Atheroscler Thromb* 2012; **19**: 570-6.
14) Sugiura T, Dohi Y, Takagi Y, Yoshikane N, Ito M, Suzuki K, et al. Relationships of Obesity-Related Indices and Metabolic Syndrome with Subclinical Atherosclerosis in Middle-Aged Untreated Japanese Workers. *J Atheroscler Thromb* 202 ; **27**: 342-352.
15) Krakauer NY, Krakauer JC. A new body shape index predicts mortality hazard independently of body mass index. *PLoS One* 2012; **7**: e39504.
16) Anoop S, Krakauer J, Krakauer N, Misra A. A Body shape index significantly predicts MRI-defined abdominal adipose tissue depots in non-obese Asian Indians with type 2 diabetes mellitus. *BMJ Open Diabetes Res Care* 2020; **8**: e001324.

The relationship between Cardio-ankle vascular index (CAVI) and metabolism-related vascular diseases in China

Hongyu Wang

It is estimated that about 330 million patients suffer from cardiovascular disease (CVD) in China, of which 13 million are stroke, 11 million are coronary heart disease, 5 million are cor pulmonale, 4.5 million are heart failure, 2.5 million are rheumatic heart disease, and 2 million are congenital heart disease. The mortality rate of CVD in rural areas has exceeded and continued to be higher than that in urban areas since 2009, and 2 out of 5 deaths are due to CVD.

Arterial system diseases are systemic diseases. Obstruction of blood flow leads to insufficient nutrition of the heart, brain, kidneys, lungs, etc., and thus to various clinical events. Arteries are like vascular trees in the human body. Arterial blood supplies nutrients to various organs. Large elastic arteries have a buffering function, which undergo structural changes in their walls with aging. The fundamental principles of vascular pathophysiology are that pulse waves travel faster in stiffer arteries. The arterial wall belongs to a class of substances that are said to be viscoelastic, in that it possesses a combination of properties belonging to both elastic solids and viscous liquids[1]. Arterial stiffness progressively increases from the heart to the periphery. Although the mechanisms of diffuse and focal atherosclerosis are not the same, the decreased elasticity of the large arteries is an important factor that leads to increased pulse pressure and increased arterial load. This plays an important role in arterial endothelial dysfunction, intima injury, mid-layer rupture and vascular degeneration. Arterial stiffness reflects the elasticity of large arteries. Regarding these large artery functions, there are concepts such as arterial distensibility and arterial compliance. Thus, Cardio-Ankle Vascular Index (CAVI), as one of parameters for reflecting vascular health, not only can reflect the arterial stiffening but also can evaluate vascular-related function. This chapter will introduce the principles and clinical research results of CAVI, explain what CAVI is, and look forward to how it can open a new chapter in vascular function evaluation, and CAVI as an index to evaluate metabolism-related vascular diseases in China.

Establishment of Early Vascular Disease Evaluation System in China

Over the past 20 years, our team established an early detection system for vascular lesions. We created the first vascular medicine professional clinical diagnosis and treatment center---Peking University Shougang Hospital Vascular Medicine Center. We introduced our experience and cooperated with experts from medical institutions nationwide to conduct a series of studies on vascular function series of studies on the evaluation of arterial stiffness in China (CASE)[2-3]. CASE researches included the evaluation of vascular function under different disease states, the study of biomarkers and vascular function, the study of ultrasound technology to evaluate vascular function, the study of vascular function status of different regions and ethnic groups, and the study of the effect of drugs and lifestyle on vascular function[4]. The concept of "Early Vascular Disease Detection System" is to use non-invasive methods to detect subclinical vascular diseases and take effective intervention to prevent serious vascular events. In 2004, the Ministry of Health of the People's Republic of China approved a project to popularize the early detection of vascular disease (Chinese Heart Vascular Health Promotion Project, CHVHPP) as part of the national 10-year health plan. In 2006, our team organized the formulation of the first international vascular lesion early detection technology application guideline. Some new vascular assessment techniques were added to the guideline in 2011 and 2018, and the updated guideline was promoted nationwide[4-7]. The guideline introduced technologies that comprehensively evaluated the structure and function of large arteries, which can be easily used and promoted. In July 2015, our team proposed the Beijing Vascular Health Stratification (BVHS)[8], which classifies the population according to different vascular health conditions. The new vascular health classification, based on traditional risk factors, superimposed the vascular structure and function evaluation indicators recommended in the guidelines, directly regarding the whole body blood vessel as the target, and conducted the grading management, to comprehensively assess vascular health status[9].

Vascular Health Research Center, PKU Health Science Center (VHRC-PKUHSC), Peking University (PKU) Shougang Hospital, Beijing, China.

The principle of Cardio-ankle vascular index (CAVI) and its application in China

Pulse wave velocity (PWV) measures segmental arterial stiffness. There are several methods for measuring PWV, including carotid-femoral PWV, heart-femoral PWV, brachial-ankle PWV, but it is greatly affected by the internal pressure of the aorta. CAVI is a new index of arteriosclerosis, which is significantly related to cardiovascular risk factors such as age, hypertension, dyslipidemia, and diabetes, not affected by the blood pressure (BP) level at measuring time. Also, CAVI can be easily measured. The principle of CAVI is described in a specific chapter of this book. Recent studies suggest that CAVI is a better index for evaluating arterial stiffness than other indexes[13].

We have evaluated the arterial function of the Chinese Miao population and analyzed the influencing factors and found that CAVI is related to age, body mass index (BMI), uric acid and systolic blood pressure (Table 1).

CAVI is not only related to age, but also related to metabolic factors. Some examples of metabolism-related diseases are hypertension, hyperlipidemia, hyperhomocysteinemia (HHcy), hyperuricemia, and diabetes mellitus (DM)[10]. The main pathophysiological mechanism of lesions are arteriosclerosis, atherosclerosis, stenosis, and occlusion, which lead to impaired vascular function and structure and further lead to cardiovascular diseases and complications. Therefore, early evaluation and comprehensive management of vascular diseases are imperative. Our study on CAVI and biomarkers in vascular-related diseases[11] showed that increase of arterial stiffness is the manifestation of arteriosclerosis, and that it is a strong predictor of future cardiovascular events and all-cause mortality[12]. Arterial stiffness is significantly correlated with endothelial dysfunction. Our study showed that the level of CAVI was significantly lower in Chinese healthy persons than that in Japanese in each age subgroup (Fig. 1A and Fig. 1B)[14].

How does blood lipid level affect CAVI?

Dyslipidemia is characterized by elevated levels of triglycerides (TG) and LDL-C and reduced levels of HDL-C. Our study showed that CAVI was negatively correlated with HDL-C in the entire group and in the healthy group[24,15]. However, there was negative tendency between CAVI and HDL-C in hypertension subjects without significant difference[16]. Maybe the effects of HDL-C on the endothelial function could be highly heterogeneous.

Our results showed that there was positive correlation between CAVI and TC and TG, while CAVI was negatively correlated with HDL-C[12]. CAVI was negatively correlated with HDL-C in the entire group and in healthy subjects. However, there was negative tendency between CAVI and HDL-C in the nonhealthy group without significant difference (**Table 2**). Thus, HDL-C might lose its beneficial effects on endothelial function under DM, or hypertension conditions.

Hypertension and vascular function

Hypertension is an important risk factor for the development of a variety of cardiovascular disorders[17]. Decreased arterial compliance is the main characteristic functional change of the hypertensive aorta. These changes are mainly due to the thickening of the vessel wall, the proliferation of collagen, the fatigue and fracture of elastic fibers, and the activation of local renin and angiotensin systems. Decreased aortic compliance leads to increased systolic blood pressure, decreased diastolic blood pressure, and increased pulse pressure. Normally, there is a significant difference in systolic pressure between the brachial artery and the aorta. The brachial artery has a higher systolic pressure than the aorta. The decreased compliance of the aorta reduces or even eliminates this difference, the systolic pressure of the aorta increases and can cause instability of blood flow, vortex or reflux. In hypertension, the inner diameter of the lumen of small arteries decreases, and the wall/cavity ratio increases, but the outer diameter and cross-sectional area of the lumen remain unchanged.

Pathological mechanism of vascular disease in hypertension

The morphological changes of vascular endothelial cells and smooth muscle cells in hypertension may be the

Table1. Relationship with CAVI and other factors, results from multicariable Logistic regressions.

Arterial stiffness	Impact factors	*p*-value
R-CAVI	Age	<0.001
	SBP	<0.001
	UA	0.002
	BMI	0.001
	Hct	0.047
L-CAVI	Age	<0.001
	SBP	<0.001
	UA	<0.001
	BMI	0.001

Abbreviations: SBP, systolic blood pressure; BMI, body mass index; UA, uric acid; Hct, hematocrit. (From Kang Liu, Shengli Long, Jian Huang et al. Chinese arterial stiffness evaluation study (CASE)-2 Evaluation of arterial function in Chinese Miao tribe population and analysis of its influential factors)

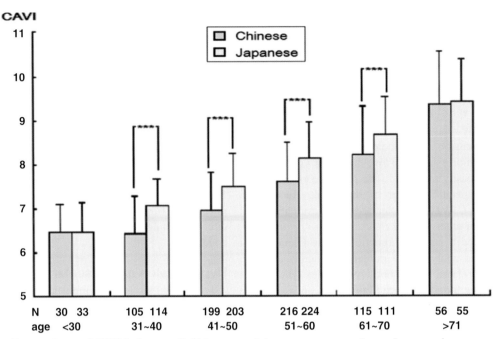

Fig. 1A. **Comparison of CAVI between all Chinese and Japanese women in each age subgroup.**
(from Wang H, Shirai K, Liu J, et al. Comparative study of cardio-ankle vascular index between Chinese and Japanese healthy subjects. Clin Exp Hypertens 2014, 36(8): 596-601.)

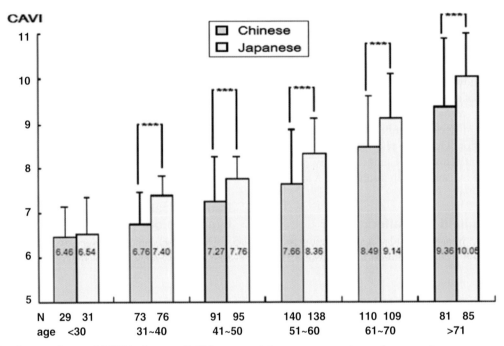

Fig. 1B. **Comparison of CAVI between all Chinese and Japanese men in each age subgroup.**
(from Wang H, Shirai K, Liu J, et al. Comparative study of cardio-ankle vascular index between Chinese and Japanese healthy subjects. Clin Exp Hypertens 2014, 36(8): 596-601.)

structural basis of vasospasm and increased vascular tone. Vascular remodeling is a dynamic process of vascular configuration changes caused by cell proliferation, necrosis, and synthesis and degradation of extracellular mechanisms. Vascular remodeling is the basic pathological process common to hypertension and many diseases.

CAVI could show the real effect of hypertension on the proper stiffness of the arterial wall. Our study found that the

level of CAVI was higher in patients with hypertension[18-21] (Table 3). This stiffness gradient disappeared or became inverse, leading to insufficiently dampening and transmission of pulsatile pressure, thus damaging the microcirculation.

We have investigated the vascular function and structure of Fujians who could take good care of themselves even at the age of over 80. We found that the SBP of the elderly was even higher, but they did not have symptoms of dizziness or

Table 2. Clinical characteristics in different groups. Multiple linear regression analysis for the relationship between CAVI and study variables among entire study group. healthy group, and non-healthy group.

	Entire Group (N = 1063)		Healthy Group (N = 639)		Non-healthy Group (N = 424)	
	β	P Value	β	P Value	β	P Value
Age	0.699	<.001	0.605	<.001	0.636	<.001
BMI	−0.189	.001	−0.234	.003	−0.134	.131
PP	0.029	.638	0.084	.293	−0.113	.235
Heart rate	0.064	.268	0.097	.227	0.013	.885
FPG	0.106	.287	0.100	.221	0.148	.094
HbAlc %	0.144	.015	0.150	.067	0.119	.189
UA	−0.068	.237	−0.044	.595	−0.095	.307
TC	−0.053	.379	−0.094	.236	−0.091	.310
HDL-C	−0.136	.019	−0.163	.036	−0.061	.496
LDL-C	−0.084	.149	−0.078	.323	−0.164	.071
TG	−0.022	.718	0.022	.783	−0.038	.670

BMI, body mass index; CAVI, cardio-ankle vascular index; DBP, diastolic blood pressure; FPG, fasting plasma glucose; LDL-C, low-density lipoprotein cholesterol; HDL-C, high-density lipoprotein cholesterol; PP, pulse pressure; SBP, systolic blood pressure; TC, cholesterol; TG, triglycerides; UA, uric acid. (From Wang H, Liu J, Zhao H, et al. Arterial stiffness evaluation by cardio-ankle vascular index in hypertension and diabetes mellitus subjects. J Am Soc Hypertens 2013, 7(6): 426-431.)

Table 3. Clinical characteristics in different groups.

Characterisitics	Healthy (N = 639)	Hypertension (N = 312)	DM (N = 58)	Hypertension + DM (N = 54)	P
Age (years)	47.04 ± 12.50	54.93 ± 11.20*	54.86 ± 9.61*	59.69 ± 9.76*	<.001
Male/female	304/335	167/145	36/22	26/28	.110
BMI	24.16 ± 3.12	25.92 ± 3.35*	24.46 ± 3.26[†]	25.88 ± 3.39*	<.001
CAVI	7.23 ± 1.10	7.94 ± 1.33*	8.25 ± 1.41*	8.59 ± 1.08*·[†]	<.001
SBP (mm Hg)	133.42 ± 18.29	146.41 ± 19.34*	135.31 ± 18.23[†]	146.56 ± 15.21*·[‡]	<.001
DBP (mm Hg)	83.82 ± 10.37	90.73 ± 11.42*	83.48 ± 9.46[†]	89.02 ± 9.83*·[‡]	<.001
PP (mm Hg)	49.60 ± 11.94	55.69 ± 14.48*	51.83 ± 13.39	57.54 ± 11.03*·[‡]	<.001
Heart rate	69.60 ± 10.90	69.55 ± 10.68	71.27 ± 9.37	72.54 ± 11.23	.190
FPG (mmol/L)	5.27 ± 0.54	5.68 ± 0.80*	8.78 ± 3.04*·[†]	7.41 ± 1.73*·[†‡]	<.001
HbAlc %	5.48 ± 0.38	5.69 ± 0.42*	7.15 ± 1.02*·[†]	6.93 ± 0.81*·[†]	<.001
UA	314.07 ± 86.75	366.73 ± 84.90*	306.44 ± 99.33[†]	347.79 ± 80.08	<.001
TC (mmol/L)	5.22 ± 1.06	5.38 ± 1.14	5.28 ± 1.12	5.56 ± 1.04	.282
HDL-C (mmol/L)	1.42 ± 0.39	1.23 ± 0.36*	1.27 ± 0.36*	1.17 ± 0.28*	<.001
LDL-C (mmol/L)	2.95 ± 0.81	3.05 ± 0.89	2.93 ± 0.75	3.13 ± 0.64	.477
TG (mmol/L)	1.46 ± 1.14	2.04 ± 1.43*	1.81 ± 0.90	2.06 ± 1.40	<.001

BMI, body mass index; CAVI, cardio-ankle vascular index; DBP, diastolic blood pressure; FPG, fasting plasma glucose; LDL-C, low-density lipoprotein cholesterol; HDL-C, high-density lipoprotein cholesterol; PP, pulse pressure; SBP, systolic blood pressure; TC, cholesterol; TG, triglycerides; UA, uric acid. The differences between groups were analyzed by one-way analysis of variance and least-significant difference (LSD). Proportions were analyzed by χ^2 test. *vs. Normal; P <.05. [†]vs. Hypertension; P <.05. [‡]vs. DM; P <.05. (From Wang H, Liu J, Zhao H, et al. Arterial stiffness evaluation by cardio-ankle vascular index in hypertension and diabetes mellitus subjects. J Am Soc Hypertens 2013, 7(6): 426-431.)

headache. Most of the elderly were detected with carotid plaques (less than 50% stenosis rate), but it did not affect the blood supply. They showed a relatively better blood vessel elasticity, which can cushion pressure and stimulation of blood vessels. Clinical pharmacology, treatment, and prognosis of hypertension are based on the reversibility of arterial stiffness and the extent of wave reflection which are increasingly important considerations, marking a major step toward the development of cardiovascular disease. Both small and large arteries are primary targets for antihypertensive therapy, and any means to specifically reduce elevated pulsatility and modify the function of blood vessels is thus likely to be highly beneficial.

Insulin resistance (IR)/Hyperinsulinemia and vascular function

Diabetic vascular complications are the main cause of death in diabetic patients. Diabetic vascular diseases include macrovascular and microvascular disease, and its microvascular disease includes diabetic nephropathy and diabetic retinopathy. Hyperglycemia can directly act on the blood vessel wall, causing a decrease in blood vessel elasticity and an increase in CAVI value. Blood glucose status is related to vascular disease. DM complications can lead to an increase of arterial wall thickness, endothelial dysfunction, and calcification, finally leading to an increase in arterial stiffness[12]. Our team focused on research about CAVI in hypertension subjects with DM simultaneously. The results showed that the value of CAVI was significantly higher in hypertension with DM group than in healthy and hypertension group, respectively (Fig. 2)[12]. The possible mechanisms are mainly that hyperglycemia might aggravate the damage of vascular function in hypertension patients. Insulin resistance, defined as decreased sensitivity of target organs to the metabolic actions of insulin, is a pathophysiological feature of metabolic syndrome, and pre-diabetes. CAVI reflects vascular damage caused by oxidative stress, which is considered central to the pathophysiology of atherosclerosis in patients with metabolic syndrome. CAVI can identify the macroangiopathy in patients with type 2 DM and result in a significantly high value in patients with macroangiopathy complications. In all age groups, the CAVI level of patients with diabetes/glucose tolerance disorder was higher than that of the patients without diabetes/glucose tolerance disorder.

Hyperuricemia and vascular function

Serum uric acid (UA), formed from xanthine, is the major product of purine metabolism, and mainly synthesized by the hepatic tissue as the end product of purine catabolism, circulating predominantly in the form of a monovalent sodium salt (urate) and excreted by the kidney. Our study has found that subjects with higher UA had a risk tendency of higher CAVI[22]. We also found that UA was independently linearly correlated with CAVI rather than CF-PWV, ABI, and CIMT. However, higher UA was not logistically related to CIMT in both genders. Thus, we speculate that UA may mainly influence the vascular function instead of the vascular structure.

Hyperhomocysteinemia (HHcy) and vascular function

Homocysteine (Hcy), a non-protein forming amino acid, is the direct metabolic precursor of methionine. Elevated Hcy can increase oxidative stress, reduce the bioavailability of endothelial nitric oxide, and cause vascular endothelial function disorders. Hcy can cause decoupling of nitric oxide synthase by reducing the bioavailability of tetrahydrobiopterin in vascular endothelial cells, leading to oxidative stress and reduced nitric oxide production[23]. HHcy has been considered an independent risk factor for atherosclerosis, especially in the oldest, and is specifically linked to various diseases of the vasculature. CAVI was associated with Hcy and the levels of CAVI were significantly higher in Hcy ≥ 15 μmol/l group than in Hcy < 15 μmol/l group[24] (**Fig. 3 and Fig. 4**). Such a causal effect could be initiated via the combination of increased thrombogenicity, increased oxidative stress, and activation of redox inflammatory mechanisms, which lead to damage of endothelium[24]. Our study enrolled subjects with hypertension, and the result showed that CAVI was significantly higher in subjects with HHcy[25]. The level of Hcy was significantly higher in subjects with one or more vascular diseases than in those without vascular disease. Hcy was an independent influencing factor of CAVI in vascular-related diseases.

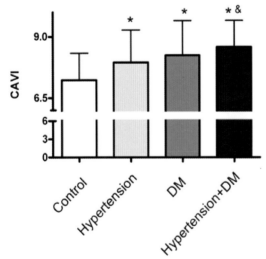

Fig. 2. Comparison of CAVI between the healthy group, hypertension group, diabetes mellitus (DM) group and hypertension patients with DM.
(From Wang H, Liu J, Zhao H, et al. Arterial stiffness evaluation by cardio-ankle vascular index in hypertension and diabetes mellitus subjects. J Am Soc Hypertens 2013, 7(6): 426-431.)

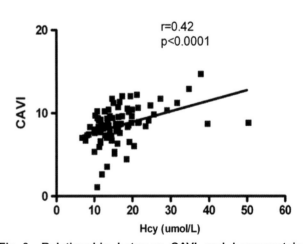

Fig. 3. Relationship between CAVI and homocysteine (Hcy) in the entire study group.
(from Wang H, Liu J, Wang Q, et al. Descriptive study of possible link between cardioankle vascular index and homocysteine in vascular-related diseases. BMJ Open 2013, 3(3):e002483)

Preliminary verification of BVHS in China

Rarely study focus on the value of multiple vascular health indicators in the same cohort. Our recent retrospective cohort study used part of the data from the Beijing Vascular Disease Population Evaluation Study (BEST study) to include subjects with at least 2 hospitalization records. We established 2 cohorts, for coronary heart disease and cerebral infarction, and the follow-up time was 1.9 and 2.1

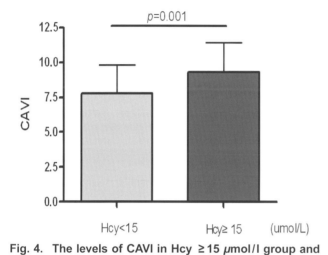

Fig. 4. **The levels of CAVI in Hcy ≥15 μmol/l group and in Hcy <15 μmol/l group.**
(from Wang H, Liu J, Wang Q, et al. Descriptive study of possible link between cardioankle vascular index and homocysteine in vascular-related diseases. BMJ Open 2013, 3(3):e002483)

years, respectively. It could be seen that even with a high level of arterial stiffness at baseline, through systematic management and treatment, severe arteriosclerosis could be delayed or even reverse the progression. Our research showed that only elevated CAVI was an independent risk factor for cerebral infarction, while the other three indicators (carotid-femoral artery PWV, carotid-radial artery PWV and ABI) were not, confirming that CAVI was a more stable indicator. It also preliminarily stated that only assessment of global vascular health status would reflect the risk of future cardiovascular events, lifelong assessment and maintenance of vascular health, thereby reducing the occurrence of cardiovascular and cerebrovascular events. Our study indicated that BVHS has predictive value for coronary heart disease (CHD), while the predictive value of cerebral infarction needs further research.

Vascular dementia and CAVI

Vascular dementia (VD) has a close relationship with hypertension, dyslipidemia, atherosclerosis, high homocysteine, heart disease, diabetes, stroke and transient ischemic attack[26]. At present, VD is the only type of dementia which can be prevented and cured. The study on risk factors and pathogenesis of VD has important clinical significance. We focused our attention on white matter prediction and CAVI. Microvascular brain disease is manifested as white matter hyperintensities and could ultimately result in cognitive impairment, including dementia. Our results showed that higher level of CAVI was independently associated with a higher prevalence of brain white matter lesions (WMLs) (Table 4)[27]. Central

Table 4. **Odds ratios (OR) and 95% confidence intervals (CI) of brain WMLs; the results of logistic regressions with the CAVI as a binary variable.**

	Brain WMLs		
	OR	95% CI	p
Variables			
Age			
(<50 years)	1	–	–
(50–59 years)	2.71	1.31 to 5.64	.008*
(60–69 years)	5.99	2.82 to 12.74	.000*
(70–79 years)	16.07	6.97 to 37.05	.000*
(≥80 years)	37.65	13.19 to 107.44	.000*
Sex			
Female	1	–	–
Male	1.84	1.21 to 2.80	.005*
SBP	1.01	1.00 to 1.02	.032*
Stroke			
No	1	–	–
Yes	7.45	4.77 to 11.64	.000*
CAVI			
CAVI ≤ 9.0	1	–	–
CAVI > 9.0	1.77	1.10 to 2.84	.018*

Multivariable adjusted for CAVI (high vs. low), age range, sex, SBP, TC, TG, HDL-C, LDL-C, CRP, Hcy, UA, BUN, Cr, hypertension, diabetes, CAD, PAD and stroke; method = forward stepwise (likelihood ratio). *indicates as $p < 0.05$ (From Liu et al. Association of brain white matter lesions with arterial stiffness assessed by cardio-ankle vascular index. The Beijing Vascular Disease Evaluation Study (BEST)[27]) artery stiffening and brain WMLs are both markers of arterial aging and they are irreversible. Thus, intervention for artery stiffening may reduce cerebrovascular disease and dementia.

Future direction

Abnormal peripheral and coronary endothelial function have been associated with increased risk of major adverse cardiovascular events (MACE) in cross-sectional retrospective and observational studies. However, the prognostic value of routine clinical evaluation, diagnosis and treatment of endothelial dysfunction on incident MACE in patients with non-obstructive coronary artery disease (NOCAD) remains unknown. We will investigate the early vascular damage such as endothelial function and its prognostic value in the Chinese population. Endothelial Function Guided Management in Patients with NOCAD (ENDOFIND) is a multicenter, randomized, patients-blinded, parallel-controlled, two-stage clinical trial evaluating the impact of routine clinical peripheral endothelial function testing on initiation and/or intensification of cardiovascular preventive therapies in Stage I, and on the risk of MACE in Stage II in patients with NOCAD. One thousand participants with NOCAD on clinically indicated coronary computed tomography or invasive angiography will be enrolled and randomized 1:1, after baseline peripheral endothelial function evaluation, to either an endothelial function guided treatment group or a standard of care control group. In Stage I, patients will be followed for 12 months and the primary outcome will be the proportion of patients receiving prescriptions for cardiovascular evidence-based lipid, blood pressure and glucose lowering medications at the clinic visit immediately after endothelial function evaluation. Secondary outcomes are change in endothelial function measured as reactive hyperemia index and patients' adherence to evidence-based medications in 12 months. The study will be extended into Stage II where sample size and follow up duration will be reevaluated to ensure statistical power, and the primary outcome will be incident MACE[29]. In summary, this study will address an unmet clinical need by providing high quality data on the value of introducing non-invasive endothelial function testing into routine clinical practice. In addition, the results of this trial will help us to better understand the mechanism of the prognosis of patients with NOCAD and whether an endothelial function-based or vascular health marker-CAVI in personalized management strategy can reduce MACE in general population.

References

1) Wang H. Vascular disease.People's Military Medical Press.2006,1-6.

2) Wang H, Hong Y, Li C, et al. A Study on relationship between homodynamic parameters and structure of common carotid artery in Fujian She nationality Chinese arterial stiffness evaluation study, CASE-4. Medical Journal of Chinese people's health 2009,21(21):2635-2638+2641.

3) Hong Y, Liu H, Wu X, et al. Vascular function and structure and related influencing factors in Fujian She nationality Chinese. Chinese Journal of Medical Imaging Technology 2016,32(08):1200-1204.

4) Wang H. Promote the concept of vascular health and promote the development of vascular medicine. Chinese Circulation Journal 2018,33(10):1026-1028.

5) Gong L, Xu Y, Zhang W, et al. Chinese guideline for early vascualr disease detection(First report). Medical Journal of Chinese people's health 2006(09):323-331.

6) Gong L, Liu L, Guan X, et al. Chinese guideline for early vascualr disease detection(Second report). China Continuing Medical Education 2011,3(07): 1-7+35.

7) Gong L, Liu L, Guan X, et al. Chinese guideline for early vascualr disease detection(Second report). Natl Med J China 2018,98(37): 2955-2967.

8) Wang H, Liu H. A new classification of vascular health and vascular medicine. Advances in Cardiovascular Diseases 2015,36(04):365-368.

9) Liu H, Wang H. Early Detection System of Vascular Disease and Its Application Prospect. Biomed Res Int 2016, **2016:** 1723485.

10) Wang H. Obesity-related metabolic syndrome and its heart and vascular damage. Advances in Cardiovascular Disease 2016,37(04):331-333.

11) Liu J, Liu H, Zhao H, et al. Descriptive study of relationship between cardio-ankle vascular index and biomarkers in vascular-related diseases. Clin Exp Hypertens. 2017,39(5):468-472.

12) Wang H, Liu J, Zhao H, et al. Arterial stiffness evaluation by cardio-ankle vascular index in hypertension and diabetes mellitus subjects. J Am Soc Hypertens 2013, **7**(6): 426-431.

13) Liu H, He Y, Liu J, et al. Predictive value of vascular health indicators on newly cardiovascular events: Preliminary validation of Beijing vascular health stratification system. Journal of Peking University(Health Sciences) 2020,52:514-519.

14) Wang H, Shirai K, Liu J, et al. Comparative study of cardio-ankle vascular index between Chinese and Japanese healthy subjects. Clin Exp Hypertens 2014, **36**(8): 596-601.

15) Zhao X, Bo L, Zhao H, et al. Cardio-ankle vascular index value in dyslipidemia patients affected by cardiovascular risk factors. Clin Exp Hypertens. 2018,40(4):312-317.

16) Wang H, Liu J, Zhao H, et al. Relationship between cardio-ankle vascular index and plasma lipids in hypertension subjects. J Hum Hypertens 2015, **29**(2): 105-108.

17) Liu J, Wang H, Zhao H, et al. Arterial stiffness is increased in healthy subjects with a positive family history of hypertension. Clin Exp Hypertens 2015, **37**(8): 622-626.

18) Wang H, Liu J, Zhao H, et al. Possible association between cardio-ankle vascular index and vascular lesion in hypertension subjects. Beijing Medical Journal 2014,36(2):81-83.

19) Wang H, Liu J, Zhao H, et al. Possible association between cardio-ankle vascular index and vascular lesion in hypertension subjects. Beijing Medical Journal 2015,23(4):400.

20) Yu Q, Li C, Chen M, et al. Study on the correlation between variability and arterial stiffness. Chinese Journal of Medicinal Guide 2017,19(03):217-220.

21) Liu H, Hong Y, Wu X, et al. Study on Inter arm difference of systolic blood pressure of bilateral upper limbs and arteriosclerosis in the She Nationality. Chinese Journal of Medicinal Guide 2016, 18(11):1081-1084.

22) Liu H, Liu J, Zhao H, et al. Relationship between Serum Uric Acid and Vascular Function and Structure Markers and Gender Difference in a Real-World Population of China-From Beijing Vascular Disease Patients Evaluation Study (BEST) Study. J Atheroscler Thromb 2018, **25**(3): 254-261.

23) Wang H, Liu J, Ma Y, et al. Possible link between

cardio-ankle vascular index and homocysteine in patients with vascular related diseases. Beijing Medical Journal 2014,36(1):15-18.

24) Wang H, Liu J, Wang Q, et al. Descriptive study of possible link between cardioankle vascular index and homocysteine in vascular-related diseases. BMJ Open 2013; **3**(3):e002438. doi: 10.1136/bmjopen-2012-002483

25) Liu J, Liu H, Zhao H, et al. Relationship between cardio-ankle vascular index and homocysteine in hypertension subjects with hyperhomocysteinemia. Clin Exp Hypertens 2016, **38**(7): 652-657.

26) Zhao X, Li H, Wang H. Research progress on risk factors of vascular dementia. Adv Cardiovasc Dis 2018, 39(3):328-331.

27) Liu H, Liu J, Zhao H, et al. Association of brain white matter lesions with arterial stiffness assessed by cardio-ankle vascular index. The Beijing Vascular Disease Evaluation STudy (BEST). Brain Imaging Behav. 2021;15:1025-1032. doi: 10.1007/s11682-020-00309-3

28) Liu H, Liu J, Huang W, et al. Association between multi-site atherosclerotic plaques and systemic arteriosclerosis: results from the BEST study (Beijing Vascular Disease Patients Evaluation Study). Cardiovasc Ultrasound 2020, 18(1): 30.

29) Liu H, Xie G, Huang W, et al. Rationale and design of a multicenter, randomized, patients-blinded two-stage clinical trial on effects of endothelial function test in patients with non-obstructive coronary artery disease (ENDOFIND). Int J Cardiol. 2020 Oct 16;S0167-5273(20)33986-3.doi: 10.1016/j.ijcard.2020.10.033

Uric acid and CAVI
—Uric acid as a cardiovascular risk—

Ichiro Tatsuno

Summary

1. Recent epidemiological studies have shown that uric acid is an independent risk factor for cardiovascular events.

2. Uric acid level is also an independent factor for increases in CAVI, which is one of the surrogate markers for arteriosclerosis.

3. The anti-arteriosclerotic effects of xanthine oxidase inhibitors were not unequivocally shown in recent large-scale intervention studies. The effect of xanthine oxidase inhibitors on CAVI should be investigated, and larger scale prospective studies are required.

Introduction

It has long been debated whether uric acid is a risk factor for arteriosclerosis, given that uric acid was reported to have contradictory effects in the body. Uric acid itself has antioxidant effects. On the other hand, oxygen is generated during production of uric acid, which has oxidative effects. Xanthine oxidase inhibitors have not unequivocally shown preventive effects against cardiovascular diseases in recent large-scale intervention studies. The cardio-ankle vascular index (CAVI), a quantitative index of arteriosclerosis, might clarify the effect of uric acid, and also that of various uric acid-lowering agents, on the progression of arteriosclerosis.

1. Hyperuricemia

Hyperuricemia, defined as a serum urate concentration exceeding the limit of solubility (about 7 mg/dL) in Japan, is a common biochemical abnormality that reflects supersaturation of the extracellular fluid with urate and predisposes affected persons to gout. Gout was a very rare disease before World War II in Japan, but the number of patients with gout has rapidly increased with the westernization of lifestyle habits. There are currently about 600,000 patients with gout in Japan.

Hyperuricemia is strongly associated with obesity. In visceral obesity, a large amount of free fatty acids is released from the visceral fat into the portal vein, which stimulates the synthesis of triglycerides in the liver and simultaneously activates the ribose-5-phosphate pathway to enhance de novo uric acid synthesis[1,2]. Moreover, hyperinsulinemia, caused by insulin resistance, which is a key factor in the pathophysiology of metabolic syndrome, causes increased Na^+ reabsorption in renal tubules and decreased excretion of uric acid[1,2], and urate production in visceral fat. In addition, the activation of xanthine oxidase, which is involved in uric acid production, has been demonstrated in visceral adipose tissue[1,2] (Fig. 1).

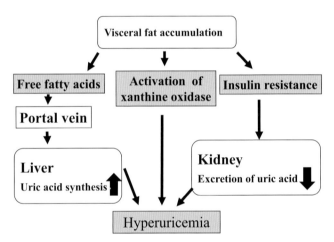

Fig. 1. Metabolic syndrome.

2. Uric acid and cardiovascular diseases

Although the cardiovascular diseases and cerebrovascular disorders have become major prognostic factors in patients with gout and hyperuricemia, large-scale epidemiological studies up to the early 1990s did not find hyperuricemia to be an independent risk factor for arteriosclerosis. Subsequently, several large-scale cohort studies, including the National Health and Nutrition Examination Survey (NHANES) I Epidemiologic Follow-up study (in which 5,926 people were observed for a mean of 16 years)[3], the Japanese Atomic Bomb Survivor Cohort study[4], and the Yamagata Cohort study[5] have demonstrated that high uric acid levels are an independent risk factor for arteriosclerosis. Interestingly, uric acid levels lower than 7 mg/dl, which is the definition of hyperuricemia[4], were reported to be more harmful in women.

3. Uric acid and CAVI

Although the vascular elasticity parameters of the CAVI

President, Chiba Prefectural University of Health Sciences, Wakaba 2-10-1, Mihama-ku, Chiba 261-0014, Japan.

have been used as a surrogate marker to determine the progression of arteriosclerosis, we reported that uric acid is an independent risk factor for an increased CAVI[5]. In this study, we analyzed data of 27,360 healthy volunteers, and found that uric acid is an independent risk factor that increases CAVI even after adjusted by the factors, including sex, age, body mass index, systolic blood pressure, high-density lipoprotein cholesterol (HDL-C), non-HDL-C, γ-GTP, creatinine, and Hba1c[5]. In addition, the effect of uric acid on the CAVI differed between men and women. The effect of uric acid on CAVI in men showed a J-shaped curve with a uric acid level of 4–4.9 mg/dL associated with the lowest CAVI (Fig. 2). On the other hand, in women the curve was linear, where the lowest level of the CAVI was observed for uric acid levels under 2.9 mg/dL (Fig. 2)[5].

4. Xanthine oxidase inhibitors and large-scale intervention studies

What mechanism is involved in the uric acid-related progression of arteriosclerosis and increase in the CAVI? Interestingly, the cardiovascular risk and the CAVI increase with uric acid even at a concentration lower than the

saturation concentration. This may suggest the important roles of xanthine oxidase, which is a key enzyme producing oxidative stress, rather than uric acid[6]. In fact, a cohort study has reported that uric acid-lowering drugs suppress cardiovascular events in hyperuricemia patients[7]. Although allopurinol requires dose-limitation in patients with renal dysfunction, such as those with CKD, due to side effects, a large-scale intervention study using febuxostat or topiroxostat, which were newly developed xanthine oxidase inhibitors with few side effects, were expected to prevent cardiovascular events.

Recently, a large-scale intervention trial of febuxostat on cardiovascular prevention unexpectedly reported higher all-cause and cardiovascular mortality in the febuxostat group than in the allopurinol group,[10]. In addition, a meta-analysis of patients with gout showed no difference in terms of cardiovascular events (major adverse cardiovascular events) between treatment with and without xanthine oxidase inhibitors, or between treatment with allopurinol and febuxostat[12]. Moreover, a randomized trial of febuxostat did not show any suppressive effect on carotid thickening in patients with asymptomatic hyperuricemia[13].

Although large-scale studies will be required to determine whether uric acid-lowering agents, such as the new xanthine oxidase inhibitors and others, have anti-arteriosclerotic effects, it is not always easy to conduct large-scale intervention studies. It is relatively easy to examine their effects on the CAVI as a surrogate marker; such studies should be useful.

Conclusions

Epidemiological studies have revealed that uric acid is an independent risk factor for arteriosclerosis, and it was also an independent risk for an increased CAVI, a surrogate marker for arteriosclerosis. Since the involvement of oxidative stress through the activation of xanthine oxidase has been considered to be the mechanism of action, anti-arteriosclerotic effects of xanthine oxidase inhibitors were expected to prevent cardiovascular disease in patients with gout and hyperuricemia; however, large-scale intervention studies with these drugs have failed to prove such effects.

It is necessary to continue to investigate whether the newly developed uric acid-lowering drugs suppress an increase in the CAVI, as a quantitative marker for arteriosclerosis, and whether this improves the associated cardiovascular events.

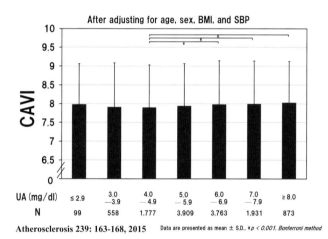

Atherosclerosis 239: 163-168, 2015　　Data are presented as mean ± S.D., *p < 0.001, Bonferroni method

Fig. 2A.　CAVI and Uric Acid (Men).
　　Cited from ref.5 【with permission of Elsevier】

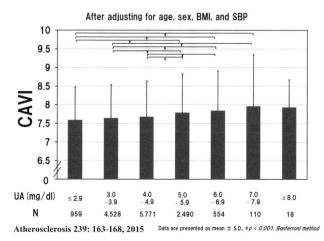

Atherosclerosis 239: 163-168, 2015　　Data are presented as mean ± S.D., *p < 0.001, Bonferroni method

Fig. 2B.　CAVI and Uric Acid (Women).
　　Cited from ref.5 【with permission of Elsevier】

References

1)　Matsuura F, Yamashita S, Nakamura T, Nishida M, Nozaki S, Funahashi T, Matsuzawa Y: Effect of visceral fat accumulation on uric acid metabolism in male obese subjects: visceral fat obesity is linked more closely to overproduction of uric acid than subcutaneous fat obesity. Metabolism 1998; 47: 929-933.

2)　Tsushima Y, Nishizawa H, Tochino Y, Nakatsuji H, Sekimoto R, Nagao Hirofumi H, Shirakura T, Kato K, Imaizumi K, Takahashi H, Tamura M, Maeda N, Funahashi T, Shimomura I: Uric acid secretion from adipose tissue and its increase in obesity. J Biol Chem 2013; 288: 27138–27149.

3) Fang J, Alderman MH: Serum uric acid and cardiovascular mortality the NHANES I epidemiologic follow-up study, 1971-1992. National Health and Nutrition Examination Survey. JAMA 2000; 283: 2404–2410.

4) Hakoda M, Oiwa H, Kasagi F, Masunari N, Yamada M, Suzuki G, Fujiwara S: Mortality of rheumatoid arthritis in Japan: A longitudinal cohort study. Ann Rheum Dis 2005; 64: 1451-1455.

5) Nagayama D, Yamaguchi T, Saiki A, Imamura H, Sato Y, Ban N, Kawana H, Nagumo A, Shirai K, Tatsuno I: High serum uric acid is associated with increased cardio-ankle vascular index (CAVI) in healthy Japanese subjects: a cross-sectional study. Atherosclerosis 2015; 239: 163-168. https://doi.org/10.1016/j.atherosclerosis.2015.01.011

6) Larsen KS, Pottegård A, Lindegaard HM, Hallas J: Effect of allopurinol on cardiovascular outcomes in hyperuricemic patients: A cohort study. Am J Med 2016; 129: 299-306.

7) Chen JH, Lan JL, Cheng CF, Liang WM, Lin HY, Tsay GJ, Yeh WT, Pan WH: Effect of urate-lowering therapy on all-cause and cardiovascular mortality in hyperuricemic patients without gout: A case-matched cohort study. PLoS One 2015;10:e0145193.

8) White WB, Saag KG, Becker MA, Borer JS, Gorelick PB, Whelton A, Hunt B, Castillo M, Gunawardhana L; CARES Investigators. Cardiovascular safety of febuxostat or allopurinol in patients with gout. N Engl J Med. 2018;378:1200-1210.

9) Al-Abdouh A, Khan SU, Barbarawi M, Upadhrasta S, Munira S, Bizanti A, Elias H, Jat A, Zhao D, Michos ED. Effects of febuxostat on mortality and cardiovascular outcomes: A systematic review and meta-analysis of randomized controlled trials. Mayo Clin Proc Innov Qual Outcomes. 2020;4:434-442.

10) Ju C, Lai RWC, Li KHC, Hung JKF, Lai JCL, Ho J, Liu Y, Tsoi MF, Liu T, Cheung BMY, Wong ICK, Tam LS, Tse G. Comparative cardiovascular risk in users versus non-users of xanthine oxidase inhibitors and febuxostat versus allopurinol users. Rheumatology (Oxford). 2020;59:2340-2349.

11) Doria A, Galecki AT, Spino C, Pop-Busui R, Cherney DZ, Lingvay I, Parsa A, Rossing P, Sigal RJ, Afkarian M, Aronson R, Caramori ML, Crandall JP, de Boer IH, Elliott TG, Goldfine AB, Haw JS, Hirsch IB, Karger AB, Maahs DM, McGill JB, Molitch ME, Perkins BA, Polsky S, Pragnell M, Robiner WN, Rosas SE, Senior P, Tuttle KR, Umpierrez GE, Wallia A, Weinstock RS, Wu C, Mauer M; PERL Study Group. Serum urate lowering with allopurinol and kidney function in type 1 diabetes. N Engl J Med 2020;382:2493-503.

Sleep Apnea and CAVI

Takatoshi Kasai

Summary

1. Since sleep apnea syndrome is sometimes associated with hypertension and/or white-coat hypertension, assessment of arterial stiffness using the CAVI, which is not dependent on blood pressure at the time of measurement, might be ideal.
2. The validity of arterial stiffness assessment by the CAVI in patients with sleep apnea has been demonstrated.
3. CPAP treatment for sleep apnea reduces the CAVI in the short-term, along with suppression of the inflammatory response and sympathetic nerve activity, which may slow progression in the CAVI due to the natural aging process over the long-term.

What Is Sleep Apnea?

In general, sleep apnea refers to obstructive sleep apnea (OSA), where the upper airway is obstructed during sleep (Fig. 1). Although the cause of OSA is multifactorial, obesity and anatomical changes and abnormalities of the upper airway morphology (tonsillar hypertrophy, micrognathia, etc.) are the main causes[1]. In particular, imbalances of boney structures and soft tissues can be contributary.

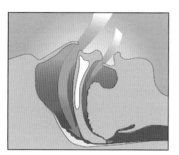

Fig. 1. Obstructive Sleep Apnea: Apnea caused by upper airway obstruction during sleep.

OSA poses a risk of cardiovascular disease development through 1) hemodynamic changes associated with negative intrathoracic pressure caused by ineffective inspiratory effort during upper airway obstruction, 2) increased sympathetic nerve activity, 3) increased oxidative stress and inflammation due to intermittent hypoxia and reoxygenation, and 4) new-onset hypertension and diabetes[2]. As a conservative treatment, continuous positive airway pressure (CPAP) is mainly used, because in radical therapy, weight reduction in obese people, is difficult to achieve and its efficacy is generally poor in the obese patient population (Fig. 2), although efficacy has varied across reports[2].

Sleep Apnea and CAVI

Pulse wave velocity (PWV), an indicator of arterial stiffness, particularly brachial-ankle (ba) PWV have been used in Japan to assess arterial stiffness and the risk of developing cardiovascular diseases. However, because high blood pressure and white coat hypertension are frequently observed in OSA patients[3], baPWV (which is affected by blood pressure at the time of measurement) is not appropriate, whereas the cardio-ankle vascular index (CAVI, which is not

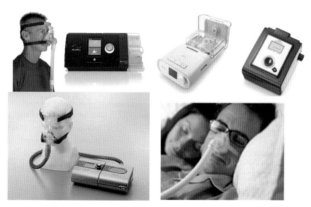

Fig. 2. Continuous positive airway pressure.
Breathing pressured air increases upper airway intramural pressure and prevents airway obstruction.

Department of Cardiovascular Medicine, Cardiovascular Respiratory Sleep Medicine, Juntendo University Graduate School of Medicine, 2-1-1 Hongo, Bunkyo-ku, Tokyo 113-8421 Japan.

affected by blood pressure) might be suitable. Therefore, to validate the use of the CAVI in OSA, we investigated the following aspects of the CAVI: 1) reproducibility in repeated measures, 2) correlations between baPWV and blood pressure values measured concurrently with the CAVI, 3) associations with carotid intima-media thickness (IMT), and 4) associations with OSA severity. The results demonstrated that use of the CAVI in studies on patients with OSA is valid, as the CAVI was highly reproducible, not affected by blood pressure than the baPWV, positively correlated with the IMT, an indicator of arteriosclerosis, and showed high value in severe OSA[4].

Furthermore, increasing OSA severity was associated with increasing blood inflammatory responses (particularly pentraxin3 levels, which are considered to reflect local vascular inflammation) and increasing CAVI values (Table 1). In addition, attenuation of OSA by CPAP treatment reduced the CAVI after 1 month of treatment, and resulted in short-term pentraxin3 level reductions[5]. These short-term effects on the CAVI were also affected by a reduction in vascular inflammation, but suppression of sympathetic

nerve activity by OSA attenuation appeared to have a stronger effect. Thus, functional changes in muscular arteries associated with sympathetic nerve activity were observed, rather than improvement in organic arteriosclerosis.

Furthermore, the effect of long-term CPAP treatment on organic arteriosclerosis was also examined[6]. Similar to the previous report, the CAVI decreased after 1 month of CPAP treatment, which was associated with lower sympathetic nerve activity as indicated by CPAP-use status and heart rate variability. On the other hand, over the course of 1 year, the CAVI rose, but the final value was similar to or less than that before CPAP treatment (Fig. 3). This change in CAVI from 1 month to 1 year after initiation of CPAP treatment correlated with CPAP use: the lower the increase in the CAVI, the better was the adherence to CPAP use. Therefore, in OSA patients, the CAVI decreased in a relatively short period, associated with a suppression of sympathetic nerve activity by CPAP treatment, but it then increased slowly with aging, but this increase might be delayed if appropriate CPAP treatment was maintained.

Table 1. OSA Severity, blood inflammatory response levels, and the CAVI.

With increasing severity of OSA, inflammatory response, particularly pentraxin3 levels, and the CAVI increased.

	Control (N = 25)	Mild OSA (N = 23)	Moderate-to-severe OSA (N = 27)
Pentraxin3, ng/ml	1.53 (1.14–2.04)	1.63 (1.15–2.05)	2.36 (1.79–2.98)[†‡]
HsCRP, mg/I	1.12 (0.58–2.17)	0.54 (0.33-1.64)	1.69 (0.97–4.30)[§]
CAVI	6.85 ± 1.22	7.00 ± 0.95	7.68 ± 1.07[†§]

[†]P < 0.01: control vs moderate-to-severe OSA, [‡]P < 0.01: mild vs moderate-to-severe OSA, [§]P < 0.05: mild vs moderate-to-severe OSA (Adapted from ref. 5) [by permission of Oxford University Press]

Future Perspectives

Recent randomized trials have shown that it may be difficult to prevent the development of cardiovascular diseases in patients with OSA by CPAP treatment, but that adherence to CPAP may be helpful. Therefore, it is important to retain the usage of CPAP, and if the risk reduction by CPAP initiation becomes easier to recognize by visualization of arteriosclerosis and cardiovascular risk by means of the CAVI, it may motivate patients to adhere to CPAP use. This may facilitate prevention of cardiovascular disease development in a larger number of cases.

Future Challenges:

1. Randomized trials testing the impact of sleep apnea treatment by CPAP on the CAVI are required.
2. Accumulation of data regarding changes in the CAVI in association with CPAP use is required.

References

1) Taranto Montemurro L, Kasai T. The upper airway in sleep-disordered breathing. UA in SDB. Minerva Med 2014; 105: 25-40.
2) Kasai T, Floras JS, Bradley TD. Sleep apnea and cardiovascular disease. a bidirectional relationship. Circulation 2012; 126: 1495-1510.
3) Garcia-Rio F, Pino JM, Alonso A et al. White coat hypertension in patients with obstructive sleep apnea–hypopnea syndrome. Chest 2004; 125:817-822.
4) Kumagai T, Kasai T, Kato M et al. Establishment of the cardio-ankle vascular index in patients with obstructive sleep apnea. Chest 2009; 136: 779-786.
5) Kasai T, Inoue K, Kumagai T et al. Plasma pentraxin3 and arterial stiffness in men with obstructive sleep apnea. Am J Hypertens 2011; 24: 401-407. https://doi.org/10.1038/ajh.2010.248
6) Kato M, Kumagai T, Naito R et al. Change in cardio-ankle vascular index by long-term continuous positive airway pressure therapy for obstructive sleep apnea. J Cardiol 2011; 58: 74-82. https://doi.org/10.1016/j.jjcc.2011.03.005

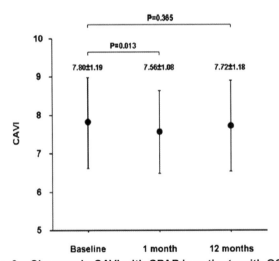

Fig. 3. Changes in CAVI with CPAP in patients with OSA.

The CAVI decreases significantly by 1 month after initiation of CPAP, then increases up to 1 year. This may be due to natural progression associated with aging, but the levels remain similar to or below those of before CPAP initiation. Dotted line (blue:) Estimated increase by aging process for patients with similar backgrounds. Cited from ref.6 [with permission of Elsevier]

Smoking

Masaaki Miyata

Summary

1. Acute and chronic effects of cigarette smoking on CAVI increase.
2. Smoking cessation reduces CAVI.

Acute effects of smoking on CAVI

We measured CAVI in 10 healthy male smokers (mean age 35 years) before and after a single cigarette to investigate the acute effects of cigarette smoking on CAVI level. As a result, a single cigarette was allowed in 5 minutes, after which CAVI levels were significantly elevated from 7.0 ± 0.9 to 7.3 ± 0.7 (P<0.01)[1]. Mechanistically, the nicotine from cigarette smoking induces activation of the central and peripheral sympathetic nervous system, which may affect not only muscular but also elastic arteries and increase CAVI levels.

Chronic effects of smoking on CAVI

We investigated the association between CAVI and risk factors for atherosclerosis, including smoking, in 160 males who underwent health checkups and were smokers (mean age 46 years)[1]. In single-regression analysis, age, triglycerides, urea nitrogen, uric acid, mean blood pressure, and Brinkman index were significantly associated with CAVI. Multivariate regression analysis of these factors demonstrated that age, triglycerides, uric acid, and Brinkman index were independently associated with CAVI, suggesting that continuous smoking increases CAVI. As a possible mechanism for the chronic effect of smoking on atherosclerosis, in addition to the aforementioned sympathetic nervous activity induced by nicotine, radical oxygen species generated by smoking might injure the arterial endothelium, while the decreased production of nitric oxide, a vascular protective factor, finally increases CAVI.

In comparison, we simultaneously measured brachial-ankle pulse wave velocity (baPWV) and found that baPWV was not independently associated with Brinkman index but

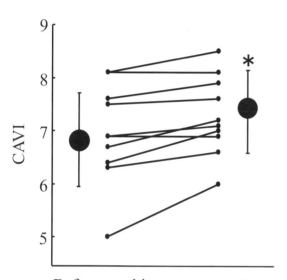

Fig. 1. Changes in CAVI levels before and after one cigarette.
* P<0.01, Adapted from ref. 1

Table 1.   Factors associated with CAVI or baPWV in smokers (multiple regression analysis).

	CAVI		PWV	
	Coefficient	P Value	Coefficient	P Value levels
Age	0.052	<0.0001	7.872	<0.0001
Triglyceride	0.002	<0.05	0.425	<0.01
Fasting glucose		0.4359		0.4037
Uric acid	0.172	<0.05	30.663	<0.05
Mean blood pressure		0.0813	7.971	<0.0001
Brinkman index	0.001	<0.05		0.4319

CAVI, cardio-ankle vascular index; baPWV, brachial-ankle pulse wave velocity
Adapted from reference 1

School of Health Sciences, Faculty of Medicine, Kagoshima University, 8-35-1 Sakuragaoka, Kagoshima City, Kagoshima 890-8544, Japan.

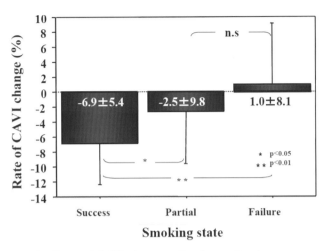

Fig. 2. Rate of CAVI change after 3 months in success, partial, and failure groups.

Success: success group of smoking cessation (22 patients), Partial: partial success group who reduced the number of cigarettes smoked (25 patients), Failure: failure group of smoking cessation (35 patients)
* P < 0.05, **P < 0.01, Adapted from reference 2

significantly associated with mean blood pressure, in contrast with CAVI[1] (Table 1).

Effects of smoking cessation on CAVI

Noike et al. examined the effects of smoking cessation on vascular stiffness by measuring CAVI in 82 smokers (mean age, 64 years; 77 men; 5 women) before and 3 months after smoking cessation education[2]. Nicotine substitution therapy was not used for smoking cessation, and smokers were divided into the success group (22 subjects, mean age 66 years), the partial success group (25 subjects, mean age 61 years) who reduced the number of cigarettes, and the failure

group (35 subjects, mean age 64 years) after 3 months. CAVI showed significantly lower values in the success group (8.6 ± 0.9) than the failure group (9.4 ± 1.2) 3 months after smoking cessation (P < 0.01). It was also shown that CAVI reduction rate after 3 months was significantly higher in the success group compared with the partial success and failure groups (Fig. 2). Furthermore, they found that the reduction rate of CAVI after 3 months was positively associated with age, years of smoking, and Brinkman index prior to smoking cessation; less years of smoking and lower Brinkman index were associated with greater improvements in vascular stiffness with smoking cessation.

Based on the above results, it seems possible to evaluate the effect of smoking cessation by measuring CAVI, which could be used as motivation for smoking cessation. Measuring CAVI during this process could be useful and I would like to recommend effectively utilizing CAVI for the smoking cessation therapy.

Future challenges

1. To integrate a lot of data in health checkups to examine differences in CAVI levels among never, former, and current smokers.
2. Further use of CAVI in smoking cessation education is desired.

References

1) Kubozono T, Miyata M, Ueyama K, et al. Acute and chronic effects of smoking on arterial stiffness. Circ J. 2011; 75: 698-702. https://doi.org/10.1253/circj.cj-10-0552
2) Noike H, Nakamura K, Sugiyama Y, et al. Changes in cardio-ankle vascular index in smoking cessation. J Atheroscler Thromb. 2010; 17: 517-525. https://doi.org/10.5551/jat.3707

CAVI during pregnancy - pregnancy-induced hypertension –

Shin-ichiro Katsuda[1], Kaori Kamijo[2], Fumihiko Yoshikawa[2], Ayano Koike[2],
Yahiro Netsu[2], Tsuyoshi Shimizu[3] and Kohji Shirai[4]

Introduction

In normal pregnancy, peripheral vascular resistance decreases to adapt to an increased blood volume, resulting in a slight decrease in blood pressure (BP)[1,2]. In hypertensive disorders of pregnancy (HDP), dysfunction of endothelium and placental angiogenesis could increase vascular resistance, thus increasing BP throughout gestation[3,4]. HDP could induce maternal complications such as preclampsia, cerebrovascular events, and renal and hepatic failures as well as fetal complications[4]. Cardio-ankle vascular index (CAVI) has been developed as a pressure-independent index of arterial stiffness[5,6], so that CAVI enables estimation of intrinsic arterial stiffness. It is important to detect cardiovascular abnormalities during pregnancy as early as possible to prevent further complications of HDP.

In the present study, we investigated changes in BP and CAVI with pregnancy progression in normal and hypertensive pregnant women to elucidate whether CAVI can be a predictor of HDP.

Methods

1. Study population

We included 197 normal pregnant women (normal group) > 35 (37.8 ± 2.0; mean ± SD) years old and 21 pregnant women with HDP (HDP group) > 35 (36.2 ± 3.8) years old who received a routine physical checkup during pregnancy at Suwa Maternity Clinic. Women with diabetes and hyperthyroidism were excluded from the present study. Table 1 shows the physical characteristics of pregnant women at 7-8 weeks of pregnancy. Body weight and body mass index (BMI) were significantly reater in the HDP

group than in the normal group. The present study was approved by the Ethics Committee of Suwa Maternity Clinic and Fukushima Medical University.

2. Measurement

The first pregnancy examination was performed at 7-8 weeks (W) of gestation. BP and CAVI were measured every 4 W (± 1 W) from 11-14 W of gestation until just before delivery (37 W) using a VaSera VA-1500AN (Fukuda Denshi Co., Ltd.). CAVI was determined by the following formula[5,6]; $CAVI = a[(2\rho/\Delta P) \times \ln(Ps/Pd) \times PWV^2] + b$ (Ps, P and, ΔP; systolic, diastolic and pulse pressures, ρ; blood density, PWV; pulse wave velocity, a and b; undisclosed coefficients). Proteinuria was measured simultaneously with BP and CAVI measurement.

Results

1. Changes in BP and CAVI in normal pregnant women

Systolic (SBP) and diastolic blood (DBP) pressures were approximately constant throughout gestation. SBP and DBP showed a slight increase at 37 W of gestation in the normal group (Fig. 1A and B). CAVI showed a significant decrease by approximately 0.6 on the left side and 0.7 on the right side after the second trimester (19 W) compared to measurements at 11-14 weeks, and then stayed relatively low until delivery (Fig. 1C and D). Heart rate (HR) increased from 66.7 at 11-14 W to 80.8 beat/min at 37 W of gestation in average similarly to that previously reported[7].

2. Changes in BP and CAVI in pregnant women with HDP

Proteinuria was observed in 7 pregnant women in the HDP group after 30 W of gestation. All pregnant women with HDP were analyzed as a group, because there was no significant difference in SBP, DBP, and CAVI between hypertensive pregnant women with and without proteinuria. SBP and DBP in pregnant women with HDP were significantly higher than those in the control group throughout the whole pregnancy. SBP and DBP tended to increase in the third trimester compared with those at 11-14 W of gestation (Fig. 1A and B). CAVI did not decrease at 19 W and tended to increase until delivery (Fig. 1C and D). HR increased from 71.4 at 11-14 W to 77.2 beat/min at 37W of gestation in average.

Table 1. Physical characteristics of pregnant women under initial prenatal screening at 7-8 weeks of pregnancy.

		Normal	HDP
Age (year)	...	37.8 ± 2.0	36.2 ± 3.8
Height (cm)	...	158.4 ± 5.2	156.9 ± 4.8
Body Weight (kg)	...	51.9 ± 6.1	55.8 ± 10.5**
BMI (kg/m²)	...	20.7 ± 2.4	22.6 ± 3.7**

**p < 0.01, BMI: body mass index, HDP: hypertensive disorders of pregnancy.

[1]Department of Cellular and Integrative Physiology, Fukushima Medical University School of Medicine, 1 Hikariga-oka, Fukushima City, Fukushima 960-1295, Japan.
[2]Suwa Maternity Clinic, Nagano 393-0077, Japan.
[3]Shimizu Institute of Space Physiology, Suwa Maternity Clinic, Nagano 393-0077, Japan.
[4]Seijinkai Mihama Hospital, Chiba 261-0013, Japan.

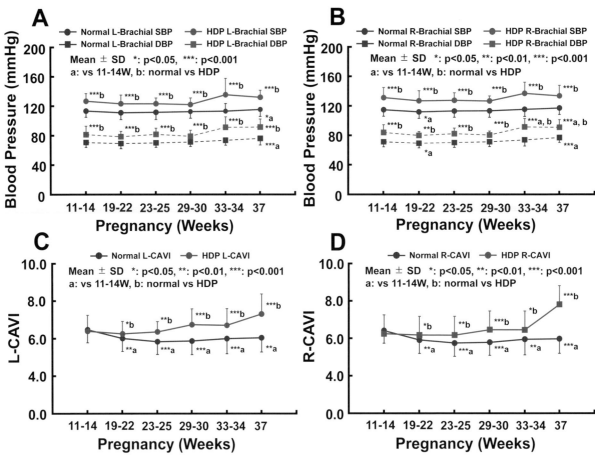

Fig. 1. Changes in left brachial SBP and DBP (A), right brachial SBP and DBP (B), left CAVI (C) and right CAVI (D) during the course of pregnancy in normal pregnant women and pregnant women with HDP.

SBP: systolic blood pressure, DBP: diastolic blood pressure, W: week, L: left, R: right. HDP: hypertension-induced pregnancy, CAVI: cardio-ankle vascular index.

Discussion

In normal pregnancy, the arteries themselves improve compliance to successfully adapt to the increased blood volume and cardiac output, which contributes to prevent blood pressure increase in the second and third trimesters[1,2]. The decreased CAVI is considered to reflect the enhanced arterial compliance in response to cardiovascular changes during pregnancy progression. In the HDP group, CAVI did not decrease during the second and third semesters and was significantly higher than in the control group at each week. These findings suggest that arteries do not appropriately respond to the increased cardiac output by ameliorating arterial elasticity. HDP may also be preceded by vascular dysfunction. More observational studies in the field of obstetrics and gynecology are required. If the relevance of CAVI as a predictor of HDP is demonstrated, CAVI may also contribute to safe maternal control.

References

1) Kaihura C, Savvidou MD, Anderson JM, McEniery CM, Nicolaides KH. Maternal arterial stiffness in pregnancies affected by preeclampsia. *Am J Physiol Heart Circ Physiol* 2009; **297**: H759-764.

2) Avni B, Frenkel G, Shahar L, Golik A, Sherman D, Dishy V. Aortic stiffness in normal and hypertensive pregnancy. *Blood Press* 2010; **19**: 11-15.

3) Watanabe K, Naruse K, Tanaka K, Metoki H, Suzuki Y. Outline of Definition and Classification of "Pregnancy induced Hypertension (PIH)". *Hypertens Res Pregnancy* 2013; **1**: 3–4.

4) Brown MA, Magee LA, Kenny LC, Karumanchi SA, McCarthy FP, Saito S, Hall DR, Warren CE, Adoyi G, Ishaku S. Hypertensive disorders of pregnancy ISSHP classification, diagnosis, and management recommendations for international practice. *Hypertension* 2018; **72**: 24-43.

5) Shirai K, Hiruta N, Song M, Kurosu T, Suzuki J, Tomaru T, Miyashita Y, Saiki A, Takahashi M, Suzuki K, Takata M. Cardio-ankle vascular index (CAVI) as a novel indicator of arterial stiffness: theory, evidence and perspectives. *J Atheroscler Thromb* 2011; **18**: 924-938.

6) Shirai K, Utino J, Saiki A, Endo K, Ohira M, Nagayama D, Tatsuno I, Shimizu K, Takahashi M, Takahara A. Evaluation of blood pressure control using a new arterial stiffness parameter, cardio-ankle vascular index (CAVI). *Curr Hypertens Rev* 2013; **9**: 66-75.

7) Koike A, Sakai M, Tatsuta M, Nakanishi M, Nagata M, Kamijo K, Yoshikawa F, Shimizu T, Netsu Y, Shirai K, Katsuda S. Assessment of arterial stiffness with CAVI during normal pregnancy. *Jpn J Clin Physiol* 2016; **46**: 139-146.

PART 5

Prognostic Values of CAVI: mortality and mobility

RAMA EGAT study: "Arterial stiffness contributes to coronary artery disease risk prediction beyond the traditional risk score"

Prin Vathesatogkit and Piyamitr Sritara

Introduction

Major cardiovascular disease prevention guidelines have recommended the use of global cardiovascular disease (CVD) risk assessment in routine clinical practice. Risk prediction tools are developed to guide healthcare professionals and individuals in their decision making regarding further management and to inform individuals about their risks of having or developing a disease in a particular period of time. Traditional risk factors for CVD that are commonly used are age, gender, smoking status, systolic blood pressure, diabetes, and blood cholesterol level. The simplicity of traditional risk score makes it possible to be implemented in a nationwide screening program with a reasonable predictive value. To improve the predictive performance, additional risk enhancers such as high-density lipoprotein cholesterol (HDL-c), family history, chronic kidney disease status or coronary calcium score are suggested in guidelines.

In recent years, researchers have demonstrated that cardio-ankle vascular index (CAVI), a novel marker of arterial stiffness, has a strong association with atherosclerotic

burden in patients with and without stable atherosclerotic cardiovascular disease[1] (ASCVD) (Fig. 1) and a modest association with incident cardiovascular disease risk[2]. Not only correlate with atherosclerotic plaque burden from coronary CT angiography, CAVI is also positively correlated with coronary artery calcium (CAC) scoring, and is considered to be a useful method to detect CAC. These observations lead to a question whether CAVI can enhance the predictive utility of traditional risk factors in an asymptomatic population.

1. Electricity Generating Authority of Thailand (EGAT) study and CAVI

In Thailand, a coronary artery disease (CAD) risk score called 'figure-EGAT score' was developed in 2008 to estimate 10-year CHD risk, using traditional risk factors [3,4]. The score was developed from a longitudinal cohort study, named Electricity Generating Authority of Thailand (EGAT) study, that primarily aimed to be a foundation of Thai cardiovascular risk estimator since 1985[5]. This score has been validated in the Thai population and was shown to be a more suitable score for evaluating cardiovascular risk in Asian subjects than the Framingham risk score[6]. The purpose of our study was to investigate the association of CAVI and coronary atherosclerosis as assessed by 64-slice multidetector CT (MDCT) coronary angiography in Thai patients with a moderate CVD risk and to determine the utility of CAVI when adding to a traditional risk score[7].

Between November 2005 to March 2006, patients referred for evaluation with 64-slice MDCT coronary angiography due to suspected CAD at a university Hospital are invited to participate in this study. CAVI was measured with a VaSera VS-1000 CAVI instrument (Fukuda Denshi Co Ltd, Tokyo, Japan) using the standard methods described in the literature in the same day as 64-slide MDCT coronary angiography. Patients with peripheral arterial disease (ankle brachial index <0.9), those who declined or had any contraindications to contrast media (previous allergic reaction to contrast media, severe renal insufficiency), those with atrial fibrillation and those who were unable to hold their breath long enough for the CT scan time were excluded

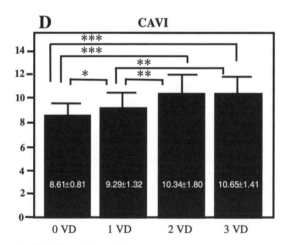

Fig. 1. Relationship between coronary angiographic findings and cardio-ankle vascular index (CAVI).
[with permission of Japanese Circulation Society][1]

Cardiology Division Department of Internal Medicine, Faculty of Medicine, Ramathibodi Hospital, Mahidol University, Bangkok, Thailand.

Table 1. Traditional risk factors (RAMA-EGAT score). (cited from Pattanaprichakul S et al. Asean Heart J. 2007;15:18-22)[3]

Score	−2	0	2	3	4	5	6	8	10
Age (years)	35−39	40−44	45−49		50−54		55−59	60−65	≥65
Gender		Female		Male					
Cholesterol (mg/dl)		<280				>280 or drug therapy			
Smoking		No	Yes						
Diabetes		No				Yes			
Hypertension		No		Yes					
Waist circumference*		Below		Above					

*Waist circumference: men ≥36 inches, women ≥32 inches.

Table 2. Characteristics of the study population and comparisons between patients with and without significant coronary artery stenosis. (cited from Yingchoncharoen T et al. Heart Asia. 2012; 4:77−82)[7]

	Significant coronary stenosis (N = 346)	No significant coronary stenosis (N = 1045)	p Value
Age (years)	62.1±8.4	56.9±9.1	<0.001
Male (%)	63	39.9	<0.001
BMI (kg/m²)	25.9±7.2	24.7±3.8	<0.001
RAMA-EGAT score	15.8±5.7	11.1±6.0	<0.001
CAC score	315.2±470.6	39.7±149.3	<0.001
Smoking (%)	9.7	6.4	0.046
HT (%)	58.5	36.5	<0.001
DM (%)	22.6	9.9	<0.001
HDL (mg/dl)	43.7±11.7	48.5±13.9	<0.001
CAVI	9.7±1.3	7.4±1.5	<0.001

BMI, body mass index; CAC, coronary artery calcium; CAVI, cardio-ankle vascular index; DM, diabetes mellitus; HDL, high density lipoprotein; HT, hypertension.

from the study. All participants were interviewed for the traditional risk factors listed in the RAMA-EGAT score[3] (Table 1). Multislice CT examinations were performed using a 64-slice CT scanner (Sensation 64, Siemens, Forchheim, Germany). Analysis of MDCT data was performed using multiplanar reconstruction. Coronary segments were analyzed by the American Heart Association classification. Significant coronary artery stenosis was defined as >= 50% of mean luminal diameter reduction in two orthogonal projections.

A total of 1391 patients completed the study. The baseline characteristics are summarized in Table 2, the mean RAMA-EGAT score differed significantly between those with and without significant coronary as well as CAC and CAVI. Patients with significant coronary artery disease have a higher risk score (15.8 vs 11.1), a higher CAC score (315.2 vs 39.7) and a higher CAVI (9.7 vs 7.4). CAVI was significantly higher in patients with single-vessel, double-vessel and triple-vessel diseases than in patients without a coronary lesion as displayed in Fig. 2. Interestingly, CAVI showed a very high predictive value for CAD, the receiver operating characteristic (ROC) curve analysis for the

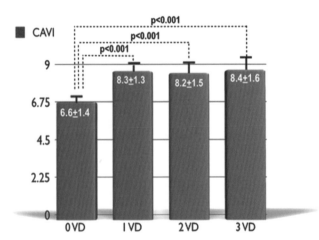

Fig. 2. Relationship between multidetector CT coronary angiography findings and cardio-ankle vascular index (CAVI): 0DV, on vessel disease; 1VD, one-vessel disease; 2VD, two-vessel disease; 3VD, three-vessel disease. Date shown as mean±SD. (cited from Yingchoncharoen T et al. Heart Asia. 2012; 4:77−82)[7]

presence of CAD was 0.87. A CAVI of >= 8 was identified as the best cut-off value for the prediction of CAD in our study (sensitivity 92%, specificity 73%, accuracy 79%).

To test the additive value of adding CAVI to the traditional risk score, the CAVI value was put into the RAMA-EGAT score with a point system. The modified RAMA-EGAT score with CAVI showed a superior performance and discrimination than our traditional RAMA-EGAT score, increasing the C-statistics from 0.72 to 0.85 (Fig. 3). Adding CAVI to traditional risk score was also improve the net reclassification improvement (NRI) by almost 28% (Table 3). Those who have CAVI >=8 can be reclassified into a higher risk group while those who have CAVI <8 reclassified to a lower risk group (Fig. 4). This means that CAVI can play an important role in predicting the long-term prognosis of patients with intermediate atherosclerotic risk factors. Moreover, a post hoc analysis of this study was conducted to evaluate the association

between CAVI and mortality[8]. The finding shows that CAVI is an independent predictor of cardiovascular events in patients with intermediate atherosclerotic risk factors and a mean CAVI of more than 8 was associated with a significant excess mortality. These findings underpinned the importance of arterial stiffness as a strong predictor of cardiovascular outcome among several candidate predictors.

Several mechanisms are proposed to explain the association between CAVI and coronary artery disease. High CAVI reflects high arterial stiffness. Arterial stiffening may lead to early pulse wave reflection resulting in an increased left ventricular load, myocardial oxygen demand and reduced ejection fraction, thereby inducing eccentric left ventricular hypertrophy[9]. Additionally, the earlier reflective wave return causes a reduction in diastolic blood pressure which may compromise coronary perfusion[10]. An elevated pulse pressure due to increased arterial stiffness may induce arterial remodeling, increased wall thickness

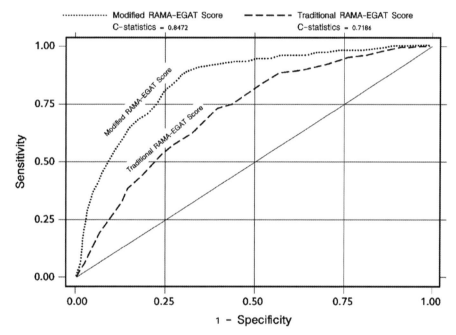

Fig. 3. Comparison of receiver operating characteristic (ROC) curve of modified RAMA-EGAT score (EGAT + cardio-ankle vascular index (CAVI)) and traditional RAMA-EGAT score (EGAT score). (cited from Yingchoncharoen T et al. Heart Asia. 2012; 4:77−82)[7]

Table 3. Calculation of Net Reclassification Improvement (NRI) for the modified RAMA-EGAT score versus the traditional RAMA-EGAT score. (cited from Yingchoncharoen T et al. Heart Asia. 2012; 4:77−82)[7]

+ Significant CAD (N=346) (Cases)	Modified RAMA-EGAT score				
RAMA-EGAT score	Risk group	Low	Intermediate	High	Cases classified upward = 4+38 (12.14%)
	Low	3	4	6	Cases classified downward = 4+17 (6.07%);
	Intermediate	4	4	38	Cases classified upward-Cases classified downward = 12.14% − 6.07% = 6.07%
	High	0	17	270	
− Significant CAD (N=1045) (Non-cases)	Modified RAMA-EGAT score				
RAMA-EGAT score	Risk group	Low	Intermediate	High	Cases classified upward = 40+121 (15.41%)
	Low	106	40	48	Cases classified downward = 109+278 (37.03%)
	Intermediate	109	81	121	Cases classified downward-Cases classified upward = 37.03% − 15.41% = 21.62%
	High	59	278	203	NRI = 6.07% + 21.62% = 27.69%

and the development of plaque[11].

2. Treatment of hypertension and CAVI

In the original EGAT study, CAVI was performed every 5 years in all participants since 2012. A study from the EGAT cohort showed that quality of hypertension treatment in those hypertensives, as measured by percent control hypertension over the period of 15 years (from 1997 to 2012) was highly correlated with CAVI in 2012[12]. Among hypertensives in 1997, those who had 100% achieving target (blood pressure < 140/90 mmHg) in all subsequent visits had the lowest CAVI followed by 75%, 50%, 25% and 0% (CAVI 8.98, 9.04, 9.09, 9.19 and 9.42 respectively, significant p for trend). Whether receiving antihypertensive medication or not was not related to CAVI. Subjects with unaware hypertension in 2012 had significantly higher CAVI than those with normotension (9.19 versus 8.78) but not different from aware hypertensives (9.19 versus 9.11). There are 2 subsequence studies on the issue of hypertension

and CAVI, focusing on the 5-year progression of CAVI from the 2007-2009 surveys to the 2012-2014 surveys[13,14]. One confirmed that uncontrolled hypertensives had a significantly higher percentage of CAVI progression than controlled group (Fig. 5). Another showed that those participants who had systolic blood pressure below 120 mmHg had a significantly slower progression of CAVI compared to those who had systolic blood pressure more than or equal to 120 mmHg (Fig. 6). These data help provide an insight why CAVI has an enormous incremental effect when adding to traditional risk factors. CAVI is not only capturing stiffness of artery, but also quantitating degrees of disease burden from those co-morbidities which are clearly not be visualized by routine clinical check up.

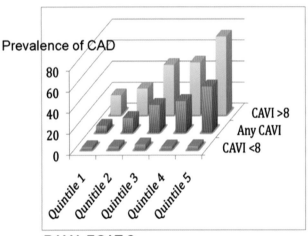

RAMA-EGAT Score

Fig. 4. Cardio-ankle vascular index (CAVI) provides additional diagnostic value at all levels of the RAMA-EGAT score. (cited from Yingchoncharoen T et al. Heart Asia. 2012; 4:77–82)[7]

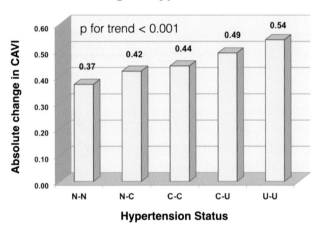

N = No HTN　　**C** = Controlled HTN　　**U** = Uncontrolled HTN

First alphabet indicates Hypertension status in 2007-8, second in 2012-3, n = 2,286

Fig. 5. Progression of CAVI in 5-year period according to hypertension status. [cited from Vutthikraivit W et al. European Heart Journal. 2016; 37 (Abstract Supplement), 1189. 15][14]

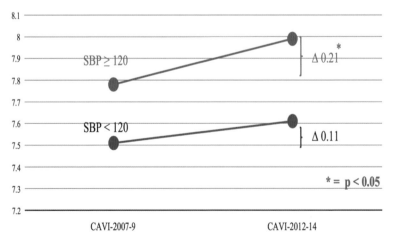

Fig. 6. Progression of CAVI in 5 year period according to SBP level at baseline. [cited from Vutthikraivit W et al. European Heart Journal. 2016; 37 (Abstract Supplement), 1189. 15][14]

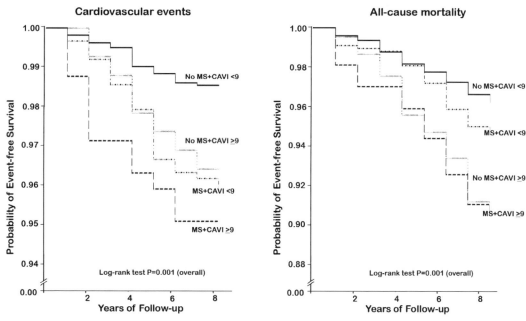

Fig. 7. Mortality outcomes stratified by CAVI and metabolic syndrome status. [with permission of ELSEVIER][15]

3. Prognostic value and CAVI in the EGAT cohort

The independence prognostic value of CAVI was also documented again in another study from the EGAT cohort[15]. This study used the CAVI data collected in 2007-2009 in more than 3,000 subjects to predict mortality outcome in 2015. CAVI is an independent risk factor for all-cause mortality after adjusted for traditional risk factors in both those with and without metabolic syndrome (Fig. 7). This finding implied that CAVI may have a role in CV prediction beyond traditional risk factors.

Summary

In summary, arterial stiffness as measured by CAVI can improve the predictive performance of a traditional risk score as shown in the RAMA-EGAT study. The ability of CAVI when adding to a traditional risk score is in a similar way with coronary calcium scan in that those with a high CAVI will be reclassified to a higher risk level and a low CAVI to an opposite direction. Measurement of CAVI give more information on subclinical atherosclerosis than using a traditional risk factor such as systolic blood pressure. High CAVI should be considered as a surrogate marker for a more intense lifestyle modification, such as tighter blood pressure control, smoking cessation, obstructive sleep apnea detection and treatment, and strict weight control. Compared to other risk enhancers e.g. CAC scan or laboratory tests that need lab setup, CAVI is technically feasible for office-based examination at low cost. CAVI is one of the most practical tools for noninvasive comprehensive cardiovascular risk assessment that give a benefit beyond traditional risk factors.

References

1) Nakamura K, Tomaru T, Yamamura S, et al. Cardio-Ankle Vascular Index is a Candidate Predictor of Coronary Atherosclerosis. Circ J 2008; 72: 598–604.

2) Matsushita K, Ding N, Kim ED, et al. Cardio-ankle vascular index and cardiovascular disease: Systematic review and meta-analysis of prospective and cross-sectional studies. J Clin Hypertens. 2019; 21:16–24.

3) Pattanaprichakul S, Jongjirasiri S, Yamwong S, et al. RAMA-EGAT risk score for predicting coronary artery disease evaluated by 64-slice CT angiography. Asean Heart J. 2007; 15:18-22.

4) Anon. [The Development of Coronary Heart Disease Assessment. Final Report.] 2005. http://thaincd.com/document/file/download/leaflet/sukit28-30-03-54.pdf

5) Vathesatogkit P, Woodward M, Tanomsup S, Ratanachaiwong W, Vanavanan S, Yamwong S, et al. Cohort profile: the electricity generating authority of Thailand study. Int J Epidemiol. 2012; 41:359–365.

6) Asia Paccific Cohort Studies Collaboration Cardiovascular risk prediction tools for populations in Asia Journal of Epidemiology & Community Health 2007;61:115-121.

7) Yingchoncharoen T, Limpijankit T, Jongjirasiri S, Laothamatas J, Yamwong S, Sritara P. Arterial stiffness contributes to coronary artery disease risk prediction beyond the traditional risk score (RAMA-EGAT score) Heart Asia. 2012; 4:77–82.

8) Yingchoncharoen T, Limpijankit T, Jongjirasiri S, Laothamatas J, Yamwong S, Sritara P. Arterial stiffness is an independent predictor of cardiac mortality in asymptomatic patients with intermediate atherosclerotic risk factors. Circulation. 2013;128(22 suppl): A11232.

9) Westerhof N, O'Rourke MF. Haemodynamic basis for the development of left ventricular failure in systolic hypertension and for its logical therapy. J Hypertens 1995; 13:943e52.

10) Watanabe H, Ohtsuka S, Kakihana M, et al. Coronary circulation in dogs with an experimental decrease in aortic compliance. J Am Coll Cardiol 1993; 21:1497e506.

11) Witteman JC, Grobbee DE, Valkenburg HA, et al. J-shaped relation between change in diastolic blood pressure

and progression of aortic atherosclerosis. Lancet 1994; 343:504e7.

12) Vathesatogkit P, Yingchoncharoen T, Thongmung N, Tatsaneeyapan A, Sritara P. Long-term blood pressure control and the severity of atherosclerosis as reflected by cardio-ankle vascular index. Eur Heart J. 2013;34 Suppl_1:P5001. https://doi.org/10.1093/eurheartj/eht310.P5001

13) Pibalyart S, Vathesatogkit P, Yingchoncharoen T, Yamwong S, Sritara P. Correlation between arterial stiffness as measured by progression of cardiac ankle vascular index and long-term hypertension control status. Eur Heart J. 2015;36 Suppl_1:817(P4672).

14) Vutthikraivit W, Vathesatogkit P, Jongyotha K, et al. Appropriate goal of systolic blood pressure to prevent rapid progression of arterial stiffness: a 5-year longitudinal follow up. Eur Heart J. 2016;37 Suppl_1:1189(5760).

15) Limpijankit T, Vathesatogkit P, Matchariyakul D, Yingchoncharoen T, Boonhat H, Sritara P. Cardio-ankle vascular index as a predictor of cardiovascular events and all-cause mortality in metabolic syndrome patients. J Am Coll Cardiol. 2018;71(11_Suppl):A1844. https://www.jacc.org/doi/pdf/10.1016/S0735-1097%2818%2932385-4

Prospective Study on CAVI - 1 - Patients with Metabolic disorders

Atsuhito Saiki

Summary

- There are a relatively few large scale prospective studies on CAVI among patients with metabolic disorders.
- In primary prevention studies, CAVI is a significant predictor of CVD events in patients with metabolic disorders.

Introduction

There are several prospective studies on mortality and morbidity about CAVI, despite CAVI having been introduced about 15 years ago. However, several studies have investigated the association between CAVI and future cardiovascular (CV) events. The participants in all studies were at high risk for cardiovascular disease (CVD), having hypertension, diabetes, obesity, chronic kidney disease (CKD), and a history of CVD. As of the summer of 2020, nine studies were from Japan, and the other two from Taiwan and Lithuania. In most studies, baseline CAVI was a predictor of future CV events. Among these trials, three were conducted in at least hundreds of Japanese patients with metabolic disorders. A comprehensive list is shown in Table 1. In this Chapter, we review the subject characteristics and results of these studies and verify the prognostic value of CAVI in Japanese patients.

A primary prevention study of 1,080 patients with metabolic disorders (Sato, et al.)[1]

Outpatients with metabolic disorders including diabetes mellitus, hypertension, and dyslipidemia at Toho University, Sakura Medical Center (Japan) between April 2004 and March 2006 were enrolled[1]. Patients who already had CV events at baseline, low ankle brachial index (ABI) (<0.9), or atrial fibrillation were excluded. Eventually, 1003 subjects (92.9% of 1,080 subjects) followed until March 2012 (follow-up duration 6.7 ± 1.6 years) were analyzed. The primary end point of this study was new-onset CV events such as myocardial infarction and stable/unstable angina pectoris. A CV event was defined as $\geq 75\%$ stenosis in an epicardial coronary artery confirmed angiographically. Baseline CAVI was 9.25 ± 1.61. For underlying diseases, 51.1% of the subjects had diabetes mellitus, 52.4% hypertension, and 62.6% dyslipidemia. During the observation period, 90 subjects had new-onset myocardial infarction or angina pectoris confirmed by angiography.

Table 1. Association of CAVI with Cardiovascular Outcomes in Prospective Studies (in Japanese Patients with Metabolic Disorders).

Author	Country	Subjects	Mean Age	Baseline CAVI	Duration of Follow-up	CV Outcomes	Incidence (%) (1000 person-years)	Prognostic Value	Cut-off Value	NRI
Sato et al. 2016[1]	Japan	1,003 subjects with CV risk factor	62.5	9.25	6.7 years	Myocardial infarction and stable/unstable angina pectoris.	13.4	CAVI was independently associated with future CV event risk (HR 1.126 per 1 unit increase).	**Not described**	Not described
Satoh-Asahara et al. 2015[2]	Japan	425 obese patients	51.5	7.6	5 years	Angina pectoris, myocardial infarction, stroke and arteriosclerosis obliterans.	15.8	CAVI was a significant predictor of CV events (HR 1.44 per 1 unit increase).	**Not described**	0.164 (p=0.066)
Kubota et al. 2011[3]	Japan	400 patients with metabolic disorders or past history of CAD	63.2-73.9	Not described	27.2 months	Coronary artery disease, stroke and death	54.0	Hazard ratio of CVD was significantly higher in CAVI ≥ 10.0 group (HR 2.25).	**9.0**	Not described

CAVI, cardio-ankle vascular index; CV, cardiovascular; CAD, coronary artery disease; CVD, cardiovascular disease; NRI, net reclassification improvement; HR, hazard ratio; SD, standard deviation.

Center of Diabetes, Endocrine and Metabolism, Toho University Sakura Medical Center, 564-1, Shimoshizu, Sakura-City, Chiba, 285-8741, Japan.

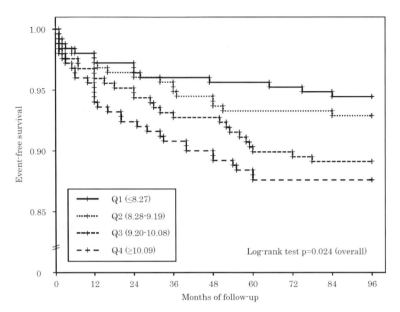

Fig. 1. Kaplan-Meier survival curves showing cardiovascular events according to quartiles of CAVI.
All subjects were stratified into quartiles by baseline CAVI (ref 1).

Table 2. Cox proportional hazards regression analysis of the association between future cardiovascular events and clinical variables (ref 1).

Variables	Hazard ratio	95% confidence interval	p value
CAVI (every 1.0 index)	1.126	1.006-1.259	0.039
Sex (male; 1, female; 0)	2.276	1.383-3.748	0.001
Elderly (Age ≧ 65; 1, <65; 0)	1.203	0.759-1.905	0.432
Obesity (BMI ≧ 25; 1, <25; 0)	0.778	0.483-1.252	0.301
Smoking (+; 1, −; 0)	1.846	1.184-2.879	0.007
Diabetes mellitus (+; 1, −; 0)	1.702	1.086-2.667	0.020
Hypertension (+; 1, −; 0)	1.682	1.073-2.636	0.023
Dyslipidemia (+; 1, −; 0)	1.376	0.875-2.165	0.167

Abbreviations are as in Table 1.

Future CV events increased with the CAVI quartile (Fig. 1). In Cox proportional hazards regression analysis, the factors independently associated with higher risk of future cardiovascular events were every 1.0 increment of CAVI, male gender, smoking, diabetes mellitus, and hypertension (Table 2).

This is currently the only primary prevention study investigating the prognostic value of CAVI in >1,000 Japanese patients. This study strongly suggests that CAVI was a predictor of future CV events, independent of traditional coronary risk factors in individuals with metabolic disorders.

Japan Obesity and Metabolic Syndrome Study (JOMS), a primary prevention study (Satoh-Asahara, et al.)[2]

It remains unclear whether CAVI can predict CVD outcomes in obese patients. Satoh-Asahara et al. reported on the Japan Obesity and Metabolic Syndrome Study (JOMS), a multicenter prospective cohort study investigating the occurrence of macrovascular complications in 425 obese Japanese outpatients followed over a 5-year period[2]. Obese subjects with a body mass index (BMI) ≥ 25 kg/m² were

recruited. The exclusion criteria were a previous history of CHD, stroke, other vascular diseases, apparent renal disease, and severe liver dysfunction. Primary outcomes of the study were the occurrence of macrovascular complication events, including the occurrence of definite coronary heart disease (CHD) (angina pectoris or myocardial infarction), stroke or arteriosclerosis obliterans. All events occurred in 28 patients, and the CVD incidence rate was 15.8 per 1000 person-years. In the analysis of adjusted models for traditional risk factors, CAVI was a significant factor for the incidence of events. In addition, high CAVI and low HDL-cholesterol were significant factors for the incidence of events in Cox stepwise multivariate analysis age- and sex-adjusted (Table 3). Interestingly, in comparison to the single model of atherosclerotic cardiovascular disease (ASCVD) score, inclusion of CAVI in the model yielded a better net reclassification improvement (NRI) of 0.164 (p = 0.066) and integrated discrimination improvement (IDI) of 0.020 (p = 0.047) in the Cox model. These results indicate that CAVI added value to the atherosclerotic CV disease risk score for predicting CVD development.

This study demonstrates for the first time that CAVI is an effective predictor of CVD events in obese patients.

Table 3. Risk factors for cardiovascular events analyzed by multivariate Cox proportional hazard models in total subjects (JOMS) (ref 2).
【with permission of Elsevier】

	HR	95% CI	p-value
Multivariate model 1:			
Male (vs. female)	1.20	0.57, 2.54	0.634
Age (per 10 years)	1.27	0.83, 1.93	0.273
CAVI (per 1)	1.49	1.04, 2.12	0.028
Multivariate model 2:			
Male (vs. female)	1.10	0.51, 2.36	0.811
Age (per 10 years)	1.03	0.99, 1.08	0.152
BMI (per 1 kg/m^2)	1.03	0.95, 1.12	0.531
Current smoking (vs. no)	2.04	0.78, 5.34	0.148
CAVI (per 1)	1.50	1.06, 2.13	0.022
Multivariate model 3:			
Male (vs. female)	1.10	0.51, 2.38	0.812
Age (per 10 years)	1.03	0.99, 1.08	0.156
BMI (per 1 kg/m^2)	1.03	0.94, 1.12	0.562
Current smoking (vs. no)	2.04	0.77, 5.46	0.154
HT (vs. non-HT)	1.12	0.44, 2.80	0.822
DL (vs. non-DL)	1.07	0.42, 2.76	0.883
DM (vs. non-DM)	0.96	0.44, 2.10	0.915
CAVI (per 1)	1.49	1.04, 2.13	0.029

Multivariate Cox proportional hazard models: model 1, age- and gender-adjusted analysis; model 2: age-, gender-, BMI-, and current smoking-adjusted analysis; model 3: age-, gender-, BMI-, current smoking-, and presence of HT-, DL-, and DM-adjusted analysis. BMI, body mass index; CAVI, cardio-ankle vascular index; HR, hazard ratio; 95% CI, 95% confidence interval; HT, hypertension; DL, dyslipidemia; DM, diabetes.

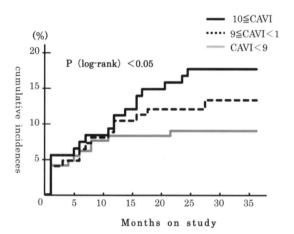

Fig. 2. Cumulative incidence of coronary artery diseases and strokes (ref 3 〔with permission of Elsevier〕).

A primary prevention study of 400 patients with metabolic disorders (Kubota, et al.)[3]

This was the first prospective study examining the association between CAVI and CVD, and demonstrated that a higher CAVI value is predictive of CVD incidence[3]. Participants with a past history of myocardial infarction, stroke, percutaneous coronary intervention for angina, or coronary artery bypass grafting for ischemic heart disease and subjects with an ABI <0.9 were excluded. CV events were defined as coronary artery disease, stroke, and death. The 400 patients were classified into 3 groups according to the CAVI score. The group with CAVI >10 showed a high incidence of CVD and stroke in 3 years (Fig. 2). A multivariate analysis showed that a significantly higher hazard ratio of CVD in this group (hazard ratio, 2.2).

Conclusions

The results of these four prospective trials in Japanese patients with metabolic disorder support that CAVI may be a significant predictor of CVD, at least for primary prevention. Currently, there are two ongoing large multicenter longitudinal studies in Japan, CAVI-J and Coupling Registry, including 3000-5000 high-risk patients[4, 5].

Future Perspective

Prospective studies are required to determine whether changes in CAVI following therapeutic interventions for metabolic disorders contribute to future CV events.

References

1) Sato Y, Nagayama D, Saiki A, et al. Cardio-ankle vascular index is independently associated with future cardiovascular events in outpatients with metabolic disorders. *J Atheroscler Thromb* 2016; **23**: 596-605. https://doi.org/10.5551/jat.31385

2) Satoh-Asahara N, Kotani K, Yamakage H, et al. Japan Obesity and Metabolic Syndrome Study (JOMS) Group: Cardio-ankle vascular index predicts for the incidence of cardiovascular events in obese patients: A multicenter prospective cohort study (Japan Obesity and Metabolic Syndrome Study: JOMS). *Atherosclerosis* 2015; **242**: 461-468. https://doi.org/10.1016/j.atherosclerosis.2015.08.003

3) Kubota Y, Maebuchim D, Takei M, et al. Cardio-Ankle Vascular Index is a predictor of cardiovascular events. Artery Res 2011; 5: 91-96. https://doi.org/10.1016/j.artres.2011.03.005

4) Miyoshi T, Ito H, Horinaka S, et al. Protocol for evaluating the cardio-ankle vascular index to predict cardiovascular events in Japan: a prospective multicenter cohort study. *Pulse* 2017; **4**(Suppl 1): 11-16.

5) Kabutoya T, Kario K. Comparative assessment of cutoffs for the cardio-ankle vascular index and brachial-ankle pulse wave velocity in a nationwide registry – a cardiovascular prognostic coupling study –. *Pulse* 2018; **6**: 131-136.

Prospective Study on CAVI - 2 - Patients with heart diseases and chronic kidney diseases

Noriaki Iwahashi

Arterial stiffness (AS) is often assessed not only in clinical research but also in medicine, because it is considered to be a good marker for the diagnosis and the prognosis of cardiovascular diseases[1, 2]. Increased AS is commonly observed in patients having atherosclerosis, hypertension, diabetes, and hyperlipidemia[3, 4]. AS measured by aortic pulse wave velocity is an independent predictor of coronary heart disease and stroke in apparently healthy subjects in the Rotterdam study[2]. AS has been shown to have an independent prognostic effect on cardiovascular disease. Although AS is used as a surrogate endpoint in many studies, and its use not so widespread in clinical practice. One of the main reasons is the need of standardized settings during measurements, and the dependency on blood pressure at the time of measurement[5]. Methodological differences make it difficult to compare populations and obtain common reference values by which individual measurements can be matched.

Cardio Ankle Vascular Index (CAVI) is a method by which AS can be evaluated and is independent of blood pressure at the time of measurement[5]. It is easy to measure and the reproducibility excellent. As expected, CAVI increases with age and reference values are higher in men. Studies have shown that CAVI is significantly related to coronary artery disease and other parameters associated with atherosclerosis. CAVI could be used in clinical practice as a new independent risk factor for outcomes.

Therefore, there are many reports about the usefulness of CAVI for prognosis prediction.

1. Primary prevention

Laucevičius et al. studied 2,106 patients with metabolic syndrome and demonstrated that higher CAVI (≥ 7.95) identified high risk patients for future cardiovascular events[6]. In this study, data on fatal and non-fatal cardiovascular events (myocardial infarction, stroke or transient ischemic attack, and sudden cardiac death) were obtained after a follow-up period >3 years.

Hitsumoto reported that a high CAVI (CAVI $=9.7$) is a predictor of primary cardiovascular events in patients with chronic kidney disease (CKD)[7]. He followed 460 outpatients with CKD for 60.1 months. The endpoint was a major adverse cardiovascular event (MACE), a composite of cardiovascular death, nonfatal myocardial infarction, nonfatal ischemic stroke and hospital admission for heart failure.

Otsuka et al. reported the serial change of CAVI in 211 patients with CHD[8]. After the second CAVI test, all 211 patients were followed for >1 year or until the occurrence of one of the following CVD events: cardiac death, non-fatal myocardial infarction, unstable angina pectoris, recurrent angina pectoris requiring coronary revascularization, or stroke. They showed that in their population, initial CAVI values were not predictive of event occurrence in univariate analysis, but a persistent impairment of CAVI was associated with future CVD events.

Below we summarize CAVI's clinical usefulness in patients with specific cardiovascular diseases.

2. HF: heart failure

Sano et al. reported its usefulness for patients with acute decompensated HF (ADHF) in clinical scenario (CS1)[9]. They analyzed the CAVI of 113 patients with CS1. TE composite end-point (cardiac death and HF rehospitalization) occurred in 25 patients during 1 year after discharge. CAVI was a stronger predictor for the composite end-point than age, liver function, anemia and left ventricular function by multivariate analysis. They analyzed receiver operating characteristic (ROC) curves to predict composite end-point.

The cut-off point was 8.65 (area under the curve 0.724, 95% confidence interval 0.614 – 0.834), and it was concluded that CAVI may be a surrogate marker for ADHF treatment.

Sato et al. explored the role of CAVI in patients with HF[10]. A total of 557 patients hospitalized because of ADHF underwent CAVI and were followed for a median 1415 days. Patients were divided to two groups by a CAVI cut-off value of 9.64. During the follow up period, 25 patients experienced stroke (18 ischemic and 7 hemorrhagic). High CAVI (≥ 9.64) was therefore an independent predictor for stroke.

3. ACS: acute coronary syndrome

Gohbara et al. explored the clinical usefulness of CAVI in patients with acute coronary syndrome[11]. They enrolled 288 patients and examined CAVI and baPWV at a stable

Cardiovascular Center, Public University Corporation Yokohama City University Medical Center, 4-57 Urafune-cho, Minami-ku, Yokohama, Kanagawa 232-0024 Japan.

Table 1.   All cut-off values for prediction of the adverse events.

Author	Subjects	Follow up	End point	cut off value of CAVI	reference
Laucevičius et al	2,106 patients with Mets	3.8 years	CV events	7.95	6
Hitsumoto	460 CKD	60.1 monts	MACE	9.7	7
Otsuka et al	211 CHD	>1 year	CVD events	NA	8
Sano et al	113 ADHF (CS1)	1 year	composite end point	8.65	9
Sato et al	557 ADHF	1,415 days	stroke	9.64	10
Gohbara et al	288 ACS	15 monts	CVD events	8.325	11
Kirigaya et al	387 ACS	5 years	CVD events	8.35	12

CHD: coronary heart disease, CV: cardiovascular, CKD: chronic kidney disease, ACS: acute coronary syndrome

phase and followed up for 15 months. The primary end point was cardiovascular death, non-fatal MI, and ischemic stroke. Nineteen patients experienced events. ROC curve analyses revealed that CAVI was stronger than baPWV in terms of predicting non-fatal stroke. Multivariate analysis demonstrated that CAVI was the strongest predictor. The CAVI cut-off value to predict the primary end point was 8.325. Their study revealed the superiority of CAVI to baPWV by DeLong's method.

Kirigaya et al. reported on 387 patients with ACS. They followed the patients for 62 months[12]. The primary end point was the occurrence of major adverse cardiovascular events (MACE: ACS, HF, CV death and stroke). They determined the CAVI cut-off point as 8.35, with high CAVI being an independent long-term predictor of MACE. Furthermore, they demonstrated that CAVI can improve risk stratification based on the Grace risk score.

Accordingly, we conclude that CAVI can have prognostic value not only for outpatients but also for hospitalized patients. However, the cut-off values were different between the populations (Table 1). Despite the many reports on the medical treatment of CAVI[13, 14], there is still no definite treatment for CAVI.

Furthermore, it is not clear if an intervention for CAVI is effective for the prevention of adverse events or not, except for the paper by Otsuka et al.[8]. Therefore, further studies are needed to confirm the usefulness of CAVI. We think the CAVI cut-off value for the incidence of cardiovascular events should be determined by large prospective cohort studies[15].

References

1) O'Rourke MF, Staessen JA, Vlachopoulos C, et al. Clinical applications of arterial stiffness; definitions and reference values. *Am J Hypertens* 2002; **15**: 426-44.
2) Mattace-Raso FU, van der Cammen TJ, Hofman A, et al. Arterial stiffness and risk of coronary heart disease and stroke: the Rotterdam Study. *Circulation* 2006; **113**: 657-63.
3) ter Avest E, Holewijn S, Bredie SJ, et al. Pulse wave velocity in familial combined hyperlipidemia. *Am J Hypertens* 2007; **20**: 263-9.
4) Benetos A, Waeber B, Izzo J, et al. Influence of age, risk factors, and cardiovascular and renal disease on arterial stiffness: clinical applications. *Am J Hypertens* 2002; **15**: 1101-8.
5) Shirai K, Utino J, Otsuka K, Takata M. A novel blood pressure-independent arterial wall stiffness parameter: cardio-ankle vascular index (CAVI). *J Atheroscler Thromb* 2006; **13**: 101-7.
6) Laucevičius A, Ryliškytė L, Balsytė J, et al. Association of cardio-ankle vascular index with cardiovascular risk factors and cardiovascular events in metabolic syndrome patients. *Medicina* (Kaunas, Lithuania). 2015; **51**: 152-8.
7) Hitsumoto T. Clinical Usefulness of the Cardio-Ankle Vascular Index as a Predictor of Primary Cardiovascular Events in Patients With Chronic Kidney Disease. *J Clin Med Res* 2018; **10**: 883-90.
8) Otsuka K, Fukuda S, Shimada K, et al. Serial assessment of arterial stiffness by cardio-ankle vascular index for prediction of future cardiovascular events in patients with coronary artery disease. Hypertens *Res* 2014; **37**: 1014-20.
9) Sano T, Kiuchi S, Hisatake S, et al. Cardio-ankle vascular index predicts the 1-year prognosis of heart failure patients categorized in clinical scenario 1. *Heart Vessels* 2020; **35**: 1537-44.
10) Sato Y, Yoshihisa A, Ichijo Y, et al. Cardio-Ankle Vascular Index Predicts Post-Discharge Stroke in Patients with Heart Failure. *J Atheroscler Thromb* 2021; **28**: 766-775.
11) Gohbara M, Iwahashi N, Sano Y, et al. Clinical Impact of the Cardio-Ankle Vascular Index for Predicting Cardiovascular Events After Acute Coronary Syndrome. *Circulation* 2016; **80**: 1420-6.
12) Kirigaya J, Iwahashi N, Tahakashi H, et al. Impact of Cardio-Ankle Vascular Index on Long-Term Outcome in Patients with Acute Coronary Syndrome. *J Atheroscler Thromb* 2020; **27**: 657-68.
13) Watanabe Y, Takasugi E, Shitakura K, et al. Administration of an angiotensin-converting enzyme inhibitor improves vascular function and urinary albumin excretion in low-risk essential hypertensive patients receiving anti-hypertensive treatment with calcium channel blockers. Organ-protecting effects independent of anti-hypertensive effect. *Clin Exp Hypertens* 2011; **33**: 246-54.
14) Ishimitsu T, Numabe A, Masuda T, et al. Angiotensin-II receptor antagonist combined with calcium channel blocker or diuretic for essential hypertension. *Hypertens Res* 2009; **32**: 962-8.
15) Miyoshi T, Ito H, Horinaka S, et al. Protocol for Evaluating the Cardio-Ankle Vascular Index to Predict Cardiovascular Events in Japan: A Prospective Multicenter Cohort Study. *Pulse* 2017; **4**(Suppl 1): 11-6.

Prospective Study on CAVI - 3 - Multicenter trial in Japan: CAVI-J

Toru Miyoshi

Purpose and Background

A prospective multicenter study was conducted to evaluate the usefulness of the cardio-ankle vascular index

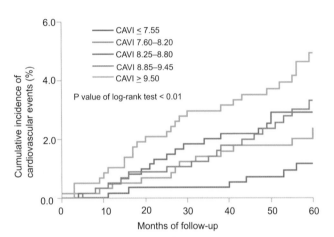

Fig. 1. Kaplan–Meyer plot of cumulative probability of cardiovascular events by quintiles of the cardio-ankle vascular index (CAVI).

The time to cardiovascular events, including cardiovascular death, nonfatal stroke, and nonfatal myocardial infarction, is shown according to baseline CAVI.

(CAVI) in Japan (CAVI-J), in terms of its utility as a predictor of cardiovascular (CV) events in patients with cardiovascular risks[1]. The study included individuals aged between 40 and 74 years with at least one of the following risk factors for CV disease: type 2 diabetes mellitus, hypertension at high-risk for cardiovascular events, metabolic syndrome, stage 3 chronic kidney disease, or a history of coronary artery disease or cerebral infarction. In total, 3,026 patients were enrolled from 48 sites between May 2013 and December 2014. The participants were followed up prospectively for 5 years from the date of the CAVI measurement. The primary outcome was a composite of CV events, including CV-related death, myocardial infarction, and stroke.

Results

The final analysis included 2,938 patients (2,001 males and 927 females; mean age, 63 years) with a median follow-up period of 4.9 years[2]. This study included 1,114 (38%) patients with a history of coronary artery disease or cerebral infarction. During the follow-up period, 82 patients experienced primary outcomes including 13 CV deaths, 44 non-fatal strokes, and 25 non-fatal myocardial infarctions. The cumulative incidence rates of the primary outcomes are

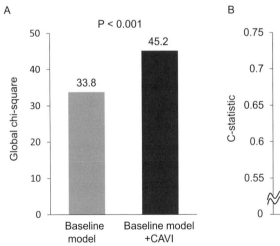

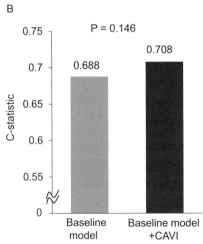

Fig. 2. Estimation of the risk assessment ability for cardiovascular events.

(A). Global chi-square and (B). C-statistic. The baseline model includes age, male sex, systolic blood pressure, type 2 diabetes mellitus, HDL-cholesterol, smoking, history of coronary artery disease or cerebral infarction, and the use of anti-hypertensive agents.

Department of Cardiovascular Medicine, Okayama University Graduate School of Medicine, Dentistry and Pharmaceutical Sciences, 2-5-1, Shikata-cho, Kita-ku, Okayama-shi, Okayama 700-8558, Japan.

shown according to the CAVI levels in Fig. 1. The rates were significantly higher in patients with a CAVI ≥ 9.50 than in patients with a CAVI ≤ 7.55 (*P* value for trend = 0.01). Every 1-point increment in the CAVI was associated with an increased risk of the primary outcomes, after adjusting for confounding factors (hazard ratio, 1.38 [95% confidence interval, 1.16–1.65]).

This study also determined the incremental value of the CAVI for predicting CV events (Fig. 2). The addition of the CAVI to a baseline model that included traditional risk factors significantly increased the global chi-square value from 33.8 to 45.2. The C-statistic was essentially unchanged (0.688–0.708, P = 0.146). The addition of the CAVI yielded a category-free net reclassification index of 0.254 (P = 0.024).

Conclusion

CAVI-J demonstrated that higher CAVI in patients with

CV risk factors indicated an elevated risk of CV events. Furthermore, adding the CAVI to a model of clinical risk factors improved the model's ability to predict the risk of CV events. These data suggest that the CAVI is clinically useful for the assessment of the risk of CV events among patients with CV risk factors.

References

1) Miyoshi T, Ito H, Horinaka S, Shirai K, Higaki J and Orimo H, Protocol for Evaluating the Cardio-Ankle Vascular Index to Predict Cardiovascular Events in Japan: A Prospective Multicenter Cohort Study, *Pulse (Basel)*, **2017**;4:11-16.
2) Miyoshi T, Prognostic Value of Cardio-ankle Vascular Index as a Marker of Arterial Stiffness for Cardiovascular Events: the CAVI-J Study, The 85th Annual Scientific Meeting of the Japanese Circulation Society. Late Breaking Cohort Studies 2, 2021 March 28.

PART 6

The Cardiac-Vascular relationship assessed with CAVI

Overview
CAVI as an index of vascular function coordinating with cardiac function

Kazuhiro Shimizu[1], Shuji Sato[1], Akihiro Ogawa[2], Masahiro Ohira[1] and Kohji Shirai[3,4]

Introduction

The systemic circulation consists of beating of the heart, transporting the blood to peripheral organs by vessels, and returning the blood to the heart. The analysis of cardiac function has already been established in various ways, and heart failure has already been classified according to the cardiac function such as ejection fraction or E/e'. On the other hand, vascular function had rarely been analyzed. This is because there were no adequate indices to reflect vascular function.

The artery dilates the caliber to receive the blood delivered by the left ventricle during systolic phase, and during left ventricular diastolic phase, the caliber contracts to send the blood to the periphery efficiently using this elasticity. This function has also been referred to as the "Windkessel function" or "diastolic pump". Furthermore, contraction of left ventricle receives reverse force from the arterial tree at each beat. The elasticity or stiffness of the artery is also involved in this reverse force as "afterload". Therefore, cardiac-Vascular relationship can easily be imagined. Pulse wave velocity (PWV) had been used as an index of arterial stiffness, but PWV is intrinsically dependent on blood pressure (BP) at the measuring time[1-3]. Therefore, PWV is inappropriate to evaluate the role of arterial stiffness as a vascular function. The cardio-ankle vascular index (CAVI) was developed as an indicator of arterial stiffness from the origin of the aorta to the ankle[4]. The feature of CAVI is its independency from blood pressure at the time of measurement[5, 6]. As a marker of vascular function, CAVI could be expected to play some role in assessing the arterial stiffness as vascular function, and the new field of "Cardiac-Vascular Interaction" might be developed.

In this chapter, we overview about CAVI as a possible index reflecting vascular function, which coordinates with cardiac functions.

1. Left ventricular function and CAVI

An increasing number of studies have referred to the interaction between heart diseases and CAVI. Zang and Ohira reported that CAVI decreased relating with increased left ventricle ejection fraction (LVEF), and decreased cardio-thoracic ratio and brain natriuretic peptide after the treatment of heart failure patients and suggested that CAVI might partially reflect the afterload[7]. Schillaci and Pucci reported that a high CAVI is associated with an inappropriately high left ventricular mass and low midwall systolic function. As a marker of the arterial diastolic-to-systolic stiffening, CAVI may have a relationship with the left ventricular structure and function that is independent of BP levels[3]. Namba reported that CAVI was significantly associated with E/e' in heart failure patients, and suggested that arterial stiffness contributed to the development of LV diastolic dysfunction[8].

As for the relationship between various left ventricular geometric patterns and CAVI, we studied about age-matched 1046 people with metabolic disorders[9].

The geometries were divided into four patterns: normal geometry, concentric remodeling (CR), concentric hypertrophy (CH) and eccentric hypertrophy (EH). As shown in Chap. 31-3, BP and CAVI were higher in the order of NG, CR and CH, but was not high in EH. EF was decreased slightly in CH and the lowest in EH. These results suggested that CR and CH could be influenced by CAVI as an afterload.

These reports strongly suggested that CAVI could be useful index to evaluate an interaction between left ventricle and arterial stiffness of the arterial tree from the origin of the aorta to the ankle.

2. Left atrial remodeling and CAVI

Osawa reported that the left atrial volume was significantly associated with high CAVI in young adults[10]. In addition, Nakamura reported that CAVI and plasma levels of N-terminal B-type natriuretic peptide were independent determinants of left atrial volume and right atrial volume in patients with atrial fibrillation[11]. They suggested that high CAVI resulted in elevated left ventricular filling pressure and could promote atrial remodeling.

[1]Department of Internal Medicine, Toho University Sakura Medical Center, 564-1 Shimoshizu, Sakura City, Chiba 285-8741, Japan.
[2]Department of Rehabilitation, Sakura Medical Center, Toho University, 564-1 Shimoshizu, Sakura City, Chiba 285-8741, Japan.
[3]Emeritus professor, Medical School, Toho university.
[4]Director, Seijinkai Mihama Hospital, 1-1-5 Utase, Mihama-ku, Chiba-shi, Chiba 261-0013, Japan.

These results suggested that CAVI could be also useful index to evaluate an interaction between left atrium and arterial stiffness of the arterial tree from the origin of the aorta to the ankle.

3. Right ventricular function and CAVI

Recently, Radchenko, et al reported that the age-adjusted patients with idiopathic pulmonary arterial hypertension (IPAH) had significantly higher CAVI than the healthy persons. CAVI correlated negatively with tricuspid annular plane systolic excursion (TAPSE) in IPAH patients. TAPSE falls with increasing severity of PAH. Moreover, they suggested that abnormal CAVI, but not PWV, could be a new independent predictor of death in the IPAH population and be used for better risk stratification in this patient population[12, 13].

Chronic thromboembolic pulmonary hypertension (CTEPH) is an intractable disease caused by organized thrombi in pulmonary artery and its prognosis is extremely poor without treatment. Sato, et al reported a case of CTEPH patient who showed increased CAVI and severe right and left ventricle dysfunctions. After riociguat administration and performing balloon pulmonary angioplasty (BPA), sigh and symptom improved associating with a decrease in CAVI[14]. Riociguat has a strong vasodilating effect.

Riociguat may work not only on the pulmonary circulation, but also systemic circulation. These results suggested that riociguat dilates both systemic peripheral arteries and the pulmonary artery and reduces the afterload on both the left and right ventricles. Additionally, BPA might not only improve the pulmonary circulation, but also improve the CAVI. The precise mechanism for this effect was not clear yet; however, the sympathetic nerve stress in CTEPH might be relieved by improving the pulmonary circulation.

In summary, the patients with pulmonary hypertension showed a high CAVI, indicating that arterial stiffness of the systemic artery increased in addition to the pulmonary artery, which may deteriorate both the right and left ventricular functions as an afterload.

4. Cardiac rehabilitation and CAVI

The increased number of patients with heart failure has become a social problem recently. Exercise tolerance is not only maintained by heart muscle, but also by vascular function and skeletal muscle functions[15]. Therefore, advanced medical therapies tried to improve not only the heart muscle itself, but also the vascular function. Then, cardiac rehabilitation became important more and more for heart failure patients. Petr Dobšák reported the exercise training or neuromuscular electrical stimulation improved CAVI significantly and also stabilized autonomic balance[16]. Ogawa and Shimizu reported that six-minute walk distance was an independent determinant factor of CAVI in elderly heart failure patients, and CAVI was higher in patients with sarcopenia than in those without sarcopenia[15]. Moreover, Watanabe reported that high CAVI (≥ 8.9) is independently associated with impaired exercise capacity and a high

cardiac event rate in heart failure patients[17].

To manage more efficient rehabilitation for patients with chronic heart failure, the exercise menu had better to adopt the plan to improve vascular functions by monitoring CAVI.

5. Leanings from continuous monitoring of CAVI -Artery is always remodeling, coordinating with cardiac function-

The continuous measurement of CAVI is useful for understanding the arterial pathophysiological response to various conditions in each case. Here, we showed three cases whose "Cardiac-Vascular Interaction" was observed during continuous monitoring of CAVI.

\<Case 1\>

A patient aged 71 years who suffered from diabetes mellitus and obstructive sleep apnea (OSA), was followed up for 8 years by measuring CAVI from age 63 (Fig. 1). He underwent coronary artery bypass grafting at age 63 years old. Just before the operation, CAVI was 11.8 on the right and 11.5 on the left. Three years later, he was found to have

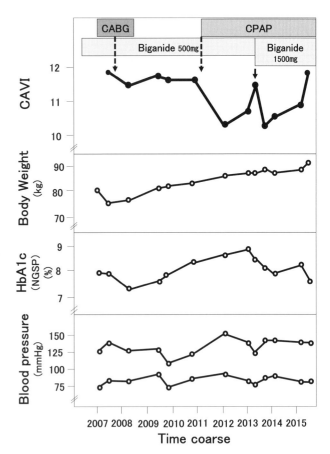

Fig. 1. Arterial stiffness, as monitored by cardio-ankle vascular index, is affected by obstructive sleep apnea, blood glucose control, and body weight -a case with 8 years follow up. International Medical Case Reports Journal 2016:9 231-235; Originally published by and used with permission from Dove Medical Press Ltd[18]

Abbreviations: CAVI: cardio ankle vascular index; CABG: coronary artery bypass grafting; CPAP: continuous positive airway pressure.

OSA and received treatment of continuous positive airway pressure (CPAP). CAVI decreased after CPAP (age 68; right 10.4, left 10.2). However, body weight gradually increased. His diabetes was difficult to control, and the CAVI increased. Subsequently, the CAVI decreased once with biguanide treatment, but increased again with an increase in the body weight. In conclusion, CAVI responded to the patient's conditions, such as obesity, diabetes mellitus, and OSA[18].

<Case 2>

A 42-year-old hypertensive woman visited our hospital complaining of shortness of breath. Her left ventricular mass index (LVMI) was observed to be increased, and CAVI was high. By treating for hypertension (HT), diabetes mellitus, and OSA, her left ventricular CH was improved, accompanied with a decrease in the CAVI (Fig. 2). These observations suggested that the arterial stiffness monitored with CAVI changed according to the change in cardiac remodeling[19].

< Case 3 >

A 65-year-old man suffered from dyspnea on exertion, and he was diagnosed as chronic thromboembolic

pulmonary hypertension (CTEPH). The mean pulmonary artery pressure (mPAP) was 51 mmHg, and the initial CAVI was 10.0, which is high for patient's age. In addition to right ventricular dysfunction, left ventricular dysfunction was observed as reduced global longitudinal strain (GLS-LV). As shown in Fig. 4, after riociguat administration, CAVI decreased to 9.1 and GLS-LV improved from −10.3% to −17.3%, although pulmonary hypertension did not completely resolve (mPAP 41 mmHg). Subsequently, five series of BPA sessions were performed. Six months after the final balloon angioplasty (BPA), mPAP decreased to 19 mmHg and GLS-LV improved to 19.3%. The patient became symptom free and his 6-minute walk distance improved from 322 m to 510 m. CAVI markedly decreased to 5.8, which is extremely low for his age[14].

In summary, clinical observations showed that arterial stiffness monitored with CAVI changed according to cardiac function and the systemic circulation composed of various arteries and veins (Fig. 3).

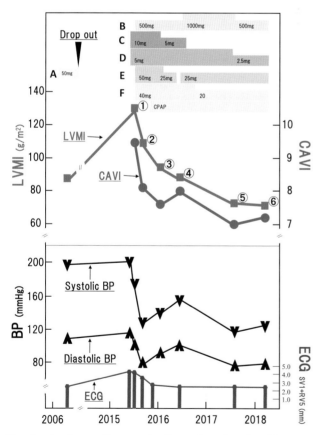

Fig. 2. A Case Demonstrating the Cardiac-Vascular Interaction by a New Cardio-Ankle Vascular Index During the Treatment of Concentric Hypertrophy. Cited from ref.19

Abbreviations: BP: blood pressure; LVMI: left ventricular mass index; CAVI: cardio ankle vascular index; ECG: Electrocardiogram. A: losartan; B: metformin; C: amlodipine; D: bisoprolol; E: spironolactone; F: telmisartan.

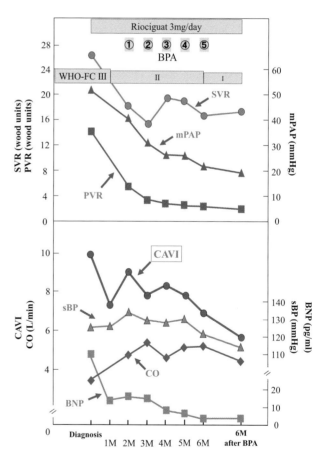

Fig. 3. Increased Arterial Stiffness in Chronic Thromboembolic Pulmonary Hypertension was improved with Riociguat and 5 times of Balloon Pulmonary Angioplasty. International Medical Case Reports Journal 2021:14 191-197; Originally published by and used with permission from Dove Medical Press Ltd[14]

Abbreviations: CAVI: cardio ankle vascular index; CO: cardiac output; SVR: systemic vascular resistance; PVR: pulmonary vascular resistance; mPAP: mean pulmonary artery pressure; sBP: systolic blood pressure; BNP: brain natriuretic peptide; BPA; balloon pulmonary angioplasty: WHO-FC; the world health organisation functional class.

Cardio-Vascular Interaction

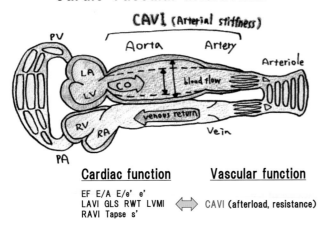

Fig. 4. Cardiac-Vascular Interaction. Systemic circulation is conducted with right ventricle, left ventricle and all vessels composing of the aorta, muscular artery, arteriole, and vein. Each artery has own function. CAVI reflects vascular function of the aorta and muscle artery, and co-ordinates with not only left ventricle, but also arteriole and right ventricle in various physio-pathological conditions.

Abbreviations: CAVI: cardio ankle vascular index; EF: ejection fraction; E/A: peak early diastolic filling velocity (E-wave)/peak atrial filling velocity (A-wave); E/e': peak early diastolic filling velocity (E-wave)/spectral Doppler tissue velocities of the septal mitral annulus (e'); LAVI; left atria volume index; GLS: global longitudinal strain. RWT: Relative wall thickness; LVMI: left ventricular mass index; RAVI: Right atria volume index; Tapse: Ticuspid annular plane systolic excursion. S': systolic wall motion velocity.

Conclusion

The arterial stiffness of the arterial tree monitored with CAVI represents the vascular function, which coordinates with left, and right ventricles and also atriums as illustrated in Fig. 4. Furthermore, the arteries composed of the aorta (elastic artery), muscular artery, arteriole and micro-vessels, may coordinate each other to maintain proper systemic circulation. Monitoring the CAVI in various pathophysiological conditions would be useful to understand the cross-talk of the whole circulation system and to seek better therapeutics for heart failure and vascular failure.

References

1) Cecelja M, Chowienczyk P. Dissociation of aortic pulse wave velocity with risk factors for cardiovascular disease other than hypertension: a systematic review. Hypertension. 2009; 54: 1328–1336.

2) Schillaci G, Pucci G, Pirro M, Settimi L, Hijazi R, Franklin SS, Mannarino E. Combined effects of office and 24-hour blood pressure on aortic stiffness in human hypertension. J Hypertens. 2011; 9: 869–875.

3) Schillaci G, Battista F, Settimi L, Anastasio F, Pucci G. Cardio-ankle vascular index and subclinical heart disease. Hypertens Res. 2015; 38: 68–73.

4) Shirai K, Utino J, Otsuka K, Takata M. A noble blood pressure-independent arterial wall stiffness parameter; cardio-ankle vascular index (CAVI). J Atheroscler Thromb. 2006; 13:101-107.

5) Shirai K, Song M, Suzuki J, Kurosu T, Oyama T, Nagayama D, et al. Contradictory effects of β1-and α1-adrenergic receptor blockers on cardio-ankle vascular stiffness index (CAVI)–CAVI is independent of blood pressure. J Atheroscler Thromb. 2011; 18: 49-55.

6) Takahashi M, Shiba T, Hirano K, Hitsumoto T, Shirai K. Acute decrease of cardio-ankle vascular index with the administration of beraprost sodium. J Atheroscler Thromb. 2012; 19: 479-484.

7) Zhang C, Ohira M, Iizuka T, Mikamo H, Nakagami T, Suzuki M, Hirano K, et al. Cardio-ankle vascular index relates to left ventricular ejection fraction in patients with heart failure. A retrospective study. Int Heart J. 2013; 54:216-221.

8) Namba T, Masaki N, Matsuo Y, Sato A, Kimura T, Horii S, et al. Arterial stiffness is significantly associated with left ventricular diastolic dysfunction in patients with cardiovascular disease. Int Heart J. 2016; 57: 729-735.

9) Shimizu K, Tabata T, Sasaki T, et al. The Relationship Between Various Left Ventricular Geometries and the Cardio Ankle Vascular Index. Journal of Cardiology and Vascular Medicine. 2020; 8: 1-11.

10) Osawa K, Nakanishi R, Miyoshi T, et al. Correlation of Arterial Stiffness With Left Atrial Volume Index and Left Ventricular Mass Index in Young Adults: Evaluation by Coronary Computed Tomography Angiography. Heart Lung Circ. 2019;28:932-938.

11) Nakamura K, Takagi T, Kogame N, et al. The Association of Cardio-Ankle Vascular Index (CAVI) with Biatrial Remodeling in Atrial Fibrillation. J Atheroscler Thromb. 2020 Aug 29. doi: 10.5551/jat.57737. Online ahead of print.

12) Radchenko GD, Zhyvylo IO, Titov EY, Sirenko YM. Systemic Arterial Stiffness in New Diagnosed Idiopathic Pulmonary Arterial Hypertension Patients. Vascular Health and Risk Management 2020;16:29–39.

13) Radchenko GD and Sirenko YM. Prognostic Significance of Systemic Arterial Stiffness Evaluated by Cardio-Ankle Vascular Index in Patients with Idiopathic Pulmonary Hypertension. Vascular Health and Risk Management 2021;17:77–93.

14) Sato S, Shimizu K, Ito T, et al. Increased Arterial Stiffness in Chronic Thromboembolic Pulmonary Hypertension Was Improved with Riociguat and Balloon Pulmonary Angioplasty: A Case Report. International Medical Case Reports Journal 2021;14:191–197.

15) Ogawa A, Shimizu K, Nakagami T, et al. Physical Function and Cardio-Ankle Vascular Index in Elderly Heart Failure Patients. Int Heart J 2020; 61: 769-775.

16) Dobšák P, Tomandl J, Spinarova L, et al. Effects of Neuromuscular Electrical Stimulation and Aerobic Exercise Training on Arterial Stiffness and Autonomic Functions in Patients With Chronic Heart Failure. Artif Organs. 2012;36:920-30.

17) Watanabe K, Yoshihisa A, Sato Y, et al. Cardio-Ankle Vascular Index Reflects Impaired Exercise Capacity and Predicts Adverse Prognosis in Patients With Heart Failure. Front Cardiovasc Med. 2021 Mar 29; 8:631807. https://doi.org/10.3389/fcvm.2021.631807.

18) Shimizu K, Yamamoto T and Shirai K. Arterial stiffness, as monitored by cardio–ankle vascular index, is affected by obstructive sleep apnea, blood glucose control, and body weight –a case with 8 years follow up. International Medical Case Reports Journal. 2016; 9. 231–235.

19) Shimizu K, Tabata T, Kiyokawa H, et al. A Case Demonstrating the Cardio-Vascular Interaction by a New Cardio-Ankle Vascular Index During the Treatment of Concentric Hypertrophy. Cardiol Res 2019; 10:54-58.

Associations of Cardio-Ankle Vascular Index with Left Ventricular Function and Geometry

Iftikhar J. Kullo

Introduction

Left ventricular (LV) contraction in systole causes a rapid increase in aortic pressure and flow that generates a forward-traveling wave propagating to the periphery at a speed mainly dependent on aortic wall stiffness[1]. This wave encounters zones of impedance mismatch at arterial branch points, regional changes in stiffness, or change in lumen area, resulting in reflection of the incident wave back towards the heart. Incident and reflected pressure waves depend on pulse wave velocity (PWV), the traveling distance of pressure waves, and the duration of ventricular ejection and interact along the arterial circuit to give rise to the local pressure wave[1, 2]. The amplitude and shape of the measured aortic BP wave are determined by the amplitudes and phase relationship (timing) between the two component waves[2, 3].

Arterial stiffness increases with age and in the presence of elevated blood pressure (BP)[4], leading to faster transmission of both forward-traveling and reflected waves. There is a growing body of literature highlighting the association between arterial stiffness and cardiac function and structure[2, 3]. Arterial stiffness increases LV afterload, eventually leading to LV hypertrophy, fibrosis, diastolic dysfunction[5], concentric LV geometry[6-8], and adverse cardiovascular events in different populations[9, 10]. The determinants of LV afterload vary in systole. Whereas systemic vascular resistance is an important determinant of wall stress throughout systole, characteristic aortic impedance affects early systole and peak systolic wall stress, and wave reflections and arterial compliance affect myocardial stress in mid and late systole[11]. This chapter summarizes the associations of arterial stiffness with cardiac function and structure, with a focus on CAVI.

Cardio-ankle vascular index (CAVI) as a measure of arterial stiffness

Multiple indices have been used to describe aortic stiffness. PWV is the most commonly used and is defined by the Moens-Korteweg relation: $PWV = (Yh/2\rho r)^{1/2}$, where Y is Young's modulus of the arterial wall, h is the aortic wall thickness, r is the end-diastolic diameter of the artery and ρ is blood density[1]. Aortic PWV can be reproducibly measured by tonometry, ultrasonography or oscillometry. Cardio-ankle vascular index (CAVI) is a measure of global arterial stiffness calculated from heart-ankle PWV (ha-PWV), aortic wall stiffness β and BP[12]. It is a cuff-based measure, accounting for the time of the pulse wave arrival at the ankle relative to the proximal aorta by placing a phonocardiogram on the chest. CAVI is calculated by the device automatically based on the following equation: CAVI = a [2ρ / (systolic BP − diastolic BP) × Ln (systolic BP/diastolic BP) × PWV^2] + b, where ρ is blood density, PWV is pulse wave velocity from the aortic valve to ankle, a and b are coefficients[12, 13]. It is highly correlated with brachial-ankle PWV (ba-PWV) and carotid femoral PWV (cf-PWV) and is easily assessed in the office setting with good reproducibility and without the need for groin exposure[13]. In contrast to cf-PWV[14], it may also capture the elastic properties of the proximal aorta.

Determinants of CAVI

To better understand the association of CAVI with LV structure and function, it is important to be aware of potential confounding factors. Variables associated with CAVI have been reported in several cohorts without cardiovascular disease including 1380 Koreans[15], 1014 Japanese[16] and 600 white individuals referred for echocardiography[6]. In these studies, older age, male sex, lower BMI, higher systolic BP were independently associated with higher CAVI in multivariable regression analysis. In the white cohort, a multivariable linear regression model explained 56% of the inter-individual variation in CAVI[6]. Chronic kidney disease was more strongly associated with CAVI than hypertension, hyperlipidemia, smoking or diabetes. The directionality of the association with chronic kidney disease is unclear. Arterial stiffening could lead to renal dysfunction by increased renal pulsatility that can damage glomeruli[17, 18]. Conversely, impaired renal function by leading to endothelial dysfunction, increased oxidative stress, and the activation of the renin-angiotensin-aldosterone system[19] could increase arterial stiffness.

Arterial stiffness and diastolic function

Late systolic loading induces more pronounced LV hypertrophy and fibrosis in an animal model, than early

Department of Cardiovascular Medicine and the Gonda Vascular Center, Mayo Clinic, 200 First Street Southwest, Rochester, Minnesota 55905, USA.

systolic loading, at identical peak LV pressure levels[20]. In humans, higher late-systolic loading affects left atrial-LV gradient and diastolic pressure decay time, leading to prolonged LV relaxation and higher LV filling pressure, and is associated with greater LV mass and concentric remodeling, systolic and diastolic myocardial dysfunction[11, 21-23]. Premature wave reflection, by increasing mid-to-late systolic load may lead to diastolic dysfunction[2, 24, 25]. Higher aortic characteristic impedance was associated with worse global longitudinal strain and diastolic dysfunction in a cohort of older hypertensives without heart failure (HF)[26-28].

Arterial stiffness (determined using ba-PWV or cf-PWV) was independently associated with LV diastolic dysfunction in a number of settings including in patients undergoing echocardiography[28], in older Chinese adults with a normal LV ejection fraction (LVEF)[29], in elderly women[30], in a population study[7] and in patients with heart failure (HF) or HF risk factors who had a normal ejection fraction[31] as well as a meta-analysis of 27 studies in 6,626 patients[32].

Ye and colleagues[6] performed CAVI in individuals referred for transthoracic echocardiography (TTE) at Mayo Clinic to assess associations of CAVI with LV function and geometry in individuals without atherosclerotic cardiovascular diseases, LV systolic dysfunction or structural cardiac disease. They investigated whether CAVI was associated with worse LV systolic function, diastolic relaxation, and with LV mass and concentric geometry (assessed by relative wall thickness, RWT). CAVI was assessed at rest on the day of the TTE examination, using a VaSera VS-1500® device (Fukuda Denshi Co., Japan). The average of early diastolic velocity (e') at medial and lateral wall was used to estimate early diastolic relaxation, using tissue Doppler; the ratio of early transmitral filling velocity (E) and e' (E/e') was used to estimate LV filling. Multivariable-adjusted log-e' based on quartiles of CAVI are shown in **Fig. 1**. Higher CAVI was associated with worse diastolic relaxation assessed by tissue Doppler, independent of BP and conventional risk factors; there was

a stronger association of higher CAVI with greater early diastolic filling in men than women.

The association of higher CAVI with worse log-e' was consistent with results of the Framingham heart study[33]. Interestingly, despite the association of higher CAVI with worse e' in both sexes, the association of CAVI with E/e' was stronger in men than women. Increased diastolic filling as assessed by E/e' is an adaptive response of LV to compensate for impaired diastolic relaxation (as assessed by e'). A weaker association of CAVI with early diastolic filling in women than men as opposed to similar association with diastolic relaxation in both sexes, suggests women are more susceptible to altered diastolic relaxation with increase in arterial stiffness. CAVI has been reported to be associated with diastolic dysfunction in additional settings: in patients with hypertension[34], in patients with clinical cardiovascular disease[35], cardiovascular risk factors[36], in hypertensive patients[37], in subjects referred for echocardiography[38], and in patients with heart failure with reduced EF[39]. In a meta-analysis CAVI correlated with the E/A ratio and e'[32].

Arterial stiffness and systolic function

Higher aortic characteristic impedance, lower arterial compliance and increased wave reflection, all have been associated with subclinical LV dysfunction[6, 8, 23, 26, 27]. For example, greater aortic characteristic impedance, a determinant of pulsatile arterial load, was associated with worse global longitudinal strain in a cohort of older hypertensives without heart failure[26, 27] and with worse LV longitudinal strain in adults from hypertensive families[26]. A study in healthy women showed that cf-PWV was significantly correlated with global circumferential strain, apical rotation and LV twist (after adjustment for age, body mass index, BP and heart rate)[40].

In the study by Ye et al[6], higher CAVI was associated with worse LV longitudinal movement as measured by s', independent of age, sex and LVEF. Multivariable-adjusted log-s' based on quartiles of CAVI are shown in **Fig. 2**. Results highlight the effect of arterial stiffness on LV

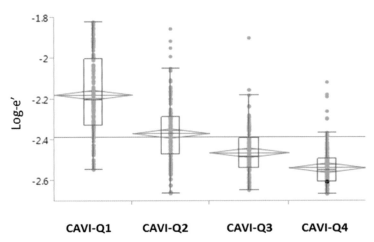

Fig. 1. Multivariable-adjusted log-e' according to quartiles of CAVI in 600 individuals without cardiovascular disease, referred for echocardiograph. Q1: CAVI ≤ 7.35; Q2: 7.35 < CAVI ≤ 8.51; Q3: 8.51 < CAVI ≤ 9.46; Q4: CAVI > 9.46. P for ANOVA < 0.001 [with permission of SAGE Publishing][6]

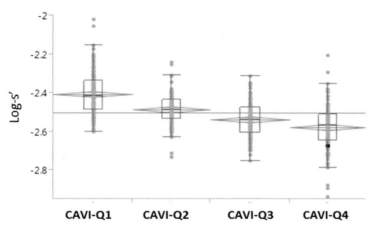

Fig. 2. Multivariable-adjusted log-s' according to quartiles of CAVI in 600 individuals without cardiovascular disease, referred for echocardiograph. Q1: CAVI ≤ 7.35; Q2: 7.35 < CAVI ≤ 8.51; Q3: 8.51 < CAVI ≤ 9.46; Q4: CAVI > 9.46. P for ANOVA < 0.001. [With permission of SAGE publishing][6]

longitudinal function in the setting of preserved EF. The LV response to chronic increases in hemodynamic load may differ in women and men. Women may be more susceptible to the effect of arterial stiffness on diastolic dysfunction. In a cohort of older hypertensive individuals[27] arterial elastance was higher in women than men mainly due to greater aortic characteristic impedance and lower arterial compliance in women. This may result in divergent arterial elastance to ventricular elastance ratio and changes in LV function that predispose to heart failure with preserved EF in women[22, 41]. Increased aortic stiffness and pulsatile load during early systole may decrease the efficiency of the cardiovascular system in women resulting in deranged coupling and exaggerated diastolic stiffness with aging in women and therefore predispose to heart failure with preserved EF[8, 26, 42].

Associations of CAVI with LV geometry

Increased arterial stiffness and pulsatile load (mainly due to increased reflected wave magnitude) have been associated with increased LV mass and the risk of developing LV concentric geometry[43] and increased LV wall thickness[44, 45]. The associations of BP and measures of arterial load with LV structure have been previously reported[21, 23, 33, 42, 46-48]. A study in healthy women showed that cf-PWV was significantly associated with relative wall thickness (RWT) after adjustment for age, body mass index, BP and heart rate[40].

In a study of 133 patients with coronary heart disease, CAVI was independently associated with LVEF, LV mass index (LVMI) and left atrial diameter[49]. The LVMI has been shown to be an independent determinant of diastolic dysfunction[50]. In the study by Ye et al.[6] higher CAVI was associated with greater LVMI and RWT; the association with LVMI was stronger in women than men; in women, CAVI, BMI, diabetes were associated with higher LVMI; in men, CAVI was not associated with LVMI after stepwise regression. Variables independently associated with RWT were body mass index, diastolic BP, HR, hyperlipidemia, type 2 diabetes, chronic kidney disease, and CAVI.

Kaess et al.[33] reported that the association of cf-PWV with LVMI and LV wall thickness was not independent of BP in participants of the Framingham Heart Study, as did a study of hypertensive families in which cf-PWV was not associated with LVMI or sex difference in the association[42]. CAVI reflects global arterial stiffness and includes the proximal aortic segment which is not accounted for by cf-PWV. This may explain differences in the results of these studies. Of note, the association of CAVI with LV mass and RWT in the study is similar to that of proximal aortic stiffness measured by MR in previous reports[8, 47], suggesting that the elastic property of proximal aorta may not be captured by cf-PWV. Ohyama et al.[47] reported a significant association of higher aortic arch PWV with greater LVMI and LV concentricity (ratio of LV mass over volume) in participants of the Multi-Ethnic Study of Atherosclerosis (MESA). A similar association of proximal aortic wall stiffness with LVMI was reported in participants of the AGES-Reykjavik study[8].

Clinical usefulness of determining arterial stiffness for cardiovascular risk assessment

As a measure of global arterial stiffness including the proximal aorta, CAVI can be used to assess the impact of LV afterload on cardiac function and structure. The potential use of measurement of arterial stiffness to identify patients at risk for structural heart disease was highlighted in a number of studies including one of individuals without known cardiovascular disease[6]. Higher CAVI was associated with worse systolic function and worse diastolic relaxation, independent of BP and other conventional risk factors. The association of arterial stiffness with altered left ventricular structure and function and vascular ventricular interaction suggests that arterial stiffness may represent a therapeutic target in heart failure with preserved EF[51, 52].

REFERENCES

1)   Nichols WW, O'Rourke MF and Vlachopoulos C. McDonald's

blood flow in arteries. *London: Hodder Arnold.* 2011.

2) Chirinos JA, Segers P, Hughes T and Townsend R. Large-artery stiffness in health and disease. *J Am Coll Cardiol.* 2019;74:1237-1263.

3) Mitchell GF. Arterial stiffness and wave reflection: biomarkers of cardiovascular risk. *Artery Res.* 2009;3:56-64.

4) Kullo IJ and Malik AR. Arterial ultrasonography and tonometry as adjuncts to cardiovascular risk stratification. *J Am Coll Cardiol.* 2007;49:1413-26.

5) Schillaci G, Battista F, Settimi L, Anastasio F and Pucci G. Cardio-ankle vascular index and subclinical heart disease. *Hypertens Res.* 2015;38:68-73.

6) Ye Z, Pellikka PA and Kullo IJ. Sex differences in associations of cardio-ankle vascular index with left ventricular function and geometry. *Vasc Med.* 2017;22:465-472.

7) Cauwenberghs N, Knez J, Tikhonoff V, D'Hooge J, Kloch-Badelek M, Thijs L, Stolarz-Skrzypek K, Haddad F, Wojciechowska W, Swierblewska E, Casiglia E, Kawecka-Jaszcz K, Narkiewicz K, Staessen JA and Kuznetsova T. Doppler indexes of left ventricular systolic and diastolic function in relation to the arterial stiffness in a general population. *J Hypertens.* 2016;34:762-71.

8) Bell V, Sigurdsson S, Westenberg JJ, Gotal JD, Torjesen AA, Aspelund T, Launer LJ, Harris TB, Gudnason V, de Roos A and Mitchell GF. Relations between aortic stiffness and left ventricular structure and function in older participants in the Age, Gene/Environment Susceptibility--Reykjavik Study. *Circ Cardiovasc Imaging.* 2015;8:e003039.

9) Kullo IJ, Malik AR, Santos S, Ehrsam JE and Turner ST. Association of cardiovascular risk factors with microvascular and conduit artery function in hypertensive subjects. *Am J Hypertens.* 2007;20:735-42.

10) Townsend RR, Wilkinson IB, Schiffrin EL, Avolio AP, Chirinos JA, Cockcroft JR, Heffernan KS, Lakatta EG, McEniery CM, Mitchell GF, Najjar SS, Nichols WW, Urbina EM and Weber T. Recommendations for improving and standardizing vascular research on arterial stiffness: A scientific statement from the American Heart Association. *Hypertension.* 2015;66:698-722.

11) Chirinos JA, Segers P, Gillebert TC, Gupta AK, De Buyzere ML, De Bacquer D, St John-Sutton M and Rietzschel ER. Arterial properties as determinants of time-varying myocardial stress in humans. *Hypertension.* 2012;60:64-70.

12) Hayashi K, Yamamoto T, Takahara A and Shirai K. Clinical assessment of arterial stiffness with cardio-ankle vascular index: theory and applications. *J Hypertens.* 2015;33:1742-57; discussion 1757.

13) Lim J, Pearman M, Park W, Alkatan M and Tanaka H. Interrelationships among various measures of central artery stiffness. *Am J Hypertens.* 2016;29:1024-8.

14) Ben-Shlomo Y, Spears M, Boustred C, May M, Anderson SG, Benjamin EJ, Boutouyrie P, Cameron J, Chen CH, Cruickshank JK, Hwang SJ, Lakatta EG, Laurent S, Maldonado J, Mitchell GF, Najjar SS, Newman AB, Ohishi M, Pannier B, Pereira T, Vasan RS, Shokawa T, Sutton-Tyrell K, Verbeke F, Wang KL, Webb DJ, Hansen TW, Zoungas S, McEniery CM, Cockcroft JR and Wilkinson IB. Aortic pulse wave velocity improves cardiovascular event prediction: an individual participant meta-analysis of prospective observational data from 17,635 subjects. *J Am CollCardiol.* 2014;63:636-646.

15) Choi SY, Oh BH, Bae Park J, Choi DJ, Rhee MY and Park S. Age-associated increase in arterial stiffness measured according to the cardio-ankle vascular index without blood pressure changes in healthy adults. *J Atheroscler Thromb.* 2013;20:911-23.

16) Kadota K, Takamura N, Aoyagi K, Yamasaki H, Usa T, Nakazato M, Maeda T, Wada M, Nakashima K, Abe K, Takeshima F and Ozono Y. Availability of cardio-ankle

vascular index (CAVI) as a screening tool for atherosclerosis. *Circ J.* 2008;72:304-8.

17) Baumann M, Pan CR, Roos M, Von Eynatten M, Sollinger D, Lutz J and Heemann U. Pulsatile stress correlates with (micro-)albuminuria in renal transplant recipients. *Transplant International.* 2010;23:292-298.

18) Hashimoto J and Ito S. Central pulse pressure and aortic stiffness determine renal hemodynamics: pathophysiological implication for microalbuminuria in hypertension. *Hypertension.* 2011;58:839-46.

19) Safar ME, London GM and Plante GE. Arterial stiffness and kidney function. *Hypertension.* 2004;43:163-8.

20) Kobayashi S, Yano M, Kohno M, Obayashi M, Hisamatsu Y, Ryoke T, Ohkusa T, Yamakawa K and Matsuzaki M. Influence of aortic impedance on the development of pressure-overload left ventricular hypertrophy in rats. *Circulation.* 1996;94:3362-8.

21) Zamani P, Bluemke DA, Jacobs DR, Jr., Duprez DA, Kronmal R, Lilly SM, Ferrari VA, Townsend RR, Lima JA, Budoff M, Segers P, Hannan P and Chirinos JA. Resistive and pulsatile arterial load as predictors of left ventricular mass and geometry: the multi-ethnic study of atherosclerosis. *Hypertension.* 2015;65:85-92.

22) Borlaug BA, Redfield MM, Melenovsky V, Kane GC, Karon BL, Jacobsen SJ and Rodeheffer RJ. Longitudinal changes in left ventricular stiffness: a community-based study. *Circ Heart Fail.* 2013;6:944-52.

23) Russo C, Jin Z, Palmieri V, Homma S, Rundek T, Elkind MS, Sacco RL and Di Tullio MR. Arterial stiffness and wave reflection: sex differences and relationship with left ventricular diastolic function. *Hypertension.* 2012;60:362-8.

24) Chirinos JA. Deep phenotyping of systemic arterial hemodynamics in HFpEF (Part 2): Clinical and therapeutic considerations. *J Cardiovasc Transl Res.* 2017;10:261-274.

25) Weber T and Chirinos JA. Pulsatile arterial haemodynamics in heart failure. *Eur Heart J.* 2018;39:3847-3854.

26) Ye Z, Coutinho T, Pellikka PA, Villarraga HR, Borlaug BA and Kullo IJ. Associations of alterations in pulsatile arterial load with left ventricular longitudinal strain. *Am J Hypertens.* 2015;28:1325-31.

27) Coutinho T, Borlaug BA, Pellikka PA, Turner ST and Kullo IJ. Sex differences in arterial stiffness and ventricular-arterial interactions. *J Am Coll Cardiol.* 2013;61:96-103.

28) Hsu PC, Tsai WC, Lin TH, Su HM, Voon WC, Lai WT and Sheu SH. Association of arterial stiffness and electrocardiography-determined left ventricular hypertrophy with left ventricular diastolic dysfunction. *PLoS One.* 2012;7:e49100.

29) Xu L, Jiang CQ, Lam TH, Yue XJ, Lin JM, Cheng KK, Liu B, Li Jin Y, Zhang WS and Thomas GN. Arterial stiffness and left-ventricular diastolic dysfunction: Guangzhou Biobank Cohort Study-CVD. *J Hum Hypertens.* 2011;25:152-8.

30) Kim HL, Lim WH, Seo JB, Chung WY, Kim SH, Kim MA and Zo JH. Association between arterial stiffness and left ventricular diastolic function in relation to gender and age. *Medicine (Baltimore).* 2017;96:e5783.

31) Luers C, Trippel TD, Seelander S, Wachter R, Hasenfuss G, Lindhorst R, Bobenko A, Nolte K, Pieske B and Edelmann F. Arterial stiffness and elevated left ventricular filling pressure in patients at risk for the development or a previous diagnosis of HF-A subgroup analysis from the DIAST-CHF study. *J Am Soc Hypertens.* 2017;11:303-313.

32) Chow B and Rabkin SW. The relationship between arterial stiffness and heart failure with preserved ejection fraction: a systemic meta-analysis. *Heart Fail Rev.* 2015;20:291-303.

33) Kaess BM, Rong J, Larson MG, Hamburg NM, Vita JA, Cheng S, Aragam J, Levy D, Benjamin EJ, Vasan RS and Mitchell GF. Relations of central hemodynamics and aortic stiffness with left ventricular structure and

function: The Framingham Heart Study. *J Am Heart Assoc.* 2016;5:e002693.

34) Kim H, Kim HS, Yoon HJ, Park HS, Cho YK, Nam CW, Hur SH, Kim YN and Kim KB. Association of cardio-ankle vascular index with diastolic heart function in hypertensive patients. *Clin Exp Hypertens.* 2014;36:200-5.

35) Namba T, Masaki N, Matsuo Y, Sato A, Kimura T, Horii S, Yasuda R, Yada H, Kawamura A, Takase B and Adachi T. Arterial stiffness is significantly associated with left ventricular diastolic dysfunction in patients with cardiovascular disease. *Int Heart J.* 2016;57:729-735.

36) Mizuguchi Y, Oishi Y, Tanaka H, Miyoshi H, Ishimoto T, Nagase N and Oki T. Arterial stiffness is associated with left ventricular diastolic function in patients with cardiovascular risk factors: early detection with the use of cardio-ankle vascular index and ultrasonic strain imaging. *J Card Fail.* 2007;13:744-51.

37) Masugata H, Senda S, Okuyama H, Murao K, Inukai M, Hosomi N, Yukiiri K, Nishiyama A, Kohno M and Goda F. Comparison of central blood pressure and cardio-ankle vascular index for association with cardiac function in treated hypertensive patients. *Hypertens Res.* 2009;32:1136-42.

38) Sakane K, Miyoshi T, Doi M, Hirohata S, Kaji Y, Kamikawa S, Ogawa H, Hatanaka K, Kitawaki T, Kusachi S and Yamamoto K. Association of new arterial stiffness parameter, the cardio-ankle vascular index, with left ventricular diastolic function. *J Atheroscler Thromb.* 2008;15:261-8.

39) Noguchi S, Masugata H, Senda S, Ishikawa K, Nakaishi H, Tada A, Inage T, Kajikawa T, Inukai M, Himoto T, Hosomi N, Murakami K, Noma T, Kohno M, Okada H, Goda F and Murao K. Correlation of arterial stiffness to left ventricular function in patients with reduced ejection fraction. *Tohoku J Exp Med.* 2011;225:145-51.

40) Zhang J, Chowienczyk PJ, Spector TD and Jiang B. Relation of arterial stiffness to left ventricular structure and function in healthy women. *Cardiovasc Ultrasound.* 2018;16:21.

41) Redfield MM, Jacobsen SJ, Borlaug BA, Rodeheffer RJ and Kass DA. Age- and gender-related ventricular-vascular stiffening: a community-based study. *Circulation.* 2005;112:2254-62.

42) Coutinho T, Pellikka PA, Bailey KR, Turner ST and Kullo IJ. Sex differences in the associations of hemodynamic load with left ventricular hypertrophy and concentric remodeling. *Am J Hypertens.* 2016;29:73-80.

43) Cauwenberghs N, Knez J, D'hooge J, Thijs L, Yang W-Y, Wei F-F, Zhang Z-Y, Staessen JA and Kuznetsova T. Longitudinal changes in LV structure and diastolic function in relation to arterial properties in general population. *JACC: Cardiovascular Imaging.* 2017;10:1307-1316.

44) Cohen DL and Townsend RR. Update on pathophysiology and treatment of hypertension in the elderly. *Curr Hypertens Rep.* 2011;13:330-7.

45) Mitchell GF. Arterial stiffness and hypertension: chicken or egg? *Hypertension.* 2014;64:210-4.

46) Chirinos JA, Segers P, Raina A, Saif H, Swillens A, Gupta AK, Townsend R, Emmi AG, Jr., Kirkpatrick JN, Keane MG, Ferrari VA, Wiegers SE and St John Sutton MG. Arterial pulsatile hemodynamic load induced by isometric exercise strongly predicts left ventricular mass in hypertension. *Am J Physiol Heart Circ Physiol.* 2010;298:H320-30.

47) Ohyama Y, Ambale-Venkatesh B, Noda C, Chugh AR, Teixido-Tura G, Kim JY, Donekal S, Yoneyama K, Gjesdal O, Redheuil A, Liu CY, Nakamura T, Wu CO, Hundley WG, Bluemke DA and Lima JA. Association of aortic stiffness with left ventricular remodeling and reduced left ventricular function measured by magnetic resonance imaging: The multi-ethnic study of atherosclerosis. *Circ Cardiovasc Imaging.* 2016;9:e004426.

48) Abhayaratna WP, Barnes ME, O'Rourke MF, Gersh BJ, Seward JB, Miyasaka Y, Bailey KR and Tsang TS. Relation of arterial stiffness to left ventricular diastolic function and cardiovascular risk prediction in patients > or =65 years of age. *Am J Cardiol.* 2006;98:1387-92.

49) Miyoshi T, Doi M, Hirohata S, Sakane K, Kamikawa S, Kitawaki T, Kaji Y, Kusano KF, Ninomiya Y and Kusachi S. Cardio-ankle vascular index is independently associated with the severity of coronary atherosclerosis and left ventricular function in patients with ischemic heart disease. *J Atheroscler Thromb.* 2010;17:249-58.

50) Kimura H, Takeda K, Tsuruya K, Mukai H, Muto Y, Okuda H, Furusho M, Ueno T, Nakashita S, Miura S, Maeda A and Kondo H. Left ventricular mass index is an independent determinant of diastolic dysfunction in patients on chronic hemodialysis: a tissue Doppler imaging study. *Nephron Clin Pract.* 2011;117:c67-73.

51) Redfield MM. Heart failure with preserved ejection fraction. *N Engl J Med.* 2016;375:1868-1877.

52) Marti CN, Gheorghiade M, Kalogeropoulos AP, Georgiopoulou VV, Quyyumi AA and Butler J. Endothelial dysfunction, arterial stiffness, and heart failure. *J Am Coll Cardiol.* 2012;60:1455-69.

Left ventricular function and CAVI in hypertensive patients

Giacomo Pucci[1,2] and Gaetano Vaudo[1,2]

This chapter is dedicated to the memory of Giuseppe Schillaci, distinguished Professor, commendable Mentor and outstanding Researcher of the University of Perugia, Italy

The progression from hypertension to left ventricular dysfunction

Hypertension is the major cardiovascular risk factor responsible worldwide for the highest number of deaths and disability related to cardiovascular (CV) disease[1]. The main feature to generate such a dubious distinction stands on its prolonged and asymptomatic course between the time of diagnosis and the development of clinically overt CV disease. This is the main reason why hypertension is defined with the nickname of "silent killer". In this context, the prediction of CV damage in any individual with hypertension, particularly if diagnosed at an early, asymptomatic and potentially reversible stage, is of paramount importance.

Heart failure (HF) is one of the main CV diseases caused by hypertension, especially if unknown or sub-optimally treated. Hypertension precedes the clinical development of HF in virtually all patients, particularly if the clinical phenotype of HF is characterized by preserved ejection fraction (HFpEF)[2]. In hypertensive individuals, diastolic dysfunction (DD) is the sub-clinical asymptomatic stage that paves the way to overt HF. In general parlance, DD may be defined as the cardiac remodelling in response to pressure left ventricular (LV) afterload. More strictly, DD is the result of a series of processes related to impaired ventricular-arterial cross-talk, which physiologically ensures LV emptying and an adequate tissue perfusion at the lowest energetic expenditure[3].

The stiffness of large arteries, such as the aorta and its major branches, is a fundamental determinant of LV external work. A stiff artery lose its ability to accumulate potential energy during wall distension and return it in form of kinetic energy during diastole. This increases flow pulsatility and causes several damage at the level of peripheral tissues. The process of arterial stiffnening, which occurs under the effect of ageing and is accelerated by the concurrence of other CV risk factors such as hypertension, obesity, diabetes and smoking, ultimately increases impedance to LV outflow and elevates the energetic expense required to pump the blood volume centrifugally during systole[4].

Many theoretical and experimental studies attempted to characterize the essential components of the ventricular-vascular interactions during the cardiac cycle. The three-element Windkessel model has been largely adopted as a validated theoretical construct to describe the impedance to the blood flow caused by aortic stiffness during the LV ejection phase[5]. One of the main components is named aortic characteristic impedance (Zc). When a forward pulsatile flow is injected into an elastic tube, such as the aorta, the amount of pressure rise vs. flow rise for any given amount of imparted energy, is determined by the aortic Zc which, in turn, depends on its elastic properties[4].

In untreated hypertensives, an increased aortic Zc was shown to predict the presence of LV hypertrophy and concentric remodelling[6]. Moreover, an impaired arterial loading sequence characterized by high aortic Zc was also found to be major determinant of less efficient LV longitudinal strain and myocardial relaxation during diastole[7]. These and other aspects have been very well detailed in numerous studies showing that arterial stiffness is a major predictor of the occurrence of DD in general population, among hypertensive subjects and across different disease categories[8,9].

Under this perspective, it is important to take into due account that systolic BP cannot be considered a measure of the mechanical load opposing to LV ejection *tout court*, as usually done in clinical practice. Systolic BP corresponds to intra-cavity pressure of the ejecting LV during systole, and should be accounted as a measure of the overall interplay between LV contractility and arterial distensibility[10]. Therefore, any measure of arterial stiffness which is sensitive to measured systolic BP levels does not fully reflect the fact that LV and arterial mechanics during systole are closely related each others. To this purpose, measures of arterial stiffness that are independent from systolic BP might have the potential to better describe and quantify how much of the LV mechanical efficiency is determined by arterial load.

Aortic Zc is a more complex concept than a single BP value. Moreover, it is a time-varying phenomenon, because the arterial load that the heart overcomes as a pump actually varies at varying conditions during the systolic phase, reaching a peak during the early ejection phase, when systolic BP reaches its maximum value, and then decreasing.

---

[1]Department of Medicine and Surgery, University of Perugia, Perugia, Italy.
[2]Unit of Internal Medicine, Terni University Hospital, Terni, Italy.

Therefore, aortic characteristic impedance influences early systolic aortic pulse pressure rise in a time-varying manner during systole[11]. This important phenomenon could be less effectively described by static measures of arterial stiffness, e.g. pulse wave velocity measured at the diastolic BP level, which do not properly account for the stiffening of the arterial wall during the cardiac cycle.

The relationship between CAVI and LV structure and function in hypertension

The cardio-ankle vascular index (CAVI) is a non-invasive measure of arterial stiffness in which pulse wave velocity (PWV) was made independent from arterial pressure changes during the cardiac cycle based on the non-linearity of the relationship between pressure and diameter, described by the stiffness index beta (β)[12]. As a result, CAVI is independent from systolic BP at the time of measurement[13]. Moreover, given its dependence from β, CAVI is a surrogate expression of the increase in arterial stiffness occurring from end-diastole to end-systole (namely diastolic-to-systolic 'stiffening'), and incorporates information on arterial properties during the entirety of systole. Finally, CAVI includes measures of stiffness of the proximal ascending aorta, whereas other measures of arterial stiffness, such as carotid-femoral (cf-PWV) or brachial-ankle pulse wave velocities (ba-PWV) do not. Based on these above premises, CAVI is a promising tool to study the relationship between aortic function and LV mechanical properties.

Noteworthy, the relationship between CAVI and measures of LV structure and function in hypertension has been the subject of extensive research. In a study conducted on 133 Italian individuals with hypertension or high-normal BP, CAVI, recorded using a VaSera VS-1500 vascular screening system (Fukuda Denshi, Tokyo, Japan) with the patient resting in a supine position, was shown to be significantly higher in subjects with inappropriately high LV mass than in subjects with appropriate LV mass (9.1 vs 7.9, respectively; p<0.001)[14]. This measure, that could be easily assessed by echocardiography, reflects how much LV mass exceeds the levels needed to compensate for hemodynamic load[15], that is for arterial impedance. Interestingly, such difference was not shown by measures of arterial properties incorporating pressure-dependent components of aortic stiffness, such as cf-PWV, that did differ between subjects with appropriate and inappropriate LV mass. Finally, higher CAVI levels among individuals with inappropriately high LV mass remained significant even after adjustment for other determinants of inappropriate LV mass such as body mass index. In the same population, we also showed an interesting inverse correlation between CAVI and LV midwall fractional shortening (r=-0.41, p<0.001). This is a measure of sub-clinical LV systolic dysfunction, defined as a low afterload-adjusted fractional shortening assessed at the midwall level, according to a geometric model that takes into account the non-uniform systolic thickening of the LV wall[16,17]. Once again, such inverse relationship was not observed when cf-PWV replaced CAVI as a measure of arterial stiffness. Interestingly, both these measures are largely known to be significantly

and independently associated with future CV events in hypertension[15,18]. Moreover, changes in LV inappropriate mass following the optimization of antihypertensive treatment were found to be significantly associated to reduced risk of future overt CV disease among hypertensive subjects[19]. Taken together, these results suggest that the baseline assessment of CAVI and the timed optimization of anti-hypertensive treatment could delay or even revert the transition from asymptomatic to symptomatic heart disease in hypertension.

This hypothesis is largely supported by the results of other studies conducted on hypertensive population. In a study performed on 136 treated hypertensives (mean age 69 years), Masugata et al.[20] evaluated the relationship between CAVI and markers of hypertensive heart disease, such as the diameter of the ascending aorta, and the E/E' ratio, a measure of DD assessed by Doppler echocardiography. In their population, despite rather well controlled BP (mean BP 135/81 mmHg), they found relatively high values of LV mass (on average 115 g/m²), suggesting that this population was at high CV risk despite optimal treatment. Results showed that CAVI was positively correlated with the diameter of ascending aorta (R=0.35, p<0.001), with the E/E' ratio (R=0.22, p<0.01), and with increased levels of brain natriuretic peptide (BNP), a bio-humoral marker of increased LV wall stress (R=0.24, p<0.004).

The relationship between CAVI and markers of DD was also confirmed in other studies. In a study of 119 patients referred for echocardiography, CAVI was showed to be independently associated with markers of DD such as E/A ratio (β=-0.25, p=0.003) and left atrial (LA) enlargement (β=0.21, p=0.003)[21]. Such association was also confirmed in a meta-analysis of 7 studies using CAVI as a measure of arterial stiffness. As compared with all the other measures of arterial stiffness, CAVI was the only measure to show low heterogenity of results among studies. Indeed, these results showed that CAVI was also correlated with e', but not with E/e' ratio. Interestingly, pressure-dependent measures of arterial stiffness did not show any superiority as compared to CAVI in their associations with indexes of DD, indicating that adding the pressure-dependent component of arterial stiffness did not result in a better prediction of cardiac damage and deterioration[22].

The potential significance of CAVI in predicting the occurrence of overt HF will be explored in two currently ongoing long-term studies which are going to evaluate the association of CAVI with future CV events in high risk patients. One is the Prospective Study of the Cardio-Ankle Vascular Index as a predictive Factor for Cardiovascular Events (CAVI-J)[23] and the other, the Cardiovascular Prognostic Coupling Study in Japan (the COUPLING Registry) to predict CV events in 3000 high-risk patients in 5 years[24].

From hypertension to heart failure. The clinical value of CAVI

CAVI demonstrated to maintain its clinical effectiveness in predicting further cardiac deterioration and CV death even in the presence of manifest heart disease. In a study that evaluated 75 hypertensive patients with HF, divided between those with HFpEF and HF with reduced EF (HFrEF), CAVI showed positive association with global longitudinal LV peak strain, a measure of LV deformation during diastole. This was observable in the sub-group of subjects with HFpEF (R = 0.60, p < 0.001), whereas the inverse relationship between CAVI and e' was found in both subjects with HFpEF (R = -0.39) and with HFrEF (R = -0.31), despite CAVI was not significantly different between these two groups (8.7 in HFpEF, 9.1 in HFrEF, p = not significant)[25].

In another study conducted in 100 patients with pre-existing CV disease, CAVI was found to be associated with e/e' in all HF categories (β = 0.252, p = 0.037) even after adjustment for confounders[26]. In a recent study [CAVI heart failure] conducted on a population of individuals with chronic HF, increased CAVI was associated with indexes of worsening physical function, such as sarcopenia, low handgrip strength, and six-minute walking distance. These results suggest that CAVI is significantly associated with indexes of reduced quality of life and adverse prognosis in HF.

In the setting of chronic HF, the acute decompensation represent a catastrophic event. This is characterized by the sudden worsening of the signs and symptoms of heart failure, which typically includes difficulty breathing (dyspnea), leg or feet swelling, and fatigue. Moreover, acute respiratory distress could complicate the clinical scenario, often leading to rapid clinical deterioration and sudden death. Observations made on a cohort of 64 patients[27] with acute decompensated HF provided interesting findings to better understand the potential detrimental link between increased arterial stiffness and cardiac function during acute HF. In this study, patients were categorized according to clinical scenario, that is depending on values of systolic BP at presentation. In subjects with high systolic BP and acute decompensed heart failure, CAVI was found as elevated. The same was not described for other clinical scenarios, such as acute decompensated HF with normal or low systolic BP, acute coronary syndrome or pulmonary hypertension, where CAVI values were lower. These results suggested that, despite apparent good residual LV pump performance, a high cardiac-arterial impedance mismatch has the potential to induce acute increases of pulmonary venous pressures leading to the occurrence of clinically detectable dyspnea or congestion.

Taken together, these results show that CAVI is a clinically useful tool to evaluate the ventricular-arterial interactions even in the presence of manifest heart disease and not only in the setting of CV risk prediction. Further studies will be aimed at evaluating if the optimization of drug treatment for HF will reduce the impact of arterial stiffness on LV function and structure, ultimately leading to a decrease in CV events and deaths.

Conclusions

The availability of non-invasive devices for the clinical assessment of the functional properties of large arteries during the cardiac cycle represents an exciting and growing opportunity to bring the evaluation of ventricular-vascular inter-connections into the field of daily clinical practice. To this aim, CAVI has the potential to be particularly attractive due to its simplicity and operator-independence for measurement. Moreover, due to its BP-independency, it has the potential to be a promising tool for the functional evaluation of the impact of elevated arterial load on LV structure and function. In the future, there is need to evaluate in appropriate studies if the reduction of CAVI values obtained by appropriate pharmacological treatment will translate into better prevention of cardiac deterioration and death in hypertension.

List of abbreviations

CV: cardiovascular
HF: heart failure
HFpEF: heart failure with preserved ejection fraction
HFrEF: heart failure with reduced ejection fraction
DD: diastolic dysfunction
LV: left ventricular
Zc: characteristic impedance
CAVI: cardio-ankle vascular index
PWV: pulse wave velocity
BP: blood pressure
BNP: brain natriuretic peptide
LA: left atrium

References

1) GBD 2019 Risk Factors Collaborators. Global burden of 87 risk factors in 204 countries and territories. 1990-2019: a systematic analysis for the Global Burden of Disease Study 2019. Lancet 2020;396:1223-1249.

2) Messerli FH, Rimoldi SF, Bangalore S. The Transition From Hypertension to Heart Failure: Contemporary Update. JACC Heart Fail 2017;5:543-551.

3) Chirinos JA, Segers P. Noninvasive evaluation of left ventricular afterload: part 1: pressure and flow measurements and basic principles of wave conduction and reflection. Hypertension 2010;56:555-562.

4) Chirinos JA, Bhattacharya P, Kumar A, Proto E, Konda P, Segers P, Akers SR, Townsend RR, Zamani P. Impact of Diabetes Mellitus on Ventricular Structure, Arterial Stiffness, and Pulsatile Hemodynamics in Heart Failure With Preserved Ejection Fraction. J Am Heart Assoc 2019;8:e011457.

5) Westerhof BE, Guelen I, Westerhof N, Karemaker JM, Avolio A. Quantification of wave reflection in the human aorta from pressure alone: a proof of principle. Hypertension 2006;48:595-601.

6) Pucci G, Hametner B, Battista F, Wassertheurer S, Schillaci G. Pressure-independent relationship of aortic characteristic impedance with left ventricular mass and geometry in untreated hypertension. J Hypertens 2015;33:153-160.

7) Chirinos JA, Segers P, Rietzschel ER, De Buyzere ML, Raja MW, Claessens T, Bacquer DD, Sutton MSJ, Gillebert TG, Asklepios Investigators. Early and late systolic wall stress differentially relate to myocardial contraction and relaxation in middle-aged adults: the Asklepios study. Hypertension 2013;61:296-303.

8) Abhayaratna WP, Srikusalanukul W, Budge MM. Aortic stiffness for the detection of preclinical left ventricular diastolic dysfunction: pulse wave velocity versus pulse

pressure. J Hypertens 2008;26:758-764.

9) Cauwenberghs N, Knez J, Boggia J, D'hooge J, Yang WY, Wei FF, Thijs L, Staessen JA, Kuznetsova T. Doppler indexes of left ventricular systolic and diastolic function in relation to haemodynamic load components in a general population. J Hypertens 2018;36:867-875.

10) O'Rourke MF. Vascular impedance in studies of arterial and cardiac function. Physiol Rev 1982;62:570-623.

11) Chirinos JA, Segers P, Gillebert TC, Gupta AK, De Buyzere ML, Bacquer DD, John-Sutton MS, Rietzschel ER, Asklepios Investigators. Arterial properties as determinants of time-varying myocardial stress in humans. Hypertension 2012;60:64-70.

12) Hayashi K, Handa H, Nagasawa S, Okumura A, Moritake K. Stiffness and elastic behavior of human intracranial and extracranial arteries. J Biomech 1980;13:175-184.

13) Shirai K, Utino J, Otsuka K, Takata M. A novel blood pressure-independent arterial wall stiffness parameter; cardio-ankle vascular index (CAVI). J Atheroscler Thromb 2006;13:101-107.

14) Schillaci G, Battista F, Settimi L, Anastasio F, Pucci G. Cardio-ankle vascular index and subclinical heart disease. Hypertens Res 2015;38:68-73.

15) de Simone G, Palmieri V, Koren MJ, Mensah GA, Roman MJ, Devereux RB. Prognostic implications of the compensatory nature of left ventricular mass in arterial hypertension. J Hypertens 2001;19:119-125.

16) Shimizu G, Hirota Y, Kita Y, Kawamura K, Saito T, Gaasch WH. Left ventricular midwall mechanics in systemic arterial hypertension. Myocardial function is depressed in pressure-overload hypertrophy. Circulation 1991;83:1676-1684.

17) Schillaci G, Verdecchia P, Reboldi G, Pede S, Porcellati C. Subclinical left ventricular dysfunction in systemic hypertension and the role of 24-hour blood pressure. Am J Cardiol 2000;86:509-513.

18) de Simone G, Devereux RB, Koren MJ, Mensah GA, Casale PN, Laragh JH. Midwall left ventricular mechanics. An independent predictor of cardiovascular risk in arterial hypertension. Circulation 1996;93:259-265.

19) Muiesan ML, Salvetti M, Paini A, Monteduro C, Galbassini G, Bonzi B, Poisa P, Belotti E, Agabiti Rosei C, Rizzoni D, Castellano C, Agabiti Rosei E. Inappropriate left ventricular mass changes during treatment adversely affects cardiovascular prognosis in hypertensive patients.

Hypertension 2007;49:1077-1083.

20) Masugata H, Senda S, Inukai M, Murao K, Himoto T, Hosomi N, Murakami K, Noma T, Kohno M, Okada H, Goda F. Association of cardio-ankle vascular index with brain natriuretic peptide levels in hypertension. J Atheroscler Thromb 2012;19:255-262.

21) Sakane K, Miyoshi T, Doi M, Hirohata S, Kaji Y, Kamikawa S, Ogawa H, Hatanaka K, Kitawaki T, Kusachi S, Yamamoto K. Association of new arterial stiffness parameter, the cardio-ankle vascular index, with left ventricular diastolic function. J Atheroscler Thromb 2008;15:261-268.

22) Chow B, Rabkin SW. The relationship between arterial stiffness and heart failure with preserved ejection fraction: a systemic meta-analysis. Heart Fail Rev 2015;20:291-303.

23) Miyoshi T, Ito H, Horinaka S, Shirai K, Higaki J, Orimo H. Protocol for Evaluating the Cardio-Ankle Vascular Index to Predict Cardiovascular Events in Japan: A Prospective Multicenter Cohort Study. Pulse (Basel) 2017;4(Suppl 1):11-16.

24) Kario K, Kabutoya T, Fujiwara T, Negishi K, Nishizawa M, Yamamoto M, Yamagiwa K, Kawashima A, Yoshida T, Nakazato J, Matsui Y, Sekizuka H, Abe H, Abe Y, Fujita Y, Sato K, Narita K, Tsuchiya N, Kubota Y, Hashizume T, Hoshide S. Rationale, design, and baseline characteristics of the Cardiovascular Prognostic COUPLING Study in Japan (the COUPLING Registry). J Clin Hypertens (Greenwich) 2020;22:465-474.

25) Noguchi S, Masugata H, Senda S, Ishikawa K, Nakaishi H, Tada A, Inage T, Kajikawa T, Inukai M, Himoto T, Hosomi N, Murakami K, Noma T, Kohno M, Okada H, Goda F, Murao K. Correlation of arterial stiffness to left ventricular function in patients with reduced ejection fraction. Tohoku J Exp Med 2011;225:145-151.

26) Namba T, Masaki N, Matsuo Y, Sato A, Kimura T, Horii S, Yasuda R, Yada H, Kawamura A, Takase B, Adachi T. Arterial Stiffness Is Significantly Associated With Left Ventricular Diastolic Dysfunction in Patients With Cardiovascular Disease. Int Heart J 2016 2;57:729-735.

27) Goto T, Wakami K, Mori K, Kikuchi S, Fukuta H, Ohte N. Vascular Physiology according to Clinical Scenario in Patients with Acute Heart Failure: Evaluation using the Cardio-Ankle Vascular Index. Tohoku J Exp Med 2016;240:57-65.

Left ventricular geometry and CAVI

Kazuhiro Shimizu[1,2] and Tsuyoshi Tabata[2]

Introduction

Left ventricular hypertrophy (LVH) is well known as a risk for cardiovascular disease[1,2]. Currently, the formula for chamber quantification of left ventricular (LV) geometry has been recommended by the American Society of Echocardiography (ASE)[3,4]. Left ventricular geometry correlates the relative wall thickness (RWT) of a ventricle to its mass, which explains the relationship between wall thickness and cavity size[5]. Using these two features, LV geometry could be classified as follows: normal geometry (NG), concentric remodeling (CR), concentric hypertrophy (CH) and eccentric hypertrophy (EH)[6].

As for the mechanism and contribution factors for LV geometry, the degree and the duration of hypertension are known to be very important factors; arterial stiffness is also thought to be important as an afterload of the heart. In the past, arterial stiffness had been measured using pulse wave velocity (PWV), such as carotid-femoral pulse wave velocity (cfPWV). However, PWV is intrinsically dependent on blood pressure (BP) at the measuring time. Therefore, it is difficult to evaluate the role of arterial stiffness measured with PWV in LV remodeling. We reported a typical case that left ventricular concentric hypertrophy was remarkably improved, accompanying with a decrease in CAVI[7]. In addition, we reported a large scale cross-sectional study on left ventricular morphology and CAVI[8].

This chapter shows the relationship between various left ventricular geometric patterns and the cardio ankle vascular index (CAVI) among patients with metabolic disorders.

Study subjects

In this retrospective observational study, patients (n = 1046) with various risk factors such as metabolic disorders (diabetes mellitus (DM), hypertension (HT) and dyslipidemia (DL)), who visited our hospital from 2007 to 2017 were enrolled. Exclusion criteria were as follows: acute myocardial infarction, acute myocarditis, open-heart surgery, atrial fibrillation, severe obesity (body mass index > 35), atherosclerosis obliterans (ankle-brachial index < 0.9) and more than moderate valve stenosis or regurgitation. There were 159 (15%) subjects with cerebrovascular disease (CVD) and 326 (31%) with coronary artery disease (CAD). As shown in Table 1, the patients (n = 1046) were divided into four groups: NG (n = 157), CR (n = 435), CH (n = 412) and EH (n = 42). Plasma brain natriuretic peptide (BNP) values were as follows; NG: 22.5pg/ml (9.9, 42.9),

CR: 28.5pg/ml (13.2, 51.0), CH: 72.1pg/ml (30.6, 212.7), and EH: 144.0pg/ml (54.3, 717.6), respectively. No significant changes were observed in the groups of patients with NG and CR type LV geometry, not in the LV geometry itself. The incidence of CH was high compared to CR (p < 0.001). EH was the highest among the four groups (NG to EH, P < 0.001, CR to EH, P < 0.001, CH to EH, P < 0.001).

The points of the study subjects

Generally, CAVI is higher in the elderly populations and men are higher compared to women. We performed the analysis at least on a similar age and gender groups.

Echocardiography measurement

The GE Vivid7, E9, S5 and S6 Ultrasound System (GE Healthcare, Boston, MA) were used for two-dimensional, M-mode, and color Doppler echocardiography. LV end-systolic and diastolic dimensions (LVEDD), septal and posterior wall thickness, LV ejection fraction (EF), and diastolic function, left ventricular mass index (LVMI) were measured according to the ASE guidelines[3,4]. All patients were classified into the following 4 groups according to the ASE guidelines: normal geometry (NG; normal LVMI and normal RWT), concentric remodeling (CR; normal LVMI and increased RWT), concentric hypertrophy (CH; increased LVMI and increased RWT) and eccentric hypertrophy (EH; increased LVMI and normal RWT).

BP, CAVI, EF and e' in various left ventricular geometries

As shown in Fig. 1, systolic BP (SBP) and diastolic BP (DBP) were significantly higher in the order of NG, CR and CH, respectively. Arterial stiffness evaluated by CAVI was higher in CR and CH than in NG. In contrast, BP and CAVI were not higher in EH compared to CH (SBP; 131 to 143, p < 0.001. DBP; 78 to 84, p < 0.001. CAVI; 8.8 to 9.4, p < 0.05). These results suggested that hypertension and high CAVI might be involved in the formation of CR and CH.

Next, cardiac functions were compared among 4 groups. EF was maintained in NG and CR, but decreased significantly in CH, and decreased further in EH. On the other hand, é decreased significantly in the order of NG, CR and CH. However, this trend was not recognized in EH. These results suggested that CR and CH was related to heart

[1]Department of Internal Medicine, Toho University Sakura Medical Center, 564-1 Shimoshizu, Sakura City, Chiba 285-8741, Japan.
[2]Department of Clinical Functional Physiology, Toho University Sakura Medical Center, 564-1 Shimoshizu, Sakura City, Chiba 285-8741, Japan.

Table 1.   Study subjects. Adapted from ref.8

	NG (n = 157)	CR (n = 435)	CH (n = 412)	EH (n = 42)	P value
Men (%)	102 (65)	313 (72)	274 (67)	31 (74)	n.s.
Age (year)	64.0 (59.0, 69.0)	66.0 (59.0, 71.0)	66.0 (58.0, 73.8)	63.0 (57.0, 71.5)	n.s.
Height (cm)	163.6 ± 8.7	163.3 ± 8.7	162.1 ± 9.3	164.2 ± 8.1	n.s.
BW (kg)	64.1 ± 12.0	66.2 ± 13.4	66.6 ± 13.1	68.3 ± 12.1	n.s.
BMI (kg/m^2)	23.6 (21.8, 25.5)	23.9 (22.1, 26.4)	25.0 (22.6, 27.6)	24.8 (21.8, 28.3)	**NG to CH
HR (bpm)	64 (58, 71)	66 (60, 76)	67 (59, 77)	67 (62, 78)	*NG to CR **NG to CH
Cre (mg/dl)	0.79 (0.67, 0.92)	0.82 (0.69, 0.96)	0.86 (0.71, 1.10)	0.88 (0.75, 1.11)	***NG to CH ***CR to CH
TC (mg/dl)	187 ± 41	196 ± 42	195 ± 45	184 ± 39	n.s.
TG (mg/dl)	144 ± 130	150 ± 110	144 ± 125	120 ± 64	n.s.
LDL (mg/dl)	106 ± 35	114 ± 36	116 ± 36	109 ± 34	*NG to CH
HDL (mg/dl)	55 ± 15	52 ± 16	51 ± 15	49 ± 15	* NG to CH

Values expressed as mean (SD) or number (%), and median (interquartile range).
*p < 0.05, **p < 0.01, ***p < 0.001

Abbreviations: NG, normal geometry; CR, concentric remodeling; CH, concentric hypertrophy; EH, eccentric hypertrophy; BW, body weight; BMI, body mass index; HR, heart rate; bpm, beats per minute; Cre, creatinine; TC, total cholesterol; TG, triglycerides; LDL, low-density lipoprotein cholesterol; HDL, high-density lipoprotein cholesterol.

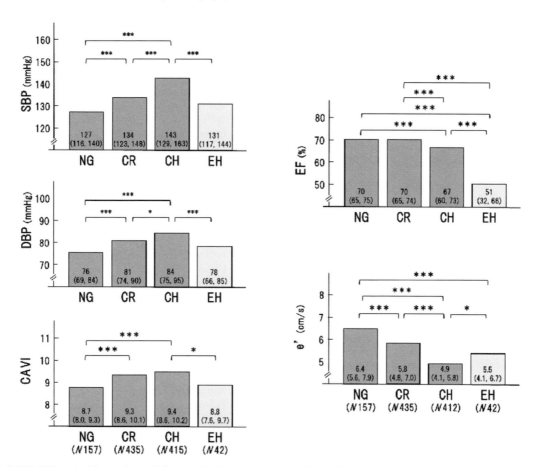

Fig. 1.   BP, CAVI, EF and e' in various left ventricular geometries. Cited from ref.8

Abbreviations: SBP: systolic blood pressure; DBP diastolic blood pressure; CAVI: cardio ankle vascular index; EF: ejection fraction; e': spectral doppler tissue velocities of the septal mitral annulus; NG: normal geometry; CR: concentric remodeling; CH: concentric hypertrophy; EH: eccentric hypertrophy.

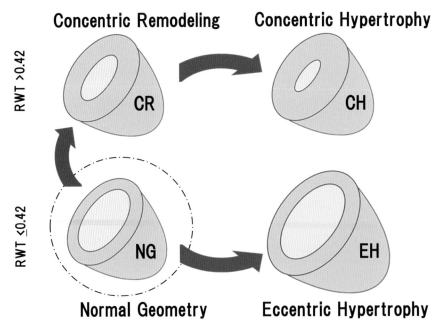

Concentric Remodeling   **Concentric Hypertrophy**

RWT >0.42   CR   CH

RWT ≤0.42   NG   EH

Normal Geometry   **Eccentric Hypertrophy**

LVMI <96 g/ m² in females, <116 g/ m² in males   LVMI ≥96 g/ m² in females, ≥116 g/ m² in males

Fig. 2. Two possible paths of left ventricular remodeling. Cited from ref.8

failure with reduced ejection fraction and preserved ejection fraction, whereas, EH was mainly related to heart failure with reduced ejection fraction.

We thought that CR and CH were apparently the same series of LV remodeling, whereas EH was seemed to be another continuum as shown in Fig. 2.

In a multiple regression analyses, CAVI was a significant factor for RWT in the NG, CR and CH groups (β 0.152, $P<0.001$) in addition to HR, SBP, Cre, LDL and HDL. In NG and EH groups, CAVI was the only significant factor (β 0.187, $P<0.01$). As for LVMI, multiple regression analysis showed that CAVI was the significant factor in the NG, CR and CH groups (β 0.068, $P<0.05$), but was not in the NG and EH groups.

Conclusion

These results supported the idea that CR and CH were apparently the same series of LV remodeling mainly affected by systolic blood pressure and CAV, whereas EH might be more related to myocardium dysfunction itself.

References

1) Dzau VJ, Antman EM, Black HR, Hayes DL, Manson JE, Plutzky J, et al. The cardiovascular disease continuum validated: clinical evidence of improved patient outcomes: part I: Pathophysiology and clinical trial evidence (risk factors through stable coronary artery disease). Circulation. 2006; 114: 2850-2870.
2) Muresan ML, Salvetti M, Monteduro C, Bonzi B, Paini A,

Viola S, et al. Left ventricular concentric geometry during treatment adversely affects cardiovascular prognosis in hypertensive patients. Hypertension. 2004; 43: 731–738.
3) Lang RM, Bierig M, Devereux RB, Flachskampf FA, Foster E, Pellikka PA, et al. Chamber Quantification Writing Group; American Society of Echocardiography's Guidelines and Standards Committee; European Association of Echocardiography. Recommendations for chamber quantification: A report from the American Society of Echocardiography's Guidelines and Standards Committee and the Chamber Quantification Writing Group, developed in conjunction with the European Association of Echocardiography, a branch of the European Society of Cardiology. J Am Soc Echocardiogr. 2005; 18: 1440–1463.
4) Lang RM, Badano LP, Mor-Avi V, Afilalo J, Armstrong A, Ernande L, et al. Recommendations for cardiac chamber quantification by echocardiography in adults: an update from the American Society of Echocardiography and the European Association of Cardiovascular Imaging. J Am Soc Echocardiogr. 2015; 28: 1–39.e14.
5) Devereux RB, Roman MJ. Left ventricular hypertrophy in hypertension: Stimuli, patterns, and consequences. Hypertens Res. 1999; 22: 1–9.
6) Koren MJ, Devereux RB, Casale PN, Savage DD, Laragh JH. Relation of left ventricular mass and geometry to morbidity and mortality in uncomplicated essential hypertension. Ann Intern Med.1991; 114: 345–352.
7) Shimizu K, Tabata T, Kiyokawa H, et al. A Case Demonstrating the Cardio-Vascular Interaction by a New Cardio-Ankle Vascular Index During the Treatment of Concentric Hypertrophy. Cardiol Res. 2019; 10:54-58.
8) Shimizu K, Tabata T, Sasaki T, et al. The Relationship Between Various Left Ventricular Geometries and the Cardio Ankle Vascular Index. Journal of Cardiology and Vascular Medicine. 2020; 8: 1-11.

Heart Failure Treatment and CAVI

Masahiro Ohira

Summary

1. CAVI levels are high in patients with impaired cardiac function.
2. In the acute stage of heart failure, CAVI shows a high value, significantly improving with heart failure treatment.

Introduction

Heart failure is "a clinical syndrome where dyspnea, malaise, and edema appear as a result of the failure of compensatory mechanism of cardiac pump function caused by organic and/or functional heart abnormalities, lowering exercise tolerance." Arterial stiffness is closely related to left ventricular afterload, and elevated afterload is a trigger of heart failure. Thus, it is easy to imagine that Cardio-Ankle Vascular Index (CAVI), an indicator of arterial stiffness, is associated with heart failure. This article reviews the relationship between cardiac function and heart failure treatment with CAVI.

Cardiac Function and CAVI

Patients with reduced left ventricular contractility have elevated CAVI even in the absence of heart failure (Fig. 1)[1]. BNP (brain natriuretic peptide) is increased in heart failure with increased wall stress, mainly due to its increased secretion in response to ventricular wall stress (stretch stress) and used in the clinic as an indicator of heart failure. In hypertensive patients without heart failure, blood BNP is significantly correlated with CAVI (Fig. 2)[2]. These results indicate that CAVI is elevated even in the absence of heart failure but with reduced left ventricular contractility or during stretch stress in the left ventricle. Although not all factors contributing to higher CAVI in these conditions are related to increased afterload, CAVI is associated with cardiac function.

Heart Failure Treatment and CAVI

CAVI is high in the acute phase of heart failure and significantly improves after heart failure treatment[3].

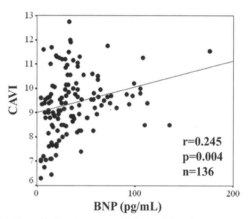

Fig. 2. Correlation between BNP and CAVI in hypertensive patients. Cited from ref.2

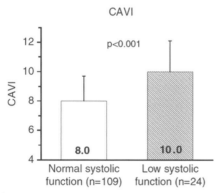

Fig. 1. CAVI in patients with normal or low left ventricular systolic function. Adapted from ref.1

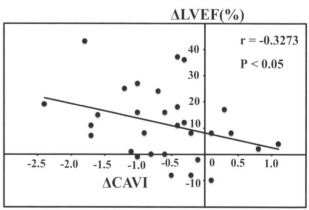

Fig. 3. Correlation between LVEF and CAVI changes with heart failure treatment.

△ change before and after heart failure treatment
LVEF: left ventricular ejection fraction, CAVI: Cardio-Ankle Vascular Index. Cited from ref.3

Division of Diabetes, Metabolism and Endocrinology, Department of Internal medicine, Toho University Ohashi Medical Center, 2-17-6 Ohashi, Meguro, Tokyo, 153-8515, Japan.

Correlations between CAVI changes after heart failure treatment and changes in blood pressure, left ventricular function, and BNP showed that changes in CAVI significantly correlated with changes in left ventricular ejection fraction (LVEF) (Fig. 3)[3]. This result probably arises from heart failure treatment reducing left ventricle afterload, resulting in improved ejection fraction. In this case, the improved CAVI may reflect an afterload reduction. However, given the various disease states other than the afterload increase involved in heart failure, CAVI changes according to heart failure type should be examined in the future.

Conclusions

CAVI is high in left ventricular dysfunction, and CAVI improvement correlated with improved left ventricular ejection fraction after heart failure treatment. As such, we could evaluate disease state by measuring CAVI in cases of left ventricular dysfunction and heart failure.

Future challenges: To clarify how CAVI changes by cause and disease state of heart failure.

References

1) Schillaci G, Battista F, Settimi L, et al. Cardio-ankle vascular index and subclinical heart disease. *Hypertens Res* 2015; **38**: 68-73. https://doi.org/10.1038/hr.2014.138

2) Masugata H, Senda S, Inukai M, et al. Association of cardio-ankle vascular index with brain natriuretic peptide levelsin hypertension. J *Atheroscler Thromb* 2012; **19**: 255-262. https://doi.org/10.5551/jat.10314

3) Zhang C, Ohira M, Iizuka T, et al. Cardio-ankle vascular index relates to left ventricular ejection fraction in patients with heart failure. A retrospective study. *Int Heart J* 2013; **54**: 216-221. https://doi.org/10.1536/ihj.54.216

Cardiac Rehabilitation and CAVI

Petr Dobšák

1. Physical Activity and Arterial Stiffness

One of the common manifestations of vascular pathologies is the decrease of arterial elasticity, which is considered a key independent risk factor for the origin of cardiovascular disease[1]. This is an actual medical problem that cannot be ignored and it is very important to study effective therapeutic interventions. Gradual growth of arterial stiffness is primarily due to aging of the organism, but this process can be significantly potentiated by the effect of identifiable cardiovascular risks, including hypo- or inactivity[1,2]. Cardiovascular diseases are typically characterized by destabilization of neurohormonal regulatory mechanisms. This is the cause of the permanent increase in tonic activity of the sympathoadrenergic system and the initiator of pathological transformational changes in the arterial wall[4]. Simultaneous inhibition of vasodilator effects makes it impossible to sufficiently antagonize excessive sympathetic activity, production of pro-inflammatory cytokines and also increased oxidative stress, which is a strong inducer of endothelial dysfunction and the atherosclerotic process[5,6]. Given the varying degrees of progression of structural-functional pathologies in the arterial system, mere pharmacological intervention appears to be debatable[7,8]. It is therefore important to pay significantly more attention to preventive issues in order to stop or slow down the process of increasing arterial stiffness at an early stage. Appropriate dietary measures, smoking cessation and, above all, adequate and regular physical activity should come into consideration. Epidemiological studies published so far have shown that there is a very tight correlation between low physical fitness or inactivity and an increase in arterial stiffness and cardiovascular mortality[9,10]. Therefore, physical activity has gained significant status and recognition in clinical medicine during the last 3-4 decades. Training programs, mainly aerobic (endurance) types, are demonstrably associated with a significant reduction in cardiovascular risk factors[11,12,13]. However, the reasons for the relatively high efficiency of physical activity have not been fully elucidated yet. Most likely it is the direct action on the vascular system through known hemodynamic stimuli, such as shear stress and transmural pressure[14]. If these stimuli are regularly repeated (regular exercise training), functional, structural and metabolic changes accrue in the cardiovascular system[15]. The essence of these changes is based on biochemical signals from endothelial cells, which have a key role in the regulation of blood flow in acute and chronic adaptive processes[15]. Exercise-induced redistribution of blood flow and systemic vasodilation ("reactive hyperemia") in the arterial bed (including coronary circulation) is mediated mainly by the increased production of nitric oxide (NO) and inhibition of vasoconstrictor stimuli[16,17]. Regular aerobic training can positively affect both the structural-functional parameters of the arterial wall and the condition of atheromatous lesions. Some experimental and clinical works suggest that regular physical activity is associated with stabilization of an atherosclerotic plaque and increased collagen and elastin content[18,19]. Regular exercise also has strong anti-inflammatory effects, stabilizes autonomous dysfunction, improves the endothelial cell state and prevents pathologic arterial wall remodeling[20,21]. Besides the improvement of the endothelial cell function by restoring the positive effects of vasoactive substances (primarily NO) the reparation of their structure also occurs. This process is mediated by endothelial progenitor cells (EPC), recruited from the bone marrow depending on the level of physical activity[22]. One recent study also showed that muscle contraction stimulates the secretion of myokines[23] which create an anti-inflammatory environment in the organism and decrease the degradation of muscle tissue and strength[23].

These data *seem* to indicate that physical exercise is an effective and cheap strategy that produces positive lifestyle changes. It increases functional capacity and improves the structural-functional characteristics of the vascular system among healthy individuals but also among individuals with a high risk of cardiovascular disease or in individuals with disease manifestation[24]. Therefore, regular monitoring of arterial system function and structure should be considered as an important tool for prevention and prediction of cardiovascular risks in this population. The current increased interest in clinical evaluation of arterial stiffness provides ideal possibilities for the use of a number of non-invasive methodologies, providing valid information on the condition of large arteries. The most commonly used method is ultrasound (US) examination of the carotid arteries, determination of the augmentation index and in particular the measurement of the pulse wave velocity (PWV). The PWV measurement is still considered by many authors as the "gold standard" in examining arterial stiffness among healthy and ill individuals[25].

2. Principles of Cardiac Rehabilitation

Impressive development and investment in state-of-the-art diagnostic and therapeutic procedures for cardiovascular

Department of Sports Medicine and Rehabilitation, St. Ann's University Hospital, Faculty of Medicine, Masaryk University Brno, Czech Republic / EU.

disease in the past few decades have substantially increased survival in industrialized countries. The current medical and social challenge is the optimization of living conditions of patients without disease progression and their active participation in social and economic life. However, the final effect cannot only be achieved automatically through modern medical interventions and pharmacotherapy, but also through cardiac rehabilitation programs[26]. The AHA and the AACVPR define cardiac rehabilitation (C-RHB) programs as: *„Coordinated, multifaceted interventions designed to optimize a cardiac patient's physical, psychological, and social functioning, in addition to stabilizing, slowing, or even reversing the progression of the underlying atherosclerotic processes, thereby reducing morbidity and mortality,,*[27]. Modern programs of C-RHB respect the individual needs and health conditions of each patient. All patients should receive complex treatment provided by a specialized team of cardiologists, nurses, dieticians, physiotherapists with specialization in cardiovascular rehabilitation and psychologists. According to current guidelines the optimal length of a C-RHB program is 8-12 weeks[28,29,30,31]. Current C-RHB usually includes 3 main phases: Phase I (in-hospital); Phase II (outpatient), which may be realized as a supervised ambulatory RHB program, spa treatment or individual home exercise program. The Phase III is the phase of stabilization and adoption of a healthy lifestyle.

Phase I (early; hospital). Ideally, the C-RHB program begins in acutely hospitalized patients. The early C-RHB program should begin with light activities such as sitting in bed, exercises that encourage normal range of joining movements, and self-care (e.g. shaving or basic hygiene). Later, the patient may be more mobilized and can start walking a short distance. The patient may also engage in activities of daily living.

Phase II (outpatient, recovery). Phase II of the C-RHB program should not be launched later than 3 weeks after an acute coronary event (as soon as possible) and not later than 6 weeks after cardiac surgery. Until then walking and scar care is recommended. Most recommended is the inclusion of the patient into a specialized rehabilitation center. Exercise during the second phase of C-RHB usually takes place at 8-12 weeks and 3 times a week in the form of group therapy. During this period, the patient gradually increases his physical fitness under careful supervision of an experienced medical team. Indications and contraindications for phase II of the RHB program are listed in the applicable international guidelines[28,29,30]. Prior to enrollment in the C-RHB program, each patient should undergo a spiroergometric test to assess functional capacity and determine training intensity. The spiroergometric test is performed using a standardized protocol and in accordance with actual expert recommendations[28,29,30,31]. The training structure during the first 2 weeks of the C-RHB program includes a warm-up period (10 min), aerobic endurance training on a bicycle ergometer (40 min) and a relaxation or "cool-down" period (10 min). The intensity of aerobic training should correspond to the level of the first ventilation threshold (VT-1) determined by spiroergometry. The total

time of one training unit is usually 60 minutes. After the first 2 weeks, it is possible to add resistance exercises and adjust the structure of the training unit to a combination of aerobic (20-25 min) and resistance training (15-20 minutes). Before the beginning of the combined training, all patients must be examined by the 1-RM test (one-repetition maximum test is defined as the maximal weight that can be lifted once by proper lifting technique on a resistance machine), informed about proper exercise techniques (including prevention of the Valsalva maneuver) and acquainted with the whole composition of the resistance training. The results of the 1-RM test (for each type of resistance exercise) are important for the determination of exercise load of 30%, 40%, 50% a 60% 1-RM. The resistance training usually consists of a variety of specific exercises, such as bench-press, leg extension, pull-down the pulley in sitting position, pull-down the pulley in standing position, etc. ECG, HR, BP and RPE are continuously monitored during the whole exercise period. Besides that, it is important to carefully watch any signs of bad tolerance of the exercise, such as excessive dyspnea, angina pectoris, significantly increased heart rate, episodes of bradycardia or arrhythmias, dizziness, signs of collapse, etc. Another important task for the C-RHB team is to recommend the patient appropriate exercise for home, such as walking, bicycling, swimming, etc. The overall goal of the outpatient program of Phase II C-RHB is not only to improve the patient's overall condition, but also to motivate the patient to adopt a healthy lifestyle, to engage in regular physical exercise, to have a healthy diet, to support their mental health, the resumption of sexual activity, social support and permanent smoking cessation. In most industrialized countries, Phase I and II costs for cardiovascular rehabilitation are covered by public health insurance.

Phase III (regeneration and stabilization). In brief, Phase III is a long-term maintenance program, something that needs to be followed for the rest of a patient's life. During this period the patient should adopt a regular exercise routine in his home environment or in a local fitness center. If the patient continues to have serious health problems, he can keep exercising in the cardio-rehabilitation center and thus stay under medical supervision. The patient continues to be educated in the fields of nutrition, lifestyle, maintaining optimal weight, etc. Maximum success is considered to be creating the lifelong habits of regular exercise and a healthy lifestyle.

3. CAVI and Supervised Exercise Training in Patients with Cardiovascular Diseases

Studies that examine the influence of physical activity on arterial stiffness among healthy individuals support the theory that aerobic and resistance training lower the PWV among individuals of all age categories[32,33]. However, despite all the evidence, recommendations and experience about the importance of physical activity in reducing cardiovascular risk, there are currently only a few controlled clinical trials, that have looked at the interactions between physical activity and arterial stiffness in patients with cardiovascular disease[34]. Despite the limited amount of information, the conclusions of these studies confirm that different types of training (aerobic, resistance or combined) in cardiac rehabilitation significantly reduce arterial stiffness, objectified mainly by the PWV or augmentation index[35,36,37]. From the point of view of general clinical practice, the measurement of PWV is suitable for the diagnosis of arteriosclerosis in any part of the arterial bed. It should however be noted that the PWV measurement may not accurately reflect the actual condition of the vascular system due to some limitations of this method[38,39]. An alternative tool of measuring arterial stiffness is currently the evaluation of the CAVI parameter, which overcomes some significant disadvantages of PWV[38,39]. However, as in the case of PWV (and other methodologies), there is actually very little experience with the use of the CAVI parameter to monitor changes in arterial stiffness due to physical activity. The known results of CAVI measurements in healthy population samples show that this recently introduced parameter very accurately reflects changes in arterial stiffness due to exercise. It confirms that regular aerobic exercise may be important for reducing arterial stiffness in young healthy individuals[40], as well as in middle-aged and older people[41,42]. An even greater information vacuum exists when the CAVI parameter is used to monitor changes in arterial stiffness due to aerobic or combined endurance training in patients with cardiac disease. One of the first information (and so far, unique) comes from a randomized clinical study from the year 2012 which measured CAVI in a cohort of patients (n = 61) with a stable form of chronic heart failure[43]. The patients were divided into two groups, one of which performed supervised aerobic training in the rehabilitation center (in a regime of 60 min/day, 3 times a week); and the second group applied low-frequency neuromuscular electrical stimulation (NMES; frequency 10Hz; maximal amplitude 60mA; working mode "20s on - 20s off") of the lower limb extensors in their home

environment (in a regime of 2x60min/day). In both groups, training of the given type lasted for a total of 12 weeks. Comparing the results of the values measured before and after the end of the training program showed that in both groups there was a significant reduction in the average value of CAVI (Fig. 1).

At the same time, there was a significant improvement in other crucial functional parameters, especially the average value of VO_{2peak}. The positive effect of both types of training was also proven by spectral analysis of the parameter HRV (heart rate variability): a decrease in sympathicotonia was found in both groups and a positive shift towards an increase in parasympathetic tone and an overall stabilization of the autonomic balance. There is a very close relationship between the parameters of functional capacity (fitness), the autonomic nervous system and arterial stiffness. Therefore, the results obtained can be considered as a valid confirmation of the positive global effectiveness of regular physical activity on the cardiovascular system in patients with chronic heart failure[43]. Between the years 2017-2020 an extensive clinical study was performed at the St. Ann´s University Hospital in Brno, Czech Republic. 223 patients with ischemic coronary artery disease or CAD (177 men; 46 women; average age 61 ± 11.5 years), underwent 12 weeks of supervised combined training in the RHB program center (the training structure was identical with the description of Phase II in the previous text). The average active participation of patients included in the final study evaluation was 88%. Based on the existing classification scheme, patients were divided into three groups according to the average baseline CAVI value and based on valid recommendations: CAVI < 8.0 is considered normal, CAVI 8 - 9 is considered borderline and in CAVI > 9.0 atherosclerosis is suspected[44]. Analysis of the results revealed a statistically significant decrease in the mean CAVI value by -0.2 (P < 0.001) after 6 weeks and by a

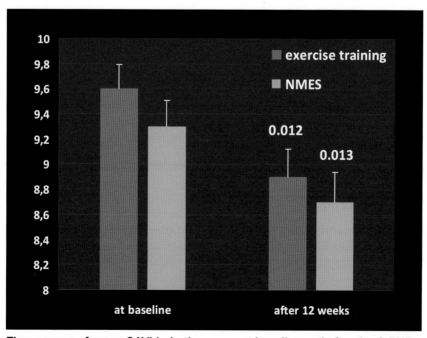

Fig. 1. Time-course of mean CAVI in both groups at baseline and after the C-RHB program.

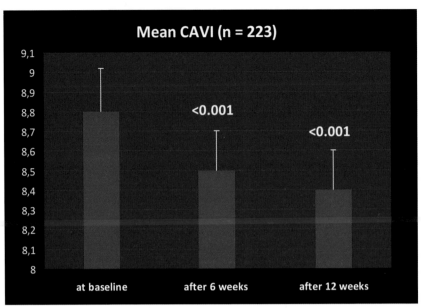

Fig. 2.   Time-course of mean CAVI change in the whole analyzed group (n = 223).

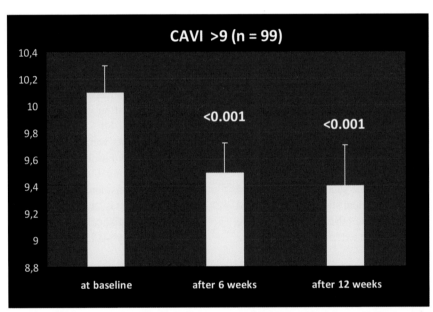

Fig. 3.   Time-course of mean CAVI change in group with CAVI > 9.0 (n = 99).

further -0.2 (P < 0.001) after 12 weeks compared to the baseline value (Fig. 2).

Statistical processing of the results also showed that the highest rate of decrease in mean CAVI was observed in the group of patients with the highest risk, i.e. with CAVI above 9 (Fig. 3). In other words, the worst affected patients benefited most from the supervised cardiovascular rehabilitation program.

A reduction in the mean CAVI value was also present in the two remaining groups, but with lower statistical significance or only with a trend to improve arterial stiffness (Fig. 4 and 5).

From the overall point of view, however, it is possible to conclude that the chosen type and length of the C-RHB program demonstrably reduces arterial stiffness as evaluated by the CAVI parameter. This finding is further supported by

a statistically significant improvement of the main functional parameters, especially the average value of VO_{2peak}/kg in the whole examined group (from 18.9 ± 4.2 to 21.2 ± 3.7 mlO_2/kg; $P < 0.002$). This clinical study is one of the first attempts to objectify changes in arterial stiffness due to controlled physical activity in a larger group of patients with CAD using the CAVI parameter. At the same time, however, it should be emphasized that the study was not randomized and a control group was absent. However, this does not diminish the clinical significance of the observations made. On the contrary, the results should motivate further intensive study of the effects of regular physical activity on arterial stiffness, not only in patients with cardiovascular disease. *The results of this study have not been published anywhere so far*.

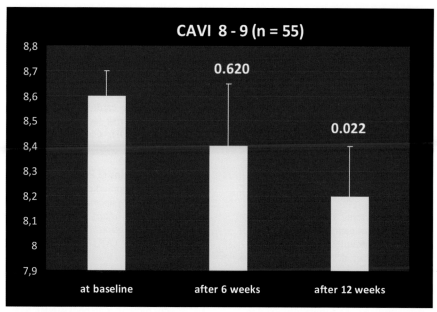

Fig. 4.   Time-course of mean CAVI change in group with CAVI 8.0 - 9.0 (n = 55).

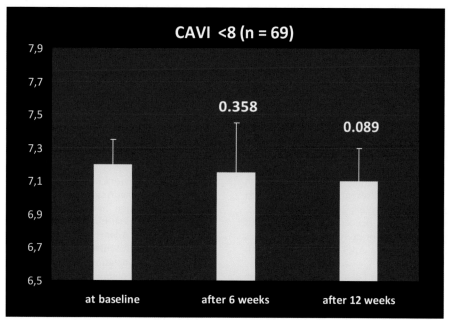

Fig. 5.   Time-course of mean CAVI change in group with CAVI < 8.0 (n = 69).

Conclusion

Aerobic training combined with training containing resistance elements can significantly lower arterial stiffness. This is objectified by the CAVI parameter in patients with cardiovascular disease. Regular physical activity is not only a traditional auxiliary tool of preventing the negative effects of aging, but also an unquestionable therapeutic intervention and evolutionary stimulus to maintain a healthy vascular system. Many questions, however, still remain unanswered. In particular, it is not entirely clear how to accurately determine the optimal length, type and intensity of exercise training needed to achieve the greatest benefit to the structural-functional properties of the arterial wall. Thus, the future creation and clinical application of exercise training programs should focus on a detailed identification of the

mechanisms that initiate positive changes in the arterial wall. The expected result would be not only a beneficial effect on the structure and remodeling of the arterial wall but also a global reduction of the emergence of cardiovascular pathologies.

Bibliography

1) Arnett DK, Evans GW, Riley WA. Arterial stiffness: A new cardiovascular risk factor? Am J Epidemiol 1994; 140: 669-82.

2) Lacolley P, Challande P, Osborne-Pellegrin M, Regnault V. Genetics and pathophysiology of arterial stiffness. Cardiovasc Res 2009; 81: 637-48.

3) Lavie CJ, Arena R, Swift DL et al. Exercise and the

cardiovascular system: clinical science and cardiovascular outcomes. Circ Res 2015; 117: 207-19.

4) Palombo C, Kozakova M. Arterial stiffness, atherosclerosis and cardiovascular risk: Pathophysiologic mechanisms and emerging clinical indications. Vascul Pharmacol 2016; 77: 1-7.

5) Yang X, Li Y, Li Y et al. Oxidative stress-mediated atherosclerosis: Mechanisms and therapies. Front Physiol 2017; 8: 600.

6) Marchio P, Guerra-Ojeda S, Vila JM et al. Targeting early atherosclerosis: A focus on oxidative stress and inflammation. Oxid Med Cell Longev 2019; 2019: 8563845.

7) Alvim RO, Santos PCJL, Bortolotto LA et al. Arterial Stiffness: Pathophysiological and genetic aspects. Int. J. Cardiovasc. Sci 2017; 30: 433-41.

8) Sakuragi S, Abhayaratna WP. Arterial stiffness: methods of measurement, physiologic determinants and prediction of cardiovascular outcomes. Int J Cardiol 2010; 138: 112-18.

9) Warren TY, Barry V, Hooker SP et al. Sedentary behaviors increase risk of cardiovascular disease mortality in men. Med Sci Sports Exerc 2010; 42: 879–85.

10) Smulyan H, Lieber A, Safar ME. Hypertension, diabetes type II, and their association: Role of arterial stiffness. Am J Hypertens 2016; 29: 5-13.

11) Woodcock J, Franco OH, Orsini N et al. Non-vigorous physical activity and all-cause mortality: systematic review and meta-analysis of cohort studies. International journal of epidemiology 2011; 40: 121-38.

12) Howden EJ, Sarma S, Lawley JS et al. Reversing the cardiac effects of sedentary aging in middle age; A randomized controlled trial: Implications for heart failure prevention. Circulation 2018; 137: 1549–60.

13) Piepoli MF, Hoes AW, Agewall S et al. 2016 European Guidelines on cardiovascular disease prevention in clinical practice: The Sixth Joint Task Force of the European Society of Cardiology and Other Societies on Cardiovascular Disease Prevention in Clinical Practice (constituted by representatives of 10 Societies and by invited experts) developed with the special contribution of the European Association for Cardiovascular Prevention & Rehabilitation (EACPR). Atherosclerosis 2016; 252: 207–74.

14) Laughlin MH, Newcomer SC, Bender SB. Importance of hemodynamic forces as signals for exercise-induced changes in endothelial cell phenotype. J Appl Physiol 2008; 104: 588–600.

15) Green DJ, Hopman MTE, Padilla J et al. Vascular adaptation to exercise in humans: Role of hemodynamic stimuli. Physiol Rev 2017; 97: 495–528.

16) Maiorana A, O'Driscoll G, Taylor R et al. Exercise and the nitric oxide vasodilator system. Sports Med 2003; 33: 1013–35.

17) Maeda S, Miyauchi T, Kakiyama T et al. Effects of exercise training of 8 weeks and detraining on plasma levels of endothelium-derived factors, endothelin-1 and nitric oxide, in healthy young humans. Life Sci 2001; 69: 1005-16.

18) Shimada K, Mikami Y, Murayama T et al. Atherosclerotic plaques induced by marble-burying behavior are stabilized by exercise training in experimental atherosclerosis. Int J Cardiol 2011; 151: 284–89.

19) Madssen E, Moholdt T, Videm V et al. Coronary atheroma regression and plaque characteristics assessed by grayscale and radiofrequency intravascular ultrasound after aerobic exercise. Am J Cardiol 2014; 114: 1504–11.

20) Sallam N, Laher I. Exercise modulates oxidative stress and inflammation in aging and cardiovascular diseases. Oxid Med Cell Longev 2016; 7239639.

21) Scheffer DDL, Latini A. Exercise-induced immune system response: Anti-inflammatory status on peripheral and central organs. Biochim Biophys Acta Mol Basis Dis 2020; 1866: 165823.

22) Cavalcante SL, Lopes S, Bohn L et al. Effects of exercise on endothelial progenitor cells in patients with cardiovascular disease: A systematic review and meta-analysis of randomized controlled trials. Rev Port Cardiol 2019; 38: 817-27.

23) Fiuza-Luces C, Santos-Lozano A, Joyner M et al. Exercise benefits in cardiovascular disease: beyond attenuation of traditional risk factors. Nat Rev Cardiol 2018; 15: 731-43.

24) Thijssen DH, Cable NT, Green DJ. Impact of exercise training on arterial wall thickness in humans. Clin Sci 2012; 122: 311-22.

25) Vlachopoulos C, Xaplanteris P, Aboyans V et al. The role of vascular biomarkers for primary and secondary prevention. A position paper from the European Society of Cardiology Working Group on peripheral circulation. Endorsed by the Association for Research into Arterial Structure and Physiology (ARTERY) Society. Atherosclerosis 2015; 241: 507-32.

26) Tessler J, Bordoni B. Cardiac Rehabilitation. [Updated 2020 Sep 13]. In: StatPearls [Internet]. Treasure Island (FL): StatPearls Publishing; 2020. Available from: https://www.ncbi.nlm.nih.gov/books/NBK537196/

27) Leon AS, Franklin BA, Costa F et al. Cardiac rehabilitation and secondary prevention of coronary heart disease: an American Heart Association scientific statement from the Council on Clinical Cardiology (Subcommittee on Exercise, Cardiac Rehabilitation, and Prevention) and the Council on Nutrition, Physical Activity, and Metabolism (Subcommittee on Physical Activity), in collaboration with the American association of Cardiovascular and Pulmonary Rehabilitation. Circulation 2005; 111: 369-76.

28) Mezzani A, Hamm LF, Jones AM et al. European Association for Cardiovascular Prevention and Rehabilitation; American Association of Cardiovascular and Pulmonary Rehabilitation; Canadian Association of Cardiac Rehabilitation. Aerobic exercise intensity assessment and prescription in cardiac rehabilitation: A joint position statement of the European Association for Cardiovascular Prevention and Rehabilitation, the American Association of Cardiovascular and Pulmonary Rehabilitation and the Canadian Association of Cardiac Rehabilitation. Eur J Prev Cardiol 2013; 20: 442-67.

29) Guazzi M, Adams V, Conraads V et al. European Association for Cardiovascular Prevention & Rehabilitation; American Heart Association. EACPR/AHA Scientific Statement. Clinical recommendations for cardiopulmonary exercise testing data assessment in specific patient populations. Circulation 2012; 126: 2261-74.

30) Piepoli MF, Corra U, Benzer W et al. Cardiac Rehabilitation Section of the European Association of Cardiovascular Prevention and Rehabilitation. Secondary prevention through cardiac rehabilitation: from knowledge to implementation. A position paper from the Cardiac Rehabilitation Section of the European Association of Cardiovascular Prevention and Rehabilitation. Eur J Cardiovasc Prev Rehabil 2010; 17: 1-17.

31) Sietsema KE, Sue DY, Stringer WW et al. Wasserman & Whipp's Principles of Exercise Testing and Interpretation: Including Pathophysiology and Clinical Applications. 6th ed. Philadelphia Lippincott Williams Wilkins, 2020. 572 p.

32) Ashor AW, Lara J, Siervo M et al. Effects of exercise modalities on arterial stiffness and wave reflection: a systematic review and meta-analysis of randomized controlled trials. PLoS One 2014; 9: e110034.

33) Okamoto T, Masuhara M, Ikuta K. Low-intensity resistance training after high-intensity resistance training can prevent the increase of central arterial stiffness. Int J Sports Med 2013; 34: 385-90.

34) Oliveira NL, Alves AJ, Ruescas-Nicolau MA et al. Arterial

Stiffness is Associated With Moderate to Vigorous Physical Activity Levels in Post-Myocardial Infarction Patients. J Cardiopulm Rehabil Prev 2019; 39: 325-330.

35) Oliveira NL, Ribeiro F, Silva G et al. Effect of exercise-based cardiac rehabilitation on arterial stiffness and inflammatory and endothelial dysfunction biomarkers: a randomized controlled trial of myocardial infarction patients. Atherosclerosis 2015; 239: 150-7.

36) Montero D, Vinet A, Roberts CK. Effect of combined aerobic and resistance training versus aerobic training on arterial stiffness. Int J Cardiol 2015; 178: 69-76.

37) Zhang Y, Qi L, Xu L et al. Effects of exercise modalities on central hemodynamics, arterial stiffness and cardiac function in cardiovascular disease: Systematic review and meta-analysis of randomized controlled trials. PLoS One 2018; 13: e0200829.

38) Saiki A, Sato Y, Watanabe R et al. The Role of a novel arterial stiffness parameter, cardio-ankle vascular index (CAVI), as a surrogate marker for cardiovascular diseases. J Atheroscler Thromb 2016; 23: 155-68.

39) Shirai K, Utino J, Otsuka K et al. A novel blood pressure-independent arterial wall stiffness parameter; cardio-ankle vascular index (CAVI). J Atheroscler Thromb 2006; 13: 101–7.

40) Wang H, Zhang T, Zhu W et al. Acute effects of continuous and interval low-intensity exercise on arterial stiffness in healthy young men. Eur J Appl Physiol 2014; 114: 1385-92.

41) Endes S, Caviezel S, Schaffner E et al. Associations of Novel and Traditional Vascular Biomarkers of Arterial Stiffness: Results of the SAPALDIA 3 Cohort Study. PLoS One 2016; 11: e0163844.

42) Kobayashi R, Kasahara Y, Ikeo T et al. Effects of different intensities and durations of aerobic exercise training on arterial stiffness. J Phys Ther Sci 2020; 32: 104-9.

43) Dobsak P, Tomandl J, Spinarova L et al. Effects of neuromuscular electrical stimulation and aerobic exercise training on arterial stiffness and autonomic functions in patients with chronic heart failure. Artif Organs 2012; 36: 920-30.

44) Saiki A, Ohira M, Yamaguchi T, Nagayama D, Shimizu N, Shirai K, Tatsuno I. New Horizons of Arterial Stiffness Developed Using Cardio-Ankle Vascular Index (CAVI). J Atheroscler Thromb 2020; 27: 732-748.

Cardiac Rehabilitation and CAVI

Akihiro Ogawa

In the past, rest was the mainstay in the treatment of heart failure. However, in recent years, exercise therapy has been shown to be effective, and exercise methods and frequency have been explored. Aerobic exercise and resistance training are now recommended; however, the evidence is still insufficient. Not only is the heart involved in systemic circulation, but arteries also supposedly play a role. Accordingly, the involvement of "vascular function" has been assumed, but it has not been fully understood.

Recently, the Cardio-Ankle Vascular Index (CAVI) was developed as an indicator of arterial stiffness[1] and was shown to be related to cardiac function. In addition, it has been shown that the improvement in cardiac ejection fraction correlates with the degree of CAVI improvement during chronic heart failure treatment[2], allowing analysis of the mechanism by which cardiac function and vascular function cooperate and complement each other.

We report below our findings on the significance of CAVI measurements as a vascular elastic function in cardiac rehabilitation.

1. Sarcopenia and CAVI in elderly heart failure patients

Skeletal muscle dysfunction, such as muscle weakness and muscle atrophy, are considered part of the pathophysiology of heart failure, and increased cardiac load and decreased oxygen uptake during exercise due to skeletal muscle dysfunction may prevent improvement in the pathophysiology of heart failure[3].

To clarify the presence of sarcopenia in heart failure patients, we investigated 100 heart failure patients aged ≥ 65 years who underwent cardiac rehabilitation for sarcopenia complications using the Asian Sarcopenia Diagnostic Criteria[4]. The results showed that 47.0% of patients presented with sarcopenia. CAVI values were significantly higher in patients with sarcopenia, even after adjusting for age, sex, atrial fibrillation, and ischemic cardiomyopathy (Fig. 1). Furthermore, we found age and physical function, such as 6-minute walk distance as factors associated with CAVI in these patients with heart failure (Table 1). Finally, multiple regression analysis showed that the main contributing factor to CAVI was the 6-minute walk distance ($\beta = -0.334$, $p < 0.001$)[5].

This suggests that sarcopenia leads to impaired arterial stiffness and that physical function contributes to CAVI.

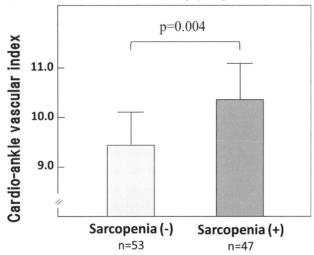

Fig. 1. CAVI in Elderly Heart Failure Patients with or without Sarcopenia. Cited from ref.5

Table 1. Correlation between CAVI and Clinical Parameters in Elderly Heart Failure Patients.
Adapted from ref.5

| | | n = 100 |
Variable	Spearman's rank correlation coefficient (ρ)	p-value
Age	0.252	0.011*
BMI	-0.017	0.867
Alb	0.067	0.511
Cre	0.184	0.066
BNP	-0.007	0.945
EF	-0.047	0.698
E/e'	0.148	0.250
sBP	0.112	0.267
dBP	0.017	0.864
HR	0.005	0.957
SMI	-0.144	0.169
Handgrip strength	-0.204	0.043*
5MWS	0.216	0.035*
5RSST	0.328	0.003**
6MWD	-0.347	0.001**

Department of Rehabilitation, Toho University Sakura Medical Center, 564-1 Shimoshizu, Sakura City, Chiba 285-8741, Japan.

2. Peak oxygen uptake and CAVI in patients with myocardial infarction

Exercise, a major pillar of cardiac rehabilitation, has many benefits, such as improving muscle strength and endurance, oxygen uptake, and inhibiting the development of atherosclerosis[6]. Oxygen uptake can be measured by the cardiopulmonary exercise test, which is an important prognostic indicator for patients with cardiac disease and an indicator of physical fitness mainly determined by cardiac function (cardiac output) and skeletal muscle function (tissue oxygenation)[7].

We investigated the relationship between oxygen uptake and CAVI values at hospital discharge in 60 patients with myocardial infarction. As shown in Fig. 2, we found a relationship between high CAVI and low oxygen uptake, further demonstrating that CAVI can act as indicator of arterial stiffness.

Therefore, we consider that exercise prescriptions based on CAVI improvement may be more effective in improving oxygen intake in exercise therapy.

3. Changes in CAVI during isometric contraction of the quadriceps

Despite the above results suggesting that CAVI improvement may lead to improved physical function, we examined whether the resistance training used in cardiac rehabilitation could actually improve CAVI.

Therefore, we investigated whether isometric contraction of the quadriceps muscle affects CAVI. We performed isometric contraction exercises on the right side of the quadriceps in 61 patients with heart failure and investigated the changes in CAVI before and after the exercises. As shown in Fig. 3, there was a significant decrease in CAVI on the right side (exercise side) immediately after exercise. In the left side, there was also a decrease in CAVI, although not significant. After 5 minutes of exercise, CAVI returned

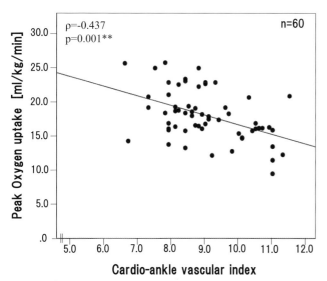

Fig. 2. CAVI and Clinical Parameters in Acute Myocardial Infarction Patients.

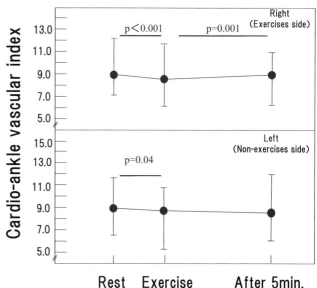

Fig. 3. Changes in CAVI with Isometric Contraction Exercises in Heart Failure Patients.

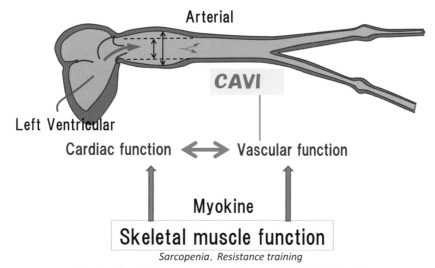

Sarcopenia, Resistance training

Fig. 4. Cardio-Vascular Coupling and Skeletal Muscle.

to its pre-exercise value. This means that short-term isometric contraction exercises may temporarily improve CAVI, and if continued for longer, the functional bullet vessel performance could be improved. Dobsak[8] reported an improvement in CAVI in heart failure patients after 12 weeks of aerobic exercise and electrical stimulation of muscle contraction.

CAVI measurements showed that exercise therapy is effective in improving muscle strength and physical function in patients with heart failure, accompanied by an improvement in vascular function. This improvement in vascular function may contribute to the corresponding one in cardiac function by decreasing cardiac afterload, suggesting that skeletal muscle function is involved in the cardio-vascular coupling (Fig. 4).

In conclusion, exercise therapy aimed to improve CAVI, as an indicator of vascular function, may be useful in future cardiac rehabilitation.

References

1) Shirai K, Utino J, et al. A novel blood pressure-independent arterial wall stiffness parameter; cardio-ankle vascular index (CAVI). *J Atheroscler Thromb* 2006; **13**: 101-7.

2) Zhang C, Ohira M, et al. Cardio-ankle vascular index relates to left ventricular ejection fraction in patients with heart failure. A retrospective study. *Int Heart J* 2013; **54**: 216-21.

3) Okita K, Kinugawa S, et al. Exercise Intolerance in Chronic Heart Failure – Skeletal Muscle Dysfunction and Potential Therapies – (REVIEW). *Circulation* 2013; **77**: 293 –300.

4) Chen LK, Liu LK, et al; Sarcopenia in Asia: Consensus Report of the Asian Working Group for Sarcopenia. *JAMDA* 2014; **15**: 95-101.

5) Ogawa A, Shimizu K, et al. Physical Function and Cardio-Ankle Vascular Index in Elderly Heart Failure Patients. *Int Heart J* 2020; **61**: 769-775. https://doi.org/10.1536/ihj.20-058

6) JCS Joint Working Group. Guidelines for rehabilitation in patients with cardiovascular disease (JCS 2012). *Circ J* 2014; **78**: 2022-93.

7) Myers J, Prakash M, et al; Exercise capacity and mortality among men referred for exercise testing. *N Engl J Med* 2002; **346**: 793-801.

8) Dobsak P, Tomandl J, et al; Effects of neuromuscular electrical stimulation and aerobic exercise training on arterial stiffness and autonomic functions in patients with chronic heart failure. *Artif Organs* 2012; **36**: 920-30.

Pulmonary Hypertension and CAVI

Yuriy Sirenko, Ganna Radchenko and Iryna Zhyvilo

Pulmonary arterial hypertension (PAH) is a rare chronic and progressive disease with unfavorable outcomes[1]. The main reason for PAH development is a proliferative and fibrotic lesion of the small pulmonary vessels caused by endothelial cell dysfunction with secretion of vasoconstrictive, inflammatory and proliferative substances with simultaneously impaired vasodilatory mechanisms (nitric oxide, prostacycline etc.). This imbalance leads to a pulmonary artery lesion accompanied by reduced vessel compliance, vasoconstriction, proliferation, remodeling and microthrombosis.

Systemic arterial stiffness in patients with pulmonary hypertension was evaluated in some studies. The objectives of these studies were well summarized in the review of N. Nickel et al.[2] It is well known that endothelial dysfunction plays a role in the development of the PAH and is the target for specific drugs in treatment of PAH patients[5]. But it is hard to imagine the isolated damage of the pulmonary arteries and no changes in the systemic arteries. Indeed, now we have some evidence indicating the systemic artery changes in pulmonary hypertension: the tendency to increase coronary heart disease prevalence in PAH patients[3, 4], the reduction in brachial artery dilation in 2.7% of patients with IPAH and 6.3% of patients with scleroderma and PAH[5], the lower cerebral blood flow at rest and with exercise in patients with PAH during the measuring of mean flow velocity in the middle cerebral artery[6], the significant albumin excretion (as marker of the endothelial dysfunction) in 15–23% of patients with PAH without known kidney disease and traditional CV risk factors[7], the morphological changes in nailfold capillaries and sublingual vessels[8].

These systemic artery changes could be mediated by some factors. The first one is genetic. The bone morphogenetic protein receptor type 2 (BMPR2) mutation could be found in 75% heritable PAH[9] and its presence was associated with proteinuria and increased C-reactive protein level in NP. Nickel et al. study[7]. The authors considered that BMPR2 signaling has an impact on vascular homeostasis through the expression of collagen 4, ephrin A1, endothelial nitric oxide, caveolin-1 and others[10, 11] and therefore, reduced BMPR2 signaling could influence the renal perfusion and protein handling (leads to albuminuria), cytokine circulation.

The second factor is systemic inflammation. A study by E. Soon and colleagues found increased levels of tumor necrosis factor-α, interferon-γ and some interleukins in patients with IPAH and HPAH compared to the control group[12]. The patients with elevated interleukin-6 had worse survival[12]. In the review by N. Nickel et al.[2] it was indicated that the systemic inflammation can be triggered by bacterium and their product translocation from the gastrointestinal tract into the systemic circulation. A M. Valentova's et al. study demonstrated that PAH patients have a high correlation of macrophage activation markers and circulating LPS concentrations, suggesting chronic bacterial translocation[13]. The role of inflammation markers in impairing of the aorta stiffness was reported in many publications[14-16]. Therefore, if PAH patients have increased inflammation factors in circulation it could lead to systemic artery damage.

The third factor is metabolic disorders mediated by peripheral circulation worsening, hypoxia and thyroid disorders. Poor peripheral circulation as a result of reduced cardiac output and sedentary life of PAH patients might lead to the skeletal muscle dysfunction and insulin resistance[17]. The hypoxia and thyroid dysfunction (the subclinical hypothyroidism rate in PAH ranges from 20 to 49.1% [18-20]) are associated with lipid disorders, increased oxidative stress and the circulation of proinflammation factors, that correlated with PAH parameters (PVR, right ventricle function). Thus in PAH patients the same metabolic disturbances could be found as in patients of high cardiovascular risk and they might be linked with increased systemic artery stiffness[21-26].

Systemic arterial stiffness could be evaluated by different methods[45]. The current gold standard is PWV assessment based on measurements of the time of the pulse wave passage between two points. This time depends on arterial stiffness and blood pressure. CAVI is a more direct measure of systemic artery stiffness and it has some advantages: blood pressure independence of arterial elasticity, the longer evaluated arterial segment (includes the ascending aorta and ankle) and relative simplicity with low cost. The two indices (the stiffness parameter β and the Bramwell-Hill formula) were combined for CAVI calculation[27-29]. The weak correlation with systolic blood pressure and significant better reproducibility compared to brachial-ankle PWV was demonstrated before[27, 30]. The PWV is dependent on gender and heart rate also, which is not reported for CAVI. A study of G.Schillaci et al. showed that CAVI, but not PWV, was associated with inappropriately high left ventricular masses for a given cardiac workload and with low midwall systolic function[31]. It means that CAVI may have a relationship to the left ventricular structure and function that is independent of blood pressure levels and is more sensitive than PWV. One more important feature of the CAVI measurement is its full independence from the operator.

CAVI has a very strong correlation with the stiffness

SI NSC "MD Strazhesko Institute of Cardiology" of NAMS, Kiev, Ukraine.

parameter β that was measured by transesophageal EchoCG[32] and ECG-gated multidetector CT scan[33]. The stiffness parameter β represents the logarithmic change in blood pressure required to increase the arterial diameter. That is why it is relatively independent of blood pressure. But this parameter evaluation is difficult in practice, because it needs synchronous, precise assessment of both pressure and diameter changes in a given artery[28]. Furthermore these measurements are obtained by assessing only a local segment of the artery, while CAVI reflects the artery stiffness from the origin of the aortic valve to the ankle region and blood pressure is measured at the upper arm.

The method, flow-mediated vasodilation in the brachial artery, was used in some studies for the evaluation of endothelium dysfunction in PAH[5, 34]. Abnormal brachial artery dilation was found in 2.7% of patients with IPAH and 6.3% of patients with scleroderma and the severity of the impairment significant correlated with the clinical and hemodynamic parameters of PAH patients[34]. But it is necessary to note that the flow-medicated vasodilation method reflects endothelium dysfunction, but not arterial stiffness. In contrast, in the American Heart Association recommendations CAVI obtained a rating of "Class I, level of evidence B" for evaluation of systemic arterial stiffness[35].

Thus the vascular changes in the patients with PAH are not limited to the lungs. We have a lot of evidence of vascular dysfunction in different organs, not only in the pulmonary arteries and the right heart. These systemic manifestations could be realized through metabolic disorders, inflammation activation and genetic origin-based injury which leads to systemic vascular dysfunction. That is why it is important to find these abnormalities, to evaluate their significance in the risk stratification, to manage them and improve the PAH patient survival. CAVI is a very simple parameter with good reproducibility and sensitivity for systemic arterial stiffness evaluation that was not used in PAH patients before.

Recently we published the results of our study comparing arterial stiffness parameters in patients with idiopathic PAH, systemic hypertension and healthy people who were adjusted to age[36]. The main results of this study are

presented in Table. We established that mean CAVI was the highest in the group with systemic hypertension, but did not differ significantly in comparison with mean CAVI in the group of the newly diagnosed idiopathic PAH.

The healthy persons had significant lower CAVI, PWVm and PWVe values than patients with IPAH, in spite of the comparable office and aortic blood pressure. Thus these data confirmed the primary hypothesis about increasing systemic artery stiffness in patients with pulmonary hypertension and we were the first to use CAVI for the systemic arterial stiffness evaluation in IPAH patients.

The results of our study about abnormalities in the systemic arteries of PAH patients were in agreement with other reports. Thus, N. Chamorro et al. detected the impairment of the endothelial function and increased arterial stiffness which were assessed as the reduced flow mediated dilation of the brachial artery and higher PWVe in patients with PAH in comparison with adjusted health subjects - 10.6 ± 3.9 vs 7.5 ± 6.3 (p< 0.05) and 8.4 ± 2.5 vs

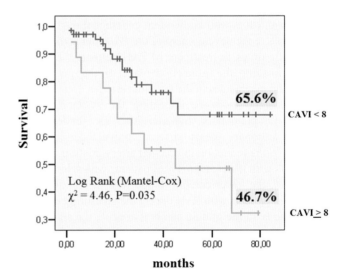

Fig. Kaplan-Meier survival of idiopathic pulmonary arterial hypertension patients (n = 89) in relation to cardio-ankle vascular index (CAVI).
[with permission of Dove Medical Press][39]

Table. Central blood pressure and arterial stiffness characteristics in groups (M ± SD).
[with permission of Dove Medical Press][36]

Patterns	Group 1 (Idiopathic PAH) n = 45	Group 2 (arterial hypertension) n = 32	Control group n = 35
Aortic SBP, mmHg	99.3 ± 10.6*	128.1 ± 20.1	101.6 ± 9,3
AIx, %	13.2 ± 10.6**	21.6 ± 17.8	13.6 ± 16.3
AIx@75, %	13.5 ± 10.6	18.4 ± 15.3	11.2 ± 9.3
PWVm, m/s	8.1 ± 1.9***#	10.3 ± 1.5	6.63 ± 1.34*
PWVe, m/s	8.49 ± 1.92*##	11.42 ± 1.70	7.29 ± 0.87*
CAVI on right side	7.40 ± 1.32###	7.19 ± 0.78	5.91 ± 0.99*
CAVI on left side	7.22 ± 1.32###	7.2 ± 1.1	5.98 ± 0.87*

* - significance P < 0.001 in comparison with group 2; ** - P < 0.033, *** - P < 0.003
\# - significance P < 0.003 in comparison with control group; ## - P < 0.008, ### - P < 0.001
CAVI - cardio-ankle vascular index, PWVm – pulse wave velocity of muscular type arteries, PWVe – pulse wave velocity of elastic type arteries, AIx – augmentation index, AIx@75 – augmentation index adjusted to heart rate 75, SBP- systolic blood pressure

7.3 ± 1.6 m/s (p < 0.05), respectively[37]. Also in patients with chronic thromboembolic pulmonary hypertension, M. Sznajder et al. found significant higher PWVe than in a control group that was matched to age, gender and concomitant diseases[38].

In the study by N.Peled et al. it was shown that endothelial dysfunction was present in idiopathic PAH and in PAH associated with scleroderma, but the peripheral arterial stiffness was normal in PAH and not correlated with PAH per se and only a tendency to be higher was found in patients with scleroderma, unrelated to the presence of PAH[34]. The differences between our and N. Peled et al. study results could be explained by the different method of the arterial stiffness evaluations. We evaluated the aorta segment stiffness, but not peripheral arterial stiffness (by finger plethysmography). The peripheral circulation could be poor in PAH patients and methods for the peripheral arterial stiffness evaluation should be less sensitive to identify its changes.

In both studies by N. Chamorro et al. and M. Sznajder et al.[37, 38] it was suggested that increased systemic arterial stiffness could be associated with poor prognosis in pulmonary hypertension, but only in our new study we tested this suggestion and confirmed that increased CAVI is associated with a higher rate of death independently from other traditional risk factors – HR = 1.13, CI 1.001-1.871. In Figure are presented Kaplan-Meier survival of IPAH patients (n = 89) in relation to CAVI level. CAVI ≥ 8 increased significantly the risk of mortality by 2.34 times (CI 1.04-5.28, P = 0.041) compared to CAVI < 8. In non-survived patients the mean CAVI was significantly higher than in survived patients – 7.8 ± 1.56 vs 6.8 ± 1.2, P = 0.004, while PWVe and PWVm did not differ significantly and were not associated with prognosis. Considering the G. Schillaci et al. study[40] results of the more prominent and strong relations of CAVI with left ventricle structure compared to PWV we could conclude that CAVI is more sensitive for the evaluation of the arterial stiffness changes in PAH patients and should be a preferable marker for survival risk stratification. However, CAVI had a significant correlation with PWV both in our study and in the G. Schillaci et al. report[36, 40].

The key question for discussion is how systemic arterial stiffness could be associated with prognosis. The one point of view is the hypothesis of reverse causality. Patients with more severe PAH course could have more enhanced endothelia dysfunction, inflammation activity and metabolic disorders that lead to an increase of systemic artery damage and the poor prognosis is mediated by not this artery damage but by the processes that were the cause of it. From the other side arterial stiffness links with the left ventricle structure and function[39, 40]. Diastolic dysfunction could be diagnosed before the left ventricle hypertrophy development in hypertensives and correlated with arterial stiffness[41]. The left ventricle function is very important for PAH patients. Usually the left ventricle suffers because of the reduced preload and the compression by the enlarged right ventricle. The rise of systemic arterial stiffness could lead to an increase of the left ventricle afterload and its functional and

structural changes. In our study we found significant correlations between CAVI and the diastolic function parameters in PAH patients that give us a reason to suggest the direct impact of increased systemic artery stiffness on the left ventricle and in this way on prognosis.

Thus for new-diagnosed idiopathic PAH population CAVI could be an independent predictor of survival as well as some other conventional and commonly accepted parameters. In future it is necessary to provide larger multicentral trials to validate this parameter as a novel predictor of death and for evaluation of its changes on treatment and their connections with prognosis.

References

1) Galiè N., Humbert M., Vachiery J.L. et al. 2015 ESC/ERS Guidelines for the diagnosis and treatment of pulmonary hypertension: The Joint Task Force for the Diagnosis and Treatment of Pulmonary Hypertension of the European Society of Cardiology (ESC) and the European Respiratory Society (ERS): Endorsed by: Association for European Paediatric and Congenital Cardiology (AEPC), International Society for Heart and Lung Transplantation (ISHLT). Eur Heart J.2016; 37(1): 67-119 doi: 10.1093/eurheartj/ehv317

2) Nickel N., Yuan K., Dorfmuller P. et al. Beyond the Lungs: Systemic Manifestations of Pulmonary Arterial Hypertension. Am J Respir Crit Care Med. 2020; 201 (2): 148-157 https://doi.org/10.1164/rccm.201903-0656CI

3) Shimony A, Eisenberg MJ, Rudski LG, Schlesinger R, Afilalo J, Joyal D, et al. Prevalence and impact of coronary artery disease in patients with pulmonary arterial hypertension. Am J Cardiol 2011;108:460–464. doi: 10.1016/j.amjcard.2011.03.066

4) Anand V, Roy SS, Archer SL, Weir EK, Garg SK, Duval S, et al. Trends and outcomes of pulmonary arterial hypertension-related hospitalizations in the United States: analysis of the nationwide inpatient sample database from 2001 through 2012. JAMA Cardiol 2016;1:1021–1029. doi: 10.1001/jamacardio.2016.3591

5) Hughes R, Tong J, Oates C, Lordan J, Corris PA. Evidence for systemic endothelial dysfunction in patients and first-order relatives with pulmonary arterial hypertension. Chest 2005;128(6, Suppl):617S. doi: 10.1378/chest.128.6_suppl.617S

6) Malenfant S, Brassard P, Paquette M, Le Blanc O, Chouinard A, Nadeau V, et al. Compromised cerebrovascular regulation and cerebral oxygenation in pulmonary arterial hypertension. J Am Heart Assoc 2017;6:e006126. doi: 10.1161/JAHA.117.006126

7) Nickel NP, de Jesus Perez VA, Zamanian RT, Fessel JP, Cogan JD, Hamid R, et al. Low-grade albuminuria in pulmonary arterial hypertension. Pulm Circ 2019;9 (2): 1-9. https://doi.org/10.1177/2045894018824564

8) Riccieri V, Vasile M, Iannace N, Stefanantoni K, Sciarra I, Vizza CD, et al. Systemic sclerosis patients with and without pulmonary arterial hypertension: a nailfold capillaroscopy study. Rheumatology (Oxford) 2013;52:1525–1528. doi: 10.1093/rheumatology/ket168

9) Soubrier F, et al. Genetics and genomics of pulmonary arterial hypertension. J Am Coll Cardiol 2013; 62: D13–D21. doi: 10.1016/j.jacc.2013.10.035

10) Rhodes CJ, et al. RNA sequencing analysis detection of a novel pathway of endothelial dysfunction in pulmonary arterial hypertension. Am J Respir Crit Care Med 2015; 192: 356–366. doi: 10.1164/rccm.201408-1528OC

11) Austin ED, et al. Whole exome sequencing to identify a

novel gene (caveolin-1) associated with human pulmonary arterial hypertension. Circ Cardiovasc Genet 2012; 5: 336–343. doi: 10.1161/CIRCGENETICS.111.961888

12) Soon E, Holmes AM, Treacy CM, et al. Elevated levels of inflammatory cytokines predict survival in idiopathic and familial pulmonary arterial hypertension. Circulation. 2010; 122: 920–927. doi: 10.1161/CIRCULATIONAHA.109.933762

13) Valentova M, von Haehling S, Bauditz J, Doehner W, Ebner N, Bekfani T, et al. Intestinal congestion and right ventricular dysfunction: a link with appetite loss, inflammation, and cachexia in chronic heart failure. Eur Heart J 2016; 37:1684–1691. doi: 10.1093/eurheartj/ehw008

14) Desjardins M., Sidibé A., Fortier C., Mac-Way F., Marquis K., De Serres S., Larivière R., Agharazii M. Association of interleukin-6 with aortic stiffness in end-stage renal disease. JASH. 2018; 12 (1): 5-13. https://doi.org/10.1016/j.jash.2017.09.013

15) Du B., Ouyang A., Eng J, Fleenor B. Aortic perivascular adipose-derived interleukin-6 contributes to arterial stiffness in low-density lipoprotein receptor deficient mice. Am J Physiol Heart Circ Physiol. 2015; 308(11): H1382–H1390.

16) Reiss A., Siegart N., De Leon J. Interleukin-6 in atherosclerosis: atherogenic or atheroprotective? Clinical Lipidology. 2017; 12 (1): 14-23. https://doi.org/10.1080/17584299.2017.1319787

17) Zamanian RT, Hansmann G., Snook S., Lilienfeld D., Rappaport KM, Reaven GM, Rabinovitch M., Doyle R.L. Insulin resistance in pulmonary arterial hypertension. Eur Respir J 2009; 33: 318–324. doi: 10.1183/09031936.00000508

18) Vakilian F, Attaran D, Shegofte M, Lari S, Ghare S. Assessment of Thyroid Function in Idiopathic Pulmonary Hypertension. Res Cardiovasc Med. 2016 Mar 5;5(2):e29361. doi: 10.5812/cardiovascmed.29361

19) Li JH, Safford RE, Aduen JF, Heckman MG, Crook JE, Burger CD. Pulmonary hypertension and thyroid disease. Chest 2007;132: 793–797. doi: 10.1378/chest.07-0366

20) Udovcic M, Pena RH, Patham B, Tabatabai L, Kansara A. Hypothyroidism and the heart. Methodist DeBakey. Cardiovasc J 2017;13:55–59. doi: 10.14797/mdcj-13-2-55

21) Rodríguez-Iturbe B, Pons H, Quiroz Y, Lanaspa MA, Johnson RJ. Autoimmunity in the pathogenesis of hypertension. Nat Rev Nephrol. 2014; 10:56–62. doi: 10.1038/nrneph.2013.248

22) Caillon A, Schiffrin EL. Role of inflammation and immunity in hypertension: recent epidemiological, laboratory, and clinical evidence. Curr Hypertens Rep. 2016; 18:21. doi: 10.1007/s11906-016-0628-7

23) McMaster WG, Kirabo A, Madhur MS, Harrison DG. Inflammation, immunity, and hypertensive end-organ damage. Circ Res. 2015; 116: 1022–1033. doi: 10.1161/CIRCRESAHA.116.303697

24) Chen TH, Gona P, Sutherland PA, et al. Long-term C-reactive protein variability and prediction of metabolic risk. Am J Med. 2009; 122: 53–61. doi: 10.1016/j.amjmed.2008.08.023

25) Tomiyama H., Shiina K., Matsumoto-Nakano C., et al. The Contribution of Inflammation to the Development of Hypertension Mediated by Increased Arterial Stiffness. Journal of the American Heart Association. 2017; 6: e005729. Available from: https://doi.org/10.1161/JAHA.117.005729

26) Mozos I, Malainer C, Horbańczuk J, Gug C, Stoian D, Luca CT, Atanasov AG. Inflammatory Markers for Arterial Stiffness in Cardiovascular Diseases. Front. Immunol. 2017; 8:1058. doi: 10.3389/fimmu.2017.01058

27) Miyoshi T., Ito H. Assessment of Arterial Stiffness Using the Cardio-Ankle Vascular Index. Pulse (Basel). 2016; 4(1): 11–23. doi: 10.1159/000445214

28) Hayashi K, Handa H, Nagasawa S, Okumura A, Moritake

K: Stiffness and elastic behavior of human intracranial and extracranial arteries. J Biomech 1980; 13: 175–184. https://doi.org/10.1016/0021-9290(80)90191-8

29) Bramwell JC, Hill AV: The velocity of the pulse wave in man. Proc R Soc B Biol Sci 1922; 93: 298–306. https://doi.org/10.1098/rspb.1922.0022

30) Kubozono T, Miyata M, Ueyama K, Nagaki A, Otsuji Y, Kusano K, Kubozono O, Tei C: Clinical significance and reproducibility of new arterial distensibility index. Circ J 2007; 71: 89–94. doi: 10.1253/circj.71.89

31) Schillaci G, Battista F, Settimi L, Anastasio F, Pucci G: Cardio-ankle vascular index and subclinical heart disease. Hypertens Res 2015; 38: 68–73. DOI: 10.1038/hr.2014.138

32) Takaki A, Ogawa H, Wakeyama T, Iwami T, Kimura M, Hadano Y, Matsuda S, Miyazaki Y, Matsuda T, Hiratsuka A, Matsuzaki M: Cardio-ankle vascular index is a new noninvasive parameter of arterial stiffness. Circ J 2007; 71: 1710–1714. https://doi.org/10.1253/circj.71.1710

33) Horinaka S, Yagi H, Ishimura K, Fukushima H, Shibata Y, Sugawara R, Ishimitsu T: Cardio-ankle vascular index (CAVI) correlates with aortic stiffness in the thoracic aorta using ECG-gated multi-detector row computed tomography. Atherosclerosis 2014; 235: 239–245. doi.org/10.1016/j.atherosclerosis.2014.04.034

34) Peled N, Shitrit D, Fox BD, Shlomi D, Amital A, Bendayan D, et al. Peripheral arterial stiffness and endothelial dysfunction in idiopathic and scleroderma associated pulmonary arterial hypertension. J Rheumatol 2009;36:970–975. doi:10.3899/jrheum.081088

35) Townsend RR, Wilkinson IB, Schiffrin EL, Avolio AP, Chirinos JA, Cockcroft JR, Heffernan KS, Lakatta EG, McEniery CM, Mitchell GF, Najjar SS, Nichols WW, Urbina EM, Weber T: Recommendations for improving and standardizing vascular research on arterial stiffness: a scientific statement from the American Heart Association. Hypertension 2015; 66: 698–722. doi.org/10.1161/HYP.0000000000000033

36) Radchenko G., Zyvilo I., Titov E., Sirenko Yu. Systemic Arterial Stiffness in New Diagnosed Idiopathic Pulmonary Arterial Hypertension Patients. Vasc Health Risk Manag. 2020;16:29-39. doi: 10.2147/VHRM.S230041

37) Chamorro N, Del Pozo R., García-Lucio J., et al. Peripheral arterial stiffness and endothelial dysfunction in pulmonary arterial hypertension. European Respiratory Journal. 2015; 46: PA2452. DOI: 10.1183/13993003.congress-2015.PA2452

38) Sznajder M., Dzikowska-Diduch O., Kurnicka K., Roik M., Wretowski D., Pruszczyk P., Kostrubiec M. Increased systemic arterial stiffness in patients with chronic thromboembolic pulmonary hypertension. Cardiol J. 2018; 7:e009459. doi: 10.5603/CJ.a2018.0109

39) Radchenko GD, Sirenko YM. Prognostic Significance of Systemic Arterial Stiffness Evaluated by Cardio-Ankle Vascular Index in Patients with Idiopathic Pulmonary Hypertension. Vasc Health Risk Manag. 2021;17:77-93. doi: 10.2147/VHRM.S294767

40) Schillaci G, Mannarino MR, Pucci G, Pirro M, Helou J, Savarese G, Vaudo G, Mannarino E. Age-specific relationship of aortic pulse wave velocity with left ventricular geometry and function in hypertension. Hypertension. 2007 Feb; 49(2):317-21. doi: 10.1161/01.HYP.0000255790.98391.9b

41) Hu Y, Li L, Shen L, Gao H The relationship between arterial wall stiffness and left ventricular dysfunction. Neth Heart J. 2013 May; 21(5):222-7. doi: 10.1007/s12471-012-0353-z

42) Kim HL, Lim WH, Seo JB, Chung WY, Kim SH, Kim MA, Zo JH. Association between arterial stiffness and left ventricular diastolic function in relation to gender and age. Medicine (Baltimore). 2017;96(1):e5783. doi: 10.1097/MD.0000000000005783

Changes in functional arterial stiffness monitored with cardio-ankle vascular index (CAVI) during hemodialysis

Shuji Sato[1], Osamu Nagakawa[2], and Junji Utino[3]

Abstract

At the time of blood pressure dropping during hemodialysis, two different responses according to CAVI fluctuations were observed. One was CAVI rising and the other was CAVI dropping, and it was considered due to different vascular responses for hemodynamic changes. Thus, monitoring arterial stiffness evaluated by CAVI during hemodialysis may make it possible to differentiate the cause of blood pressure dropping. In addition, it may help to select appropriate treatments for hypotension during hemodialysis. Measuring CAVI may play a key role in keeping a stable blood pressure during hemodialysis.

Background

Cardiac function and vascular functions are constantly changing to maintain systemic hemodynamics. Additionally, vascular functions are regulated by the central nervous system, sympathetic nervous system, and renin-angiotensin-aldosterone system. In daily clinical practice, we identify the interaction of these functions by measuring blood pressure and pulse rate without knowing vascular function itself.

Cardio-ankle vascular index (CAVI) was developed as a new blood pressure-independent arterial stiffness index by applying the stiffness parameter β theory. CAVI reflects arterial stiffness from the origin of the aorta to the ankle as a whole, and is independent from the blood pressure at measuring time. Recently, it is shown that CAVI reflects functional stiffness due to smooth muscle contraction or relaxation in addition to organic arterial stiffness[1].

During hemodialysis, the hemodynamics change due to water removal. The cardiac output decreases and systemic blood pressure usually drops due to reduced blood volume, following which, various vasoconstrictive reactions occur. Theoretically, vascular function plays an important role in maintaining constant general circulation. Considering the property of CAVI, it is assumed that CAVI might increase the reflecting contracture of the arterial smooth muscle cells by various blood pressure raising factors to keep blood pressure constant. Therefore, we measured the CAVI of hemodialysis patients during therapy, and the obtained complicated results were discussed.

Subjects and Methods

The subjects were 25 dialysis patients who received 4-hour dialysis therapy, for a total of 57 dialysis sessions at Mihama Sakura Clinic. Blood pressure (BP), heart rate (HR), CAVI, and stroke volume (SV) were measured every 30 to 60 minutes during hemodialysis. BP, HR, and CAVI were measured. Simultaneously, SV was non-invasively measured using an impedance cardiac output meter. The systemic vascular resistance (SVR) was calculated from the ratio of mean blood pressure to minute cardiac output (CO). Changes in various parameters were observed at three points: at the start of dialysis, at the maximum blood pressure dropping time (Max BDT), and after blood return.

Results

Twenty-five dialysis patients (57 dialysis sessions) were included in this study, with 68% of them being men, and median age of 67.0 years. The median dialysis duration was 7.5 years, percentage of incidence of diabetes mellitus was 28%, with 48% having a history of coronary artery disease. The mean CAVI value was 9.0 ± 1.0. The dialysis duration was 4 hours in all hemodialysis sessions, with a mean total water removal volume (TWRV) of 3129.6 ± 746.9 mL and a median Max BDT of 240.0 minutes. Echocardiographic findings showed that the mean left ventricular ejection fraction was $68.6 \pm 8.1\%$, and median E/e' was 17.4, which is suggestive of left ventricular diastolic dysfunction.

Changes in CAVI and various circulatory parameters in all the hemodialysis sessions are shown in Fig. 1. In all hemodialysis sessions, CAVI at the max BDT significantly increased compared with that at the start (CAVI: 9.0 ± 1.0-

[1]Division of Cardiovascular Medicine, Toho University Sakura Medical Center, 564-1 Shimoshizu, Sakura City, Chiba 285-8741, Japan.
[2]Seijinkai Mihama Sakura Clinic, 602-1 Shimosizu, Sakura City, Chiba 285-0841, Japan.
[3]Seijinkai Mihama Hpspital, 1-1-5 Utase, Mihatra-ku, Chiba City, Chiba 261-0013, Japan.

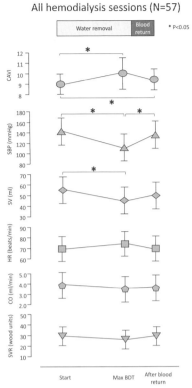

All hemodialysis sessions (N=57)

Fig. 1. Changes in CAVI and various circulatory parameters during hemodialysis in all hemodialysis sessions.

CAVI: cardio-ankle vascular index; SBP: systolic blood pressure; SV: stroke volume; HR: heart rate; CO: cardiac output; SVR: systemic vascular resistance; max BDT: maximum blood pressure dropping time.

10.0 ± 1.6; $p < 0.05$; Fig. 1). SBP and SV decreased significantly at the max BDT (SBP: 142.2 ± 25.9-110.0 ± 22.8 mmHg; SV: 55.0 ± 14.2-46.8 ± 13.1 mL; $p < 0.05$; Fig. 1). During this time, HR tended to increase and CO and SVR tended to be maintained. After blood return, SBP significantly increased; at the same time, SV increased and CAVI decreased (Fig. 1).

We expected that CAVI would increase in all hemodialysis sessions, but, about 30% dialysis sessions did not show CAVI increase. Consequently, according to CAVI fluctuation at the max BDT, 43 dialysis sessions were divided into the rising CAVI group and 14 dialysis sessions were divided into the dropping CAVI group. Changes in CAVI and various circulatory parameters in both groups are shown in Fig. 2. CAVI increased significantly from 8.9 ± 1.0 to 10.4 ± 1.6 in the rising CAVI group, whereas CAVI decreased from 9.3 ± 0.7 to 8.7 ± 0.8 in the dropping CAVI group at the max BDT (Fig. 2a and 2b). In both groups, SV tended to decrease and HR tended to increase, and CO and SVR tended to be maintained at the max BDT. Changes in SBP between both groups were not significantly different, but those of the Dropping CAVI group tended to be larger (Fig. 2c).

Correlating factors for -$\triangle$SBP during hemodialysis in the rising CAVI group and the dropping CAVI group were shown in Table 1. In the rising CAVI group, $\triangle$SV (r = 0.31, p = 0.04), and $\triangle$SVR (r = 0.51, p = 0.0005), TWRV (r = 0.51, p = 0.0004) and max BDT (r = -0.32, p = 0.03) significantly correlated with -$\triangle$SBP in the single linear analysis.

$\triangle$CAVI was not correlated with -$\triangle$SBP. In the multiple

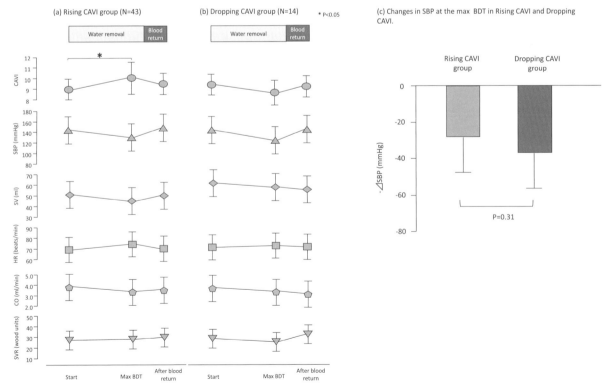

Fig. 2. Changes in CAVI and various circulatory parameters during hemodialysis in Rising CAVI group and Dropping CAVI group.

CAVI: cardio-ankle vascular index; SBP: systolic blood pressure; SV: stroke volume; HR: heart rate; CO: cardiac output; SVR: systemic vascular resistance; max BDT: maximum blood pressure dropping time.

Table 1. Correlating factors for -△SBP during hemodialysis in Rising CAVI group and Dropping CAVI group.

(a) Rising CAVI group (N = 43)

	Single linear analysis		Multiple regression analysis		
	R	P-value	β	T-value	P-value
△HR (bpm)	-0.15	0.35			
△SV (mL)	0.31	0.04	0.49	3.9	0.0004
△CO (L/min)	0.01	0.93			
△SVR (Wood units)	0.51	0.0005	0.58	4.8	<0.0001
△CAVI	-0.26	0.1			
TWRV (mL)	0.51	0.0004	-0.3	-2.8	0.008
Max BDT (min)	-0.32	0.03	-0.04	-0.35	0.73

R2 = 0.62, F-value 15.5, P<0.0001

(b) Dropping CAVI (N = 14)

	Single linear analysis		Multiple regression analysis		
	R	P-value	β	T-value	P-value
△HR (bpm)	-0.31	0.28			
△SV (mL)	0.68	0.007	0.49	1.9	0.09
△CO (L/min)	0.06	0.83			
△SVR (Wood units)	0.42	0.14			
-△CAVI	0.62	0.02	0.32	1.2	0.25
TWRV (mL)	0.26	0.48			
Max BDT (min)	-0.35	0.36			

R2 = 0.53, F-value 6.2, P=0.02

SBP: systolic blood pressure; CAVI: cardio-ankle vascular index; HR: heart rate; SV: stroke volume; CO: cardiac output; SVR: systemic vascular resistance; TWRV: total water removal volume; max BDT: maximum blood pressure dropping time.

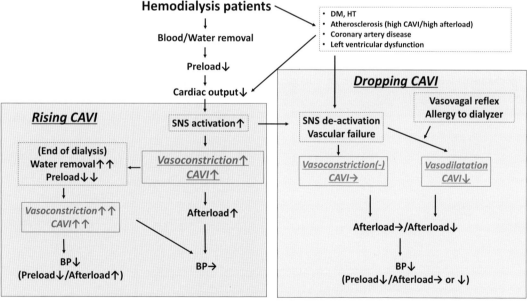

Fig. 3. The role of CAVI on maintaining hemodynamics during hemodialysis.
CAVI: cardio-ankle vascular index; DM: diabetes mellitus; HT: hypertension; SNS: sympathetic nerve system; BP: blood pressure.

regression analysis, △SV and △SVR were selected as independent contributing factors for -△SBP in the Rising CAVI group. (Table 1a).

In the dropping CAVI group, △SV (r = 0.68, p = 0.007) and -△CAVI (r = 0.62, p = 0.02) were significantly correlated with -△SBP in single linear analysis. However, in the multiple regression analysis, these were not selected as

independent contributing factors for -△SBP in the Dropping CAVI group (Table 1b).

Discussion

In this study, changes in hemodynamics and CAVI during hemodialysis were observed. The role of vascular function evaluated by CAVI on circulatory regulation mechanism was evaluated by grouping according to the fluctuation of CAVI at the max BDT. About three quarter hemodialysis sessions in the subjects were divided into the rising CAVI group, the other one quarter hemodialysis sessions were divided into the dropping CAVI group. These results suggest that there are two different blood pressure dropping mechanisms according to CAVI fluctuation.

In the rising CAVI group, independent contributing factors for $-\triangle$SBP were decrement of SV and SVR along with TWRV. This means that the direct cause of the blood pressure dropping in the rising CAVI group was the decrease in the cardiac output and vascular resistance due to water removal. As a result of the blood pressure dropping, some vasoconstrictive reactions occurred; resultantly, CAVI increased. This CAVI increment may be explained by sympathetic nerve activation against a reducing preload. Moreover, CAVI reacted differently from SVR and SBP at the max BDT. This result suggests that CAVI could reflect vascular conditions more sensitively than conventional afterload indicators such as SBP and SVR. Thus, CAVI could be quantified using vasoconstrictive reactions even in the low preload state during hemodialysis. In contrast, SBP and SV increased after blood return, and at the same time, CAVI decreased. These reactions could be explained by increment of shear stress on the vessel wall due to volume loading and subsequent increase NO production.

In the dropping CAVI group, CAVI decreased at the max BDT and changes in BP tended to be larger than those of the rising CAVI group. These results suggest that, there are some antagonistic mechanisms for vasoconstrictive reactions during hemodialysis. Although the contributing factor for $-\triangle$SBP in the dropping CAVI group was not identified, strong correlations were observed between $-\triangle$CAVI and $-\triangle$SBP. Presumably, some vasodilating reactions may occur, and possible mechanisms were presumed to be an allergic reaction to dialyzers and vasovagal reflex.

Shimizu et al. reported that functional stiffness was preserved in patients with cardiovascular disease with advanced atherosclerosis. Considering that CAVI could change during hemodialysis in this study, functional stiffness was preserved in hemodialysis patients who have advanced atherosclerosis. However, it is not clear whether this theory could be applied for all dialysis patients. As a hypothesis, there may be patients with vascular failure in whom functional stiffness was not preserved and CAVI did not change with hemodynamic changes. To clarify the potential mechanisms for preservation of functional stiffness in dialysis patients, further investigations are required.

The results of this study suggested that vascular function evaluated by CAVI plays an important role in maintaining hemodynamics during hemodialysis (Fig. 3). In any case, by measuring CAVI during dialysis as performed in this study, it may be possible to distinguish the pathophysiological conditions during blood pressure dropping, and the appropriate treatment for hypotension during hemodialysis could be selected by evaluating CAVI fluctuations. Further studies are necessary to establish the concept of vascular function in the circulatory regulation mechanism during hemodialysis.

References

1) Shirai K, Song M, Suzuki J, Kurosu T, Oyama T, Nagayama D, et al. Contradictory effects of β1- and α1-adrenergic receptor blockers on cardio-ankle vascular stiffness index (CAVI): CAVI is independent of blood pressure. J Atheroscler Thromb. 2011;18:49−55.
2) Shimizu K, Yamamoto T, Takahashi M, Sato S, Noike H, Shirai K. Effect of nitroglycerin administration on cardio-ankle vascular index. Vasc Health Risk Manag. 2016;12:313−9.

Effects of Nitroglycerin administration on CAVI in Patients with Coronary artery disease

Kazuhiro Shimizu[1] and Tomoyuki Yamamoto[2]

Introduction

Nitric oxide (NO) released from the vascular endothelium has a major influence on basal arteriolar tone and blood pressure[1,2]. The salutary effects of nitroglycerin (NTG) in patients with angina pectoris are thought to be the result of the widespread action of the drug as a smooth muscle vasodilator[3]. It has been suggested that NTG not only dilates the veins but also increases the dilation of peripheral muscular arteries and may decrease systemic resistance. Until the advent of Cardio Ankle Vascular Index (CAVI), it was not possible to properly evaluate the vasoactive agents on arterial stiffness. This is because Pulse wave velocity (PWV) is strongly influenced by blood pressure at the time of measurement. On the other hand, CAVI is independent from BP at the time of measurement[4]. This chapter shows the difference between effects of NTG on the functional stiffness in patients with and without coronary artery disease (CAD) using CAVI.

Nitroglycerin stress test and study subjects

The procedure for the nitroglycerin stress test is as follows[5]. After resting for 10 minutes in supine position on a bed, CAVI was measured at baseline. Next, a tablet of NTG (0.3 mg) was administered sublingually and CAVI was measured every 5 minutes for 20 minutes using a VaSela 1500 (Fukuda Denshi Co., Ltd, Tokyo, Japan).

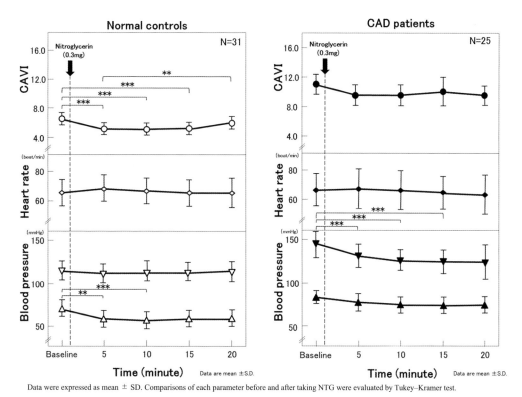

Data were expressed as mean ± SD. Comparisons of each parameter before and after taking NTG were evaluated by Tukey–Kramer test.

Fig. 1.   The Changes of CAVI, HR, BP after sublingual administration of nitroglycerin.
Vascular Health and Risk Management   2016;12:313–319; Originally published by and used with permission from Dove Medical Press Ltd[5]

[1]Department of Internal Medicine, Toho University Sakura Medical Center, 564-1 Shimoshizu, Sakura City, Chiba 285-8741, Japan.
[2]Biological Information Analysis Section, Fukuda Denshi Co.,Ltd, Tokyo, Japan.

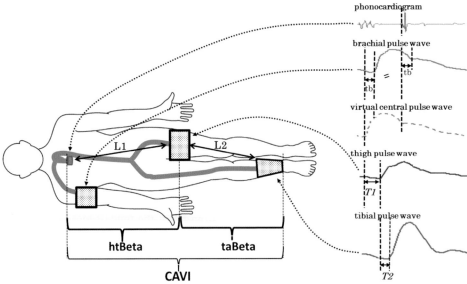

$$CAVI = a \times 2\rho \, \ln(Psys / Pdia) / (Psys - Pdia) \{ (L1 + L2) / (T1 + T2) \}^2 + b$$

$$htBeta = 2\rho \, \ln(Psys / Pdia)/(Psys\text{-}Pdia) (L1/T1)^2$$

$$taBeta = 2\rho \, \ln(Psys / Pdia) / (Psys \text{-}Pdia)(L2/T2)^2$$

Fig. 2.　A diagram showing the measurement of arterial stiffness of various portions of the arterial tree with the cardio-ankle vascular index, htBeta and taBeta. Cited from ref.6

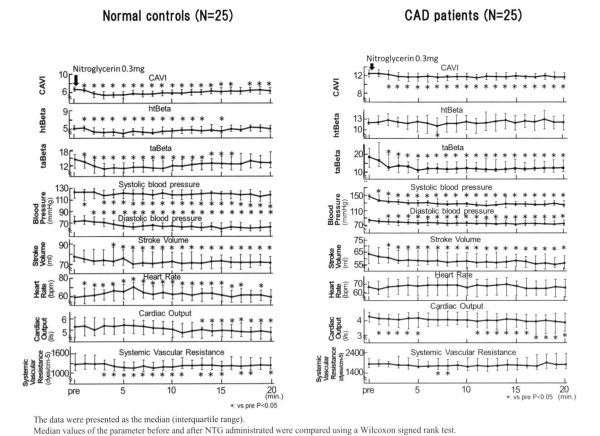

The data were presented as the median (interquartile range).
Median values of the parameter before and after NTG administrated were compared using a Wilcoxon signed rank test.

Fig. 3.　The change of CAVI, htBeta, taBeta, blood pressure, stroke volume, heat rate, cardiac output, and systemic vascular resistance during the administration of nitroglycerin. Adapted from ref.6

　　The normal controls were 31 healthy volunteers (males 21; females 10) aged 24–50 years (mean ± standard deviation [SD], 31.1 ± 1.3 years), who came to our institute responding to our public announcement. They had no medical history and were not on regular medications. The CAD subjects were 25 patients (males 20; females 5) aged

60–84 years (mean ± SD, 73.0±5.9 years). The CAD patients comprised 19 with angina pectoris and six with old myocardial infarction; 17 patients underwent percutaneous coronary intervention, and eight patients had coronary artery bypass grafting.

The Effect of Nitroglycerin on Arterial Stiffness of the Aorta and the Femoral-Tibial Arteries

Yamamoto T devised a method for measuring arterial stiffness in segments and used it to perform a nitroglycerin stress test[6]. In order to measure arterial stiffness of the aorta as an elastic artery, and of the femoral-tibial arteries as muscular arteries separately, we applied the stiffness parameter β theory to those arteries by utilizing Bramwell-Hill's equation in the same way as it is applied when measuring CAVI (Fig. 2). In this way, the stiffness of the aortic artery is called heart to thigh Beta (htBeta), and that of femoral-tibial arteries is called thigh to ankle Beta (taBeta). htBeta which indicates the stiffness of the aorta, was calculated by measuring pulse wave velocity from the origin of the aorta to the upper portion of the femoral artery, and blood pressure at the upper brachial artery. taBeta which indicates the stiffness of the femoral-tibial arteries, was calculated by measuring pulse wave velocity from the upper portion of the femoral artery to the ankle, and blood pressure at the upper brachial artery. These parameter values were introduced into the equation without "a" and "b" constants of the CAVI formula as stated above. htBeta and taBeta values were thus obtained.

In this study, measurement of cardiac stroke volume and cardiac output, and calculation of the systemic vascular resistance was follows. The changes of cardiac stroke volume and cardiac output/min were continuously monitored using the Aesculon mini machine (Osypka medical, California, USA)[7]. Systemic vascular resistance (SVR) was calculated by dividing the mean brachial blood pressure minus constant central venous pressure with cardiac output. Central venous pressure was supposed to be 5 mmHg in this case.

The nitroglycerin stress test using CAVI depicted organic and functional arterial stiffness

When arteriosclerosis is progression, one of the major vascular qualitative changes is the calcification of the artery. The smooth muscle cells are even present in an advanced arteriosclerotic artery. The smooth muscle cells relax or contracture functionally. It is difficult to distinguish this organic state and functional state strictly. But we might be able to evaluate this phenomenon as the baseline of CAVI and the rapid changes of CAVI in both healthy people and CAD patients. Baseline of CAVI indicates arteriosclerotic condition in each individual. And ΔCAVI of baseline may indicate the potential for functional vascular elasticity (Fig. 1 and Fig. 3).

Conclusion

After NTG administration, the stiffness of the arteries from the origin of the aorta to the ankle as measured by CAVI decreased in both the healthy volunteers and CAD patients.

It is noteworthy that muscular arteries in arteriosclerotic patients maintained their responsiveness to NTG much more than those in healthy people. The response of the arterial smooth muscle cells to NO is preserved even in CAD patients under medications.

References

1) Vallance P, Collier J, Moncada S. Effects of endothelium-derived nitric oxide on peripheral arteriolar tone in man. Lancet. 1989; 2: 997–1000.

2) Haynes WG, Noon JP, Walker BR, et al. Inhibition of nitric oxide synthesis increases blood pressure in healthy humans. J Hypertens. 1993; 11: 1375–1380.

3) Smulyan H, Mookherjee S, Warner RA. The effect of nitroglycerin on forearm arterial distensibility. Circulation. 1986; 73: 1264–1269.

4) Shirai K, Song M, Suzuki J, et al. Contradictory effects of β1-and α1-aderenergic receptor blockers on cardio-ankle vascular stiffness index (CAVI)–CAVI is independent of blood pressure. J Atheroscler Thromb. 2011;18: 49-55.

5) Shimizu K, Yamamoto T, Takahashi M, Sato S, Noike H, Shirai K. Effect of nitroglycerin administration on cardio-ankle vascular index. Vasc Health Risk Manag. 2016;12:313–319.

6) Yamamoto T, Shimizu K, Takahashi M, Tatsuno I, Shirai K. The Effect of Nitroglycerin on Arterial Stiffness of the Aorta and the Femoral-Tibial Arteries. J Atheroscler Thromb. 2017;24:1048–1057.

7) Zoremba N, Bickenbach J, Krauss B, Rossaint R, Kuhlen R, Schälte G. Comparison of electrical velocimetry and thermodilution techniques for the measurement of cardiac output. Acta Anaesthesiol Scand. 2007;51:1314-1319.

Effects of PGI2 analog, Beraprost Sodium Administration on CAVI

Mao Takahashi

Summary

The cardio-ankle vascular index (CAVI) is known to reflect the organic stiffness of the arterial tree; however, there is inadequate information on whether the CAVI reflects the functional stiffness of the arterial tree. Beraprost sodium (BPS), a prostaglandin I_2 analog, is a drug that relaxes the vascular smooth muscle cells but has little effect on the blood pressure. We monitored CAVI for 4 hrs after the administration of BPS. This is to avoid readers interpreting it as BPS was administered for 4 hrs. When BPS was administered to healthy volunteers, the CAVI decreased; however, the blood pressure did not change. These results suggest that the CAVI reflected functional stiffness caused by the contraction and relaxation of the vascular smooth muscle cells.

Introduction

The cardio-ankle vascular index (CAVI) is an index of stiffness of the large arteries and is reported to reflect changes of arteriosclerotic diseases and chronic kidney disease[1] and disorders of the eyes[2]. An increase in the

CAVI suggests the progression of cardiovascular disease and microvascular complications. Thus, the CAVI could reflect the organic stiffness of the arterial tree. However, arterial stiffness is known to adapt to maintain the systemic circulatory condition by contraction and relaxation of the

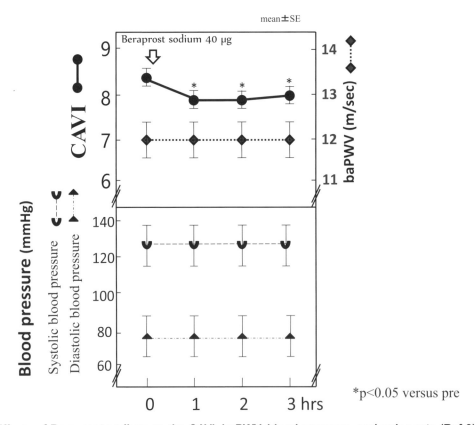

Fig. 1. Effects of Beraprost-sodium on the CAVI, baPWV, blood pressure, and pulse rate (Ref 3).
Beraprost sodium (40μg) was administered to 18 men. The CAVI, baPWV, systolic blood pressure, diastolic blood pressure, and pulse rate were measured every hour for 3 hours.

Cardiovascular center, Toho University Sakura Medical Center, 564-1, Shimoshizu, Sakura-City, Chiba, 285-8741, Japan.

arterial smooth muscle cells. However, it is not completely clear whether the CAVI could reflect the functional stiffness of the arteries adequately. Beraprost sodium (BPS), a prostaglandin I_2 analog, has a potent vasodilating effect and has been used for the treatment of peripheral arterial diseases such as arteriosclerosis obliterans and pulmonary hypertension and has little effect on the blood pressure.

We investigated the acute change in the CAVI in response to vasodilation by administering BPS to healthy volunteers for 4 hours after administration of BPS[3].

Can the CAVI be an indicator of peripheral vascular function?

Healthy male volunteers ($n = 18$, 46.3 ± 4.2 years) were enrolled in this study and administered BPS (40 μg). The CAVI and brachial-ankle pulse wave velocity (baPWV) were measured every hour for 4 hours. When BPS was administered to the volunteers, the systolic and diastolic blood pressure fluctuated slightly; however, the mean BP did not change. The CAVI significantly decreased in the 1st hour from 8.3 ± 0.34 (mean $\pm$ SE) to 7.9 ± 0.34 ($p < 0.05$), and this decrease persisted for 3 hours, while baPWV did not change significantly. ΔbaPWV was significantly

Correlations between ΔbaPWV and ΔBlood pressure 3 hours after the administration of Beraprost sodium

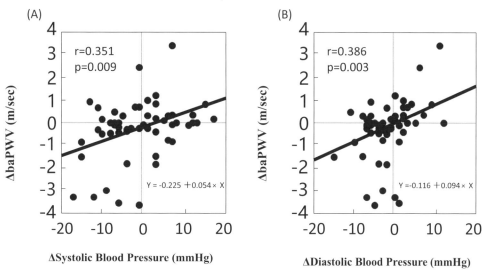

Correlations between ΔCAVI and ΔBlood pressure 3 hours after the administration of Beraprost sodium

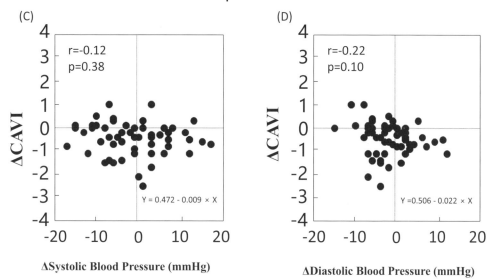

Fig. 2. Correlations between ΔCAVI or ΔbaPWV and Δ blood pressure during Beraprost sodium administration (Ref 3).

Differences in the vascular parameters (Δ) before and each hour after Beraprost sodium administration were calculated and their correlations are shown.
A, B: Correlations among ΔbaPWV, Δsystolic blood pressure (A) and Δdiastolic blood pressure (B) during Beraprost sodium administration. C, D: Correlations among ΔCAVI, Δ systolic blood pressure (C) and Δdiastolic blood pressure (D) during Beraprost sodium administration.

correlated with both Δsystolic blood pressure and Δdiastolic blood pressure at each time point; however, ΔCAVI showed no correlation with either Δsystolic blood pressure ($r = -0.12$, $p = 0.38$) or Δdiastolic blood pressure ($r = -0.22$, $p = 0.10$). These results suggest that CAVI reflected functional stiffness of the arterial tree independent of the changes in blood pressure.

Summary

On administration of BPS to healthy volunteers, the CAVI decreased, whereas blood pressure showed no changes. baPWV decreased, and the changes were correlated with blood pressure. These results suggested that the CAVI could reflect the functional stiffness of the arterial wall based on the smooth muscle tone in addition to the organic stiffness of the arterial matrix component.

References

1) Nakamura K, Iizuka T, Takahashi M, et al. Association between cardio-ankle vascular index and serum cystatin C levels in patients with cardiovascular risk factor. J Atheroscler Thromb. 2009;16:371-9.

2) Taniguchi H, Shiba T, Takahashi M, et al. Cardio-ankle vascular index elevation in patients with exudative age-related macular degeneration. J Atheroscler Thromb. 2013;20:903-10.

3) Takahashi M, Shiba T, Hirano K, et al. Acute decrease of cardio-ankle vascular index with the administration of beraprost sodium. J Atheroscler Thromb. 2012;19:479-84. https://doi.org/10.5551/jat.9266

Effects of Vaso Dilating Agents, Riociguat on CAVI in patients with chorionic thromboembolic pulmonary hypertension

Shuji Sato

Abstract

Arterial stiffness as evaluated by CAVI was enhanced in patients with chorionic thromboembolic pulmonary hypertension (CTEPH), potentially deteriorating cardiac function because of enhanced afterload. Riociguat administration improved CTEPH pathophysiology partly by decreasing CAVI.

Introduction

Riociguat, a soluble guanylate cyclase (sGC) stimulator, is a pulmonary vasodilator directly stimulating sGC independently of nitric oxide (NO) and increasing the sGC sensitivity to NO. Recently, riociguat has been applied for pulmonary arterial hypertension (PAH) and chorionic thromboembolic pulmonary hypertension (CTEPH). CTEPH is classified as group 4 pulmonary hypertension (PH), and its predominant cause is pulmonary artery obstruction due to organized thrombi in the large pulmonary arteries. Radchenko et al. reported that arterial stiffness as evaluated by CAVI was significantly higher in PAH patients than in healthy subjects[1]. Therefore, arterial stiffness may play an important role in the pathophysiology of CTEPH as well as PAH. In this chapter, we present two CTEPH cases where enhanced CAVI was improved after riociguat administration and focus on riociguat's effect on CTEPH, including arterial stiffness (CAVI).

Case 1:

Case 1 was a man in his 60s with mean pulmonary arterial pressure (mPAP) of 50 mmHg, which indicates severe PH, and a cardiac index (CI) of 1.8 $L/min/m^2$ at CTEPH diagnosis (Fig. 1). The initial CAVI value was 10.0, which is high for his age. Right ventricle (RV) enlargement was detected by echocardiography, which oppressed the interventricular septum which was shifted leftward. Although the left ventricular ejection fraction (LVEF) was within the normal range, the global longitudinal strain on the left ventricle (GLS-LV) was -10.3% indicating that LV dysfunction, and longitudinal strain (LS) impairment was observed in both septal and non-septal LV segments. After riociguat administration, mPAP improved to 40 mmHg, but PH and RV overload remained. Whereas CAVI decreased to 9.1 and CI increased to 2.6 $L/min/m^2$. The enlarged RV remained, but the LV oppression was released and GLS-LV improved to the normal range.

Case 2:

Case 2 was a woman in her 80s with mPAP 32 mmHg, CI 1.7 $L/min/m^2$, whose CAVI increased to 10.5 at CTEPH diagnosis (Fig. 2). Although echocardiography showed PH, RV enlargement was mild and LV oppression not observed. LVEF was normal, but GLS-LV was impaired to -8.2%. Unlike the first case, the LS impairment was observed only in non-septal LV segments. After riociguat administration, mPAP remained stable, but CAVI decreased to 9.7 and the CI improved to 2.4 $L/min/m^2$. Thereafter, GLS-LV improved to the normal range (-19.2%).

Discussion

Important findings in both cases were: 1) enhanced CAVI at CTEPH diagnosis, 2) LV dysfunction detected as a GLS-LV impairment before riociguat administration, and 3) improved CAVI and LV function after riociguat administration despite of remaining PH.

Initial CAVI values were increased in the present cases. This finding usually suggests advanced organized atherosclerosis. However, considering that enhanced CAVI improved after riociguat administration, functional stiffness was also enhanced due to smooth muscle contraction in those CTEPH patients. This functional stiffness increase may be explained by sympathetic nerve activation according to reduced cardiac output due to severe PH and enhanced physical and/or mental stress caused by severe dyspnea and hypoxia.

Enhanced arterial stiffness is thought to result in high afterload on the LV, which could deteriorate LV function. Recently, Kishiki et al. reported that PAH patients had LV dysfunction detected as reduced GLS-LV and LV diastolic

Division of Cardiovascular Medicine, Toho University Sakura Medical Center, 564-1 Shimoshizu, Sakura City, Chiba 285-8741, Japan.

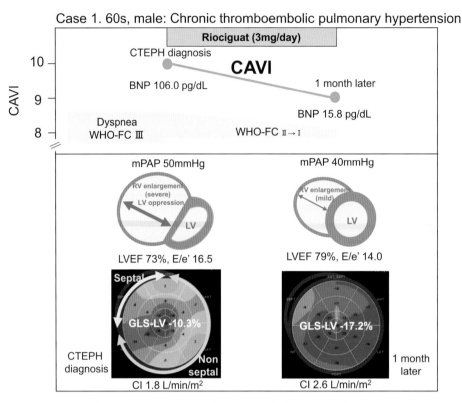

Fig. 1.   Changes in CAVI and clinical parameters after riociguat administration in case 1.

CTEPH: chronic thromboembolic pulmonary hypertension; CAVI: cardio-ankle vascular index; BNP: brain natriuretic peptide; WHO-FC: world health organization functional class; mPAP: mean pulmonary arterial pressure; RV: right ventricle; LV: left ventricle; LVEF: left ventricular ejection fraction; E: peak early diastolic transmitral flow velocity; e': peak early diastolic annular velocity; E/e': ratio of E to e'; GLS-LV: global longitudinal strain on left ventricle; CI: cardiac index.

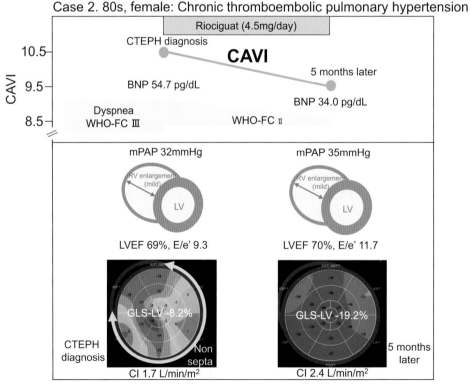

Fig. 2.   Changes in CAVI and clinical parameters after riociguat administration in case 2.

CTEPH: chronic thromboembolic pulmonary hypertension; CAVI: cardio-ankle vascular index; BNP: brain natriuretic peptide; WHO-FC: world health organization functional class; mPAP: mean pulmonary arterial pressure; RV: right ventricle; LV: left ventricle; LVEF: left ventricular ejection fraction; E: peak early diastolic transmitral flow velocity; e': peak early diastolic annular velocity; E/e': ratio of E to e'; GLS-LV: global longitudinal strain on left ventricle; CI: cardiac index.

dysfunction in addition to right heart dysfunction[2]. They also reported impaired LS in both septal and non-septal LV segments, suggesting that the LV dysfunction was caused not only by interventricular effects due to RV pressure and/or volume overload but also by other factors affecting LV function in PAH patients. In the first case, LS impairment was also detected in both septal and non-septal LV segments, whereas in the second case, the impairment was detected only in non-septal LV segments. After riociguat administration, PH and RV enlargement persisted, whereas the enhanced CAVI decreased and CI increased. In addition, GLS-LV was markedly improved. Potentially, high CAVI may deteriorate LV function by increased afterload on the LV.

Riociguat has a strong vasodilating effects, but the PH improvement for inoperable CTEPH patients by riociguat is reportedly limited[3]. The vasodilating effect of riociguat may work on systemic circulation, predominantly in inoperable CTEPH patients whose pulmonary circulation was impaired due to organized thrombi, which remains in most pulmonary arteries. Similarly, in the present cases, it is possible that riociguat predominantly dilated systemic peripheral arteries and reduced afterload on the LV,

improving cardiac dysfunction and pulmonary circulation.

In summary, these observations suggested that arterial stiffness as evaluated by CAVI was increased in CTEPH, potentially deteriorating cardiac function because of higher afterload. The mechanism of CAVI increase in cases of CTEPH was unclear; however, riociguat administration might improve the pathophysiology of CTEPH partly by decreasing CAVI.

References

1) Radchenko GD, Zhyvylo IO, Titov EY, Sirenko YM. Systemic arterial stiffness in new diagnosed idiopathic pulmonary arterial hypertension patients. *Vasc Health Risk Manag* 2020; **16**: 29–39.
2) Kishiki K, Singh A, Narang A, Gomberg-Maitland M, Goyal N, Maffessanti F, et al. Impact of severe pulmonary arterial hypertension on the left heart and prognostic implications. *J Am Soc Echocardiogr* 2019; **32**: 1128-37.
3) Ghofrani HA, D'Armini AM, Grimminger F, Hoeper MM, Jansa P, Kim NH, Mayer E, et al. Riociguat for the treatment of chronic thromboembolic pulmonary hypertension. *N Engl J Med* 2013; **369**: 319-29.

PART 7

The role of Arterial stiffness in vascular function - From animal studies -

Overview
The role of Arterial stiffness in vascular function -From animal studies

Akira Takahara

Cardio-ankle vascular index (CAVI) was developed to assess vascular functions more precisely in clinical practice. The index can estimate the arterial stiffness of the arterial tree from the origin of the aorta to the tibial artery quantitatively[1]. The equation of the CAVI is determined from combination of the theory of stiffness parameter β, which expresses the changes of inner pressure requiring some extension of the caliber of the arterial wall[2], together with the equation of Bramwell-Hill[3]. Based on several clinical observations as revealed in the previous chapters of this book, it is recognized that higher values of CAVI in patients are associated with the presence of atherosclerotic diseases including coronary artery disease, cerebral infarction, chronic kidney disease, and thickening of the carotid intima–media thickness, and coronary risk factors, such as hypertension, diabetes mellitus, uric acid disorders, sleep apnea syndrome, smoking, and obesity in several cross-sectional studies. Although the stiffness of the artery measured by CAVI is assumed to be composed of organic stiffness and functional stiffness based on clinical observations, there is a few basic research on CAVI.

Measuring system of CAVI in anesthetized rabbit

Recently, we established the measuring system of CAVI in anesthetized rabbits[★] to analyze the physiological regulation of vascular function by comparing responses of vasoactive drugs to stiffness of large conduit arteries with those to resistant arteries. We can measure CAVI continuously via direct measurement of brachial and tibial blood pressures in this measurement system, which enables us to obtain physiological and pharmacological responses to CAVI in seconds or in minutes[4,5,6]. Using this system, we confirmed that the intravenous administration phenylephrine increased CAVI at hypertensive doses (Fig. 1), suggesting that α1-adrenoceptors on the vascular smooth muscle cells contribute to control vascular stiffness[4]. Also, a vasoactive peptide angiotensin II is confirmed to increase CAVI via activation of angiotensin II type 1 receptors[5]. Importantly, intravenous administration of doxazosin, an α1-adrenoceptor blocker, significantly decreases CAVI at a hypotensive dose (Fig. 1), which is in accordance with clinical observations[7]. In another animal study[6], we have shown that acetylcholine-induced decrement of CAVI was completely suppressed by a nitric oxide synthase inhibitor L-NAME, whereas the inhibitor did not affect the CAVI at a hypertensive dose, suggesting that the arterial stiffness in rabbits is independent from homeostatic production of nitric oxide; however, it can be decreased by large amounts of nitric oxide that are intrinsically produced by exogenously administered acetylcholine. The experimental system measuring CAVI is expected to bridge the gap between basic research and clinical observation.

Differences of arterial functions among the vascular regions

We further examined histological features of the arterial trees that corresponded to CAVI in rabbits. As shown in Fig. 2, each section of isolated arterial vessels from a rabbit was stained by Elastica van Gieson staining, resulting in the visualization of black-brown nuclei, black-stained elastic fibers, red collagen and yellow-stained muscles. Elastic fibers are rich in the media of the ascending and thoracic aortae, whereas vascular smooth muscle was wholly observed in the media of the iliac and tibial arteries. The observation raises an intriguing question on whether intravenously administered phenylephrine and angiotensin II equally affected vascular stiffness both in the aortic and femoral regions. More importantly, vasoactive drugs have been demonstrated to act unequally on the vascular beds of the intestine, kidney, and legs, as shown in Fig. 3, where a hypertensive dose of α1-adrenoceptor agonist methoxamine hardly affected the mesenteric arterial blood flow despite the marked decrement of the renal and iliac arterial blood flow. It should be noted that angiotensin II hardly affected the iliac arterial blood flow despite the marked decrement of the mesenteric and renal arterial blood flow. Therefore, it is important to analyze functional stiffness from the origin of the aorta to the tibial artery based on the knowledge regarding tissue selective action of vasoactive drugs, leading to newly establishing "pharmacology of arterial stiffness."

We have begun new experiments that simultaneously measure the aortic ß and femoral ß (Fig. 2). Intravenous administration of angiotensin II increased the blood pressure and femoral ß, but decreased the aortic ß, as described in the

---

[★] using modified device 'VaSera', Fukuda Co., Ltd. Tokyo

Department of Pharmacology and Therapeutics, Faculty of Pharmaceutical Sciences, Toho University, Funabashi, Chiba 274-8510, Japan.

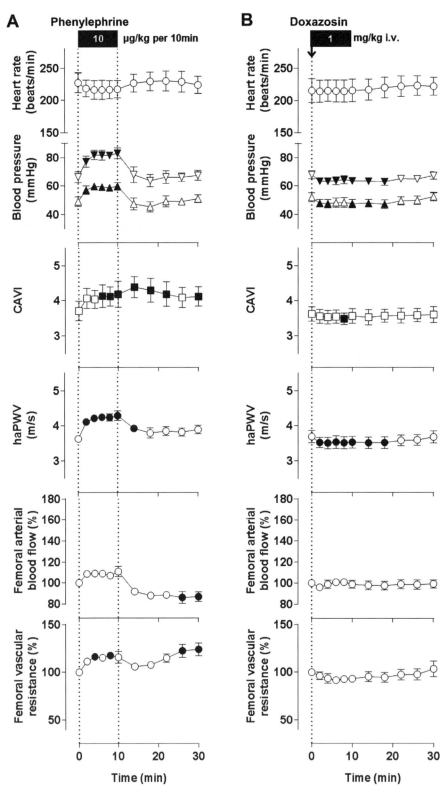

Fig. 1. Time courses of the effects of phenylephrine (A) and doxazosin (B) on the heart rate, systolic (inverted triangles) and diastolic (triangles) brachial arterial blood pressures, CAVI, haPWV, femoral arterial blood flow and femoral vascular resistance. Each value of femoral arterial blood flow and vascular resistance is expressed as a percentage compared with that at 0 min (=100%). Data are presented as mean ± S.E.M. (n=6). The closed symbols represent significant differences from corresponding control value of each parameter by $p < 0.05$.

(cited from Chiba T et al., J Pharmacol Sci. 2015; 128:185-192) 【with permission of Elsevier】[4]

Chapter 40, which supports existence of a functional co-relationship between large and small arteries. This study will be important to understand the precise roles of arterial stiffness on the efficiency of blood circulation at physiological as well as various pathophysiological conditions.

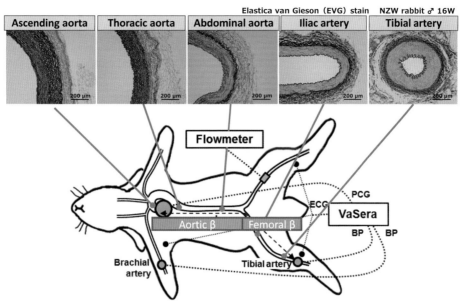

Fig. 2. Histological features of the arterial trees corresponded to CAVI in rabbits. Each section of isolated arterial vessels from a rabbit was stained by Elastica van Gieson staining, resulting in the visualization of black-brown nuclei, black-stained elastic fibers, red collagen and yellow-stained muscles. The stiffness parameter ß can be estimated in each section of aorta or femoral artery (aortic ß or femoral ß). Notably, the pharmacological effects of angiotensin II on aortic ß and femoral ß are markedly different, which are described in Chapter 40.

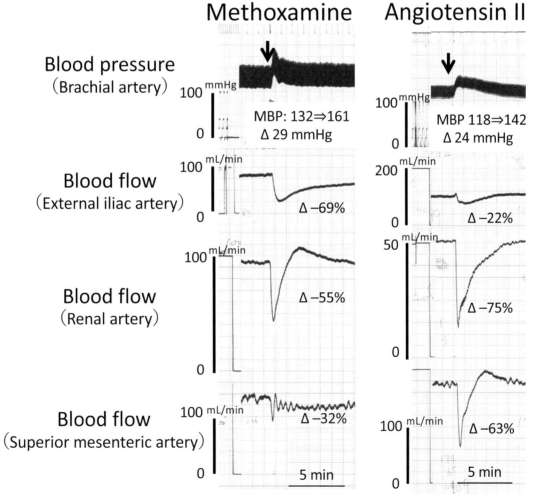

Fig. 3. Different vascular actions of methoxamine and angiotensin II in anesthetized dogs. Intravenous injection of methoxamine (50 μg/kg) markedly decreased the renal and iliac arterial blood flow, whereas that of angiotensin II (0.1 μg/kg) markedly decreased the renal and mesenteric blood flow.

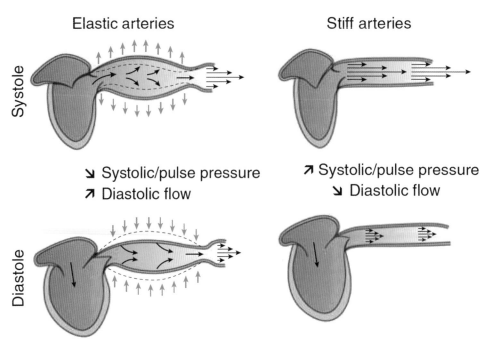

Fig. 4. Schematic representation of the role of arterial stiffness in ensuring blood flow through the peripheral circulation.
(cited from Briet M et al., Kidney International 2012; 82, 388–400) 【with permission of Elsevier】[8]

Distribution of the blood to the key organs through the aorta

It is well recognized that intrinsic elasticity of the arterial wall relates propagation of the pressure wave along the arterial tree, and more importantly, aortic elasticity also contributes to ensuring continuous blood flow[8]. As shown in Fig. 4, the blood from the ventricle is forwarded directly to the peripheral tissues during ventricular contraction, and part of the blood is momentarily stored in the aorta and central arteries by stretching the arterial walls, leading to store of energy in the vessel walls. During diastole, the stored energy recoils the aorta, propelling the accumulated blood forward into the peripheral tissues, ensuring continuous flow, which is known as the Windkessel function. When the arterial system is rigid and/or cannot be stretched, the entire stroke volume flows through the arterial system and peripheral tissues only during systole with two consequences: intermittent flow and short capillary transit time, with reduced metabolic exchanges. Since CAVI is an index reflecting cardiac ejection-associated changes in arterial diameter in part, monitoring of CAVI evokes blood distribution to the key organs including the heart and kidney.

Aortic impedance is an index of afterload that varies continuously during ejection. Since the index is the aortic blood pressure divided by the aortic flow at that instant, a high arterial blood pressure or aortic valve stenosis will increase impedance and hence afterload when the function of the cardiac muscle is intact. Importantly, physiological or pathophysiological changes in cardiac function may alter aortic performance. Thus, the evaluation of aortic function will be especially important when measured simultaneously with echocardiology, which can help us understanding the existence of the functional co-relationship between the heart and large arteries, as well as that between large and small

arteries. Further understanding of the physiological as well as the pathophysiological characteristics of CAVI will offer a paradigm for clinical emergency therapy as well as treatment of cardiovascular diseases in the new era.

References

1) Shirai K, Utino J, Otsuka K, Takata M. A novel blood pressure-independent arterial wall stiffness parameter; cardio-ankle vascular index (CAVI). J Atheroscler Thromb. 2006;13:101-107.

2) Hayashi K, Handa H, Nagasawa S, Okumura A, Moritake K. Stiffness and elastic behavior of human intracranial and extracranial arteries. J Biomech. 1980;13: 175-184.

3) Bramwell JC, Hill AV. The velocity of the pulse wave in man. Proc R Soc B Biol Sci. 1922;93:298-306.

4) Chiba T, Yamanaka M, Takagi S, et al. Cardio-ankle vascular index (CAVI) differentiates pharmacological properties of vasodilators nicardipine and nitroglycerin in anesthetized rabbits. J Pharmacol Sci. 2015;128:185-192. https://doi.org/10.1016/j.jphs.2015.07.002

5) Sakuma K, Shimoda A, Shiratori H, Komatsu T, Watanabe K, Chiba T, Aimoto M, Nagasawa Y, Hori Y, Shirai K, Takahara A. Angiotensin II acutely increases arterial stiffness as monitored by cardio-ankle vascular index (CAVI) in anesthetized rabbits. J Pharmacol Sci. 2019;140:205-209.

6) Chiba T, Sakuma K, Komatsu T, Cao X, Aimoto M, Nagasawa Y, Shimizu K, Takahashi M, Hori Y, Shirai K, Takahara A. Physiological role of nitric oxide for regulation of arterial stiffness in anesthetized rabbits. J Pharmacol Sci. 2019;139:42-45.

7) Shirai K, Song M, Suzuki J, Kurosu T, Oyama T, Nagayama D, Miyashita Y, Yamamura S, Takahashi M. Contradictory effects of β_1- and α_1-aderenergic receptor blockers on cardio-ankle vascular stiffness index (CAVI). –CAVI independent of blood pressure. J Atheroscler Thromb. 2011;18:49-55.

8) Briet M, Boutouyrie P, Laurent S, London GM: Arterial stiffness and pulse pressure in CKD and ESRD. Kidney Int 2012;82:388-400. https://doi.org/10.1038/ki.2012.131

CAVI during bleeding

Yoshinobu Nagasawa

For several years, the role of arterial stiffness in the vascular function had been less understood because the conventional indices used for the evaluation of arterial stiffness, such as the pulse wave velocity (PWV), were intrinsically influenced by the blood pressure at the time of measurement[1]. Conversely, the cardio-ankle vascular index (CAVI), a novel index for the evaluation of arterial stiffness, is theoretically independent of the blood pressure at the measuring time, and that property has been verified experimentally[2,3]. We think that CAVI may be a useful index for analyzing the vascular function under the various pathophysiological conditions accompanying the reduction in blood pressure. In this chapter, we discussed the arterial stiffness monitored by CAVI during the blood removal and blood return in rabbits.

Effects of the blood removal on arterial stiffness monitored by CAVI and haPWV in rabbits

Introduction

Severe bleeding elicits a hemorrhage shock that results in life-threatening multiple organ failure. To maintain the vital functions of the organs during the hemorrhage shock, various hemodynamic defense reactions are evoked in the body. Typically, the reduction in the total blood volume and blood pressure activates the sympathetic nervous system,

resulting in potent vasoconstriction[4]. Although arterial stiffness may change during the hemorrhage shock, the actual effects of the reduction of the total blood volume on arterial stiffness have not been investigated.

Aim

Thus, we assessed the effects of blood removal and subsequent blood re-transfusion on blood pressure and CAVI in rabbits. Heart-ankle pulse wave velocity (haPWV) was also measured in this study to clarify the difference

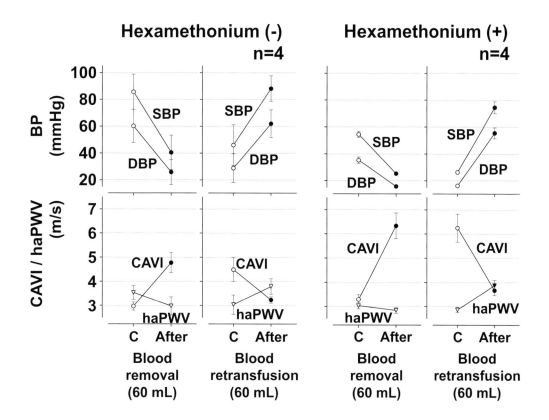

C: Control, After: after each procedure   Closed symbol: p<0.05 v.s. C

Fig. 1. The effects of blood removal and retransfusion on the blood pressure (BP), CAVI, and haPWV under the absence and presence of hexamethonium.

Department of Pharmacology and Therapeutics, Faculty of Pharmaceutical Sciences, Toho University, Funabashi, Chiba 274-8510, Japan.

between CAVI and PWV[5-7].

Furthermore, the effect of the ganglion blocker, hexamethonium on these parameters during hemorrhagic shock was also studied to clarify the involvement of the sympathetic nerve function in this condition.

Methods

Under isoflurane-anesthesia, 60 ml of blood (40% of the total blood volume, 4 ml/minutes) was withdrawn from the brachial artery of rabbits, and the blood was subsequently re-transfused at the same speed. To assess the involvement of the autonomic nervous system, we also conducted the experiment mentioned above under the presence of the ganglion blocker, hexamethonium.

Results

As shown in Fig. 1 (left side), the blood removal decreased the blood pressure gradually and increased the CAVI. In contrast, haPWV was slightly decreased, paralleling the decrease in blood pressure. When the blood began to be returned, the blood pressure began to increase and CAVI decreased to the basal level. A decreased haPWV also returned to the baseline.

As shown in Fig. 1 (right side), even in the presence of hexamethonium, blood removal decreased the blood pressure and haPWV, and increased the CAVI. Blood retransfusion returned all parameters to the baseline.

Discussion

Our experimental study demonstrated that the reduction in the circulatory blood volume induced by blood removal increases the arterial stiffness monitored with CAVI.

The relationship between the reduction of circulatory blood volume and arterial stiffness had not been fully understood until recently. Ögünc H et al. previously reported that PWV used for the evaluation of arterial

stiffness decreased during a single hemodialysis session, in which the circulatory blood volume is decreased by the removal of water[8]. We think that the reduction in the PWV during hemodialysis in their study may not reflect the actual changes in the arterial stiffness, because the PWV is intrinsically influenced by the blood pressure at measuring time[1]. Our previous data in the rabbits demonstrated that the cardioactive agent, metoprolol, that reduces the myocardial contractility and cardiac output, increased CAVI[5]. The increase in CAVI induced by metoprolol was also observed in humans[9]. In addition, our preliminary experiment using high-resolution ultrasonography showed that arterial wall motion against the pulse pressure was dulled after the blood removal, reflecting an increase in the arterial stiffness (manuscript under preparation). These results indicate that the reduction in the circulatory blood volume increases the arterial stiffness, and the use of CAVI is an appropriate approach to evaluate the vascular function under the pathophysiological conditions accompanying blood pressure reduction, such as hemorrhagic shock.

Notably, the blood removal increased the CAVI even though the autonomic reflex was inhibited by the ganglion blocker, hexamethonium. These results suggest that the arterial stiffness may be modulated via both the neurological (e.g. autonomic nervous system) and non-neurological pathway during the hemorrhage shock, although further studies are needed to clarify the detailed mechanisms for the regulation of arterial stiffness (Fig. 2).

Clinical implication

Our experimental study demonstrated that CAVI reflects the state of arterial smooth muscle cell contraction induced by hypovolemia with blood removal. These findings might suggest that enhanced CAVI can be an additional indicator for the diagnosis of hemorrhagic shock in addition to low blood pressure.

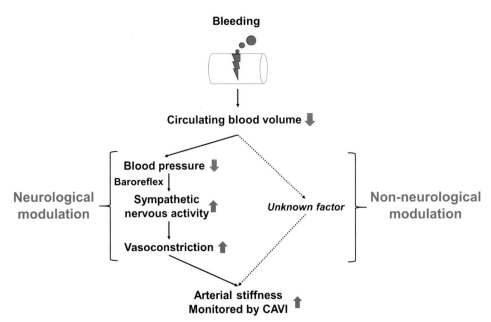

Fig. 2. Schema of proposal mechanisms of the increase in arterial stiffness monitored by CAVI during hemorrhage shock.

Conclusion

The acute reduction in the circulatory blood volume increases the CAVI, which may be evoked via both the neurological and non-neurological pathways.

References

1) Takahashi K et al., The Background of Calculating CAVI: Lesson from the Discrepancy Between CAVI and CAVI$_0$. *Vasc Health Risk Manag*, 2020;16;193-201.

2) Shirai K et al., A novel blood pressure-independent arterial wall stiffness parameter; cardio-ankle vascular index (CAVI). *J Atheroscler Thromb*, 2006;13;101-107.

3) Hayashi K et al., Analysis of constitutive laws of vascular walls by finite deformation theory. *Iyodenshi To Seitai Kogaku*, 1975;13;293-298.

4) Arnold M. Katz. **Physiology of the Heart 4th ed**. Lippincott Williams & Wilkins, Philadelphia, PA, U.S.A, 2006.

5) Chiba T et al., Cardio-ankle vascular index (CAVI) differentiates pharmacological properties of vasodilators nicardipine and nitroglycerin in anesthetized rabbits. *J Pharmacol Sci*, 2015;128;185-192.

6) Chiba T et al., Physiological role of nitric oxide for regulation of arterial stiffness in anesthetized rabbits. *J Pharmacol Sci*, 2019;139;42-45.

7) Sakuma K et al., Angiotensin II acutely increases arterial stiffness as monitored by cardio-ankle vascular index (CAVI) in anesthetized rabbits. *J Pharmacol Sci*, 2019;140;205-209.

8) Ögünc H et al., The effects of single hemodialysis session on arterial stiffness in hemodialysis patients. *Hemodial Int*, 2015;19;463-471.

9) Shirai K et al., Contradictory effects of β_1- and α_1- adorenergic receptor blockers on cardio-ankle vascular stiffness index (CAVI)--CAVI independent of blood pressure. *J Atheroscler Thromb*, 2011;18;49-55.

Effects of nitroglycerin on CAVI in Rabbits

Tatsuo Chiba

Background and purpose

The cardio-ankle vascular index (CAVI) has been clinically utilized for assessments of the arterial stiffness to estimate the progress of arteriosclerosis[1]. While it is assumed that the stiffness of the artery measured by CAVI is composed of organic stiffness and functional stiffness

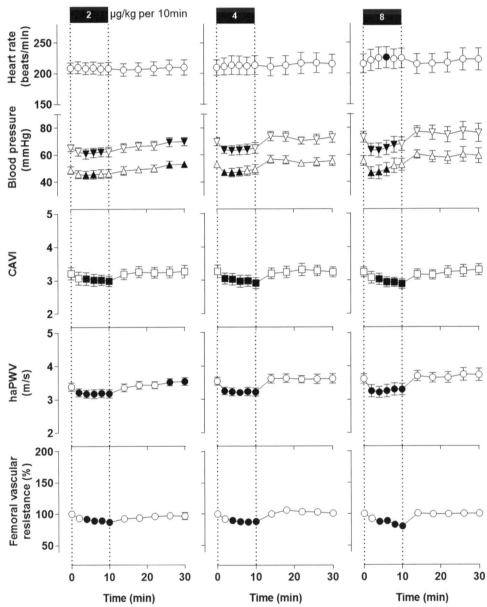

Fig. 1. Effects of nitroglycerin on the heart rate, brachial blood pressure, CAVI, haPWV, and femoral vascular resistance. The value of femoral vascular resistance is expressed as a percentage compared with that at 0 min (= 100%). Data are presented as mean ± S.E.M. (n = 6). The closed symbols represent significant differences from the corresponding control value of each parameter by p < 0.05.

Adapted from ref.5 〖with permission of Elsevier〗

Department of Pharmacy, Toho University Ohashi Medical Center, 2-17-6 Ohashi, Meguro, Tokyo, 153-8515, Japan.

based on clinical observations[2], the concept is required to be further strengthened by pharmacological approaches in animals.

Nitroglycerin is known to dilate the large conductance artery and coronary artery[3]. Shimizu and Yamamoto reported that nitroglycerine administration decreased CAVI in men[4,5]. We established the measuring system of CAVI in rabbits and studied the effect of nitroglycerin administration on CAVI[6].

Animals and methods

New Zealand White rabbits weighing 3–4 kg were initially anesthetized with ketamine (35 mg/kg, i.m.) and xylazine (5 mg/kg, i.m.). After intubation of the tracheal cannula, 0.5% halothane vaporized with 100% oxygen was inhaled with a ventilator (SN-480-7, Shinano, Tokyo).

For measurements of the heart-ankle pulse wave velocity (haPWV) and CAVI, the signals of electrocardiogram, phonocardiogram, and blood pressure were fed to VaSera VS-1500 (Fukuda Denshi Co. LTD, Tokyo)[1]. The effects of nitroglycerin (2, 4, and 8 μg/kg) were assessed. The femoral vascular resistance was calculated using the basic equation: mean blood pressure/femoral arterial blood flow.

Results and Discussion

As shown in Fig. 1, the administration of nitroglycerin decreased the systolic and diastolic blood pressure, CAVI, haPWV, and femoral vascular resistance dose-dependently. PWV is known to depend on the blood pressure at the measuring time. Therefore, the change in haPWV accompanied the blood pressure decrease in this study. The measurement of haPWV has no meaning as an index of the functional stiffness in this kind of study.

We found that the CAVI could change at least on the minute time scale during the administration of nitroglycerin. Arterial stiffness essentially correlates with arterial structural changes, including collagen accumulation, elastin fragmentation and degeneration, and thickening of the arterial wall. In addition to those structural changes, arterial stiffness is affected by vascular smooth muscle contraction, and this functional stiffness could be monitored with CAVI.

The decrease in CAVI was coordinated with the vascular resistance during the administration of nitroglycerin, suggesting that CAVI might reflect a part of peripheral arterial resistance.

Summary

Pharmacological studies using nitroglycerin in rabbits indicated that CAVI reflected the functional arterial stiffness mediated by arterial smooth muscle dilatation and might contribute as an index to understand the role of vascular function in the regulation of systemic circulation.

References

1) Shirai K., Utino J., Otsuka K., & Takata M. A novel blood pressure-independent arterial wall stiffness parameter; cardio-ankle vascular index (CAVI). *Journal of Atherosclerosis and Thrombosis* 2006; 13, 101–107. https://doi.org/10.5551/jat.13.101

2) Shirai K., Song M., Suzuki J. et al. Contradictory effects of β1- and α1- aderenergic receptor blockers on cardio-ankle vascular stiffness index (CAVI)--CAVI independent of blood pressure. *Journal of Atherosclerosis and Thrombosis* 2011; 18, 49–55. https://doi.org/10.5551/jat.3582

3) McGregor M. The nitrates and myocardial ischemia. *Circulation* 1982; 66, 689e692.

4) Shimizu K., Yamamoto T., Takahashi M. et al. Effect of nitroglycerin administration on cardio-ankle vascular index. *Vascular Health and Risk Management* 2016; 12, 313–319. https://doi.org/10.2147/VHRM.S106542

5) Yamamoto T., Shimizu K., Takahashi M. et al. The effect of nitroglycerin on arterial stiffness of the aorta and the femoral-tibial arteries. *Journal of Atherosclerosis and Thrombosis* 2017; 24, 1048–1057. https://doi.org/10.5551/jat.38646

6) Chiba T., Yamanaka M., Takagi S. et al. Cardio-ankle vascular index (CAVI) differentiates pharmacological properties of vasodilators nicardipine and nitroglycerin in anesthetized rabbits. *Journal of Pharmacological Sciences* 2015; 128, 185–192. https://doi.org/10.1016/j.jphs.2015.07.002

Effects of angiotensin II infusion on CAVI, aortic Beta and femoral Beta in rabbits; the presence of crosstalk between elastic artery and muscular artery

Kiyoshi Sakuma[1,2]

Background and Purpose

Angiotensin II, which is the predominant bioactive peptide in the renin–angiotensin system, promotes the maintenance of systemic pressure through various mechanisms in the cardiovascular and renal systems. This peptide is also implicated more specifically in vascular smooth muscle contraction. The degree of arteriosclerosis progression can be evaluated by measuring arterial stiffness, for which pulse wave velocity (PWV) has been used as an index. It was reported that angiotensin II increased PWV in anesthetized rabbits[1]. However, PWV essentially depends on the blood pressure at the time of measurement. Therefore, raised arterial stiffness measured by PWV does not necessarily imply a true increase in arterial stiffness.

The cardio-ankle vascular index (CAVI) was developed as an index reflecting arterial stiffness of the arterial tree, from the origin of the aorta to the ankle, and it is independent from blood pressure at the measurement time-point. We developed a system to measure the CAVI of anesthetized rabbits[2] and attempted to study the effect of angiotensin II

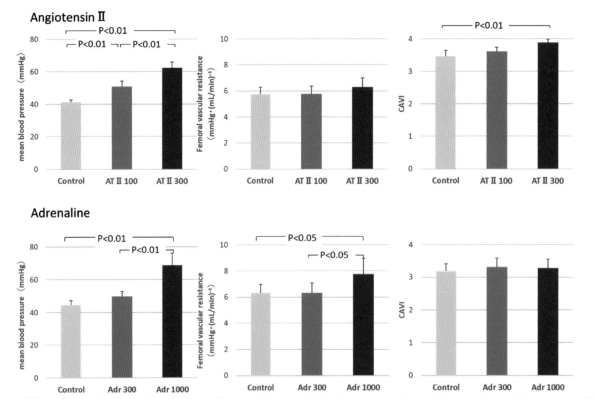

Fig. 1. Effects of angiotensin II and adrenaline on the mean blood pressure, femoral vascular resistance and CAVI.

[1]Department of Pharmacology and Therapeutics, Faculty of Pharmaceutical Sciences, Toho University, Funabashi, Chiba 274-8510, Japan.
[2]Department of Pharmacy, Toho University Sakura Medical Center, Sakura-shi, Chiba 285-8741, Japan.

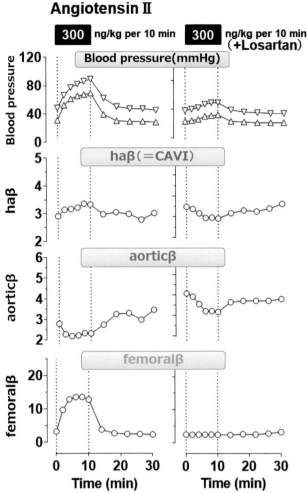

Fig. 2. Time courses of the effects of angiotensin II on the systolic and diastolic brachial arterial blood pressures, heart-ankleβ (=CAVI), aorticβ and femoralβ.

on the CAVI in the rabbit. Furthermore, we applied CAVI theory to the aortic segment (aortic Beta) and the iliac femoral arterial segment (femoral Beta), and studied the effect of angiotensin II on both Beta segments.

Effect of angiotensin II on CAVI in rabbits

The effect of angiotensin II infusion on the CAVI was investigated in rabbits. Blood pressure and the pulse wave of the right brachial artery and right tibial artery, electrocardiogram, and phonocardiogram of NZW rabbits were recorded under isoflurane anesthesia, and the CAVI was obtained in the same way as in humans. The femoral arterial blood flow was measured using an ultrasonic blood flowmeter. Angiotensin II (100 and 300 ng/kg) was intravenously administered over 10 min, and each cardiovascular parameter was sequentially measured until 30 min after the start of drug infusion (partly shown in Ref 3).

The results are shown in Fig. 1. Angiotensin II increased

the CAVI, and also increased the brachial artery blood pressure and femoral vascular resistance. These results suggested that angiotensin II contracted the arterial tree from the origin of the aorta to the femoral artery, raising the blood pressure.

Effect of angiotensin II on arterial stiffness of the aorta and femoral artery

Angiotensin II was shown to increase arterial stiffness of the whole arterial tree from the origin of the aorta to the tibial artery. This arterial tree is composed of elastic arteries and muscular arteries, which differ not only in terms of the composition of smooth muscle cells, elastic fibers, and collagen fibers, but may also be different in their response to vasoconstrictive agents. However, the precise effect of angiotensin II on arterial stiffness of the aorta and femoral artery had not been studied. We developed a method for measuring arterial stiffness of the aorta and femoral artery by applying CAVI theory. Additionally, the effects of angiotensin II on arterial stiffness (β value) in the aortic (aortic β) and femoral artery (femoral β) were studied.

Methods: To determine the β values (aortic β, femoral β) of each artery, the pulse wave at the bifurcation of the left common iliac artery was measured, in addition to using the conventional measurement method.

Results and discussion

The results are shown in Fig. 2. When angiotensin II was administered, femoral β increased with the increase in brachial artery blood pressure, whereas aortic β decreased, and CAVI increased. These responses were interpreted as follows: Angiotensin II constricted the arterial smooth muscle cells of the femoral artery, and raised arterial stiffness along with the increase in blood pressure. The decrease in aortic β was unexpected. This reaction of the aorta may be associated with increased internal pressure of the aortic wall, leading to relaxing of the stiffness of this arterial wall. This may indicate the presence of cross-talk between the elastic artery and muscular artery. Further studies on the meaning of and the mechanism underlying reciprocal reactions to angiotensin II between the aorta and the muscular artery are required.

References

1) Obara S, Hayashi S, Hazama A, Muraoka M, Katsuda S. Correlation between augmentation index and pulse wave velocity in rabbits. J Hypertens. 2009;27:332-340.
2) Chiba T, Yamanaka M, Takagi S, et al. Cardio-ankle vascular index (CAVI) differentiates pharmacological properties of vasodilators nicardipine and nitroglycerin in anesthetized rabbits. J Pharmacol Sci. 2015;128:185-192.
3) Sakuma K, Shimoda A, Shiratori H, et al. Angiotensin II acutely increases arterial stiffness as monitored by cardio-ankle vascular index (CAVI) in anesthetized rabbits. J Pharmacol Sci. 2019;140:205-209.

The changes of Aortic stiffness monitored with hrBETA during clamping the abdominal aorta

Aya Saito

Background and objective

Clamping the aorta is a very common maneuver to obtain a bloodless field during cardiovascular surgery. Abdominal aortic surgery is one of the major procedures requiring an aortic clamping maneuver, and appropriate hemodynamic management is crucial to avoid malperfusion injury distal to the clamping site. Abrupt blood pressure changes and intravascular volume shifts are thought to occur with the aortic clamp; however, precise vascular wall responses to those changes have not been clearly observed or understood. In this report, we sought to clarify the vascular wall compliance capacity by directly measuring heart–renal aortic stiffness (hrBeta), based on beta theory, using animal experiments

Animal and methods

New Zealand White Rabbits were intubated and anesthetized with isoflurane. An arterial blood pressure (BP) monitoring line was secured at the right axillar artery and right renal artery (under laparotomy). The hrBeta was calculated from the well-established basic equations with variables obtained from the axillar and renal blood pressure (AxBP and RBP) and phonocardiogram. Hemodynamic parameter monitoring, data collection, and data calculation were carried out using VaSera vs-1500 (Fukuda Denshi Co. Ltd., Tokyo, Japan). The abdominal aorta was secured and a cross-clamp was applied for 15 minutes, followed by 10 minutes of releasing the clamp ("declamp"A maneuver), and 2 sets of clamp/declamp maneuvers were applied to each rabbit. Other standard hemodynamic parameters (heart rate, central venous pressure [CVP], pulse-wave velocity [PWV]) were also measured. CVP was used as the reference of the volume status of the systemic circulation. The above experimental model is presented in Fig. 1.

Baseline values (AxBP, RBP, hrBETA, PWV, and systemic vascular resistance [SVR]) were defined as the average of 3 sets of measurement before aortic clamping. Values are expressed as the difference between each

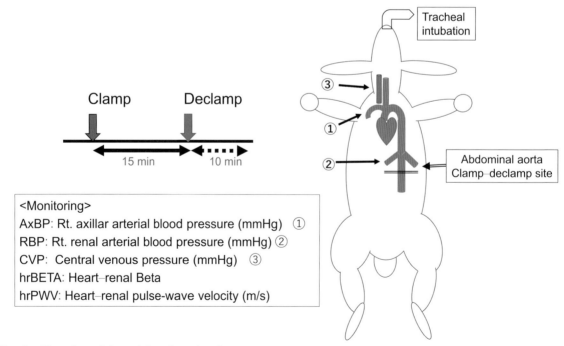

Fig. 1. Experimental model and protocol.
Hemodynamic monitoring sites during abdominal aortic clamp/declamp maneuvers are demonstrated in the figure.

Division of Cardiovascular Surgery, Toho University Sakura Medical Center, 564-1 Shimoshizu, Sakura City, Chiba 285-8741, Japan.

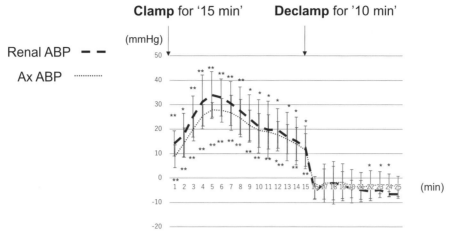

Fig. 2-1. Shows parallel change in renal and axial arterial pressures in accordance with aortic clamp/declamp maneuvers.

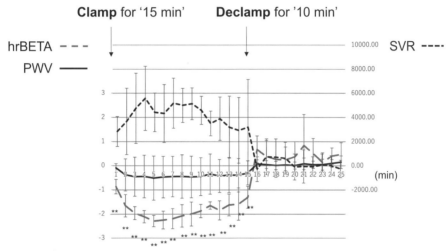

Fig. 2-2. Shows paradoxical changes in SVR and hrBETA, while no response in PWV in accordance with clamp/declamp maneuvers.

Fig. 2   Results for hemodynamic changes and vascular tonus changes are shown.

measurement and its baseline value.

Results

Fig. 2-1. presents changes in the AxBP and RBP after abdominal aortic clamping for 15 minutes, followed by declamping (i.e., releasing the clamp), and continuous monitoring for another 10 minutes. The clamp maneuver induced abrupt increases in both AxBP and RBP, peaking at 5–6 minutes after the clamp maneuver. BP measurements during the whole 15 minutes of the clamp procedure were significantly higher than the baseline BP. Both AxBP and RBP showed a gradual decrease until declamping, at which point both parameters abruptly decreased to levels even lower than baseline throughout the 10-minute observation period.

Fig. 2-2. presents changes in hrBETA, PWV, and SVR. HrBeta presented a rapid response occurring at the time of aortic clamping: a significant decrease from the baseline value. The declamp maneuver resulted in rapid recovery of hrBETA to a level similar to that at baseline. In contrast, the SVR increased (although non-significantly) following aortic

clamping, and normalized to baseline values immediately after declamping. PWV did not show any apparent response to the clamp/declamp maneuver throughout the whole 25-minute procedure.

Comments

Abrupt BP and simultaneous reciprocal changes in hrBETA following the aortic clamp/declamp maneuver may indicate the underlying potential of the hemodynamic system to achieve homeostasis in vascular stiffness. The mechanism of vascular stiffness regulation is not yet fully understood. Possible explanations include sympathetic nerve regulation and unknown autocrine/paracrine regulation, considering the rapid response of the hemodynamic parameters measured in our experiment. Involvement of chemical mediators is less likely because of the immediacy of these changes.

Further investigation is needed to elucidate the mechanism of vascular stiffness regulation, to seek an ideal management of blood pressure control.

Intracranial pressure enhancement and CAVI

Chikao Miyazaki

Introduction

An increase in blood pressure is frequently associated with the onset of stroke[1-3]. Brainstem ischemia has been suggested as a potential mechanism by which blood pressure rises in response to increased intracranial pressure[4]. It is possible that this may occur due to the involvement of arterial stiffness, which, in turn, causes vascular resistance, but the details of the underlying mechanism is not well understood[5].

Conventionally, pulse wave velocity (PWV) has been used as an index of arterial elasticity, which is proportional related to arterial stiffness. However, it has been pointed out that PWV changes, depending on the blood pressure at the time of measurement[6-9]. Therefore, it is difficult to know whether PWV is appropriate as an analytical index of arteries in the context of stroke.

We encountered the case of a patient with subarachnoid hemorrhage in whom a high cardio-ankle vascular index (CAVI) was found. This case suggested that the role of arterial elasticity in hemodynamics during increased

intracranial pressure can be elucidated by using the CAVI, which does not depend on blood pressure. We used a rabbit model to confirm this mechanism.

1. CAVI as an analytical index for a subarachnoid hemorrhage case

A 39-year-old male was diagnosed with subarachnoid hemorrhage (WFNS grade 2, Fisher grade 3) due to arterial elasticity and impaired consciousness after emergency transportation. Cerebrovascular three-dimensional computed tomography angiography examination confirmed the presence of a cerebral aneurysm, for which the patient was surgically treated the next day. The blood pressure (BP) and the CAVI were measured to be 124/77 mmHg and 6.7, respectively (Unfortunately, the pre-symptomatic values have not been measured). Although both increased thereafter, they decreased by about 3 weeks after the onset (Fig. 1).

Upon detailed study of the BP and CAVI values during this period, we observed a difference of about 1 week in the

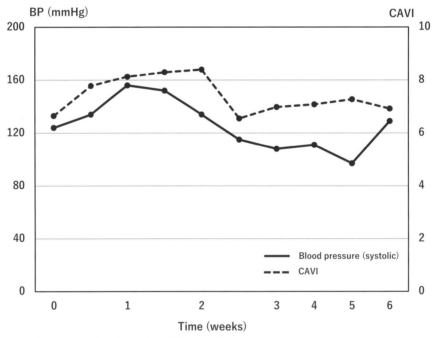

Fig. 1. Changes in a case of subarachnoid hemorrhage.
Blood pressure (BP) shows a gradual upward trend after surgery and peaks in about 1 week. On the other hand, it shows an upward trend from after surgery and peaks in about 2 weeks. Both blood pressure and CAVI improved to the level before surgery in about 3 weeks.

Department of Neurosurgery, JCHO Tokyo Kamata Medical Center, 2-19-2 South Kamata, Ota-ku, Tokyo, 144-0035, Japan.

timing of their peak values, with BP peaking before the CAVI. This result suggests that the extent of arterial stiffness may affect BP control, although other mechanisms may also exist. In order to reduce the sequelae of stroke, it is necessary to elucidate the role of arterial stiffness in this type of BP fluctuation, and then to establish a control method.

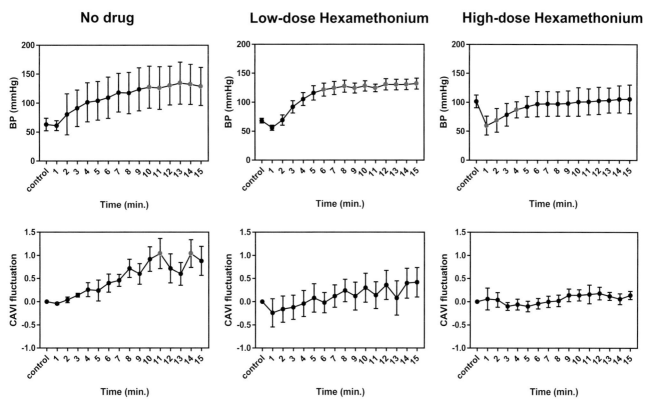

Fig. 2. Blood pressure and CAVI (value changes) during increased intracranial pressure in rabbits.

BP was significantly increased (p < 0.05) by raising intracranial pressure up to 10 mmHg for 5~15 minutes with saline injection into the cisterna magna. The upward tendency of BP is completely suppressed by the use of high dose hexamethonium due to autonomic nerve blockade with preadministration. CAVI also shows a significant upward tendency due to an increase in intracranial pressure. The autonomic nerve blockade suppresses the upward tendency of CAVI in a concentration-dependent manner. The red dot is a situation where the change is statistically significantly different compared to the control.

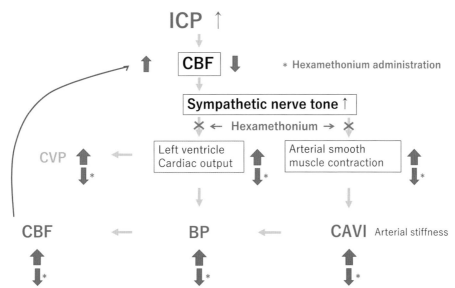

Fig. 3.   All parameters showed a concentration-dependent suppression tendency with respect to hexamethonium.

ICP; Intracranial pressure; CBF; cerebral blood flow, BP; blood pressure, CAVI; cardio ankle vascular index, CVP; central venous pressure. Quoted from 10)

2. Change in BP and CAVI due to raised intracranial pressure demonstrated in a rabbit model

In order to further investigate the relationship between intracranial pressure and BP, ventilator management was performed after induction of anesthesia in rabbits. Brachial BP and the CAVI were measured in the animals. By inserting a cannula into the foramen magnum and injecting saline, the intracranial pressure was increased upto 100 mmHg and was maintained for 5~15 min. We observed that, with the rise in intracranial pressure, the brachial BP as well as the CAVI increased (Fig. 2) [11]. Subsequently, we found that pre-administration of the autonomic ganglionic blocker hexamethonium suppressed the increase in the CAVI and BP. Furthermore, this tendency in the CAVI was clearly observed when hexamethonium was used at a low concentration, suggesting its usefulness.

Summary

We observed in both our observational and experimental studies that BP as well as the CAVI increased prominently with an increase in intracranial pressure. Pre-administration of hexamethonium suppressed these variations in rabbits. This suggests that the rise of BP in cases of subarachnoid hemorrhage is associated with increased intracranial pressure, which causes contraction of vascular medial smooth muscle cells by stimulation of the sympathetic nervous system[10]. In addition, a blood pressure control site is assumed to be present in the brainstem (Fig. 3) [11]. It is necessary to establish a post-stroke BP control method, considering the enhancement of arterial stiffness monitered with CAVI.

References

1) Qureshi Adnan I, et al.: Prevalence of elevated blood pressure in 563,704 adult patients with stroke presenting to the ED in the United States. Am J Emerg Med 2007; 25: 32-38.

2) Willmot Mark, Jo Leonardi-Bee, Philip M W Bath. High blood pressure in acute stroke and subsequent outcome: A systematic review. Hypertension 2004; 43: 18-24.

3) Bath Philip et al.: International Society of Hypertension (ISH): statement on the management of blood pressure in acute stroke. J Hypertens 2003; 21: 665-672.

4) Harvey Cushing: Concerning a definitive regulatory mechanism of the vasomotor center which controls blood pressure during cerebral compression. Bull Johns Hopkins Hosp 1901; 12: 290-292.

5) Gasecki, D., Rojek, A., Kwarciany, M., Kubach, M., Boutouyrie, P., Nyka, W., Laurent, S., & Narkiewicz, K. Aortic stiffness predicts functional outcome in patients after ischemic stroke. Stroke, 2012; 43, 543–544.

6) Bramwell J.C.,Downing A. C., Hill A.V.: The effect of blood pressure on the extensibility of the human artery. Heart 1923; 10: 289-300.

7) Nye E.R.: The effect of blood pressure alteration on the pulse wave velocity. Br Heart J 1964; 26: 261-265.

8) Van Bortel Luc M, et al.: Clinical Applications of arterial stiffness, Task force III: Recommendations for User Procedures. Am J Hypertens 2002; 15: 445-452.

9) Laurent Stephane, et al.: Expert consensus document on arterial stiffness: methodological issues and clinical applications. Eur Heart J 2006; 27: 2588-2605.

10) Chiba Tatsuo, Mari Yamanaka, Sachie Takagi, Kazuhiro Shimizu, Mao Takahashi, Kohji Shirai, Akira Takahara: Cardio-ankle vascular index (CAVI) differentiates pharmacological properties of vasodilators nicardipine and nitroglycerin in anesthetized rabbits. J Pharmacol Sci 2015; 128: 185-192.

11) Miyazaki Chikao et al.: Effects of enhanced intracranial pressure on blood pressure and the cardio-ankle vascular index in rabbits. J Atheroscler Thromb in press. http://doi.org/10.5551/jat.59451

Effect of Phentolamine and Atenolol on aortic Beta and iliac-femoral Beta - The presence of crosstalk between elastic-artery and muscular-artery -

Shin-ichiro Katsuda

Background and Purpose

Antihypertensive drugs have been used to prevent cerebrovascular and cardiovascular disorders. It has been reported that the cardiovascular preventive events differ among drugs, even if their antihypertensive effect is similar[1]. The mechanism underlying the difference is not yet clear. Although arterial stiffness has been assumed to result in functional changes during administration of antihypertensive drugs, it has not yet been investigated what type of vascular function change actually occurs. Pulse wave velocity (PWV) has been used as a direct measure of arterial stiffness[2]. It is dependent on blood pressure (BP) at the time of measurement[3], and hence, the effects of antihypertensive agents on vascular inherent elastic performance was not verified.

The cardio-ankle vascular index (CAVI) has recently been developed as a blood pressure-independent index of arterial stiffness, which now makes it possible to measure elasticity over the length of the entire artery [4, 5]. The arteries consist of the aorta (an elastic artery), thick and thin arteries (muscular arteries), and arterioles. It remains unclear whether each type of artery responds uniformly to antihypertensive drugs. We obtained the arterial stiffness index of the aorta (aortic Beta; aBeta) and the common iliac–femoral artery (iliac-femoral Beta; ifBeta), respectively, by applying the CAVI theory to the elastic artery (entire aorta) and muscular arteries (common iliac and femoral arteries).

In the present study, we investigated changes in aBeta and ifBeta to clarify the intrinsic response of the aorta and iliac–femoral arteries in rabbits when a non-selective α-adrenergic receptor blocker, phentolamine, and a β_1-adrenergic receptor blocker, atenolol, were administered intravenously (iv).

Methods

Twenty-five male Japanese white rabbits, aged 10–12 months, were anesthetized by administration of pentobarbital (30 mg/kg, iv) and fixed in a supine position. Butorphanol tartrate (0.3 mg/kg, intramuscular) was injected to reduce pain. Pressure waves were recorded at the origin of the aorta

(oA), the distal abdominal aorta (dA), and the distal end of the left femoral artery (fA), simultaneously with flow waves at oA when phentolamine (50 µg/kg/min) and atenolol (10 mg/kg/min) were infused for 2 min, respectively. PWV was determined by the difference in rising time of the two pressure waves and the distance between the two pressure sensors. Beta was calculated using the following equation: Beta = 2ρ / PP $\times$ ln(SBP / DBP) $\times$ PWV^2 (ρ: blood density, SBP: systolic blood pressure, DBP: diastolic blood pressure; PP: pulse pressure). aBeta, ifBeta, and aifBeta were calculated based on PWV in the entire aorta (aPWV), from dA to fA (ifPWV), and from oA to fA (aifPWV), respectively.

Results

SBP and DBP decreased significantly during the administration of phentolamine (Fig. 1A) and atenolol (Fig. 1B). Cardiac output increased significantly and decreased during the infusion of phentolamine and atenolol, respectively[6]. Total peripheral vascular resistance significantly decreased due to the administration of phentolamine, while it did not change significantly in response to the atenolol administration[6]. aBeta increased significantly despite the decrease in BP, while ifBeta decreased during the administration of phentolamine (Fig. 1C). aifBeta showed a slight but significant increase at 4 min after the infusion of phentolamine (Fig. 1C). On the other hand, aBeta, ifBeta, and aifBeta showed no significant change during atenolol infusion (Fig. 1D). aPWV, ifPWV, and aifPWV declined significantly concomitant with the decrease in BP during the infusion of phentolamine (Fig. 1E) and atenolol (Fig. 1F). aBeta and aifBeta showed a significant negative correlation with SBP and DBP, whereas ifBeta showed a significant positive correlation with SBP and DBP in response to the infusion of phentolamine (Table 1).

Discussion

The present study revealed that the elastic and muscular arteries showed contradictory responses to the intravenous infusion of phentolamine: that is, the aorta stiffened functionally, whereas the iliac–femoral arteries softened. To

Department of Cellular and Integrative Physiology, Fukushima Medical University, School of Medicine, 1 Hikariga-oka, Fukushima City, Fukushima 960-1295, Japan.

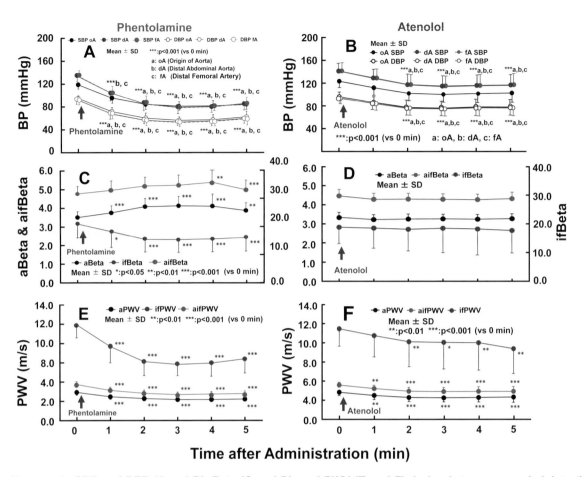

Fig. 1. Changes in SBP and DBP (A and B), Beta (C and D), and PWV (E and F) during intravenous administration of a non-selective α-adrenergic receptor blocker, phentolamine, and a β1-adrenergic receptor blocker, atenolol.

BP: blood pressure, SBP: systolic blood pressure, DBP: diastolic blood pressure, oA: origin of the aorta, dA: distal abdominal aorta, fA: distal end of the femoral artery, aBeta: aortic Beta, ifBeta: iliac–femoral Beta, aifBeta: aortic-iliac-femoral Beta, aPWV: aortic pulse wave velocity, ifPWV: iliac–femoral pulse wave velocity, aifPWV: aortic-iliac–femoral pulse wave velocity, 0 min: before administration (control). Phentolamine and atenolol were intravenously administered for 2 min using a syringe pump in doses of 50 μg/kg/min and 10 mg/kg/min, respectively. Adapted from ref.6

Table 1. Correlation coefficients between SBP and Beta, between DBP and Beta, between SBP and PWV, and between DBP and PWV during the intravenous administration of phentolamine and atenolol.

		Beta	ifBeta	aifBeta	aPWV	ifPWV	aifPWV
Phentolamine	SBP	- 0.523[***]	0.380[***]	- 0.381[***]	0.845[***]	0.778[***]	0.884[***]
	DBP	- 0.586[***]	0.405[***]	- 0.424[***]	0.801[***]	0.793[***]	0.864[***]
Atenolol	SBP	0.111	0.050	0.156	0.916[***]	0.403[***]	0.902[***]
	DBP	0.006	0.278	0.220	0.868[***]	0.611[***]	0.924[***]

[***]p < 0.001. See the legend of Fig. 1.

date, arteries were thought to respond to some vasoactive drugs uniformly; however, the difference in the response of different arterial sites to vasoactive drugs produced contradictory changes in elastic performance. Yamamoto et al.[7] previously reported that the arterial response to nitroglycerin was different between the aorta to femoral arteries and the femoral to tibial artery segments. The vasodilatory response in the femoral to tibial artery segment is prominent in artherosclerotic subjects as compared with that in healthy subjects. It is necessary to verify whether conflicting arterial responses to phentolamine could occur in humans. This raises questions as to how this phenomenon was reflected in atherosclerosis progression after long-term administration of vasoactive drugs, and how it was involved in the occurrence of cardiovascular events. Clinical observational studies are needed in future.

Conclusion

The aorta and iliac–femoral arteries showed conflicting responses to decreased BP induced by phentolamine, but not by atenolol. These results indicated that the arterial wall stiffness is separately regulated in the elastic and muscular arteries. That is, it might be suggested that there existed cross-talk between both arteries. The precise mechanism needs further studies.

Acknowledgement

The author wants to express gratitude to Dr. Kohji Shirai for his kind instructions and to Ms. Yuko Horikoshi, Dr. Yuko Fujikura, and Mr. Haruyuki Wago for their kind support for the present study.

References

1) Williams B, Lacy PS, Thom SM, Cruickshank K, Stanton A, Collier D, Hughes AD, Thurston H, O'Rourke M. Differential impact of blood pressure-lowering drugs on central aortic pressure and clinical outcomes: principal results of the Conduit Artery Function Evaluation (CAFE) study. Circulation 2006; 113: 1213-1225.

2) Laurent S, Cockcroft J, Van Bortel L, Boutouyrie P, Giannattasio C, Hayoz D, Pannier B, Vlachopoulos C, Wilkinson I, Struijker-Boudier H. Expert consensus document on arterial stiffness: methodological issues and clinical applications. Eur Heart J 2006; 27: 2588-2605.

3) Spronck B, Heusinkveld MH, Vanmolkot FH, Roodt JO, Hermeling E, Delhaas T, Kroon AA, Reesink KD. Pressure-dependence of arterial stiffness: potential clinical implications. J Hypertens 2015; 33: 330-338.

4) Shirai K, Hiruta N, Song M, Kurosu T, Suzuki J, Tomaru T, Miyashita Y, Saiki A, Takahashi M, Suzuki K, Takata M. Cardio-ankle vascular index (CAVI) as a novel indicator of arterial stiffness: theory, evidence and perspectives. J Atheroscler Thromb 2011; 18: 924-938.

5) Shirai K, Utino J, Saiki A, Endo K, Ohira M, Nagayama D, Tatsuno I, Shimizu K, Takahashi M, Takahara A. Evaluation of blood pressure control using a new arterial stiffness parameter, cardio-ankle vascular index (CAVI). Curr Hypertens Rev 2013; 9: 66-75.

6) Katsuda S, Fujikura Y, Horikoshi Y, Hazama A, Shimizu T, Shirai K. Different responses of arterial stiffness between the aorta and the ilio-femoral artery during the administration of phentolamine and atenolol in rabbits. J Atheroscler Thromb 2021; 28: 611-621.

7) Yamamoto T, Shimizu K, Takahashi M, Tatsuno I, Shirai K: The effect of nitroglycerin on arterial stiffness of the aorta and the femoral-tibial arteries. J Atheroscler Thromb 2017; 24: 1048-1057.

PART 8

Various applications of CAVI in Clinical usage

Cardio-Ankle Vascular Index Values of Koreans

Jeong Bae Park[1,2]

The aging process is associated with elevation of blood pressure and metabolic changes in glucose, cholesterol, and weight, depending on genetic background, in the healthy population. A change in arterial function, such as increased stiffness with structural remodeling, is indicative of progressive aging. In the case of cardiovascular risks such as hypertension, dyslipidemia, metabolic syndrome, and diabetes, the aging-associated vascular alterations are accelerated[1]. This is particularly true in Korea now because the aging progress in the Korean population is rapid. Therefore, understanding the pathophysiology of the aging process is important to distinguish accelerated aging from healthy aging. Among aging-associated changes, arterial stiffening is a key process in aging-driven changes in

atherosclerotic occlusive cardiovascular events, pulse wave encephalopathy, nephropathy, and dementia (Fig. 1).

The cardio-ankle vascular index (CAVI) was introduced in 2006 to evaluate arterial stiffness. CAVI applied the stiffness parameter beta (arterial distensibility at one point) in all arterial segments from heart to ankle using pulse wave velocity (PWV). The technique improved blood pressure dependency of the measurement of PWV, and CAVI is now widely used in clinical settings. Since the first publication on CAVI in 2013[2], 31 studies in Korea have been published, as identified in a search of PubMed (www.pubmed.gov). This brief review aims to summarize the CAVI articles published under diverse conditions from the healthy population to the patients with cardiovascular risk and

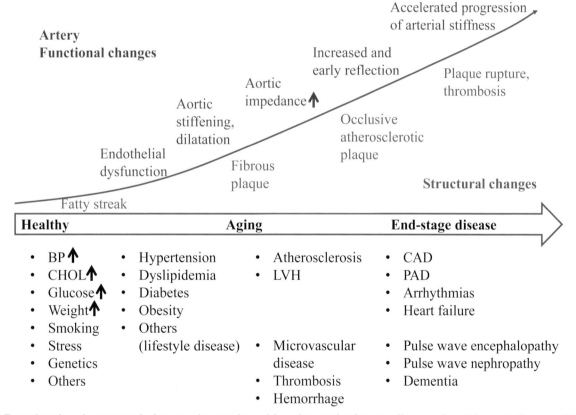

Fig. 1. Functional and structural changes in arteries with aging and other cardiovascular risks and disease. BP, blood pressure; CHOL, cholesterol; LVH, left ventricular hypertrophy; CAD, coronary artery disease; and PAD, peripheral artery disease.

[1]Director of JB lab and clinic, Seoul, Korea.
[2]Department of Precision Medicine and Biostatistics, Yonsei University, Wonju College of Medicine, Seoul, Korea.

disease among Koreans. This will lead to a better understanding of cardiovascular-risk–driven changes in arterial stiffness with age.

CAVI in Healthy Asymptomatic Koreans

The first paper evaluated the effect of age on arterial stiffness using CAVI in asymptomatic and apparently healthy Koreans between 20–80 years of age[2]. CAVI showed a linear increase with age compared with systolic or diastolic blood pressure and pulse pressure. The slightly higher CAVI value in men than in women less than 60 years of age disappeared in subjects older than 60 years. Whereas

Table 1.   Key reference studies for clinical application of CAVI in Koreans.

Category	Subjects	Findings	references
General population	Asymptomatic healthy Koreans	▪ Age- and sex-stratified value of CAVI in healthy Koreans ▪ Clinical application of CAVI in healthy Koreans ▪ A high hsCRP level as a predictor of high CAVI in healthy adult females ▪ Epicardial fat reflects arterial stiffness ▪ Nonalcoholic fatty liver disease as a risk factor for arterial stiffness in an apparently healthy population ▪ Association of coronary artery calcification or stenosis in asymptomatic subjects ▪ Association between arterial stiffness and obstructive sleep apnea in the elderly ▪ Association of metabolic syndrome with CAVI in an asymptomatic Korean population ▪ Association of cerebral small-vessel disease in healthy young and middle-aged subjects ▪ *Helicobacter pylori* infection and arterial stiffness, CAVI ▪ Association of controlled attenuation parameter of liver steatosis with CAVI in the general population ▪ Association between muscle mass deficits and arterial stiffness in middle-aged men ▪ Association of urine 6-sulfatoxymelatonin levels with arterial stiffness in post-menopausal women	2, 3, 4, 5, 6, 7, 8, 9, 13, 15, 16, 17, 18
Patients with disease	Diabetes	▪ Association of diabetic peripheral neuropathy with arterial stiffness ▪ Association of microvascular complication with CAVI ▪ Association of changes in retinal and choroidal microvasculature with CAVI ▪ Surrogate marker of early atherosclerotic cardiovascular disease ▪ Association between CAVI and coronary atherosclerosis ▪ Association of FAM19A5, a novel secreted adipokine, with CAVI ▪ Relationship between systemic vascular characteristics and retinal nerve-fiber layer loss ▪ Serum bone morphogenetic protein 4 levels in relation to arterial stiffness and carotid atherosclerosis	10, 11, 12, 19, 20, 21, 22, 23
	Kidney disease	▪ Predictive value of CAVI for end-stage renal disease ▪ Association of serum albumin and homocysteine levels and CAVI ▪ Association of the ratio of osteoprotegerin to fetuin-A and vascular stiffness ▪ Cinacalcet effect on endothelial dysfunction and arterial stiffness	14, 24, 25, 26
	Other	▪ Association or clinical implication of other diseases such as polycystic ovary syndrome, Turner syndrome, psoriasis, preeclampsia, critical limb ischemia, and Tai Chi exercise effects on arterial stiffness in elderly women with rheumatoid arthritis	27, 28, 29, 30, 31, 32

CAVI, cardio-ankle vascular index; hsCRP, high-sensitivity C-reactive protein

blood pressure in men less than 60 years of age was much higher than in women of the same age, this difference was not observed after 60 years. This implies that arterial stiffness is a better parameter of age-driven vascular changes than blood pressure, a long-standing traditional tool. CAVI is probably the most consistent parameter of aging, particularly vascular aging, irrespective of gender[3]. The usefulness of CAVI was demonstrated by its identification of the close association of arterial stiffness with high-sensitivity C-reactive protein in women[4] and epicardial adipose tissue[5], non-alcoholic fatty liver[6], coronary calcification[7], and sleep apnea in the elderly[8]. These observations suggest that CAVI can be used as a screening tool to assess cardiovascular risk and subclinical disease in an apparently healthy population[3]. In Korea, there is no CAVI cutoff point for high cardiovascular risk. The categorization as low (CAVI < 8), moderate (8 ≤ CAVI < 9), and high (CAVI ≥ 9) are generally well accepted, and it appears that CAVI ≥ 8 may be a more generally accepted cutoff value for the early detection of arteriosclerosis in a high-risk population.

CAVI in Metabolic Syndrome and Diabetes

Metabolic syndrome is a cluster of metabolic cardiovascular risks such as hypertension, diabetes, dyslipidemia, and obesity. The more metabolic risk factors were closely associated with high CAVI values and, among risk factors, blood pressure with age and in men independently predicted CAVI in an asymptomatic Korean population[9]. In patients with diabetes, an advanced form of metabolic disease, CAVI was the most sensitive surrogate marker compared to carotid intima-media thickness and ankle-brachial index for the prediction of future atherosclerotic cardiovascular disease[10]. Two papers dealt with micro- and macro-complications of diabetes with arterial stiffness, with most data showing a significant association between the two[11, 12]. In a diabetes clinic setting, monitoring of arterial stiffness will help identify patients with early atherosclerotic cardiovascular disease and its complications and to monitor the effects of therapy in those patients.

CAVI with Small-Vessel Disease in Brain

Cerebral small-vessel disease increases the risk of stroke and cognitive impairment. In a study on arterial stiffness and small-vessel disease in the brain, 4.1% of asymptomatic young and middle-aged subjects had silent cerebral small-vessel disease[13]. The highest quartile, CAVI > 7.65 compared to other quartiles, was independently associated with cerebral small-vessel disease after adjustment for pulse pressure (odds ratio 1.889, p = 0.002), an indirect component of arterial stiffness. This study showed the possibility of arterial stiffness as a surrogate marker of subclinical small-vessel disease in the brain.

CAVI and the Risk of End-Stage Renal Disease

A 7-year follow-up in a total of 8701 patients, with mostly diabetes and hypertension, cerebrovascular disease, or peripheral vascular disease at baseline showed 203 and 1071 patients with end-stage renal disease and mortality retrospectively[14]. This demonstrated that patients in the highest quartile of CAVI showed a higher risk of end-stage renal disease than those in the lowest quartile, with an adjusted hazard ratio of 2.35. The predictive value of CAVI for end-stage renal disease in this study was independent of death risk and other relevant risk factors such as age, sex, renal function, and drug use. Progression of kidney disease is associated with the progression of arteriosclerosis and atherosclerosis, and the detection of subclinical arterial changes might improve cardiovascular risk prediction. Therefore, continuous monitoring of CAVI in diabetic patients may be suggested to monitor the risk of chronic kidney disease and end-stage renal disease.

In conclusion, the clinical application of CAVI, a measure of arterial stiffness that is independent of blood pressure, was evaluated in asymptomatic healthy subjects as a predictor of hypertension, metabolic syndrome, and diabetes. The prediction of future atherosclerotic cardiovascular disease, subclinical coronary atherosclerosis, and end-stage renal disease was highly accurate (Table 1). Approval of continuous monitoring of CAVI after treatment is needed to allow wider use in a clinical setting.

Key references

1) Kim SA, Park JB, O'Rourke MF. Vasculopathy of Aging and the Revised Cardiovascular Continuum. Pulse (Basel). 2015;3:141-7.

2) Choi SY, Oh BH, Bae Park JB, Choi DJ, Rhee MY, Park S. Age-associated increase in arterial stiffness measured according to the cardio-ankle vascular index without blood pressure changes in healthy adults. J Atheroscler Thromb. 2013;20:911–923.

3) Choi SY. Clinical Application of the Cardio-Ankle Vascular Index in Asymptomatic Healthy Koreans. Pulse (Basel). 2017;4(Suppl 1):17-20.

4) Yang JY, Nam JS, Choi HJ. Association between high-sensitivity C-reactive protein with arterial stiffness in healthy Korean adults. Clin Chim Acta. 2012;413:1419-23.

5) Park HE, Choi SY, Kim HS, Kim MK, Cho SH, Oh BH. Epicardial fat reflects arterial stiffness: assessment using 256-slice multidetector coronary computed tomography and cardio-ankle vascular index. J Atheroscler Thromb. 2012;19:570-6.

6) Chung GE, Choi SY, Kim D, Kwak MS, Park HE, Kim MK, Yim JY. Nonalcoholic fatty liver disease as a risk factor of arterial stiffness measured by the cardioankle vascular index. Medicine (Baltimore) 2015;94:e654.

7) Park JB, Park HE, Choi SY, Kim MK, Oh BH. Relation between cardio-ankle vascular index and coronary artery calcification or stenosis in asymptomatic subjects. J Atheroscler Thromb. 2013;20:557-67.

8) Kim T, Lee CS, Lee SD, Kang SH, Han JW, Malhotra A, Kim KW, Yoon IY. Impacts of comorbidities on the association between arterial stiffness and obstructive sleep apnea in the elderly. Respiration. 2015;89:304-11.

9) Nam SH, Kang SG, Lee YA, Song SW, Rho JS. Association of Metabolic Syndrome with the Cardioankle Vascular Index in Asymptomatic Korean Population. J Diabetes Res. 2015;328585.

10) Kim ES, Moon SD, Kim HS, Lim DJ, Cho JH, Kwon HS, Ahn CW, Yoon KH, Kang MI, Cha BY, Son HY. Diabetic peripheral neuropathy is associated with increased arterial

stiffness without changes in carotid intima-media thickness in type 2 diabetes. Diabetes Care. 2011;34:1403-5.

11) Kim KJ, Lee BW, Kim HM, Shin JY, Kang ES, Cha BS, Lee EJ, Lim SK, Lee HC. Associations between cardio-ankle vascular index and microvascular complications in type 2 diabetes mellitus patients. J Atheroscler Thromb. 2011;18:328-36.

12) Kim M, Kim RY, Kim JY, Park YH. Correlation of systemic arterial stiffness with changes in retinal and choroidal microvasculature in type 2 diabetes. Sci Rep. 2019;9:1401.

13) Choi SY, Park HE, Seo H, Kim M, Cho SH, Oh BH. Arterial stiffness using cardio-ankle vascular index reflects cerebral small vessel disease in healthy young and middle aged subjects. J Atheroscler Thromb. 2013;20:178-85.

14) Jeong JS, Kim JH, Kim DK, Oh KH, Joo KW, Kim YS, Cho YM, Han SS. Predictive value of cardio-ankle vascular index for the risk of end-stage renal disease. Clin Kidney J. 2020;14:255-260.

15) Choi JM, Lim SH, Han YM, Lee H, Seo JY, Park HE, Kwak MS, Chung GE, Choi SY, Kim JS. Association between Helicobacter pylori infection and arterial stiffness: Results from a large cross-sectional study. PLoS One. 2019 Aug 29;14:e0221643.

16) Park HE, Lee H, Choi SY, Kwak MS, Yang JI, Yim JY, Chung GE. Usefulness of controlled attenuation parameter for detecting increased arterial stiffness in general population. Dig Liver Dis. 2018;50:1062-1067.

17) Im IJ, Choi HJ, Jeong SM, Kim HJ, Son JS, Oh HJ. The association between muscle mass deficits and arterial stiffness in middle-aged men. Nutr Metab Cardiovasc Dis. 2017;27:1130-1135.

18) Lee JY, Lee DC. Urine 6-sulfatoxymelatonin levels are inversely associated with arterial stiffness in post-menopausal women. Maturitas. 2014;78:117-22.

19) Park SY, Chin SO, Rhee SY, Oh S, Woo JT, Kim SW, Chon S. Cardio-Ankle Vascular Index as a Surrogate Marker of Early Atherosclerotic Cardiovascular Disease in Koreans with Type 2 Diabetes Mellitus. Diabetes Metab J. 2018;42:285-295.

20) Park HE, Choi SY, Kim MK, Oh BH. Cardio-ankle vascular index reflects coronary atherosclerosis in patients with abnormal glucose metabolism: assessment with 256 slice multi-detector computed tomography. J Cardiol. 2012;60:372-6.

21) Lee YB, Hwang HJ, Kim JA, Hwang SY, Roh E, Hong SH, Choi KM, Baik SH, Yoo HJ. Association of serum FAM19A5 with metabolic and vascular risk factors in human subjects with or without type 2 diabetes. Diab Vasc Dis Res. 2019;16:530-538.

22) Jeon SJ, Park HL, Lee JH, Park CK. Relationship between Systemic Vascular Characteristics and Retinal Nerve Fiber Layer Loss in Patients with Type 2 Diabetes. Sci Rep. 2018;8:10510.

23) Son JW, Jang EH, Kim MK, Baek KH, Song KH, Yoon KH, Cha BY, Son HY, Lee KW, Jo H, Kwon HS. Serum BMP-4 levels in relation to arterial stiffness and carotid atherosclerosis in patients with Type 2 diabetes. Biomark Med. 2011;5:827-35.

24) Lee JA, Kim DH, Yu SJ, Oh DJ, Yu SH. Association of serum albumin and homocysteine levels and cardio-ankle vascular index in patients with continuous ambulatory peritoneal dialysis. Korean J Intern Med. 2006;21:33-8.

25) Kim HR, Kim SH, Han MJ, Yoon YS, Oh DJ. The ratio of osteoprotegerin to fetuin-a is independently associated with vascular stiffness in hemodialysis patients. Nephron Clin Pract. 2013;123:165-72.

26) Choi SR, Lim JH, Kim MY, Hong YA, Chung BH, Chung S, Choi BS, Yang CW, Kim YS, Chang YS, Park CW. Cinacalcet improves endothelial dysfunction and cardiac hypertrophy in patients on hemodialysis with secondary hyperparathyroidism. Nephron Clin Pract. 2012;122:1-8.

27) Kim J, Choi SY, Park B, Park HE, Lee H, Kim MJ, Kim SM, Hwang KR, Choi YM. Arterial stiffness measured by cardio-ankle vascular index in Korean women with polycystic ovary syndrome. J Obstet Gynaecol. 2019;39:681-686.

28) Heo YJ, Jung HW, Lee YA, Shin CH, Yang SW. Arterial stiffness in young women with Turner syndrome using cardio-ankle vascular index. Ann Pediatr Endocrinol Metab. 2019;24:158-163.

29) Choi BG, Kim MJ, Yang HS, Lee YW, Choe YB, Ahn KJ. Assessment of Arterial Stiffness in Korean Patients With Psoriasis by Cardio-Ankle Vascular Index. Angiology. 2017;68:608-613.

30) Kim S, Lim HJ, Kim JR, Oh KJ, Hong JS, Suh JW. Longitudinal change in arterial stiffness after delivery in women with preeclampsia and normotension: a prospective cohort study. BMC Pregnancy Childbirth. 2020;20:685.

31) Kim D, Cho DJ, Cho YI. Reduced amputation rate with isovolemic hemodilution in critical limb ischemia patients. Clin Hemorheol Microcirc. 2017;67:197-208.

32) Shin JH, Lee Y, Kim SG, Choi BY, Lee HS, Bang SY. The beneficial effects of Tai Chi exercise on endothelial function and arterial stiffness in elderly women with rheumatoid arthritis. Arthritis Res Ther. 2015;17:380.

Application of CAVI as a Vascular Biomarker in Environmental Research and Clinical Studies in Taiwan

Ta-Chen Su[1,2,3,4]

Abstract

Cardio-ankle vascular index (CAVI), an index of arterial stiffness, can be noninvasively measured and applied as a simple subclinical marker of vascular damage and cardiovascular disease. CAVI can be a sensitive vascular index in investigating the health effects of air pollution exposure, particularly fine particulate matter (PM) and transition metal components in PM. CAVI also can be applied in clinical studies, including subjects with prediabetes, patients with hemodialysis and renal transplantation, and women with overactive bladder syndrome. The clinical utility and usefulness of CAVI measurement in environmental cardiology also indicate its advantage in preventive cardiology.

Introduction

Cardiovascular diseases (CVDs) are the leading causes of mortality and a major disease burden worldwide, particularly among Asian populations in Taiwan and China[1-2]. In recent decades, environmental pollution and climate change issues became more and more critical, and studies show such issues are associated with CVDs and related risk factors. Scientific evidence has shown that air pollution is associated with cardiovascular mortality and morbidity; a consensus report was published in American Heart Association/ American College of Cardiology[3]. In addition to traditional major risk factors, such as diabetes, hypertension, hypercholesterolemia, smoking habit, obesity, and family history, air pollution is also recognized as a contributing factor of CVDs[3-6].

Arterial stiffness was a surrogate marker of CVDs and related risk factors[7-8]. Cardio-ankle vascular index (CAVI), indicative of aortic, femoral and tibial arterial stiffness, can be noninvasively measured simply by wrapping the four extremities with blood pressure cuffs, and it serves as a simple marker of vascular damage and cardiovascular disease[9-11]. CAVI represents the changes in vascular tone and is correlated with the left ventricular function in patients with ischemic heart disease[11]. Thus, using the biomarker of arterial stiffness to investigate the association between CAVI and air pollution may shed light on the hazardous effects of environmental pollution. Clinical studies using CAVI can also provide an advantageous tool in investigating vascular health outcomes.

CAVI and Air pollution

In a review article that summarized previous studies conducted in the Asia Pacific area[12], important cardiovascular biomarkers related to air pollutants were discussed[13-16]. Among them, CAVI was first documented to be positively associated with ozone (O_3) and fine particulate matter (PM) exposure[16]. In addition, CAVI was also shown to be significantly associated with transition metals in fine PM exposure[17].

In this panel study of seventeen mail carriers, the participants were followed for 5−6 days while delivering mail outdoors. We analyzed the component- and source-specific health effects on heart rate variability (HRV) indices and CAVI using mixed models. Researchers reported that an interquartile range (IQR) increase in personal exposure to O_3 and $PM_{1.0-2.5}$ was associated with a 4.8% and 2.5% increase in CAVI but not with HRV change among young, healthy mail carriers in Fig. 1[16].

Personal filter samples of $PM_{2.5-1.0}$ and $PM_{0.25}$ were analyzed for their elemental concentrations. The source-specific exposures were further estimated using absolute principal factor analysis. Further investigation of the association between element carbon and arterial stiffness in the same study subjects also demonstrated some transition metals are significantly positively correlated with CAVI[17]. The source apportionment results were applied in the mixed models analyses. It was found that an IQR increase in personal exposure to $PM_{2.5-1.0}$ from regional sources was significantly associated with a 3.3% (95% CI: 1.5%−5.1%) increase of CAVI. This significant effect remained with 3.35% (1.62%−5.11%) after controlling for the O_3

[1]Department of Environmental and Occupational Medicine, National Taiwan University Hospital, Taipei, Taiwan.
[2]Department of Internal Medicine and Cardiovascular Center, National Taiwan University Hospital, Taipei, Taiwan.
[3]Institute of Environmental and Occupational Health Sciences, College of Public Health, National Taiwan University, Taipei, Taiwan.
[4]The Experimental Forest, National Taiwan University, Nantou, Taiwan.

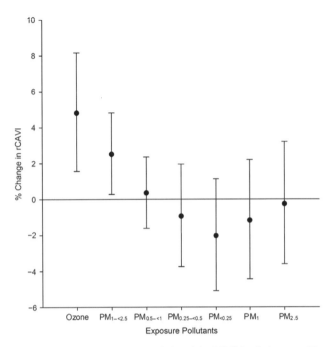

Fig. 1. Percent change in right-side CAVI for interquartile range changes of ozone and particulate matter exposures in single-pollutant models, Taipei County, Taiwan, February–March, 2007.
[Adapted with permission of Oxford University Press from Wu et al.][16)

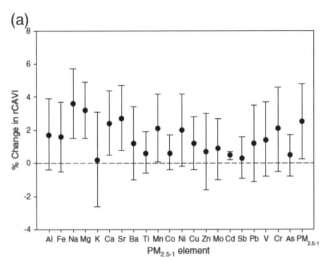

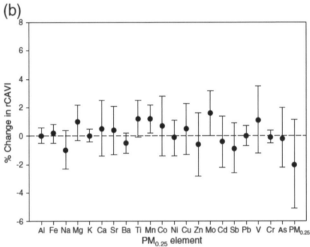

Fig. 2. Percent changes in rCAVI indices for an IQR of (a) $PM_{2.5-1}$ element and (b) $PM_{0.25}$ element levels in single-pollutant, mixed-effects models. [Adapted with permission of Elsevier from Chang-fu et al.][17)

exposures[17).

For $PM_{2.5-1.0}$ transition metals, an IQR increase in exposures to sodium (Na), magnesium (Mg), calcium (Ca), strontium (Sr), manganese (Mn), and cadmium (Cd), significantly increased the CAVI by 3.6% (95% CI: 1.5%–5.7%), 3.2% (1.5%–4.9%), 2.4% (0.5%–4.4%), 2.7% (0.8%–4.7%), 2.1% (0.4%–4.2%) and 0.5% (0.2%–0.7%), respectively. However, Mn and Molybdenum (Mo) were the only two elements having significant impacts on CAVI for the $PM_{0.25}$ elements (Fig. 2)[17). This series of studies indicates that arterial stiffness may be more sensitive to air pollutants than the autonomic balance and CAVI can be used as a novel marker of cardiovascular effects while investigating exposure to air pollution[18).

We also used CAVI as an indicator of subclinical cardiovascular disease in assessing the effects of long-term exposure to a forest environment[19). Although there was no significant difference in CAVI measurements between workers in the Xitou forest environment and office workers in Taipei, there was a trend of higher CAVI values in urban office workers.

Clinical studies

1. Prediabetes

Postprandial hyperglycemia and diabetes have been shown to be associated with CVDs[20-22). Even after controlling for traditional risk factors, diabetics still exhibit a two- to four-fold increased risk compared to non-diabetic subjects[20). Increasing evidence suggests that postprandial hyperglycemia is a direct and independent risk factor for CVD[21, 22). Studies support that the pathogenesis of vascular

diseases in diabetes partly comes from stiffness in affected arteries[23).

Our previous study in healthy adults showed that the post-challenge hyperglycemic spike is significantly associated with CAVI[24). In addition, we also demonstrated that this non-invasive assessment is easily performed and highly reliable among Taiwanese, with an inter-observer correlation coefficient of 0.85 for mean CAVI[24). Thus, applying CAVI measurement for pre-diabetic subjects and diabetic patients can provide important information regarding subclinical CVDs.

2. Chronic Renal Failure

Arterial stiffness is an independent predictor of all-cause and cardiovascular mortality, particularly in patients with end-stage renal disease (ESRD). Studies in Japan had proved that CAVI is a prognostic predictor for CVDs in hemodialysis patients[25-26). Shen et al. followed up 59 dialysis patients without initial arterial stiffness for one year and found that *de novo* arterial stiffness in dialysis patients as determined by CAVI was significantly associated with age and initial serum phosphorus[27].

Recent studies have noted that B-type natriuretic peptide (BNP) acts as a local paracrine molecule that modulates endothelial permeability and regeneration[28]. The serum fasting N-terminal pro-BNP level is associated with arterial stiffness in renal transplant recipients[29]. The clinical utility of measurement of CAVI was confirmed in patients with ESRD not only among Japanese but also in Taiwanese.

3. Other clinical trials

Overactive bladder syndrome (OAB), with or without urge incontinence, is characterized by urinary urgency, frequency, and nocturia[30]. The overall prevalence of OAB is not rare, with an estimated 16.9% in women[31]. A higher prevalence of CVDs in OAB women has been reported[32]. In a clinical trial in Taiwan, we studied the anti-muscarinics related effects in female OAB patients, and found that tolterodine could improve arterial stiffness, indexed by decreasing the CAVI[33]. However, tolterodine may improve arterial stiffness but may deteriorate autonomic dysfunction to more sympathetic predominance. In this study, CAVI serves as a vascular marker in clinical outcome studies.

Conclusions

CAVI is an easy-to-use and highly reliable measure for the diagnosis of subclinical CVDs, particularly in patients with pre-diabetes and ESRD, and can be applied as a sensitive vascular marker for clinical trials. The clinical utility and usefulness of CAVI measurement in environmental cardiology also indicate its advantage in preventive cardiology.

References

1) Reddy KS. Cardiovascular disease in non-Western countries. N Engl J Med 2004;350:2438-2440.
2) He J, Gu D, Wu X, Reynolds K, Duan X, Yao C, et al. Major causes of death among men and women in China. N Engl J Med. 2005;353:1124-1134.
3) Brook RD, Rajagopalan S, Pope III CA, Brook JR, Bhatnagar A, Diez-Roux AV, et al. American Heart Association council on epidemiology and prevention, council on the kidney in cardiovascular disease, and council on nutrition, physical activity and metabolism. Particulate matter air pollution and cardiovascular disease: an update to the scientific statement from the American Heart Association. Circulation 2010;121: 2331-2378.
4) Ito K, Mathes R, Ross Z, Na´das A, Thurston G, Matte T. Fine particulate matter constituents associated with cardiovascular hospitalizations and mortality in New York City. Environ Health Perspect. 2011;119: 467-473.
5) Silva R, West JJ, Zhang Y, Anenberg SC, Lamarque JF, Shindell DT, et al. Global premature mortality due to anthropogenic outdoor air pollution and the contribution of past climate change. Environ Res Lett. 2013;8:03400514.
6) Su TC, Hwang JJ, Shen YC, Chan CC. Carotid intima-media thickness and long-term exposure to traffic-related air pollution in middle-aged residents of Taiwan: A cross-sectional study. Environ Health Perspect. 2015;123:773-8.
7) Amar J, Ruidavets JB, Chamontin B, Drouet L, Ferrières J. Arterial stiffness and cardiovascular risk factors in a population-based study. J Hypertens. 2001;19:381-7.
8) Najjar SS, Scuteri A, Lakatta EG. Arterial aging: is it an immutable cardiovascular risk factor? Hypertension 2005 Sep;46(3):454-62.
9) Shirai K, Utino J, Otsuka K, Takata M. A novel blood pressure-independent arterial wall stiffness parameter; cardio-ankle vascular index (CAVI). J Atheroscler Thromb. 2006;13:101-7.
10) Shirai K, Hiruta N, Song M, Kurosu T, Suzuki J, Tomaru T, et al. Cardio-ankle vascular index (CAVI) as a novel indicator of arterial stiffness: theory, evidence and perspectives. J Atheroscler Thromb. 2011;18:924-38.
11) Miyoshi T, Doi M, Hirohata S, Sakane K, Kamikawa S, Kitawaki T, et al. Cardio-ankle vascular index is independently associated with the severity of coronary atherosclerosis and left ventricular function in patients with ischemic heart disease. J Atheroscler Thromb. 2010;17;249-258.
12) Su TC, Chen SY, Chan CC. Progress of ambient air pollution and cardiovascular disease research in Asia. Prog Cardiovasc Dis. 2011;53:369-78.
13) Su TC, Chan CC, Liau CS, Lin LY, Kao HL, Chuang KJ. Urban air pollution increases plasma activator inhibitor-1 and fibrinogen levels in susceptible patients. Eur J Cardiovasc Prev Rehabil. 2006;13: 849-852.
14) Chuang KJ, Chan CC, Chen NT, Su TC, Lin LT. Effects of particle size fractions on reducing heart rate variability in cardiac and hypertensive patients. Environ. Health Perspect. 2005;113:1693-1697.
15) Chuang KJ, Chan CC, Su TC, Lee CT, Tang CS. The effect of urban air pollution on inflammation, oxidative stress, coagulation, and autonomic dysfunction in young adults. Am J Respir Crit Care Med. 2007;176:370-6.
16) Wu CF, Kuo IC, Su TC, Li YR, Lin LY, Chan CC, Hsu SC. Effects of personal exposure to particulate matter and ozone on arterial stiffness and heart rate variability in healthy adults. Am J Epidemiol. 2010;171:1299-309.
17) Wu CF, Li YR, Kuo IC, Hsu SC, Lin LY, Su TC. Investigating the association of cardiovascular effects with personal exposure to particle components and sources. Sci Total Environ. 2012;431:176-82.
18) Hoffmann B, Moebus S, Kroger K, Stang A, Möhlenkamp S, Dragano N, et al. Residential exposure to urban pollution, ankle-brachial index, and peripheral arterial disease. Epidemiology 2009; 20:280-288.
19) Tsao TM, Tsai MJ, Wang YN, Lin HL, Wu CF, Hwang JS, et al. The health effects of a forest environment on subclinical cardiovascular disease and health-related quality of life. PLoS One 2014 Jul 28;9(7):e103231.
20) Stamler J, Vaccaro O, Neaton J, Wentwirth D. For the Multiple Risk Factor Intervention Trial Research Group. Diabetes, other risk factors, and 12-year cardiovascular mortality for men screened in the Multiple Risk Factor Intervention Trial. Diabetes Care 1993; 16: 434-444.
21) Donahue RP, Abbott RD, Reed DM, Yano K. Postchallenge glucose concentration and coronary heart disease in men of Japanese ancestry. Honolulu Heart Program. Diabetes 1987; 36: 689–692.
22) The DECODE study group on behalf of the European Diabetes Epidemiology Group. Glucose tolerance and mortality: comparison of WHO and American Diabetes Association diagnostic criteria. Lancet 1999; 354: 617–621.
23) Grundy SM, Benjamin IJ, Burke GL, Chait A, Eckel RH, Howard BV, et al. Diabetes and cardiovascular disease: a statement for healthcare professionals from the American Heart Association. Circulation 1999; 100: 1134–1146.
24) Huang CL, Chen MF, Jeng JS, Lin LY, Wang WL, Feng MH, et al. Post-challenge hyperglycemic spike associate with arterial stiffness. Int J Clin Pract 2007; 61: 397-402.
25) Ichihara A, Yamashita N, Takemitsu T, Kaneshiro Y, Sakoda

M, Kurauchi-Mito A, Itoh H. Cardio-ankle vascular index and ankle pulse wave velocity as a marker of arterial fibrosis in kidney failure treated by hemodialysis. Am J Kidney Dis. 2008;52:947-955.

26) Ueyama K, Miyata M, Kubozono T, Nagaki A, Hamasaki S, Ueyama S, Tei C. Noninvasive indices of arterial stiffness in hemodialysis patients. Hypertens Res 2009;32:716-720.

27) Shen TW, Wang CH, Lai YH, Hsu BG, Liou HH, Fang TC. Use of cardio-ankle vascular index in chronic dialysis patients. Eur J Clin Invest 2011;41:45-51.

28) Kuhn M. Endothelial actions of atrial and B-type natriuretic peptides. Br J Pharmacol. 2012;166:522-31.

29) Chen YC, Lee MC, Lee CJ, Ho GJ, Yin WY, Chang YJ, Hsu BG. N-terminal pro-B-type natriuretic peptide is associated with arterial stiffness measured using the cardio-ankle vascular index in renal transplant recipients. J Atheroscler Thromb. 2013;20:646-53.

30) Haylen BT, de Ridder D, Freeman RM, Swift SE, Berghmans B, Lee J, et al. An international Urogynecological Association (IUGA)/International Continence Society (ICS) joint reporton the Terminology for female pelvic floor dysfunction. Int Urogynecol J 2010;21:5–26.

31) Stewart WF, Van Rooyen JB, Cundiff GW, Abrams P, Herzog AR, Corey R, et al. Prevalence and burden of over-active bladder in the United States. World J Urol 2003;20:327–36.

32) Andersson KE, Sarawate C, Kahler KH, Stanley EL, Kulkarni AS. Cardiovascular morbidity, heartrates and use of antimuscarinics in patients with overactive bladder. BJU Int 2010;106:268–74.

33) Hsiao SM, Su TC, Chen CH, Chang TC, Lin HH. Autonomic dysfunction and arterial stiffness in female overactive bladder patients and antimuscarinics related effects. Maturitas. 2014 Sep;79(1):65-9.

How to use the cardio-ankle vascular index (CAVI) in routine clinical practice

Takashi Hitsumoto

Summary

1. CAVI is a prognostic indicator for patients with chronic heart failure and chronic kidney disease.
2. There is a significant relationship between CAVI and novel risk factors such as oxidative stress, hypotestosteronemia, and advanced glycation end products.
3. By utilizing CAVI in daily practice, custom-made treatment for patients with lifestyle-related diseases becomes possible.

Introduction

Hitsumoto medical clinic sees patients with lifestyle-related diseases and cardiovascular diseases as a general clinic. In addition to the routine tests such as body weight measurement, blood pressure assessment, biochemical tests, electrocardiography, and cardiac ultrasonography, we measured arterial stiffness using the cardio-ankle vascular index (CAVI), periodically. This has been helpful to make a diagnosis of the stage of systemic arteriosclerosis, and also to quantify the progression speed of systemic arteriosclerosis. Furthermore, CAVI measurement enables us to investigate new risk factors beyond the classical risks for arteriosclerosis, and also helps us understand the validity of various treatments for each patient.

In this chapter, we explore our studies on the relationship between prognosis of the patients with chronic heart failure (CHF) and chronic kidney disease (CKD) and CAVI. Furthermore, as a candidate of another new risk beyond ordinary coronary risks, the relationship between serum testosterone values and CAVI will also be elaborated. Additionally, we will demonstrate how to use CAVI in seeing patients with lifestyle-related diseases by discussing three cases.

1. What we learned from our experience treating outpatients

With the rapid increase in the elderly population in Japan, the incidence of age-related diseases such as CHF and CKD has gradually increased. Even without the typical signs and symptoms, many biochemical blood examinations and, echocardiography reveal the presence of CHF and CKD among elderly patients. Therefore, the management of patients with CHF and CKD has become important for clinicians.

1) Prospective study on patients with CHF and CKD

In order to confirm the usefulness of the CAVI as a prognostic index for patients with CHF and CKD, we conducted a prospective prognostic survey among outpatients and found that the CAVI is an index for predicting initial hospitalization for heart failure in elderly

Table 1. Multivariate cox regression analysis for heart failure hospitalization.

A

	HR	95%CI	P value
Stage C	7.67	2.82-20.84	<0.001
CAVI ($\geq$ 10)	2.71	1.34-5.50	0.006
Group H	2.26	1.21-3.52	0.014
Diabetes mellitus	2.21	1.18-4.17	0.017
hs-CRP ($\geq$ 0.1mg/dL)	2.23	1.14-4.24	0.019
E/e' ($\geq$ 15)	2.10	1.01-4.44	0.049
BNP ($\geq$ 200pg/ml)	1.32	0.96-2.62	0.076
Age ($\geq$ 70years)	2.04	0.91-4.62	0.085
eGFR ($<$ 60ml/min/1.73m^2)	1.89	0.88-4.09	0.104
Current smoker	1.62	0.85-3.07	0.142
β-blocker	0.41	0.09-1.75	0.229

B

	HR	95%CI	P value
CAVI ($\geq$ 10)	2.85	1.33-6.09	0.007
Group H	2.36	1.15-4.86	0.019
hs-CRP ($\geq$0.1mg/dL)	2.30	1.14-4.63	0.020
Diabetes mellitus	2.09	1.14-4.24	0.034
E/e' ($\geq$ 15)	2.11	1.01-4.46	0.048
BNP ($\geq$ 200pg/ml)	1.85	0.96-3.56	0.066
eGFR ($<$ 60ml/min/1.73m^2)	1.70	0.86-3.58	0.127
Age ($\geq$ 70years)	1.67	0.72-3.54	0.144
β-blocker	0.25	0.03-1.91	0.183
Current smoker	1.20	0.47-3.07	0.227

A: Analysis in all patients, B: Analysis in patients with stage C

Hitsumoto T. Cardiol Res. 2020;11:247-255.

Hitsumoto Medical Clinic, 2-7-7 Takezakicho, Shimonoseki City, Yamaguchi 750-0025, Japan.

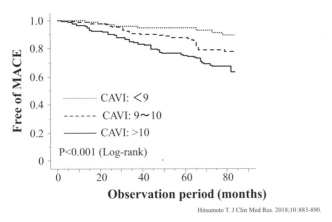

Hitsumoto T. J Clin Med Res. 2018;10:883-890.

Fig. 1. Major adverse cardiovascular events and CAVI in patients with chronic kidney disease.

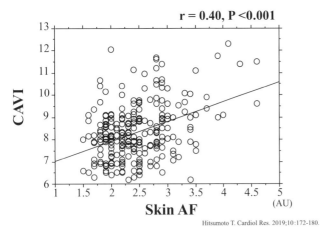

Hitsumoto T. Cardiol Res. 2019;10:172-180.

Fig. 2. Correlation between skin autofluorescence and CAVI in metabolic syndrome.

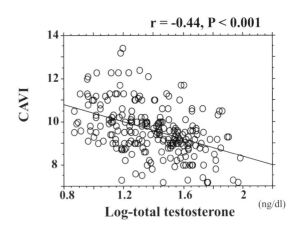

Hitsumoto T. Cardiol Res. 2019;10(1):9-17.

Fig. 3. Correlation between blood total testosterone concentrations and CAVI in Japanese females.

patients with CHF (**Table 1**)[1]; Furthermore, we found that the CAVI is related to the onset of cardiovascular events (primary event) in CKD patients[2] (**Fig. 1**). CHF and CKD are considered to be diseases with poor prognosis in patients across the globe. Many treatments to lower CAVI have been reported as described in other chapters (see chapter 55). The aforementioned results of our research have already might indicate that various treatments which a lower CAVI at an earlier stage could contribute to improve the prognosis of patients with CHF and CKD. Interventional studies to prove this are currently underway.

CAVI might be useful in identifying several patients with heart failure, and during follow up for various treatments.

2) The new risks found by CAVI

Recent studies have shown that inflammation and oxidative stress, in addition to the conventional risk factors of atherosclerosis, such as hypertension, diabetes mellitus, dyslipidemia, smoking, and obesity are deeply involved in the progression of atherosclerosis[3]. An examination of the relationship of inflammation and oxidative stress with arteriosclerosis using the d-ROMS test, which is a test for the oxidative stress marker, confirmed a significant relationship with CAVI[4]. Furthermore, the author also

reported that advanced glycation end products that are closely related to aging are significantly related to the CAVI[5] (**Fig. 2**).

The male hormone testosterone is also attracting attention as a novel risk factor for arteriosclerosis, and the importance of hypotestosteronemia in the onset of cardiovascular disease has been reported. We examined the relationship between blood testosterone levels and the CAVI in male patients who had risk factors for atherosclerosis and found a significant negative correlation between the two indicators. It is noteworthy that hypotestosteronemia was significantly associated with an elevated CAVI in female patients[6] (**Fig. 3**). However, the author has discovered the meaning and usefulness of 7-ketocholesterol as a new arteriosclerosis-promoting factor, lipoprotein lipase mass as a marker of insulin sensitivity, and high sensitivity troponin T as a marker of myocardial injury[3,7-10]. In the future, it is hoped that the relationship between CAVI and novel atherosclerosis risk factors will be examined from various aspects.

Thus, CAVI could help clinicians to resolve the issues faced in daily clinical practice.

2. Optimal usage of the CAVI during medical treatment

CAVI changes during the long term in each patient due to various conditions. **Fig. 4** shows the data of three patients with a history of hypertension over a long period of time (10 years).

Case A: 65 years old man: Improved CAVI during life style after retirement

Case A was an apparently healthy patient who retired and then began physical exercises such as mountain climbing and table tennis. He maintained a healthy body weight, and did not smoke. After 10 years of his hospital visit, the CAVI was measured again. As shown in Fig. 4, the CAVI value had improved significantly, compared to the value measured 10 years before. Usually, the CAVI increases with age in many patients; however, in patients who exercised regularly and consumed a healthy diet, as did patient A, and we observed a decrease in CAVI over a long period of time.

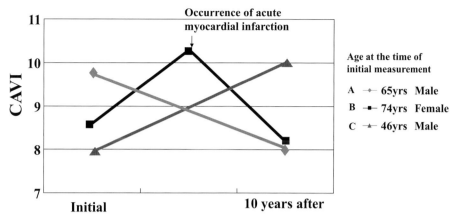

Fig. 4.   Long-term fluctuation of CAVI.

Therefore, practitioners and clinic staff should encourage patients with lifestyle-related diseases to perform regular exercise and consume a healthy diet by monitoring CAVI. We realized that good lifestyle habits are important for maintaining arterial stiffness.

Case B: 74 years old man.: Myocardial infarction after increased CAVI

In case B, the CAVI at the time of the initial measurement was slightly lower than that for the actual age; however, after 5 years, the CAVI increased sharply compared to the previous value. This patient suffered from acute myocardial infarction shortly thereafter. Fortunately, the patient survived by undergoing a coronary angioplasty and was recovering. Consequently, he was put on a continued course of statins at our outpatient department. As a result, the CAVI after 10 years was much lower than that recorded previously. Therefore, even if the patient develops a cardiovascular disease, secondary events can be prevented by continuing solid treatment including drugs and lifestyle modification with monitoring CAVI.

Case C: 46 year-old man; Heavy smoker

Case C was of a patient who was a heavy smoker, did not exercise regularly, and was obese with visceral fat accumulation. There was no significant change in the patient's subjective symptoms, and his blood pressure was controlled well. However, the CAVI value after the long-term follow-up was considerably higher than that measured previously. Moreover, the patient's mother had died of myocardial infarction. We explained to the patient the risk of a raised CAVI value and strongly persuaded to him quit smoking, exercise and reduce his body weight.

Previous reports have shown that smoking elevates the CAVI, and smoking cessation improves the CAVI. A long-term study at our hospital also confirmed that the CAVI of smokers rises faster than that of nonsmokers. Therefore, at the author's clinic, we provide smoking cessation guidance (for 3 months) using drug treatment and by providing counseling to patients who wish to quit smoking. While some patients successfully quit smoking with these treatments, some patients did not (smoking cessation success rate: 40%–60%). Sometimes, several patients drop

out during the treatment, because of no improvement of subjective symptoms. In order to encourage these patients to quit smoking, while periodically measuring CAVI periodically (during and after treatment) and showing them that an improved CAVI value might be useful.

Conclusion

At our clinic, we have outlined our novel findings and the appropriate treatment system that we have developed using regular CAVI measurements. The data obtained at our clinic show that CAVI could be a useful indicator to control asymptomatic silent diseases in which CAVI raises in daily clinical practice. Furthermore, it is expected that new knowledge or insight can be obtained by monitoring CAVI during medical treatment.

Commentary from the Editor

Dr. Takashi Hitsumoto, MD, PhD. is a cardiologist and is now a president of the private clinic. He established a cardiovascular laboratory in the clinic, and follow-up system for all patients. As demonstrated above, he has performed many cross-sectional and longitudinal studies using CAVI, and has published many valuable papers. He has been "learning from the patients." We express our sincere respect for his earnest and strenuous efforts for research. We are very happy that CAVI could contribute to his studies.

In the future, many new insights and theories can be discovered by monitoring the CAVI in various patients even in the clinics, if the doctor retains a research-oriented mind.

References

1) Hitsumoto T. Skin Autofluorescence as a Predictor of First Heart Failure Hospitalization in Patients With Heart Failure With Preserved Ejection Fraction. Cardiol Res. 2020;11:247-255. https://doi.org/10.14740/cr1097
2) Hitsumoto T. Clinical Usefulness of the Cardio-Ankle Vascular Index as a Predictor of Primary Cardiovascular Events in Patients With Chronic Kidney Disease. J Clin Med Res. 2018;10:883-890. https://doi.org/10.14740/jocmr3631
3) Hitsumoto T, Takahashi M, Iizuka T, Shirai K. Clinical significance of serum 7-ketocholesterol concentrations in the progression of coronary atherosclerosis. J Atheroscler

Thromb. 2009;16:363-370.

4) Hitsumoto T. Clinical Significance of Cardio-Ankle Vascular Index as a Cardiovascular Risk Factor in Elderly Patients With Type 2 Diabetes Mellitus. J Clin Med Res. 2018;10:330-336.

5) Hitsumoto T. Relationships Between Skin Autofluorescence and Cardio-Ankle Vascular Index in Japanese Male Patients With Metabolic Syndrome Cardiol Res. 2019;10:172-180. https://doi.org/10.14740/cr878

6) Hitsumoto T. Clinical Impact of Blood Testosterone Concentration on Cardio-Ankle Vascular Index in Female Patients With Type 2 Diabetes Mellitus. Cardiol Res. 2019;10:9-17. https://doi.org/10.14740/cr827

7) Hitsumoto T, Ohsawa H, Noike H, et al. Preheparin serum lipoprotein lipase mass is negatively related to coronary atherosclerosis. Atherosclerosis 2000;153:391-396.

8) Hitsumoto T, Yoshinaga K, Aoyagi K, et al. Association between preheparin serum lipoprotein lipase mass and acute myocardial Infarction in Japanese men. J Atheroscler Thromb 2002;9:163-169.

9) Hitsumoto T, Takahashi M, Iizuka T, Shirai K. Relationship between metabolic syndrome and early stage coronary atherosclerosis. J Atheroscler Thromb. 2007;14:294-302.

10) Hitsumoto T, Shirai K. Factors affecting high-sensitivity cardiac troponin T elevation in Japanese metabolic syndrome patients. Diabetes Metab Syndr Obes. 2015;8:157-162.

Labor conditions and CAVI

Tomonori Sugiura

Introduction

Obesity has become a global health care problem with the increasing prevalence of the Western lifestyle and is associated with cardiovascular disease and all-cause death[1]. In particular, visceral fat obesity often complicates high blood pressure (BP), lipid metabolism disorder, and glycemic metabolism disorder and leads to the development of multiple metabolic disorders, or metabolic syndrome[2]. Metabolic syndrome, hypertension, dyslipidemia, and diabetes mellitus are related to unhealthy lifestyles and have been shown to be associated with a poor prognosis[3]. These lifestyle-related diseases and smoking are considered to be established cardiovascular risk factors.

These cardiovascular risk factors induce sustained vascular impairment with increased oxidative stress and promotion of inflammatory activation in the vascular wall[4]. Persistent vascular impairment causes systemic vascular damage, leading to atherosclerosis, which is a chronic inflammatory disease of the vascular wall[5]. Thus, obesity and lifestyle-related disease could subclinically promote vascular damage and atherosclerosis, which is characterized by functional and structural alterations in the vascular systems[6]. In a clinical setting, the extent of subclinical atherosclerosis is mainly evaluated in large arteries by non-invasive examinations, such as the cardio-ankle vascular index (CAVI) and carotid intima-media thickness (IMT). The CAVI is a functional index that indicates arterial stiffness, which is pathologically characterized by decreased arterial elasticity, whereas the carotid IMT is a morphological index of atherosclerotic vascular damage that reflects pathological thickening in the vascular wall. Moreover, complications of cardiovascular risk factors may influence work conditions and could be considered a serious problem in occupational health. Therefore, employees have periodically evaluated their visceral fat accumulation and subclinical atherosclerosis in our institutes. In this chapter, we explain how lifestyle and work-style affect the presence of atherosclerosis and obesity in middle-aged Japanese workers, and the usefulness of the CAVI for their assessment, as compared to the carotid IMT.

Participants

In Japan, all employees must receive annual medical examinations in accordance with the Industrial Safety and Health Law of Japan. Notably, the Toyota Motor Corporation (Toyota, Japan) recommends that their employees attend their special physical check-ups every 4 years in the Health Support Center WELPO, the company's healthcare institute established in 2008. We report the results mainly focusing on the influence of lifestyle and work-style, and the usefulness of the CAVI and carotid IMT based on data obtained in 2008[8,9].

We instructed all participants to fast overnight before the medical examination. The physical examination included body height, body weight, and percentage body fat, measured using an automated BF-220 instrument equipped with a bioelectrical impedance analyzer system (Tanita, Tokyo, Japan). Waist circumference was measured at the umbilicus level in a standing position while breathing normally (at the end of expiration while breathing gently). Systolic and diastolic BP were measured using a validated oscillometric technique, with the subject in a seated position. Blood samples were taken from the antecubital vein on the morning for the blood test. Metabolic syndrome was diagnosed by the combination of visceral obesity (visceral fat area [VFA] $\geq$ 100 cm^2) and 2 or more of the following 3 criteria: (1) triglycerides $\geq$ 150 mg/dL and/or high-density lipoprotein cholesterol $<$ 40 mg/dL; (2) systolic BP $\geq$ 130 mmHg, and/or diastolic BP $\geq$ 85 mmHg; and (3) fasting blood glucose $\geq$ 110 mg/dL[10]. Then, the CAVI, carotid ultrasound, and computed tomography (CT) examinations were performed to measure arterial stiffness, carotid IMT, and visceral fat accumulation.

Measurement of CAVI and carotid IMT

CAVI was examined by using an automated system after the subject had rested in the supine position. After the measurement of the CAVI, carotid IMT and plaque were assessed by well-trained clinical laboratory technicians, who were blinded to other clinical information, using an ultrasound apparatus. The carotid IMT and plaque presence were evaluated manually using a 7.5-MHz frequency probe, and all subjects were examined in the supine position. Common carotid artery IMT was measured in the far wall at ~20 mm from the carotid bifurcation using recorded images of the carotid artery. Plaques were identified as elevated lesions with a maximum thickness $\geq$ 1.1 mm and with a point of inflection on the surface of the intima-media complex in the common carotid artery, carotid bulb, and internal carotid artery.

Assessment of visceral fat area

VFA was measured by the assessment of CT images, in accordance with the guidelines for obesity treatment set by the Japan Society for the Study of Obesity. Modified measurement levels were adopted in cases of apparently low

Department of Cardiology, Nagoya City University Graduate School of Medical Sciences, 1, Kawasumi, Mizuho-cho, Mizuho-ku, Nagoya-shi, Aichi 467-8601, Japan.

umbilical body type. Image analysis software was used at an attenuation range from -70 to -160 Hounsfield units to quantify abdominal areas of adipose tissue. The VFA was defined as intra-abdominal fat bound by the parietal peritoneum or transversalis fascia.

Assessment of labor conditions and lifestyle habits

We evaluated the labor conditions by the point-of-work contents, in which subjects were categorized into physical workers or office workers, according to their job category. Additionally, because circadian rhythm could also have impacts on vascular health, work-style was also divided into fixed daytime work or shift work. Regarding labor conditions, subjects were categorized into fixed daytime workers or shift workers (including subjects working with an irregular schedule, outside of daytime hours, or at night). Fixed daytime workers were defined as subjects working mainly during daytime hours, while shift workers were defined as subjects working outside of daytime hours, or at night, with or without an irregular schedule. Part-time daytime workers were defined as fixed daytime workers. All employees were instructed to perform a self-reported questionnaire regarding lifestyle behaviors, called the Standard Questionnaire for Health Examination[11]. We evaluated lifestyle behavior in each individual from several important points based on information obtained from the questionnaire.

Among the lifestyle habits, overeating is classically linked with body weight gain and obesity among daily lifestyle factors. Moreover, eating breakfast was also associated with metabolic factors, such as daily energy intake, dietary efficiency, and appetite regulation. On the other hand, irregular dietary habits, such as skipping breakfast or nighttime eating, were deemed unfavorable due to their association with the acceleration of overweight and obesity, and metabolic disorder. Furthermore, alcohol drinking increases the risk of obesity, while habitual smoking is an accepted risk factor for atherosclerosis. Sleeping and working hours were also assessed to evaluate the health condition of each individual. Thus, we administered the following questionnaire items to assess the lifestyle and medical history of individuals: 1) eating breakfast without skipping, 2) nighttime eating (eating a meal within 2 hours of bedtime), 3) regular exercise more than 30 minutes per day, 4) habitual drinking, 5) habitual smoking, 6) sleeping hours (hours/day), and 7) working hours (hours/day). We thus aimed to assess how lifestyle

and shift work affect the accumulation of visceral fat and the presence of atherosclerosis in middle-aged workers.

Evaluation of visceral fat and subclinical atherosclerosis in different labor conditions

Based on the information obtained, we investigated labor conditions and the individual's lifestyle habits that might influence the prevalence of visceral fat obesity and the presence of subclinical atherosclerosis in the employees. Multivariable regression and logistic regression analyses identified that regular exercise were negatively associated with VFA, while fixed daytime work was positively associated with VFA. Multivariable regression and logistic regression analyses also showed that habitual smoking was positively associated with the increased CAVI after adjustment for possible confounding factors. Similarly, multivariable regression and logistic regression analyses showed that habitual smoking was positively associated with increased carotid IMT after adjustment for possible confounding factors, but that work-style had no significant association with the IMT. In subgroup analyses separating physical workers and office workers, lifestyle and work-style were not consistently associated with VFA. However, habitual smoking was consistently associated with increased both CAVI and carotid IMT in both groups. The other lifestyle and work shift factors showed partial, but not necessarily consistent, associations with these indices of atherosclerosis. Thus, reduced regular exercise and fixed daytime work was significantly associated with visceral fat accumulation, while habitual smoking was consistently and independently associated with increased CAVI and carotid IMT. This finding indicates that smoking may functionally and structurally accelerate the atherosclerotic process and was concordant with smoking as a major risk factor of atherosclerotic cardiovascular disease.

On the other hand, regression analyses between obesity-related indices and subclinical atherosclerosis showed that VFA was positively correlated with the CAVI, while other obesity-related indices, including body mass index and percentage body fat, were negatively correlated with this index. However, the CAVI was negatively associated with obesity-related indices, while the IMT was positively associated with obesity-related indices in the logistic regression analyses, with the endpoint of "obesity" for each obesity-related index (Table 1). Although the details of the underlying mechanisms are not clearly understood, a negative association was considered as a physiological adaptation to the hyperemic state of obesity and a transient

Table 1. Results of logistic regression analysis with the endpoint of "obesity" based on each obesity-related criterion in middle-aged untreated employees (*n* = 7,750).

Variable	Abdominal obesity		Visceral fat obesity	
	Odds ratio (95% confidence interval)	*P* value	Odds ratio (95% confidence interval)	*P* value
CAVI, per 1.0	0.637 (0.589–0.690)	< 0.0001	0.853 (0.773–0.942)	< 0.0001
Carotid IMT, per 0.1 mm	1.408 (1.377–1.482)	< 0.0001	1.302 (1.222–1.387)	< 0.0001

Abdominal obesity was diagnosed by a waist circumference ≥ 85 cm for men or ≥ 90 cm for women. Visceral fat obesity was diagnosed by a visceral fat area ≥ 100 cm². CAVI and carotid IMT were simultaneously included and were adjusted for age, sex, and smoking status. Adapted from ref.9

response during this period. In contrast, in logistic regression analysis with the endpoint of metabolic syndrome, based on either waist circumference or VFA, both the CAVI and carotid IMT were positively associated with the presence of metabolic syndrome (Table 2). Metabolic syndrome is a condition with overlapping metabolic disruptions and, thus, vascular inflammation is more substantial, and cardiovascular risk is higher than in simple visceral fat obesity. Hence, metabolic syndrome may promote arterial stiffness more than simple visceral fat accumulation. These findings support the concept that the impact of obesity on the CAVI is different in healthy individuals than in patients with metabolic syndrome. In addition to the usefulness of the CAVI for detecting arterial stiffness and cardiovascular events, assessment of the CAVI could be meaningful in physical check-ups and evaluation of labor conditions.

In addition, when a combination of both chronic obstructive pulmonary disease (COPD)[12] and carotid plaque was investigated in male smokers, receiver operating characteristics curve analysis, to discriminate these subjects using the CAVI or carotid IMT, showed that the areas under the curves (AUCs) and cut-off levels were 0.747 and 7.70 and 0.740 and 0.55 mm, respectively, in middle-aged untreated male smokers (Fig. 1)[13]. Thus, measuring the CAVI might be a useful means to detect middle-aged male smoking subjects with the presence of both carotid plaque and COPD.

Summary

Habitual smoking showed a consistent association with arterial stiffness, presented by the CAVI, and carotid atherosclerosis, evaluated by the carotid IMT, whereas the work shift did not have an independent association with arterial stiffness and carotid atherosclerosis. On the other hand, the CAVI was preserved, but the carotid IMT was increased with increasing visceral fat accumulation, while both the carotid IMT and CAVI were worsened with the

Table 2. **Results of logistic regression analysis with the endpoint of metabolic syndrome in middle-aged untreated employees (*n* = 7,750).**

Variable	Based on abdominal obesity		Based on visceral fat obesity	
	Odds ratio (95% confidence interval)	*P* value	Odds ratio (95% confidence interval)	*P* value
CAVI, per 1.0	1.339 (1.197–1.499)	< 0.0001	1.188 (1.003–1.406)	< 0.05
Carotid IMT, per 0.1 mm	1.309 (1.217–1.409)	< 0.0001	1.439 (1.292–1.602)	< 0.0001

Endpoint of analysis fulfilled the criteria of metabolic syndrome, which is a combination of either abdominal obesity (waist circumference ≥ 85 cm for men and ≥ 90 cm for women) or visceral fat obesity (visceral fat area ≥ 100 cm^2) and two other risk factors from lipid metabolism disorder (triglyceride ≥ 150 mg/dL and/or high-density lipoprotein cholesterol < 40 mg/dL), high blood pressure (systolic blood pressure ≥ 130 mmHg and/or diastolic blood pressure ≥ 85 mmHg), or high fasting blood glucose (fasting blood glucose ≥ 110 mg/dL). CAVI and carotid IMT were simultaneously included and were adjusted for age, sex, and smoking status. Adapted from ref.9

a　　　　　　　　　　　　　　　　**b**

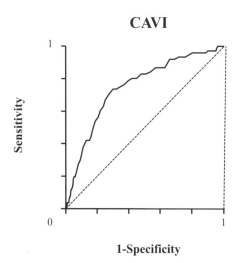

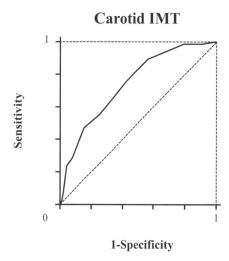

Fig. 1. **Receiver operating characteristics curve analyses to determine the area under the curve (AUC) and cut-off level in examinations of atherosclerosis for both the presence of chronic obstructive pulmonary disease (COPD) and of carotid plaque in middle-aged untreated male smokers (*n* = 3,775).**

a. The AUC, cut-off level, sensitivity, and specificity of cardio-ankle vascular index (CAVI) for the presence of both COPD and carotid plaque were 0.747 (95% confidence interval: [CI] 0.732–0.760, *p* < 0.0001), 7.70, 0.737 (95% CI 0.623–0.831), and 0.700 (95% CI 0.685–0.715), respectively.
b. The AUC, cut-off level, sensitivity, and specificity of carotid intima-media thickness (IMT) for the presence of both COPD and carotid plaque were AUC 0.740 (95% CI 0.725–0.754, *p* < 0.0001), 0.55 mm, 0.750 (95% CI 0.637–0.842), and 0.582 (95% CI 0.566–0.598), respectively. Adapted from ref.16

development of metabolic syndrome. These findings indicate that lifestyle modification has a more significant impact on health than intervention in the working life of middle-aged workers. Thus, measurement of the CAVI is useful for assessing employees' health and estimating cardiovascular risks, independent of labor conditions.

References

1) Yatsuya H, Li Y, Hilawe EH, Ota A, Wang C, Chiang C, Zhang Y, Uemura M, Osako A, Ozaki Y, Aoyama A. Global trend in overweight and obesity and its association with cardiovascular disease incidence. Circ J, 2014; 78:2807-2818.

2) Tchernof A, Després JP. Pathophysiology of human visceral obesity: An update. Physiol Rev, 2013; 93:359-404.

3) Grundy SM. Pre-diabetes, metabolic syndrome, and cardiovascular risk. J Am Coll Cardiol, 2012; 59:635-643.

4) Sugiura T, Dohi Y, Takase H, Yamashita S, Tanaka S, Kimura G. Increased reactive oxygen metabolites is associated with cardiovascular risk factors and vascular endothelial damage in middle-aged Japanese subjects. Vasc Health Risk Manag, 2011; 7:475–482.

5) Sugiura T, Dohi Y, Takase H, Yamashita S, Fujii S, Ohte N. Oxidative stress is closely associated with increased arterial stiffness, especially in aged male smokers without previous cardiovascular events: a cross-sectional study. J Atheroscler Thromb, 2017; 24:1186-1198.

6) Vanhoutte PM, Shimokawa H, Feletou M, Tang EH. Endothelial dysfunction and vascular disease—A 30th anniversary update. Acta Physiol (Oxf), 2017; 219:22-96.

7) Davignon J, Ganz P. Role of endothelial dysfunction in atherosclerosis. Circulation, 2004; 109: III27-III32.

8) Sugiura T, Dohi Y, Takagi Y, Yoshikane N, Ito M, Suzuki K, Nagami T, Iwase M, Seo Y, Ohte N. Impacts of lifestyle behavior and shift work on visceral fat accumulation and the presence of atherosclerosis in middle-aged male workers. Hypertens Res. 2019;43:235-245.

9) Sugiura T, Dohi Y, Takagi Y, Yoshikane N, Ito M, Suzuki K, Nagami T, Iwase M, Seo Y, Ohte N. Relationships of obesity-related indices and metabolic syndrome with subclinical atherosclerosis in middle-aged untreated workers. J Atheroscler Thromb. 2020;27:342-352.

10) Committee to Evaluate Diagnostic Standards for Metabolic Syndrome. Definition and the diagnostic standard for metabolic syndrome—Committee to Evaluate Diagnostic Standards for Metabolic Syndrome. *Nihon Naika Gakkai Zasshi*. 2005;94:794-809.

11) Ministry of Health, Labor, and Welfare. Standardized health checkup and intervention program. 2007. https://www.mhlw.go.jp/seisakunitsuite/bunya/kenkou_iryou/kenkou/seikatsu/dl/hoken-program2.pdf (accessed 6 November, 2020) (in Japanese).

12) Fukuchi Y, Nishimura M, Ichinose M, Adachi M, Nagai A, Kuriyama T, Takahashi K, Nishimura K, Ishioka S, Aizawa H, Zaher C. COPD in Japan: the Nippon COPD Epidemiology study. Respirology. 2004;9:458-465.

13) Sugiura T, Dohi Y, Takagi Y, Yokochi T, Yoshikane N, Suzuki K, Tomiishi T, Nagami T, Iwase M, Takase H, Seo Y, Ohte N. Close association between subclinical atherosclerosis and pulmonary function in middle-aged male smokers. J Atheroscler Thromb. 2020;27:1230-1242.

Availability of the cardio–ankle vascular index (CAVI) in general health check–up

Yuji Shimizu[1,2]

Summary

1. The CAVI, measured during general health check–ups, proved its utility as a screening tool for evaluating arterial stiffness.
2. The CAVI is useful not only as a screening test but also for health guidance and public awareness.

In general, progression of arterial stiffness (atherosclerosis) is asymptomatic until onset of severe cardiovascular disease, including sudden death, are experienced. Despite the development of modern diagnostic and therapeutic technology and better understanding of cardiovascular risk factors, cardiovascular disease remains one of the major causes of death in developed countries. Aging, hypertension, hyperglycemia, dyslipidemia, smoking, etc., are well–known cardiovascular risk factors that are also associated with development of arterial stiffness. Aging is an important and unavoidable process associated with arterial stiffness. Since Japan is known as an aged society and as the rate of aging is still increasing, preventing the development of arterial stiffness should be viewed as urgent and necessary. However, arterial stiffness is not evaluated during general health check–ups.

A non–invasive tool, such as the cardio–ankle vascular index (CAVI) is efficient in evaluating arterial stiffness during general health check–up, because it does not require particular skills. Therefore, we performed arterial stiffness evaluation in the Nagasaki study, which was attached to a general heath check–up. The purposes of this survey were not only to evaluate the risk of cardiovascular disease, which provides important data for preventive medicine research, but also provides insight into cardiovascular disease prevention among the general population.

In order to avoid the confounding effects of blood pressure when evaluating functional values of arterial stiffness, the CAVI was developed. Using ultrasonography, organic values of arterial stiffness can be evaluated, such as the carotid intima media thickness (CIMT). Therefore, even though both the CAVI and CIMT are known as indexes of arterial stiffness, their measurement methods and targets are markedly different. Accordingly, we evaluated the correlation between the CAVI and CIMT.

The correlation between the CAVI and CIMT was examined in 1,014 individuals (242 men and 772 women) over 40 years of age, without a medical history of cardiovascular diseases, who participated in the general health check–up performed by Goto City, Nagasaki Prefecture. By simple correlation analysis, a significant positive correlation was observed between the CAVI and CIMT for both men and women (simple correlation coefficient r = 0.32, p < 0.01 for men and r = 0.37, p < 0.01 for women, respectively)[1].

Even after adjustment for sex, age, abdominal circumference, systolic blood pressure, triglycerides, HDL–cholesterol, HbA1c, serum creatinine, uric acid, and homocysteine, the correlation between the CAVI and CIMT were unchanged (standardized parameter estimate [β] = 0.81, p < 0.001). This study proved the utility of the CAVI as a screening tool for arterial stiffness.

To develop organic (structural) values of arterial stiffness (increase CIMT), increased production of hematopoietic stem cell (CD34–positive cells) is necessary, because those cells are known to differentiate into sources of atherosclerosis, such as endothelial cells, foam cells, and mural cells. We found a significant positive association between yearly increased CIMT ($\geq \triangle$ 0.01 mm/year) and circulating CD34–positive cells among non–hypertensive men, but not among hypertensive men[2]. Since hypertension might cause reduction of CD34–positive cells by the number of such cells that differentiate into mature cells, such as endothelial cells, foam cells, and mural cells, hypertension might act as a strong confounding factor when increased CIMT is associated with CD34–positive cells[2].

Development of CIMT is the result of aggressive repair. However, hematopoietic activity declines during aging. Therefore, aging should be associated with low productivity of CD34–positive cells. Then, older participants with lower hematopoietic activity might not show an increase in the organic value of arterial stiffness (CIMT) but could increase

[1]Department of Cardiovascular Disease Prevention, Osaka Center for Cancer and Cardiovascular Diseases Prevention, 1-6-107 Morinomiya, Joto-ku, Osaka-shi, Osaka, 536-8588 Japan.
[2]Department of General Medicine, Nagasaki University Graduate School of Biomedical Sciences, 1-12-4 Sakamoto, Nagasaki City, Nagasaki, 852-8523 Japan.

the functional values of arterial stiffness (CAVI) because of the deficiency of endothelial repair. To clarify these associations, we performed subanalysis with men aged 60–69 years. There was a significant positive correlation between the CIMT and CAVI among those with a higher level of CD34–positive cells ($\geq$ median value), but not among those with lower CD34–positive cell levels ($<$ median value). This study also revealed a significant inverse correlation between the CAVI and CD34–positive cells, only among those with a lower level of CD34–positive cells[3]. As circulating CD34–positive cell counts might indicate endothelial repair activity, the CAVI can be an efficient tool for evaluating the influence of endothelial repair deficiency, which could not evaluated by the CIMT.

Diabetes mellitus is a known risk factor for developing arterial stiffness (atherosclerosis). The ratio of triglycerides to HDL–cholesterol (TG–HDL ratio) could act as an indicator of insulin resistance. Therefore, we used TG–HDL ratios to classify diabetes into three groups in 1,344 men aged 36–79 years. As shown in Table 1, the high TG–HDL diabetic group, which is considered to be relatively more insulin–resistant, showed a significantly positive association with atherosclerosis (CIMT $\geq$ 1.1 mm, CAVI $\geq$ 9) and early atherosclerosis ($8 \leq$ CAVI < 9). In addition, the CAVI was found to be more sensitive for this than the CIMT[4].

A previous study has reported a positive association between increased arterial stiffness, as evaluated by pulse wave velocity and hemoglobin levels (Hb) in women, but not in men[5]. However, since a significant positive relationship was recognized between Hb and hypertension[6,7], the CAVI, which is not affected by blood pressure, seemed to be the best candidate for evaluating the association between increased arterial stiffness and Hb.

The results of a study of 1,064 men and 1,886 women without anemia aged 30–79 years demonstrated that Hb levels were positively associated with arterial stiffness (CAVI $\geq$ 9) in both men and women[8]. This study also indicated that the usefulness of the CAVI in general health check–ups (Table 2).

The CAVI is a non-invasive arterial stiffness (atherosclerosis) evaluating tool that requires no special skill. Moreover, the measurement values are not affected by blood pressure at the time of measurement. Therefore, it is easy to use this tool in a general health check-up. In addition, the result of evaluating values could be shown immediately after taking examination. This is why, CAVI is not only efficient tool for screening the risk of cardiovascular disease but also an efficient tool for health guidance and enlightening the public for interest and for awareness of

Table 1. Relationships between diabetes mellitus grouped by TG−HDL ratios and atherosclerosis.

	Low TG–HDL diabetes			Intermediate TG–HDL diabetes			High TG–HDL diabetes		
	(−)	(+)	p	(−)	(+)	p	(−)	(+)	p
Atherosclerosis (CIMT $\geq$ 1.1 mm)									
No. at risk	1,301	43		1,313	31		1,288	56	
No. of cases (percentages)	279 (21)	13 (30)		284 (22)	8 (26)		269 (21)	23 (41)	
Age–adjusted OR	1.00	1.26 (0.64–2.49)	0.509	1.00	1.09 (0.47–2.53)	0.849	1.00	2.63 (1.48–4.66)	0.001
Multivariable OR	1.00	1.17 (0.52–2.63)	0.709	1.00	0.76 (0.29–2.00)	0.575	1.00	2.57 (1.32–5.02)	0.006
Early atherosclerosis ($8 \leq$ CAVI < 9)*									
No. at risk	836	20		838	18		831	25	
No. of cases (percentages)	373 (45)	9 (45)		374 (45)	8 (44)		365 (44)	17 (68)	
Age–adjusted OR	1.00	0.73 (0.29–1.81)	0.491	1.00	0.77 (0.29–2.05)	0.597	1.00	2.29 (0.95–5.52)	0.064
Multivariable OR	1.00	0.64 (0.20–1.98)	0.432	1.00	0.76 (0.25–2.36)	0.635	1.00	2.70 (1.05–6.91)	0.039
Atherosclerosis (CAVI $\geq$ 9)**									
No. at risk	928	34		939	23		923	39	
No. of cases (percentages)	465 (50)	23 (68)		475 (51)	13 (57)		457 (50)	31 (79)	
Age–adjusted OR	1.00	1.28 (0.56–2.95)	0.556	1.00	1.29 (0.47–3.50)	0.622	1.00	3.98 (1.60–9.86)	0.008
Multivariable OR	1.00	0.98 (0.38–2.50)	0.957	1.00	0.89 (0.28–2.84)	0.843	1.00	4.40 (1.52–12.75)	0.006

Multivariable OR: adjusted further for age and body mass index, smoking, alcohol intake, hypertension, antidiabetic medication use, anti-hyperlipidemic medication use, history of cardiovascular disease, serum alanine aminotransferase (ALT), and glomerular filtration rate (GFR). *Analyses were performed for participants without CAVI $\geq$ 9. **Analyses were performed for participants without $8 \leq$ CAVI < 9. Median values of TG–HDL for each types of diabetes are 1.00 for lowest TG–HDL, 2.08 for intermediate, and 4.29 for highest TG–HDL diabetes. Adapted from ref.4 [with permission of Elsevier]

Table 2. **Relationship between hemoglobin (Hb) and arterial stiffness.**

	Hemoglobin level quartiles				P for trend	1-SD increment in hemoglobin
	Q1 (low)	Q2	Q3	Q4 (high)		
Increased arterial stiffness (CAVI ≥ 9)						
Men						
No. at risk	267	279	266	252		
No. of cases (percentages)	78 (29)	73 (26)	73 (27)	72 (29)		
Age-adjusted OR	1.00	1.39 (0.91–2.13)	1.64 (1.06–2.53)	1.90 (1.22–2.96)	0.003	1.26 (1.08–1.47)
Multivariable OR	1.00	1.39 (0.89–2.16)	1.48 (0.94–2.33)	1.60 (1.00–2.56)	0.049	1.17 (1.00–1.38)
Women						
No. at risk	451	458	496	481		
No. of cases (percentages)	69 (15)	81 (18)	96 (19)	99 (21)		
Age-adjusted OR	1.00	1.24 (0.84–1.82)	1.53 (1.05–2.24)	1.65 (1.13–2.41)	0.005	1.18 (1.04–1.35)
Multivariable OR	1.00	1.22 (0.82–1.81)	1.49 (1.01–2.19)	1.62 (1.09–2.40)	0.010	1.17 (1.02–1.34)

Multivariable OR: adjusted further for age, systolic blood pressure, antihypertensive medication use, body mass index, smoking, alcohol intake, diabetes, serum triglycerides, serum alanine aminotransferase(ALT), serum γ-glutamyltranspeptidase (γ–GTP) and glomerular filtration rate (GFR). Hb levels for quartiles among non-anemic participants were 13.0–14.0 g/dL, 14.1–14.7 g/dL, 14.8–15.4 g/dL, and >15.4 g/dL for men and 12.0–12.6 g/dL, 12.7–13.1 g/dL, 13.2–13.7 g/dL, and > 13.7 g/dL for women. Cited from ref.8

cardiovascular disease prevention. At present, the follow-up study by the Nagasaki study is continuing. To achieve an efficient strategy for prevention of cardiovascular disease, elucidation the arterial stiffness-related mechanisms that underly cardiovascular disease is needed.

Future issues:

1. To elucidate the relationship between the CAVI and the development of atherosclerotic diseases (e.g., stroke and ischemic heart disease).

2. Promoting the use of the CAVI in health promotion and disease prevention activities.

References

1) Kadota K, Takamura N, Aoyagi K, Yamasaki H, Usa T, Nakazato M, Maeda T, Wada M, Nakashima K, Abe K, Takeshima F, Ozono Y: Availability of cardio–ankle vascular index (CAVI) as a screening tool for atherosclerosis. Circ J 2008; 72: 304–308.

2) Shimizu Y, Kawashiri SY, Kiyoura K, Koyamatsu J, Fukui S, Tamai M, Nobusue K, Yamanashi H, Nagata Y, Maeda T: Circulating CD34+ cells and active arterial wall thickening among elderly men: A prospective study. Sci Rep 2020; 10: 4656.

3) Shimizu Y, Yamanashi H, Noguchi Y, Koyamatsu J, Nagayoshi M, Kiyoura K, Fukui S, Tamai M, Kawashiri SY, Kondo H, Maeda T: Cardio–ankle vascular index and circulating CD34–positive cell levels as indicators of endothelial repair activity in older Japanese men. Geriatr Gerontol Int 2019; 19: 557–562.

4) Shimizu Y, Nakazato M, Sekita T, Kadota K, Yamasaki H, Takamura N, Aoyagi K, Maeda T: Association of arterial stiffness and diabetes with triglycerides–to–HDL cholesterol ratio for Japanese men: the Nagasaki Islands Study. Atherosclerosis 2013; 228: 491–495. https://doi.org/10.1016/j.atherosclerosis.2013.03.021

5) Kawamoto R, Tabara Y, Kohara K, Miki T, Kusunoki T, Katoh T, Ohtsuka N, Takayama S, Abe M. A slightly low hemoglobin level is beneficially associated with arterial stiffness in Japanese community–dwelling women. Clin Exp Hypertens 2012; 34: 92–98.

6) Shimizu Y, Nakazato M, Sekita T, Kadota K, Arima K, Yamasaki H, Takamura N, Aoyagi K, Maeda T: Association between the hemoglobin levels and hypertension in relation to the BMI status in a rural Japanese population: the Nagasaki Islands Study. Intern Med 2014; 53: 435–440.

7) Shimizu Y, Sato S, Koyamatsu J, Yamanashi H, Nagayoshi M, Kadota K, Kawashiri SY, Maeda T: Possible mechanism underlying the association between higher hemoglobin level and hypertension in older Japanese men. Geriatr Gerontol Int 2017; 17: 2586–2592.

8) Shimizu Y, Nakazato M, Sekita T, Kadota K, Yamasaki H, Takamura N, Aoyagi K, Maeda T: Association between hemoglobin levels and arterial stiffness for general Japanese population in relation to body mass index status: The Nagasaki Islands study. Geriatr Gerontol Int 2014; 14: 811–818. https://doi.org/10.1111/ggi.12171

The roles of basal CAVI and enhanced ΔCAVI during the development of Ischemic Changes in electrocardiography and hypertensive Retinal arteriosclerosis in Healthy Individuals over a three year period

Mao Takahashi[1], Kenji Suzuki[2] and Shinichi Tsuda[3]

Summary

1. Among the individuals undergoing medical examination and who had no abnormal findings, men who developed ischemic changes in electrocardiography for 3 years showed a higher cardio-ankle vascular index (CAVI) at the first visit than those who did not. However, in women, CAVI was not higher in individuals developing ischemic changes in electrocardiography.
   Both men and women who developed hypertensive retinal arteriosclerosis showed higher CAVI at the first visit than those without it.
2. Furthermore, men who developed ischemic changes in electrocardiography during 3 years showed a higher enhanced CAVI (ΔCAVI) than those who did not develop it. Women who developed hypertensive retinal artery abnormalities showed enhanced CAVI (ΔCAVI) than those who did not develop it.
   Periodic measurements of CAVI in medical examinations are useful for predicting the development of macro- and micro-vascular diseases.

Introduction

The cardio-ankle vascular index (CAVI) reflects the arterial stiffness of the arterial tree from the origin of the aorta to the ankle[1]. CAVI shows higher values with an increase in age, and men showed higher values than women. CAVI also showed high values in various arteriosclerotic patients and patients with diabetes mellitus, obesity, hypertension, and smoking, which were well known coronary risk factors[2]. In addition, it has become clear that cardiovascular events occur at a high rate in cases with high CAVI levels[3]. Therefore, CAVI may be able to identify individuals who may potentially develop cardiovascular diseases in the near future. Conversely, the significance of the variability of CAVI observed when CAVI is continuously measured has not yet been clarified. Therefore, an attempt was made to clarify the relationship between the enhancement of CAVI and the progression of macro- and micro-vascular disorders among followed-up individuals, who were diagnosed as healthy in the initial medical examination and were checked up again after 3 years at the Japan Health Promoting Foundation.

As an indicator of the vascular disorder, ischemic changes on the electrocardiogram (ECG) and hypertensive retinal arteriosclerosis with Sheie H classification were studied. Additionally, the relations between these and CAVI in the initial health check, and also the relation between these and the progression of CAVI (ΔCAVI) for 3 years were examined. Factors, such as age, body mass index (BMI), blood pressure, and various lipid values were also examined as background factors.

1. Base characteristics in developed electrocardiographic ischemic changes and retinal arteriosclerosis during 3 years

Among 9,173 individuals who underwent medical examination, individuals without ischemic changes in the ECG and Sheie H0 (n = 1,288), and whose CAVI was measured every year for 3 years were enrolled. The contributing factors for the development of ischemic changes in the ECG and of retinal arterial arteriosclerosis were studied.

[1]Cardiovascular center, Toho University Sakura Medical Center, 564-1, Shimoshizu, Sakura-City, Chiba, 285-8741, Japan.
[2]Japan Health Promoting Foundation, 1-24-4 Ebisu, Shibuya-ku, Tokyo, 150-0013, Japan.
[3]Fukuda Denshi Co. LTD.

1) Factors for the development of ischemic changes in the electrocardiogram (Table 1 (A))

The people were divided into IC group (with the ischemic change in ECG) and normal group (with no change in ECG during 3 years).

In men, age, BMI, systolic pressure, and diastolic blood pressures were higher in the IC group than in the normal group. The CAVI was higher in the IC group than that in the normal group.

In women, age and systolic blood pressure were higher in the IC group. However, BMI, diastolic pressure, high-density lipoprotein cholesterol (HDL-C), and triglyceride (TG) were not higher in the IC group; additionally, CAVI was not higher in the IC group.

2) Factors for the development of hypertensive retinal arteriosclerosis (SheieH) (Table 1 (B))

The individuals were divided into two groups, namely the group with hypertensive retinal arteriosclerosis (group B) and without it (group A) during 3 years.

In men, age, systolic and diastolic pressure, HDL-C, and CAVI were higher in the group B than in the group A.

In women, age, BMI, systolic and diastolic pressure, and CAVI were higher in group B than group A.

2. Enhancement of various factors involved in developing electrocardiographic ischemic changes and hypertensive retinal arteriosclerosis (Sheie H) during 3 years

1) Enhanced factors for developing ischemic changes in the electrocardiogram during 3 years (Table 2 (A))

The individuals were divided into the ischemic change in

Table 1. Background factors at the initial medical examination in the electrocardiographic ischemic changes and hypertensive retinal arteriosclerosis developed after 3 years.

(A) Electrocardiographic ischemic changes. (B) Hypertensive Retinal arteriosclerosis.

(A)

	Male		Female	
	Normal group (n=652)	IC group (n=18)	Normal group (n=644)	IC group (n=48)
Age	43.3 ± 11.8	53.1 ± 12.7***	44.9 ± 11.3	48.7 ± 10.7*
BMI (kg/m²)	23.4 ± 3.1	25.1 ± 3.8*	21.5 ± 3.2	20.9 ± 3.5
sBP (mmHg)	122.7 ± 13.4	132.2 ± 13.6**	113.9 ± 14.0	120.8 ± 15.9**
dBP (mmHg)	77.0 ± 9.8	85.3 ± 10.0***	71.2 ± 10.0	73.9 ± 10.6
<Serum lipid>				
HDL-C (mg/dl)	60.2 ± 16.4	56.9 ± 14.8	76.7 ± 17.3	77.4 ± 18.2
TG (mg/dl)	123.4 ± 113.1	116.0 ± 51.0	76.7 ± 52.8	75.436.4
CAVI	7.4 ± 0.9	7.9 ± 1.1*	7.3 ± 0.9	7.5 ± 1.0

Mean ± S.D. P*<0.05,p**<0.01,p***<0.001 vs normal group, respectively. Paired t-test. IC; Ischemic change in ECG. BMI: Body mass index, sBP: systolic blood pressure, dBP: diastolic blood pressure, HDL: high-density lipoprotein, TG: triglyceride

(B)

	Male		Female	
	Group A (n=621)	Group B (n=45)	Group A (n=667)	Group B (n=27)
Age	42.2 ± 11.3	57.4 ± 9.9***	44.6 ± 11.2	52.5 ± 8.3***
BMI (kg/m²)	23.4 ± 3.2	23.3 ± 2.5	21.3 ± 3.1	22.9 ± 3.1*
sBP (mmHg)	121.7 ± 12.2	138.4 ± 13.8***	113.5 ± 13.6	128.3 ± 14.9***
dBP (mmHg)	76.3 ± 9.6	87.3 ± 7.4***	70.6 ± 9.6	83.5 ± 9.8***
<Serum lipid>				
HDL-C (mg/dl)	59.8 ± 16.0	65.8 ± 19.9*	77.2 ± 17.3	75.4 ± 18.9
TG (mg/dl)	123.5 ± 88.4	117.5 ± 63.3	75.9 ± 71.6	83.2 ± 43.8
CAVI	7.3 ± 0.9	8.4 ± 0.9***	7.3 ± 0.9	7.7 ± 0.6**

Mean ± S.D. P*<0.05,p**<0.01,p***<0.001 vs group A, respectively. Paired t-test. BMI: Body mass index, sBP: systolic blood pressure, dBP: diastolic blood pressure, HDL: high-density lipoprotein cholesterol, TG: triglyceride.

Table 2. Associations with CAVI variations (ΔCAVI) and the development of electrocardiographic ischemic changes and hypertensive retinal arteriosclerosis.

(A) Predictors of incident electrocardiogram ischemic disease. (B) Predictors of new-onset hypertensive retinal arteriosclerosis (Scheie H 1-4).

(A)

(Male)

	Normal group (n=652)	IC group (n=18)	Cox-hazards-model Hazard ratio (95%CI)	P value
Age	43.3 ± 11.8	53.1 ± 12.7***	1.07 (1.02-1.11)	<0.01
Δ BMI (kg/m²)	0.1 ± 1.2	0.1 ± 1.5	-	-
Δ sBP (mmHg)	0.4 ± 10.5	0.2 ± 15.5	-	-
Δ dBP (mmHg)	1.2 ± 7.4	-0.4 ± 12.5	-	-
<Serum lipid>			-	-
Δ HDL-C (mg/dl)	-0.9 ± 10.2	-0.2 ± 12.3	-	-
Δ TG (mg/dl)	7.1 ± 98.2	-3.7 ± 51.8	-	-
Δ CAVI	0.3 ± 0.6	0.6 ± 0.7*	14.3 (1.1-181.1)	<0.05

(Female)

	Normal group (n=644)	IC group (n=48)	Cox-hazards-model Hazard ratio (95%CI)	P value
Age	44.9 ± 11.3	48.7 ± 10.7*	1.03 (1.00-1.05)	<0.05
Δ BMI (kg/m²)	0.1 ± 1.1	0.1 ± 0.9	-	-
Δ sBP (mmHg)	0.9 ± 9.9	3.2 ± 10.0**	-	-
Δ dBP (mmHg)	0.4 ± 6.8	1.8 ± 6.5	-	-
<Serum lipid>			-	-
Δ HDL-C (mg/dl)	-0.5 ± 11.1	-0.6 ± 10.5	-	-
Δ TG (mg/dl)	3.6 ± 54.6	2.2 ± 27.4	-	-
Δ CAVI	0.2 ± 0.2	0.2 ± 0.2	-	-

Mean ± S.D. P*<0.05,p**<0.01,p***<0.001 vs normal group, respectively. Unpaired t-test. IC; Ischemic change on ECG. Cox-hazards-models, Including variables were age, Δ BMI, Δ sBP, Δ HDL-c, Δ TG, Δ CAVI. Various parameters were calculated by least square methods. IC; Ischemic change in ECG. BMI: Body mass index, sBP: systolic blood pressure, dBP: diastolic blood pressure, HDL-C: high-density lipoprotein cholesterol, TG: triglyceride

(B)

(Male)

	Group A (n=621)	Group B (n=45)	Cox-hazards-model Hazard ratio (95%CI)	P value
Age	42.2 ± 11.3	57.4 ± 9.9***	1.11 (1.08-1.13)	<0.01
Δ BMI (kg/m²)	0.1 ± 0.6	0.2 ± 1.3	-	-
Δ sBP (mmHg)	0.03 ± 3.3	1.2 ± 4.7*	-	-
Δ dBP (mmHg)	0.3 ± 2.3	0.6 ± 3.2	-	-
<Serum lipid>			-	-
Δ HDL-C (mg/dl)	-0.3 ± 3.4	-0.5 ± 4.4	-	-
Δ TG (mg/dl)	2.8 ± 31.8	-1.5 ± 11.1	-	-
Δ CAVI	0.08 ± 0.6	0.11 ± 0.7	-	-

(Female)

	Group A (n=667)	Group B (n=27)	Cox-hazards-model Hazard ratio (95%CI)	P value
Age	44.9 ± 11.3	48.7 ± 10.7*	1.02 (1.03-1.13)	<0.01
Δ BMI (kg/m²)	1.2 ± 2.6	1.9 ± 3.0	-	-
Δ sBP (mmHg)	0.3 ± 3.1	2.6 ± 4.4***	1.17 (1.05-1.31)	<0.01
Δ dBP (mmHg)	0.1 ± 2.2	0.4 ± 2.0	-	-
<Serum lipid>			-	-
Δ HDL-C (mg/dl)	-0.2 ± 4.2	-0.3 ± 3.3	-	-
Δ TG (mg/dl)	1.1 ± 16.1	11.4 ± 20.2**	1.02 (1.00-1.04)	<0.05
Δ CAVI	0.07 ± 0.2	0.17 ± 0.2**	25.9 (3.2-209.7)	<0.01

Mean ± S.D. P*<0.05,p**<0.01,p***<0.001 vs normal group, respectively. Unpaired t-test. IC; Ischemic change on ECG. Cox-hazards-models, Including variables were age, Δ BMI, Δ sBP, Δ HDL-c, Δ TG, Δ CAVI. Various parameters were calculated by least square methods. BMI: Body mass index, sBP: systolic blood pressure, dBP: diastolic blood pressure, HDL-C: high-density lipoprotein cholesterol, TG: triglyceride

the ECG group (IC group) and no change group (normal group) during 3 years.

In men, only the ΔCAVI was higher in the IC group than in the normal group.

In the Cox hazard model analysis, age and ΔCAVI were significant factors for the development of ischemic changes in ECG.

In women, Δsystolic blood pressure was higher in the IC group. However, the ΔBMI, Δ diastolic pressure, ΔHDL-C, and ΔTG were not higher in the IC group; additionally, ΔCAVI was not higher in the IC group. In the Cox hazard model analysis, only age was observed as a significant factor for the development of ischemic changes in ECG.

2) Enhanced factors for developing hypertensive retinal arteriosclerosis during 3 years (Table 2 (B))

The individuals were divided into the group who developed positive retinal arteriosclerosis (Sheie H2-4, group B) and normal retinal artery group (Sheie H0, group A). Additionally, the contributions of age, Δ BMI, Δ systolic blood pressure, ΔHDL-C, ΔTG, and CAVI progression (ΔCAVI) for the development of hypertensive retinal arteriosclerosis were compared between the two groups.

In men, age and Δsystolic blood pressure were significant contributors, and the ΔCAVI was higher in group B; however, it was not significant.

In the Cox hazard model analysis, only age was significant.

In women, age, Δsystolic blood pressure, ΔTG, and ΔCAVI were significantly higher in group B when compared to group A. In the Cox hazard model analysis, age, Δsystolic blood pressure, ΔTG, and ΔCAVI were the significant contributing factors for hypertensive retinal arteriosclerosis.

Discussion

The significance of CAVI as an indicator of the vascular disorder in healthy subjects was examined.

An initial high CAVI and high enhanced ΔCAVI during 3 years were related with the progression of ischemic changes on ECG in men. However, in women, the initial CAVI and enhanced ΔCAVI during 3 years were not contributing factors for ischemic changes in the ECG. These results raised the possibility that ischemic changes (ST depression) in ECG might not indicate the progression of coronary arterial stenosis in women. This problem warrants further research.

In contrast, as for hypertensive retinal arteriosclerosis, the initial CAVI contributed to the progression of retinal arterial arteriosclerosis, both in men and women. ΔCAVI was related to retinal arterial arteriosclerosis in women.

Conclusion

These results suggested that it is important to measure the CAVI periodically and to suppress the elevation of CAVI for the prevention of macro and micro vascular disorders.

References

1) Shirai K, Song M, Suzuki J, et al. Contradictory effects of β1- and α1- aderenergic receptor blockers on cardio-ankle vascular stiffness index (CAVI)--CAVI independent of blood pressure. J Atheroscler Thromb. 2011;18:49-55.
2) Saiki A, Ohira M, Yamaguchi T, et al. New horizons of arterial stiffness developed using cardio-ankle vascular index (CAVI). J Atheroscler Thromb. 2020, 1;27:732-748.
3) Saiki A, Ohira M, Yamaguchi T, et al. New horizons of arterial stiffness developed using cardio-ankle vascular index (CAVI). J Atheroscler Thromb. 2020 Aug 1;27:732-748.

Insulin Resistance and CAVI

Nobuyuki Masaki[1], Takayuki Namba[2] and Takeshi Adachi[2]

1. Insulin resistance and endothelial dysfunction

Endothelial dysfunction is considered to be a functional cause of arterial stiffness in addition to the medial degeneration and extracellular matrix remodeling caused by mechanical arterial wall stress. The vascular tone is determined by the balance of endothelium-derived vasoactive substances that include vasodilators, such as nitric oxide (NO), prostaglandins, endothelium-derived hyperpolarizing factor, epoxyeicosatrienoic acids, and vasoconstrictors, such as angiotensin II (Ang-II), endothelin-1 (ET-1), prostanoids, and isoprostanes[1]. Among them, NO is a physiologically relevant molecule to maintain vascular homeostasis. NO exerts anti-proliferative and anti-inflammatory effects on the endothelium. NO promotes vasodilatation and prevents leukocyte adhesion[2], thrombocyte aggregation[3], and smooth muscle cell proliferation[4].

NO secreted from the endothelium activates guanylate cyclase in the vascular smooth muscle cells (VSMC), which increases cyclic guanosine monophosphate formation and reduces the intracellular VSMC Ca^{2+} concentration leading to vascular relaxation. Therefore, the deficiency of NO production increases the distensibility of the aorta and peripheral arterial resistance, which precipitates the timing of pulse wave reflection in late systole and causes additional stress on the vessel wall leading to intima-media thickening[5]. In addition, increased intrinsic stiffness of VSMC has been implicated as a mechanism distinct from extracellular matrix remodeling[6]. Endothelial NO modulates transglutaminase-2, which regulates the vascular smooth muscle cytoskeletal proteins[7,8]. The endothelial and smooth muscle crosstalk is involved in modulating arterial stiffness.

Insulin resistance is closely associated with endothelial dysfunction. It is defined as the impaired action of insulin in the organs responsible for glucose metabolism, including adipose tissue, skeletal muscle, and the liver[9]. Insulin-mediated glucose uptake is reduced in muscles and adipocytes. Moreover, hepatic gluconeogenesis and lipogenesis are elevated, whereas lipolysis occurs in adipose

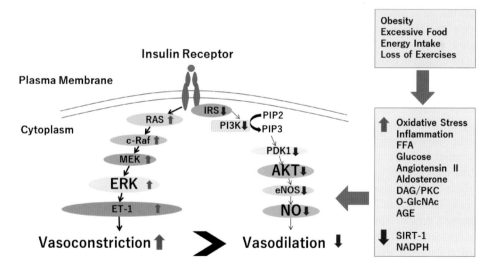

Fig. 1. Insulin pathways in endothelial cells.
There are two post-insulin receptor pathways. Insulin resistance implicates the selective loss of insulin's actions via the IRS/PI3K/Akt pathway, which reduces insulin's protective effect against atherosclerosis. FFA: free fatty acid; DAG, diacylglycerol; PKC, protein kinase C; O-GlcNAc, O-linked N-acetyl glucosamine; AGE, advanced glycation end-products; NADPH, nicotinamide adenine dinucleotide phosphate; SIRT-1, Sirtuin 1; IRS, insulin receptor substrate; PDK, phosphoinositide-dependent protein kinase; PI3K, phosphatidylinositol 3-kinase; Akt, protein kinase B; eNOS, endothelial nitric oxide synthase; NO, nitric oxide; ERK, extracellular signal-regulated kinase; MEK, MAPK kinase; ET-1, endothelin-1.
(Dr. Atsushi Sato, Department of Cardiology, National Defense Medical College, kindly provided the original figure for Fig.1.)

[1]Department of Intensive Care Medicine, National Defense Medical College, 3-2 Namiki, Tokorozawa, Saitama 359-8513, Japan.
[2]Department of Cardiology, National Defense Medical College, 3-2 Namiki, Tokorozawa, Saitama 359-8513, Japan.

tissue. The increased supply of free fatty acids into the muscles, liver, and pancreatic β cells further interferes with the metabolic action of insulin and insulin secretion[10].

In the vasculature, insulin stimulates the release of NO from the endothelium by activating insulin receptor substrate (IRS)-1, which leads to phosphatidylinositol 3-kinase (PI3K)/protein kinase B (Akt)-mediated phosphorylation of endothelial NO synthetase (eNOS). Although the receptors that sense shear forces have not been identified[11], increased mechanical forces from the blood flow directly stimulate the release of NO from the endothelium via the PI3K/Akt-mediated phosphorylation of eNOS[12–14]. Additionally, the IRS-1/PI3K/Akt signaling pathway increases the expressions of heme oxygenase-1[15] and vascular endothelial growth factor[16] and the reduces the expression of vascular cell adhesion molecule-1[17]. However, the signal transduction of the IRS-1/PI3K/Akt/eNOS pathway deteriorates in obesity, metabolic disorders, and diabetes mellitus, leading to a decrease of NO production. Instead, the activity of the Ras/Raf/mitogen-activated protein and extracellular signal-regulated kinase (MEK)/mitogen-activated protein kinase (ERK) pathway is preserved[18]. The second cascade of insulin signaling promotes vasoconstriction through ET-1 secretion[19]. Therefore, the imbalance of insulin action in the two downstream signaling pathways is involved in the pathogenesis of endothelial dysfunction.

Those endothelial dysfunctions induced by insulin resistance are expected to be reflected in the physiological property of the arterial wall. The knockout of eNOS significantly increases the pulse wave velocity (PWV) of the aorta in animal models[20,21]. However, PWV is observed to depend on the blood pressure at the measuring time. Therefore, the relationship had definitely not been clarified. Recently, the cardio-ankle vascular index (CAVI) is developed as the blood pressure-independent arterial stiffness index and it is reported that administration of the NO liberator, nitroglycerin, decreased the CAVI[22,23]. Insulin infusion diminishes the wave reflection in the aorta, which is another index of arterial stiffness, and induces peripheral vasodilation in healthy men. However, the effect is blunted when an impaired whole-body glucose uptake exists[24]. The administration of pioglitazone, an enhancer of insulin sensitivity, improves the CAVI[25]. Altogether, it is strongly suggested that the enhancement of arterial stiffness occurs as a consequence of endothelial dysfunctions due to the impairment of insulin action.

2. Insulin resistance and oxidative stress

Furthermore, insulin resistance is a condition of high oxidative stress. The oxidative stress implicates an excess production of reactive oxygen species (ROS) derived from mitochondria, xanthine oxidase, uncoupled NO synthesis, and nicotinamide adenine dinucleotide phosphate (NADPH) oxidase[26] or of impairment of antioxidant defense. In obesity-induced insulin resistance, an excessive calorie intake induces the overproduction of energy in the mitochondria. This increases the generation of superoxide in the mitochondrial electric transport chain[27]. The

oxidative stress induces endothelial function by the oxidation of tetrahydrobiopterin (BH4)[28], an enzymatic cofactor of eNOS. The nutritional, therapeutic, and endothelium-derived factors, including vitamin C, folate, and other antioxidants, enhance the endothelial BH4 bioavailability through chemical stabilization or scavenging of ROS[29]. However, oxidative stress causes the depletion of BH4 by oxidation into 7,8 dihydrobiopterin (BH2) in endothelial cells through so-called eNOS "uncoupling." In this state, $ONOO^-$, a form of ROS, is produced instead of NO[30]. The deficiency of NO accelerates the progression of arterial stiffness.

3. Mediators between insulin resistance, endothelial dysfunction, and arterial stiffness

A significant number of studies have so far been performed to identify exaggerating or ameliorating factors in the molecular mechanisms of endothelial dysfunction and arterial stiffness caused by insulin resistance. Inflammation and neurohormonal activation contribute to the pathogenesis of insulin resistance[31]. The activation of the renin-angiotensin system is a possible cause of arterial stiffness[32, 33]. Ang-II and aldosterone inhibit insulin signaling in both the endothelial cells and VSMCs. The hormones, nutrition, and cytokines activate the mammalian target of rapamycin/S6 kinase pathway and induce phosphorylation of serine residues of IRS-1 mainly due to visceral adipocyte dysfunction. The modification negatively regulates the signal transduction of the IRS-1/PI3K/Akt/eNOS pathway[34].

The metabolic axis is important to understand the vascular complication of diabetes mellitus and insulin resistance. Hyperglycemia increases the flux of minor glycolysis pathways through mitochondrial superoxide production[35]. The produced metabolites and the course of action through the pathways, such as the polyol pathway, hexosamine pathway, diacylglycerol/protein kinase C[36], and advanced glycation end-products (AGE) alter the vascular function[27]. For instance, aldose reductase reduces glucose to sorbitol, which is secondarily oxidized to fructose in the polyol pathway. The process consumes the cofactor of NADPH, which is also necessary for the recycling of the glutathione antioxidant system[37, 38]. Therefore, an increased glucose level induces NADPH deficiency leading to additional oxidative stress. O-linked N-acetyl glucosamine (O-GlcNAc) is a post-translational protein modification by binding uridine diphosphate N-acetyl glucosamine, the end-product of the hexosamine pathway with the O-link. The modification of the transcription factor Sp1 increases the expression of the transforming growth factor-β1 and plasminogen activator inhibitor-1, which enhances collagen production and decreases fibrinolysis[39]. Hyperglycemia-associated O-GlcNAc modification of eNOS causes a reciprocal decrease in O-linked serine phosphorylation at residue 1177 (p-eNOS Ser^{1177}), resulting in a decrease in eNOS activity[40].

Sirtuin 1 (SIRT-1) is a nuclear nicotinamide adenine dinucleotide-dependent nuclear deacetylase[41]. The protein deacetylase acts on histone and nonhistone proteins regulating the gene expression associated with the lifespan under calorie restriction. SIRT-1 promotes DNA damage repair and telomere stability[42]. SIRT-1 positively regulates the insulin signaling pathway in the skeletal muscle and the liver and stimulates the secretion of insulin from pancreatic cells[43]. SIRT-1 upregulates the adiponectin expression by deacetylation of the forkhead box protein O-1 that ameliorates the response to insulin in adipocytes. On the other hand, SIRT-1 exerts anti-inflammatory, antioxidant, and antiapoptotic effects on the endothelium[44,45]. The expression and activity of SIRT-1 in the arteries decreases with aging[46]. SIRT-1 protects against high fat-, high sucrose-induced arterial stiffness[47]. Activation of SIRT-1 by caloric restriction increases the eNOS expression[48]. A specific SIRT-1activator[49] or overexpression of SIRT-1 in the endothelium[50] attenuates the arterial stiffness assessed by PWV in animal models; thus, SIRT-1 maintains vascular elasticity. This might also be supported in humans. The administration of the SIRT-1 activator, resveratrol, improved the CAVI[51]. The dysregulation of SIRT-1 is involved in vascular remodeling and arterial stiffness, although a causative role remains to be established.

4. Clinical research of the CAVI for insulin resistance

The relationship between the CAVI and various markers of insulin resistance has been reported. The biomarkers of insulin resistance used in clinical practice include immunoreactive insulin (IRI), a homeostatic model assessment of insulin resistance (HOMA-IR), glucose-tolerance test, glucose clamp, triglycerides (TG) to high-density lipoprotein cholesterol (HDL-C) ratio[52,53]. The CAVI was associated with the IRI level measured at 12-hour fasting condition. The study also demonstrated that a weight reduction program was effective in decreasing the CAVI[54]. Another study of 487 subjects for annual health checks revealed that HOMA-IR was an independent determinant of the CAVI along with age, high-molecular weight adiponectin, and the amount of visceral adipose tissue[55]. The relationship of the CAVI with HOMA-IR was also reported in a study of

the skin autofluorescence reader, which detects the accumulated AGE in the skin[56]. A high TG/HDL-C ratio represented increased arterial stiffness assessed by the CAVI in the subjects with diabetes mellitus[57] and metabolic syndrome[58].

As for the body shape relating to insulin resistance and arterial stiffness, the CAVI was negatively related to the body mass index (BMI)[59,60] and the ratio of subcutaneous adipose tissue to visceral adipose tissue[61]. However, the visceral fat area, which is related to insulin resistance, is positively related to the CAVI[55,59,61].

Furthermore, the postprandial glucose levels, which refer to the presence of insulin resistance, showed a high CAVI[62]. As stated above, the administration of an insulin sensitivity enhancer, pioglitazone, improved the CAVI[24]. These results suggest that overeating and sedentary behavior cause insulin resistance and increase the CAVI.

5. Endothelial insulin resistance

A more comprehensive concept of insulin resistance includes insulin-insensitivity in organs and tissues that are regulated by insulin but not directly involved in the control of blood glucose levels[63]. Endothelial insulin resistance is an insulin-insensitivity in the vascular endothelium considered peripheral insulin resistance[64]. At present, the definition of endothelial insulin resistance is almost equal to the deterioration of IRS-1/PI3K/Akt/eNOS signaling, which can be observed only in experimental models using endothelial cells or animals[63]. The concept of endothelial insulin resistance has not been clinically established because only a small number of studies have shown an actual response to insulin in the endothelial cells of patients with metabolic disorders to date[65,66]. Thus, if possible, it is preferable to evaluate the endothelial insulin resistance for this purpose.

Several groups retrieved human forearm vein/artery endothelial cells by endovascular guide-wire abrasion to clarify the pathogenesis of vascular dysfunction. Protein kinase C[65], SIRT-1[67], and exercise-induced eNOS phosphorylation[68] were investigated previously. O-GlcNAc modification was increased in the freshly isolated endothelial

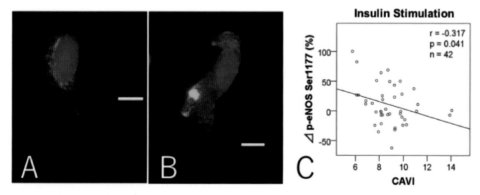

Fig. 2. Endothelial insulin sensitivity and CAVI.
Isolated endothelial cells from the radial catheter sheath were incubated with or without insulin 100 nM for 30 minutes (A: control, B: insulin). The percentage of increase was associated with the cardio-ankle vascular index (C: Ref. 70) 〖with permission from Wolters Kluwer Health, Inc.〗. Blue: 4′,6-diamidino-2-phenylindole, dihydrochloride (DAPI); Green: phosphorylated-endothelial nitric oxide synthase at Ser[1177]; Red: von Willebrand Factor. The yellow bar indicates 10 μm.

cells (FIECs) in patients with type-2 diabetes mellitus[69]. The increase of O-GlcNAc modification was associated with the endothelial insulin resistance defined as a decrease of insulin-stimulated increase of p-eNOS Ser[1177] in the study. The association of the CAVI with endothelial insulin resistance was investigated using the technique to harvest endothelial cells from radial catheter sheaths, which are disposable devices for coronary angiography. The CAVI negatively correlated with the percent increase of insulin-mediated p-eNOS Ser[1177] in the FIECs[70]. The result suggests that a high CAVI is associated with deteriorated signal transduction of the IRS1/PI3K/Akt/eNOS pathway suggesting endothelial dysfunction.

Recently, a strategy of achieving gene expression profiles of FIECs taken from the human iliac artery using a combination of fluorescence-activated cell sorting and single-cell quantitative real-time polymerase chain reaction was reported[71]. It is expected that translational research linking the molecular mechanisms to the vascular physiology will elucidate the role of endothelial insulin resistance in arterial stiffness expressed by the CAVI in the future.

References

1) Muniyappa R, Sowers JR. Role of insulin resistance in endothelial dysfunction. Rev Endocr Metab Disord. 2013;14:5-12. doi: 10.1007/s11154-012-9229-1.

2) Carreau A, Kieda C, Grillon C. Nitric oxide modulates the expression of endothelial cell adhesion molecules involved in angiogenesis and leukocyte recruitment. Exp Cell Res. 2011;317:29-41. doi: 10.1016/j.yexcr.2010.08.011. Epub 2010 Sep 8.

3) Apostoli GL, Solomon A, Smallwood MJ, Winyard PG, Emerson M. Role of inorganic nitrate and nitrite in driving nitric oxide-cGMP-mediated inhibition of platelet aggregation in vitro and in vivo. J Thromb Haemost. 2014;12:1880-9. doi: 10.1111/jth.12711. Epub 2014 Oct 1.

4) Qiu J, Zheng Y, Hu J, Liao D, Gregersen H, Deng X, Fan Y, Wang G. Biomechanical regulation of vascular smooth muscle cell functions: from in vitro to in vivo understanding. J R Soc Interface. 2013;11:20130852. doi: 10.1098/rsif.2013.0852. Print 2014 Jan 6.

5) Brandes RP, Fleming I, Busse R. Endothelial aging. Cardiovasc Res. 2005;66:286-94. doi: 10.1016/j.cardiores.2004.12.027.

6) Qiu H, Zhu Y, Sun Z, Trzeciakowski JP, Gansner M, Depre C, Resuello RR, Natividad FF, Hunter WC, Genin GM, Elson EL, Vatner DE, Meininger GA, Vatner SF. Short communication: vascular smooth muscle cell stiffness as a mechanism for increased aortic stiffness with aging. Circ Res. 2010;107:615-9. doi: 10.1161/CIRCRESAHA.110.221846. Epub 2010 Jul 15.

7) Jandu SK, Webb AK, Pak A, Sevinc B, Nyhan D, Belkin AM, Flavahan NA, Berkowitz DE, Santhanam L. Nitric oxide regulates tissue transglutaminase localization and function in the vasculature. Amino Acids. 2013;44:261-9. doi: 10.1007/s00726-011-1090-0. Epub 2011 Oct 8.

8) van den Akker J, VanBavel E, van Geel R, Matlung HL, Guvenc Tuna B, Janssen GM, van Veelen PA, Boelens WC, De Mey JG, Bakker EN. The redox state of transglutaminase 2 controls arterial remodeling. PLoS One. 2011;6:e23067. doi: 10.1371/journal.pone.0023067. Epub 2011 Aug 25.

9) Riehle C, Abel ED. Insulin signaling and heart failure. Circ Res. 2016; 118:1151-69.

10) Lteif AA, Han K, Mather KJ. Obesity, insulin resistance and the metabolic syndrome: determinants of endothelial dysfunction in whites and blacks. Circulation. 2005;112:32-8.

11) Zhang QJ, McMillin SL, Tanner JM, Palionyte M, Abel ED, Symons JD. Endothelial nitric oxide synthase phosphorylation in treadmill-running mice: Role of vascular signalling kinases. J Physiol. 2009;587:3911-20.

12) Fulton D, Gratton JP, McCabe TJ, Fontana J, Fujio Y, Walsh K, Franke TF, Papapetropoulos A, Sessa WC. Regulation of endothelium-derived nitric oxide production by the protein kinase Akt. Nature. 1999;399:597-601.

13) Montagnani M, Chen H, Barr VA, Quon MJ. Insulin-stimulated activation of eNOS is independent of Ca2+ but requires phosphorylation by Akt at Ser(1179). J Biol Chem. 2001;276:303928.

14) Gélinas DS, Bernatchez PN, Rollin S, Bazan NG, Sirois MG. Immediate and delayed VEGF-mediated NO synthesis in endothelial cells: Role of PI3K, PKC and PLC pathways. Br J Pharmacol. 2002;137:1021-30.

15) Geraldes P, Yagi K, Ohshiro Y, He Z, Maeno Y, Yamamoto-Hiraoka J, Rask-Madsen C, Chung SW, Perrella MA, King GL. Selective regulation of heme oxygenase-1 expression and function by insulin through IRS1/phosphoinositide 3-kinase/Akt-2 pathway. J Biol Chem. 2008;283:34327-36. doi: 10.1074/jbc.M807036200. Epub 2008 Oct 14.

16) Jiang ZY, He Z, King BL, Kuroki T, Opland DM, Suzuma K, Suzuma I, Ueki K, Kulkarni RN, Kahn CR, King GL. Characterization of multiple signaling pathways of insulin in the regulation of vascular endothelial growth factor expression in vascular cells and angiogenesis. J Biol Chem. 2003;278:31964-71. doi: 10.1074/jbc.M303314200. Epub 2003 May 29.

17) King GL, Park K, Li Q. Selective Insulin Resistance and the Development of Cardiovascular Diseases in Diabetes: The 2015 Edwin Bierman Award Lecture. Diabetes. 2016;65:1462-71. doi: 10.2337/db16-0152.

18) Zecchin HG, Priviero FB, Souza CT, Zecchin KG, Prada PO, Carvalheira JB, Velloso LA, Antunes E, Saad MJ. Defective insulin and acetylcholine induction of endothelial cell-nitric oxide synthase through insulin receptor substrate/Akt signaling pathway in aorta of obese rats. Diabetes. 2007;56:1014-24. doi: 10.2337/db05-1147. Epub 2007 Jan 17.

19) Kim JA, Montagnani M, Koh KK, Quon MJ. Reciprocal relationships between insulin resistance and endothelial dysfunction: molecular and pathophysiological mechanisms. Circulation. 2006;113:1888-904. doi: 10.1161/CIRCULATIONAHA.105.563213.

20) Soucy KG, Ryoo S, Benjo A, Lim HK, Gupta G, Sohi JS, Elser J, Aon MA, Nyhan D, Shoukas AA, Berkowitz DE. Impaired shear stress-induced nitric oxide production through decreased NOS phosphorylation contributes to age-related vascular stiffness. J Appl Physiol. 2006;101:1751-9. doi: 10.1152/japplphysiol.00138.2006.

21) Jung SM, Jandu S, Steppan J, Belkin A, An SS, Pak A, Choi EY, Nyhan D, Butlin M, Viegas K, Avolio A, Berkowitz DE, Santhanam L. Increased tissue transglutaminase activity contributes to central vascular stiffness in eNOS knockout mice. Am J Physiol Heart Circ Physiol. 2013;305:H803-10. doi: 10.1152/ajpheart.00103.2013. Epub 2013 Jul 19.

22) Chiba T, Yamanaka M, Takagi S, Shimizu K, Takahashi M, Shirai K, Takahara A. Cardio-ankle vascular index (CAVI) differentiates pharmacological properties of vasodilators nicardipine and nitroglycerin in anesthetized rabbits. J Pharmacol Sci. 2015;128:185-92. doi:10.1016/j.jphs.2015.07.002. Epub 2015 Jul 14. PMID: 26238254.

23) Shimizu K, Yamamoto T, Takahashi M, Sato S, Noike H, Shirai K. Effect of nitroglycerin administration on cardio-

ankle vascular index. Vasc Health Risk Manag. 2016;12:313-9. doi: 10.2147/VHRM.S106542. eCollection 2016. PMID: 27536126 Free PMC article.

24) Westerbacka J, Seppälä-Lindroos A, Yki-Järvinen H. Resistance to acute insulin induced decreases in large artery stiffness accompanies the insulin resistance syndrome. J Clin Endocrinol Metab. 2001;86:5262-8. doi: 10.1210/jcem.86.11.8047.

25) Ohira M, Yamaguchi T, Saiki A, Ban N, Kawana H, Nagumo A, Murano T, Shirai K, Tatsuno I. Pioglitazone improves the cardio-ankle vascular index in patients with type 2 diabetes mellitus treated with metformin. Diabetes Metab Syndr Obes. 2014;7:313-9. doi: 10.2147/DMSO.S65275. eCollection 2014. PMID: 25092992.

26) Mueller CF, Laude K, McNally JS, Harrison DG. ATVB in focus: redox mechanisms in blood vessels. Arterioscler Thromb Vasc Biol. 2005;25:274-8. doi: 10.1161/01. ATV.0000149143.04821.eb. Epub 2004 Oct 28.

27) Brownlee M. The pathobiology of diabetic complications: a unifying mechanism. Diabetes. 2005;54:1615-25. doi: 10.2337/diabetes.54.6.1615.

28) Luiking YC, Ten Have GA, Wolfe RR, Deutz NE. Arginine de novo and nitric oxide production in disease states. Am J Physiol Endocrinol Metab. 2012;303:E1177-89. doi: 10.1152/ajpendo.00284.2012. Epub 2012 Sep 25.

29) Shi W, Meininger CJ, Haynes TE, Hatakeyama K, Wu G. Regulation of tetrahydrobiopterin synthesis and bioavailability in endothelial cells. Cell Biochem Biophys. 2004;41:415-34. doi: 10.1385/CBB:41:3:415.

30) Crabtree MJ, Channon KM. Synthesis and recycling of tetrahydrobiopterin in endothelial function and vascular disease. Nitric Oxide. 2011;25:81-8. doi: 10.1016/j.niox.2011.04.004. Epub 2011 Apr 22.

31) Aroor AR, McKarns S, Demarco VG, Jia G, Sowers JR. Maladaptive immune and inflammatory pathways lead to cardiovascular insulin resistance. Metabolism. 2013;62:1543-52. doi: 10.1016/j.metabol.2013.07.001. Epub 2013 Aug 8.

32) Jia G, Aroor AR, Hill MA, Sowers JR. Role of Renin-Angiotensin-Aldosterone System Activation in Promoting Cardiovascular Fibrosis and Stiffness. Hypertension. 2018;72:537-48. doi: 10.1161/HYPERTENSIONAHA. 118.11065.

33) Jia G, Aroor AR, DeMarco VG, Martinez-Lemus LA, Meininger GA, Sowers JR. Vascular stiffness in insulin resistance and obesity. Front Physiol. 2015;6:231. doi: 10.3389/fphys.2015.00231. eCollection 2015.

34) Aroor AR, Demarco VG, Jia G, Sun Z, Nistala R, Meininger GA, Sowers JR. The role of tissue Renin-Angiotensin-aldosterone system in the development of endothelial dysfunction and arterial stiffness. Front Endocrinol (Lausanne). 2013;4:161. doi: 10.3389/fendo.2013.00161.

35) Nishikawa T, Edelstein D, Du XL, Yamagishi S, Matsumura T, Kaneda Y, Yorek MA, Beebe D, Oates PJ, Hammes HP, Giardino I, Brownlee M. Normalizing mitochondrial superoxide production blocks three pathways of hyperglycaemic damage. Nature. 2000;404:787-90. doi: 10.1038/35008121.

36) Geraldes P, King GL. Activation of protein kinase C isoforms and its impact on diabetic complications. Circ Res. 2010;106:1319-31. doi: 10.1161/CIRCRESAHA.110.217117.

37) Lee AY, Chung SS. Contributions of polyol pathway to oxidative stress in diabetic cataract. FASEB J. 1999;13:23-30. doi: 10.1096/fasebj.13.1.23.

38) Yan LJ. Redox imbalance stress in diabetes mellitus: Role of the polyol pathway. Animal Model Exp Med. 2018;1:7-13. doi: 10.1002/ame2.12001. Epub 2018 Apr 19.

39) Du XL, Edelstein D, Rossetti L, Fantus IG, Goldberg H, Ziyadeh F, Wu J, Brownlee M. Hyperglycemia-induced mitochondrial superoxide overproduction activates the hexosamine pathway and induces plasminogen activator inhibitor-1 expression by increasing Sp1 glycosylation. Proc Natl Acad Sci U S A. 2000;97:12222-6. doi: 10.1073/pnas.97.22.12222.

40) Du XL, Edelstein D, Dimmeler S, Ju Q, Sui C, Brownlee M. Hyperglycemia inhibits endothelial nitric oxide synthase activity by posttranslational modification at the Akt site. J Clin Invest. 2001;108:1341-8. doi:10.1172/JCI200111235.

41) Chang HC, Guarente L. SIRT1 and other sirtuins in metabolism. Trends Endocrinol Metab. 2014;25:138-45. doi: 10.1016/j.tem.2013.12.001. Epub 2013 Dec 30.

42) Rahman S, Islam R. Mammalian Sirt1: insights on its biological functions. Cell Commun Signal. 2011;9:11. doi: 10.1186/1478-811X-9-11.

43) Liang F, Kume S, Koya D. SIRT1 and insulin resistance. Nat Rev Endocrinol. 2009;5:367-73. doi: 10.1038/nrendo.2009.101. Epub 2009 May 19.

44) Zu Y, Liu L, Lee MY, Xu C, Liang Y, Man RY, Vanhoutte PM, Wang Y. SIRT1 promotes proliferation and prevents senescence through targeting LKB1 in primary porcine aortic endothelial cells. Circ Res. 2010;106:1384-93. doi: 10.1161/CIRCRESAHA.109.215483. Epub 2010 Mar 4.

45) Zarzuelo MJ, López-Sepúlveda R, Sánchez M, Romero M, Gómez-Guzmán M, Ungvary Z, Pérez-Vizcaíno F, Jiménez R, Duarte J. SIRT1 inhibits NADPH oxidase activation and protects endothelial function in the rat aorta: implications for vascular aging. Biochem Pharmacol. 2013;85:1288-96. doi: 10.1016/j.bcp.2013.02.015. Epub 2013 Feb 17.

46) Gogulamudi VR, Cai J, Lesniewski LA. Reversing age-associated arterial dysfunction: insight from preclinical models. J Appl Physiol (1985). 2018;125:1860-70. doi: 10.1152/japplphysiol.00086.2018. Epub 2018.

47) Fry JL, Al Sayah L, Weisbrod RM, Van Roy I, Weng X, Cohen RA, Bachschmid MM, Seta F. Vascular Smooth Muscle Sirtuin-1 Protects Against Diet-Induced Aortic Stiffness. Hypertension. 2016;68:775-84. doi: 10.1161/HYPERTENSIONAHA.116.07622. Epub 2016 Jul 18.

48) Nisoli E, Tonello C, Cardile A, Cozzi V, Bracale R, Tedesco L, Falcone S, Valerio A, Cantoni O, Clementi E, Moncada S, Carruba MO. Calorie restriction promotes mitochondrial biogenesis by inducing the expression of eNOS. Science. 2005;310:314-7. doi: 10.1126/science.1117728.

49) Gao D, Zuo Z, Tian J, Ali Q, Lin Y, Lei H, Sun Z. Activation of SIRT1 Attenuates Klotho Deficiency-Induced Arterial Stiffness and Hypertension by Enhancing AMP-Activated Protein Kinase Activity. Hypertension. 2016;68:1191-9. doi: 10.1161/HYPERTENSIONAHA.116.07709. Epub 2016 Sep.

50) Ding Y, Han Y, Lu Q, An J, Zhu H, Xie Z, Song P, Zou MH. Peroxynitrite-Mediated SIRT (Sirtuin)-1 Inactivation Contributes to Nicotine-Induced Arterial Stiffness in Mice. Arterioscler Thromb Vasc Biol. 2019;39:1419-31. doi: 10.1161/ATVBAHA.118.312346. Epub 2019.

51) Imamura H, Yamaguchi T, Nagayama D, Saiki A, Shirai K, Tatsuno I. Resveratrol Ameliorates Arterial Stiffness Assessed by Cardio-Ankle Vascular Index in Patients With Type 2 Diabetes Mellitus. Int Heart J. 2017;58:577-83. doi: 10.1536/ihj.16-373. Epub 2017 Jul 13.

52) McLaughlin T, Abbasi F, Cheal K, Chu J, Lamendola C, Reaven G. Use of metabolic markers to identify overweight individuals who are insulin resistant. Ann Intern Med. 2003;139:802-9. doi: 10.7326/0003-4819-139-10-200311180-00007.

53) Karelis AD, Pasternyk SM, Messier L, St-Pierre DH, Lavoie JM, Garrel D, Rabasa-Lhoret R. Relationship between insulin sensitivity and the triglyceride-HDL-C ratio in overweight and obese postmenopausal women: a MONET study. Appl Physiol Nutr Metab. 2007;32:1089-96. doi: 10.1139/H07-095.

54) Iguchi A, Yamakage H, Tochiya M, Muranaka K, Sasaki Y, Kono S, Shimatsu A, Satoh-Asahara N. Effects of weight reduction therapy on obstructive sleep apnea syndrome and arterial stiffness in patients with obesity and metabolic syndrome. J Atheroscler Thromb. 2013;20:807-20. doi: 10.5551/jat.17632. Epub 2013 Jul 25.

55) Ohashi N, Ito C, Fujikawa R, Yamamoto H, Kihara Y, Kohno N. The impact of visceral adipose tissue and high-molecular weight adiponectin on cardio-ankle vascular index in asymptomatic Japanese subjects. Metabolism. 2009;58:1023-9. doi: 10.1016/j.metabol.2009.03.005.

56) Hitsumoto T. Relationships between skin autofluorescence and cardio-ankle vascular index in Japanese male patients with metabolic syndrome. Cardiol Res. 2019;10:172-80. doi: 10.14740/cr878. Epub 2019 Jun 7.

57) Shimizu Y, Nakazato M, Sekita T, Kadota K, Yamasaki H, Takamura N, Aoyagi K, Maeda T. Association of arterial stiffness and diabetes with triglycerides-to-HDL cholesterol ratio for Japanese men: the Nagasaki Islands Study. Atherosclerosis. 2013;228:491-5. doi: 10.1016/j.atherosclerosis.2013.03.021. Epub 2013 Apr 1.

58) Kawada T, Andou T, Fukumitsu M. Relationship between cardio-ankle vascular index and components of metabolic syndrome in combination with sex and age. Diabetes Metab Syndr. 2014;8:242-4. doi: 10.1016/j.dsx.2014.09.023. Epub 2014 Oct 16.

59) Sugiura T, Dohi Y, Takagi Y, Yoshikane N, Ito M, Suzuki K, Nagami T, Iwase M, Seo Y, Ohte N. Relationships of Obesity-Related Indices and Metabolic Syndrome with Subclinical Atherosclerosis in Middle-Aged Untreated Japanese Workers. J Atheroscler Thromb. 2020;27:342-52. doi: 10.5551/jat.50633. Epub 2019 Aug 28.

60) Yue M, Liu H, He M, Wu F, Li X, Pang Y, Yang X, Zhou G, Ma J, Liu M, Gong P, Li J, Zhang X. Gender-specific association of metabolic syndrome and its components with arterial stiffness in the general Chinese population. PLoS One. 2017;12:e0186863. doi: 10.1371/journal.pone.0186863. eCollection 2017.

61) Park HE, Choi SY, Kim HS, Kim MK, Cho SH, Oh BH. Epicardial fat reflects arterial stiffness: assessment using 256-slice multidetector coronary computed tomography and cardio-ankle vascular index. J Atheroscler Thromb. 2012;19:570-6. doi: 10.5551/jat.12484. Epub 2012 Apr 4.

62) Tsuboi A, Ito C, Fujikawa R, Yamamoto H, Kihara Y. Association between the Postprandial Glucose Levels and Arterial Stiffness Measured According to the Cardio-ankle Vascular Index in Non-diabetic Subjects. Intern Med. 2015;54:1961-9. doi: 10.2169/internalmedicine.54.3596. Epub 2015 Aug 15.

63) Fulton DJ. Mechanisms of vascular insulin resistance: a substitute Akt? Circ Res. 2009;104:1035-7. doi: 10.1161/CIRCRESAHA.109.198028.

64) Muniyappa R, Sowers JR. Role of insulin resistance in endothelial dysfunction. Rev Endocr Metab Disord. 2013;14:5-12. doi: 10.1007/s11154-012-9229-1.

65) Tabit CE, Shenouda SM, Holbrook M, Fetterman JL, Kiani S, Frame AA, Kluge MA, Held A, Dohadwala MM, Gokce N, Farb MG, Rosenzweig J, Ruderman N, Vita JA, Hamburg NM. Protein kinase C-β contributes to impaired endothelial insulin signaling in humans with diabetes mellitus. Circulation. 2013;127:86-95. doi: 10.1161/CIRCULATIONAHA.112.127514. Epub 2012 Nov 30.

66) Bretón-Romero R, Feng B, Holbrook M, Farb MG, Fetterman JL, Linder EA, Berk BD, Masaki N, Weisbrod RM, Inagaki E, Gokce N, Fuster JJ, Walsh K, Hamburg NM. Endothelial Dysfunction in Human Diabetes Is Mediated by Wnt5a-JNK Signaling. Arterioscler Thromb Vasc Biol. 2016;36:561-9. doi: 10.1161/ATVBAHA.115.306578. Epub 2016 Jan 21.

67) Donato AJ, Magerko KA, Lawson BR, Durrant JR, Lesniewski LA, Seals DR. SIRT-1 and vascular endothelial dysfunction with ageing in mice and humans. J Physiol. 2011;589:4545-54. doi: 10.1113/jphysiol.2011.211219. Epub 2011 Jul 11.

68) Casey DP, Ueda K, Wegman-Points L, Pierce GL. Muscle contraction induced arterial shear stress increases endothelial nitric oxide synthase phosphorylation in humans. Am J Physiol Heart Circ Physiol. 2017;313:H854-H859. doi: 10.1152/ajpheart.00282.2017

69) Masaki N, Feng B, Bretón-Romero R, Inagaki E, Weisbrod RM, Fetterman JL, Hamburg NM. O-GlcNAcylation Mediates Glucose-Induced Alterations in Endothelial Cell Phenotype in Human Diabetes Mellitus. J Am Heart Assoc. 2020;9:e014046. doi: 10.1161/JAHA.119.014046. Epub 2020 Jun 6.

70) Masaki N, Ido Y, Yamada T, Yamashita Y, Toya T, Takase B, Hamburg NM, Adachi T. Endothelial Insulin Resistance of Freshly Isolated Arterial Endothelial Cells From Radial Sheaths in Patients With Suspected Coronary Artery Disease. J Am Heart Assoc. 2019;8:e010816. doi: 10.1161/JAHA.118.010816. https://www.ahajournals.org/journal/jaha

71) Sun Z, Lawson DA, Sinclair E, Wang CY, Lai MD, Hetts SW, Higashida RT, Dowd CF, Halbach VV, Werb Z, Su H, Cooke DL. Endovascular biopsy: Strategy for analyzing gene expression profiles of individual endothelial cells obtained from human vessels. Biotechnol Rep (Amst). 2015;7:157-65. doi: 10.1016/j.btre.2015.07.001. Epub 2015 Aug 1.

CAVI during sepsis

Daiji Nagayama[1] and Haruki Imamura[2]

Summary

1. It is debatable whether BP is the most suitable non-invasive indicator to detect hemodynamic changes in sepsis.
2. The CAVI may reflect sepsis-induced vascular changes not indicated by the change in BP and might be associated with the severity of sepsis.

1. Introduction

Critically ill patients with sepsis are prone to develop multiple organ failure and have a high risk of mortality. Sepsis develops due to a systemic inflammatory response syndrome (SIRS) to infection. Furthermore, the pathophysiologic features of sepsis result from the extensive effects of microbes and their products. These products can activate cytokines, complements, the coagulation system, plasmakinin, endorphins, and the sympathetic nervous system. In recent times, procalcitonin (PCT) has been proposed as a marker of infection, and the serum PCT level positively correlates with the severity of infection. The major benefit of PCT-guided therapy is a shorter duration of antibiotic treatment than with standard care[1].

Disseminated intravascular coagulation (DIC) is the major complication of sepsis and is characterized by the massive formation of thrombin and widespread microvascular thrombosis leading to multiple organ ischemia. Indeed, the pathophysiology of sepsis-induced circulatory failure includes not only coagulation disorders but also decreased blood flow. This hemodynamic change involves some degree of hypovolemia and a decrease in the vascular tone. Vasodilation and vascular permeability induced by pro-and anti-inflammatory cytokines released in sepsis induce peripheral circulatory failure. However, blood pressure (BP) does not necessarily reflect the pathophysiology, due to a compensated increase in the cardiac output. In other words, even when BP is within the normal range, a residual risk of circulatory failure induced by sepsis cannot be completely ruled out. It is therefore questionable whether BP is the most suitable non-invasive indicator to detect hemodynamic changes in sepsis.

We therefore examined whether the CAVI reflects hemodynamic change before and after the treatment of sepsis. Furthermore, we analyzed whether the serum PCT level as an indicator of the severity of sepsis contributes to the hemodynamic change in sepsis[2].

2. Subjects and the study methods to examine the relationship between sepsis and CAVI

The inclusion criteria for this study were the American College of Chest Physicians/Society of Critical Care Medicine consensus definitions for diagnosing SIRS and sepsis.

Resuscitation protocols related to hemodynamic management and antibiotic administration were followed in accordance with the Surviving Sepsis Campaign Guidelines 2012 (SSCG 2012). However, the Japanese guideline was followed only for the use of immunoglobulin, recombinant thrombomodulin, or antithrombin III.

3. Results of the study

We analyzed a total of 21 patients with sepsis and compared the patients' characteristics before and after one week of treatment for sepsis, as shown in Table 1. Among 21 subjects, 33.3% had hypertension and 28.6% had diabetes. The average number of SIRS criteria met at presentation was 2.43 ± 1.12. The types and proportions of infectious diseases diagnosed among the 21 participants were as follows: Pyelonephritis 9 (42.9%), Pneumonia/Lung abscess 4 (19.0%), Hepatic abscess/Cholecystitis 4 (19.0%), Iliopsoas abscess 1 (4.8%), Spondylitis 1 (4.8%), Vasculitis 1 (4.8%) and Cellulitis 1 (4.8%). All subjects received antibiotics including meropenem (33.3%), ceftriaxone (42.9%), sulbactam/ampicillin (14.3%), and tazobactam/piperacillin (9.5%). In some patients, intravenous immunoglobulin (33.3%), recombinant thrombomodulin (23.8%), or antithrombin III (14.3%). Ultimately, all subjects recovered from sepsis.

After one week of treatment for sepsis, a significant increase in the CAVI (7.9 to 9.6) and platelet (Plt) count was observed, while a decrease was seen in HR, WBC, CRP, and ln(PCT). No significant changes in systolic and diastolic BP were observed.

Correlations between hemodynamic variables or markers of the severity of sepsis were examined. The change in (Δ) CAVI was positively correlated with Δsystolic BP (SBP) (R = 0.585, P = 0.005) and negatively with the change in ln(PCT) (R = -0.546, P = 0.010). In addition, there were also a significant correlation between the ΔSBP and Δln(PCT) (R = -0.611, P = 0.003).

Additionally, we compared patients stratified by the severity of infectious disease. The subjects were divided

[1]Nagayama Clinic, 2-12-22, Tenjin-Cho, Oyama-City, Tochigi 323-0032, Japan.
[2]Hiyoshidai Hospital, 1-6-2 Hiyoshidai, Tomisato-City, Chiba 286-0201, Japan.

Table 1. **Patient characteristics before and after one week of treatment for sepsis. Vascular Health and Risk Management   2019; 019;15:509-516; Originally published by and used with permission from Dove Medical Press Ltd[2]**

Data are presented as mean ± SD. Paired *t*-test was used to compare the parameters before and after one week of treatment.

	At presentation	After one week	P value
N (male/female)	21 (14/7)	-	-
Age (years)	62.8 ± 19.0	-	-
Height (cm)	163.0 ± 9.6	-	-
Body weight (kg)	64.2 ± 17.9	-	-
BMI (kg/m^2)	24.0 ± 5.7	-	-
CAVI	7.9 ± 2.4	9.6 ± 1.8	< 0.001
SBP (mmHg)	121 ± 30	125 ± 14	0.523
DBP (mmHg)	70 ± 15	70 ± 12	0.939
HR (/min)	101 ± 16	76 ± 13	< 0.001
WBC (/μl)	17,104 ± 7,579	8,874 ± 4,090	< 0.001
Plt (/μl)	22.7 ± 11.5	31.7 ± 10.7	0.001
CRP (mg/dl)	20.9 ± 8.8	4.6 ± 3.9	< 0.001
PCT (ng/ml)	44.2 ± 102.9	0.7 ± 1.3	0.064
ln (PCT)	1.90 ± 1.94	0.39 ± 0.46	< 0.001
Hypertension (%)	7 (33.3)	-	-
Diabetesmellitus (%)	6 (28.6)	-	-

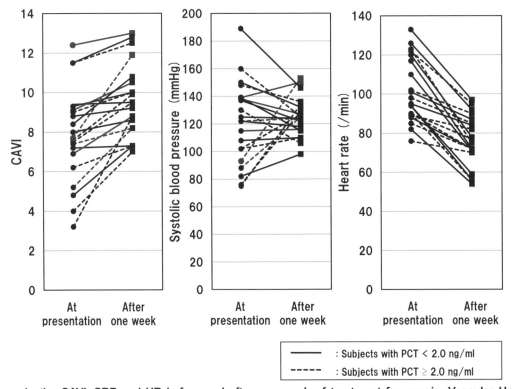

Fig. 1. **Changes in the CAVI, SBP and HR before and after one week of treatment for sepsis. Vascular Health and Risk Management   2019; 019;15:509-516; Originally published by and used with permission from Dove Medical Press Ltd[2]**

The CAVI, SBP, or HR for each participant at presentation (circles) and after one week of treatment (squares); Continuous lines indicate subjects with serum PCT < 2.0 ng/ml (N = 11), and dotted lines indicate those with PCT ≥ 2.0 ng/ml (N = 10).

into two groups by the cut-off PCT level for the severity of sepsis i.e., PCT level at presentation ≥ 2.0 ng/ml and < 2.0 ng/ml. Subjects with PCT at presentation ≥ 2.0 ng/ml had significantly higher ΔCAVI, ΔPlt count, PCT at presentation, and lower ΔPCT than those with PCT < 2.0 ng/ml at presentation. Furthermore, a notable but not significant increase in SBP was observed in subjects with PCT at presentation ≥ 2.0 ng/ml. These results indicated that a higher serum PCT level was associated with a relatively larger amplitude of hemodynamic changes after treatment.

Fig. 1 demonstrates the changes in CAVI, SBP, and HR from before to after one week of treatment for sepsis. Only 4 out of 21 subjects showed SBP below 90 mmHg at presentation, which is the cut-off value of septic shock[22]. Almost all (20 of 21) subjects, especially subjects with PCT at presentation $\geq$ 2.0 ng/ml (100%), showed an increase in CAVI (ΔCAVI, 1.7; Δ%CAVI, 20.0%) after treatment. However, the change in SBP was not uniform (ΔSBP, 4.1 mmHg; Δ%SBP, 2.9%). All subjects showed a decrease in HR after treatment, while a greater rate of change was observed in subjects with PCT at presentation < 2.0 ng/ml (-28.4 vs. -18.9%, P = 0.046).

There was no association between CAVI and SIRS score, prevalence of hypertension and diabetes, and type of infectious disease or treatment.

4. Patients with sepsis showing markedly decreased CAVI should be started on vasoconstrictor agents even if they are not yet in a hypotensive state

An analysis of all subjects in the present study showed no significant change in the BP during the treatment for sepsis, while the CAVI increased significantly. These findings suggest that even when arterial stiffness is decreased due to sepsis, BP can be maintained if the cardiac compensation is effective. Measuring the CAVI in a patient of sepsis in the emergency room therefore seems to be helpful to evaluate the risk of circulation crisis. Furthermore, for patients of sepsis with markedly decreased CAVI, initiating vasoconstrictor agents may be effective in preventing circulatory failure even if they are not in a hypotensive state. An interpretable machine learning model for the accurate prediction of sepsis has been reported recently. Variations in BP may be useful for real-time prediction of the onset of sepsis by applying artificial intelligence. In the future, an algorithm to predict the onset of sepsis may be constructed by combining CAVI and artificial intelligence.

5. Usefulness of the CAVI for managing circulatory failure in septic patients

As noted above, the CAVI may reflect sepsis-induced vascular changes not indicated by the changes in BP and is associated with the severity of sepsis. These findings suggest the usefulness of CAVI for managing circulatory failure in patients with sepsis.

References

1) Prkno A, Wacker C, Brunkhorst FM, Schlattmann P. Procalcitonin guided therapy in intensive care unit patients with severe sepsis and septic shock- a systematic review and meta-analysis. Crit Care. 2013;17:R291. doi:10.1186/cc12734

2) Nagayama D, Imamura H, Endo K, Saiki A, Sato Y, Yamaguchi T, Watanabe Y, Ohira Y, Shirai K, Tatsuno I. Marker of sepsis severity is associated with the variation in cardio-ankle vascular index (CAVI) during sepsis treatment. Vasc Health Risk Manag. 2019;15:509-516. doi: 10.2147/VHRM.S228506. eCollection 2019

CAVI during rituximab and cyclophosphamide, doxorubicin, vincristine, and prednisolone (R-CHOP) therapy

Naomi Shimizu

Summary

1. In recent times, an increased risk of atherosclerosis has been noted in cancer survivors who have undergone chemotherapy.
2. The patients treated with rituximab, cyclophosphamide, doxorubicin, vincristine, and prednisolone (R-CHOP) therapy with high vWF activity in the plasma showed cardio-ankle vascular index (CAVI elevation)
3. Plaque score and mean carotid intima-media thickness increased more significantly after the final R-CHOP therapy in the group with CAVI levels below nine.

Introduction

An increased risk of atherosclerosis has been noted in cancer survivors. However, studies focusing on the risk of atherosclerosis in patients treated with chemotherapy are scarce. Sekijima et al. reported that platinum-based chemotherapy was associated with an increased brachial-ankle pulse wave velocity in patients with gynecological malignancies[1]. Nuver et al. also reported that patients with testicular cancer who received chemotherapy showed progression of atherosclerosis[2].

B-cell lymphoma, including diffuse large B-cell lymphoma (DLBCL), is the most common subtype of malignant lymphoma. Patients with B-cell lymphoma are usually treated with a regimen comprising rituximab, cyclophosphamide, doxorubicin, vincristine, and prednisolone (R-CHOP)[3, 4], which shows complete remission (CR) rates of around 70%–90%[5]. R-CHOP is administered every 21 days for four to eight cycles depending on the stage of cancer. To date, no studies evaluating the relationship between atherosclerosis and R-CHOP therapy in a large sample of patients with malignant lymphoma have been published.

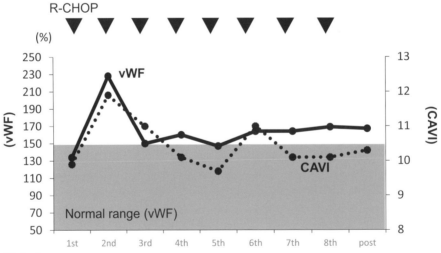

Fig. 1. Clinical course.
▼ means the R-CHOP therapy
vWF: von Willebrand factor, CAVI: Cardio-Ankle Vascular Index
Cited from ref.6

Department of Hematology, Toho University Sakura Medical Center, 564-1 Shimoshizu, Sakura City, Chiba, 285-8741, Japan.

An arterial stiffness parameter, the cardio-ankle vascular index (CAVI), was developed as a marker related to arteriosclerosis, and it is theoretically independent of blood pressure at the time of measurement. In this study, we investigated the hypothesis that the R-CHOP regimen promotes atherosclerosis by evaluating the CAVI just before each treatment cycle and by performing carotid ultrasonography at baseline and after the final treatment cycle.

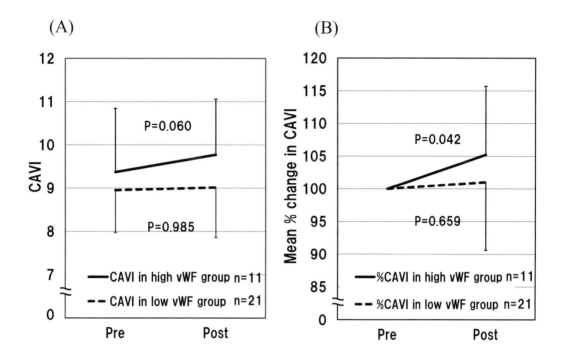

Wilcoxon signed-ranks test

Fig. 2.   Change in CAVI before and after first chemotherapy.

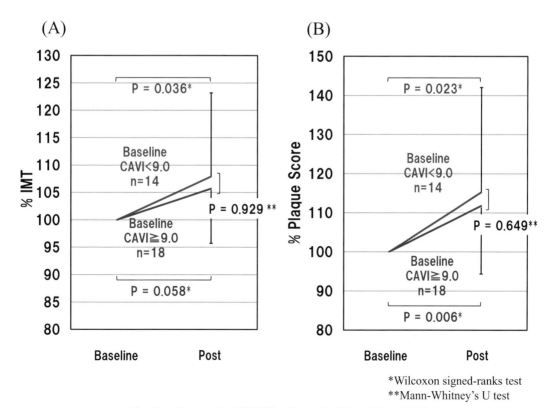

*Wilcoxon signed-ranks test
**Mann-Whitney's U test

Fig. 3.   Change in IMT/PS with and without high CAVI.

Case Presentation

We had previously reported the first case with malignant lymphoma who showed elevated CAVI coupled with plaque formation after eight cycles of R-CHOP[6]. Recently, we evaluated the von Willebrand factor (vWF) activity in plasma as a marker of endothelial damage, in addition to the CAVI levels. A 66-year-old Japanese female with multiple lymphadenopathies, follicular lymphoma, grade 1, clinical stage IVA, was treated with eight cycle R-CHOP therapy and achieved complete remission. The patient showed no complications such as diabetes mellitus (DM), hypertension (HT), and hyperlipidemia (HL) during chemotherapy. As shown in Fig. 1, CAVI levels and vWF activity increased after the first R-CHOP therapy and maintained high levels during the chemotherapy, compared with the levels just before the initiation of treatment. In addition, intima-media thickness (IMT) and plaque formation in the internal carotid artery was measured pre and post chemotherapy. After eight R-CHOP cycles, IMT and plaque score (PS) showed elevation (IMT; pre rt/lt 0.7/0.7 to post 0.71/0.71, PS; pre 3.6 to post 4.7), respectively.

Change in the CAVI after R-CHOP therapy

We evaluated the CAVI in patients with B-cell malignant lymphoma during the R-CHOP therapy. The mean age of 19 male and 13 female patients enrolled was 71 ± 6.4 years.

We divided the patients into two groups: the high vWF group comprised patients with plasma vWF activity ≥ 150 μg/ml, and the low vWF group consisted of patients with plasma vWF activity < 150 μg/ml. We analyzed the CAVI levels and mean % change in the CAVI using CAVI levels just before the first and second chemotherapy. Wilcoxon signed-rank test was used to identify differences between the two time points. As shown in Fig. 2A, there were no differences in the CAVI levels between the high and low vWF groups; however, the mean % change in the CAVI was significantly higher in the high vWF group (Fig. 2B). We speculated that the patients with high vWF activity, which indicates the progression of endothelial damage are prone to changes in CAVI by the anti-cancer drugs.

Carotid ultrasonography findings after R-CHOP therapy

We also analyzed the changes in mean carotid IMT and carotid PS in 32 patients. As shown in Fig. 3A and B, there were no significant differences in the % IMT and PS between the groups (CAVI < 9.0 and ≥ 9.0) by Mann-Whitney's U test. Following the chemotherapy, % IMT significantly increased in the patients with CAVI < 9.0 (Fig. 3A), and % PS increased significantly in both groups (Fig. 3B) by Wilcoxon signed-rank test. However, patients with CAVI < 9.0 showed a higher increase than patients with CAVI ≥ 9.0; Hence, we contemplated that the patients in whom vascular elasticity is maintained are prone to changes in CAVI by the anti-cancer drugs.

Conclusions

Our study showed that R-CHOP therapy promotes atherosclerosis with an elevation of CAVI.

Future challenges: Further studies are required to understand which anti-cancer drug(s) and what mechanism(s) promote atherosclerosis in patients undergoing R-CHOP therapy.

References

1) Sekijima T, Tanabe A, Maruoka R, Fujishiro N, Yu S, Fujiwara S, Yuguchi H, Yamashita Y, Terai Y, and Ohmichi M: Impact of Platinum-Based Chemotherapy on the Progression of Atherosclerosis. Climacteric, 2011; 14: 31-40.

2) Nuver J, Smit A J, Sleijfer D T, Van Gessel A I, Van Roon A M, Van Der Meer J, Van Den Berg M P, Burgerhof J G, Hoekstra H J, Sluiter W J, and Gietema J A: Microalbuminuria, Decreased Fibrinolysis, and Inflammation as Early Signs of Atherosclerosis in Long-Term Survivors of Disseminated Testicular Cancer. Eur J Cancer, 2004; 40: 701-6.

3) Bento L, Diaz-Lopez A, Barranco G, Martin-Moreno A M, Baile M, Martin A, Sancho J M, Garcia O, Rodriguez M, Sanchez-Pina J M, Novelli S, Salar A, Bastos M, Rodriguez-Salazar M J, Gonzalez De Villambrosia S, Cordoba R, Garcia-Recio M, Martinez-Serra J, Del Campo R, Luzardo H, Garcia D, Hong A, Abrisqueta P, Sastre-Serra J, Roca P, Rodriguez J, and Gutierrez A: New Prognosis Score Including Absolute Lymphocyte/Monocyte Ratio, Red Blood Cell Distribution Width and Beta-2 Microglobulin in Patients with Diffuse Large B-Cell Lymphoma Treated with R-Chop: Spanish Lymphoma Group Experience (Geltamo). Br J Haematol, 2020; 188: 888-97.

4) Gleeson M, Hawkes E A, Cunningham D, Chadwick N, Counsell N, Lawrie A, Jack A, Smith P, Mouncey P, Pocock C, Ardeshna K M, Radford J, Mcmillan A, Davies J, Turner D, Kruger A, Johnson P W, Gambell J, and Linch D: Rituximab, Cyclophosphamide, Doxorubicin, Vincristine and Prednisolone (R-Chop) in the Management of Primary Mediastinal B-Cell Lymphoma: A Subgroup Analysis of the Uk Ncri R-Chop 14 Versus 21 Trial. Br J Haematol, 2016; 175: 668-72.

5) Pfreundschuh M, Trumper L, Osterborg A, Pettengell R, Trneny M, Imrie K, Ma D, Gill D, Walewski J, Zinzani P L, Stahel R, Kvaloy S, Shpilberg O, Jaeger U, Hansen M, Lehtinen T, Lopez-Guillermo A, Corrado C, Scheliga A, Milpied N, Mendila M, Rashford M, Kuhnt E, and Loeffler M: Chop-Like Chemotherapy Plus Rituximab Versus Chop-Like Chemotherapy Alone in Young Patients with Good-Prognosis Diffuse Large-B-Cell Lymphoma: A Randomised Controlled Trial by the Mabthera International Trial (Mint) Group. Lancet Oncol, 2006; 7: 379-91.

6) Shimizu N, Ban N, Watanabe Y, Rikitake A, Watanabe R, Tanaka S, Sato Y, Imamura H, Kawana H, Yamaguchi T, Saiki A, Tatsuno I, and Shirai K: The Elevation of Cardio-Ankle Vascular Index in a Patient with Malignant Lymphoma Treated with a Combination Therapy of Rituximab and Cyclophosphamide, Doxorubicin, Vincristine, and Prednisolone. J Clin Med Res, 2017; 9: 729-32. https://doi.org/10.14740/jocmr3071w

CAVI after huge earthquake

Kazuhiro Shimizu

Introduction

It is known that the frequency of cardiovascular events increases just after a huge earthquake[1-4]. Arterial stiffness might provide valuable information about arterial wall conditions, which include arteriosclerosis and contraction of arterial smooth muscles. It is reported that increased arterial stiffness is an important risk factor for cardiovascular morbidity and mortality[5-7].

On March 11th, 2011, an earthquake of magnitude 9.0 occurred on the Pacific coast of Tohoku, Honshu Island, Japan, at 14:46 local time (the Great East Japan Earthquake). It was followed by a series of powerful aftershocks, with 31 earthquakes of magnitude larger than 6 in 3 days. As shown in Fig. 1, our institute (Toho University Sakura Medical Center Hospital) was situated about 300 km away from the epicenter. The building was strongly shaken and part of a

wall were collapsed. An unusual crisis occurred in our town. We started to investigate Cardio ankle vascular index (CAVI) for healthy volunteers and the patients with cardiovascular risks just after the earthquake[8].

Negative effects of emotional stress on CAVI

As shown in Fig. 1, Shimizu et al reported that CAVI was enhanced transiently just after the earthquake in healthy people and in coronary artery disease (CAD) patients. Particularly in healthy people, CAVI increased even though blood pressure was not raised significantly.

The number of patients who suffered from cerebral bleeding increased by two-fold compared to the several years before the earthquake. Furthermore, the number of deaths in our town increased in the year 2011 compared to 2009, 2010 and 2012 (Fig. 2A). We thought this increase in

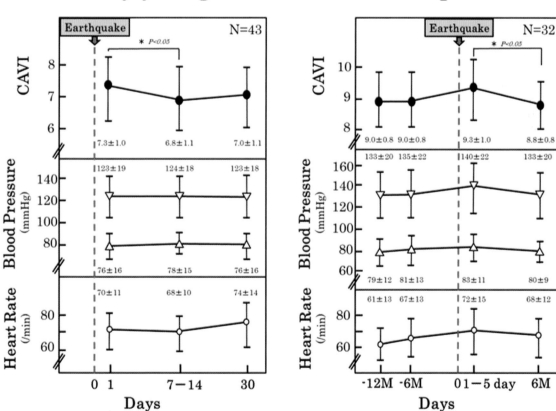

Data were expressed as mean ± SD. Comparisons of each measurements were evaluated by Tukey–Kramer test.

Fig. 1.   Changes in CAVI damaged by huge earthquake. Adapted from ref.8

Department of Internal Medicine, Toho University Sakura Medical Center, 564-1 Shimoshizu, Sakura City, Chiba 285-8741, Japan.

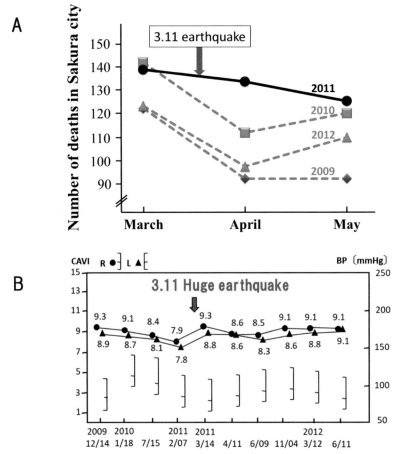

Fig. 2.   A. Changes in the fatalities of Sakura city. Cited from ref.8
     B. A case of increase in cardio-ankle vascular index (CAVI) just after the Great East Japan Earthquake (M9;
March 11, 2011). **Vascular Health and Risk Management**   2021; 17:37-47; Originally published by and used with
permission from Dove Medical Press Ltd[9]

mortality in 2011 was primarily due to psychological stress caused by the huge earthquake.

Fig. 2B shows the one case with metabolic disorder who had psychological damage such as fear and anxiety by the huge earthquake and increased CAVI. He had been treated for diabetes mellitus, hypertension and dyslipidemia in our hospital. Because his hometown was damaged by the huge earthquake and subsequent nuclear power plant troubles caused by the ensuing tsunami, he felt deep stress and his CAVI increased considerably.

Conclusion

The acute increase in arterial stiffness might be an important risk factor for cardiovascular morbidity and mortality after natural calamity. This finding could play a key role in solving the cause of cardiovascular events affected by mental stress.

References

1) Trichopoulos D, Zavitsanos X, Katsouyanni K, Tzonou A, Dalla-Vorgia P. Psychological stress and fatal heart attack: the Athens (1981) earthquake natural experiment.*Lancet.* 1983; 321: 441–444.

2) Dobson AJ, Alexander HM, Malcolm JA, Steele PL, Miles

TA. Heart attacks and the Newcastle earthquake. *Med J Aust.* 1991; 155: 757-761.

3) Leor J, Poole WK, Kloner RA. Sudden cardiac death triggered by an earthquake. *N Engl J Med.* 1996; 334: 413-419.

4) Kario K, Matsuo T, Kobayashi H, Yamamoto K, Shimada K. Earthquake-induced potentiation of acute risk factors in hypertensive elderly patients: Possible triggering of cardiovascular events after a major earthquake. *J Am Coll Cardiol.* 1997; 29: 926-933.

5) Asmar R, Rudnichi A, Blacher J, London GM, Safar ME. Pulse pressure and aortic pulse wave are markers of cardiovascular risk in hypertensive populations. Am J Hypertens. 2001; 14: 91-97.

6) Laurent S, Boutouyrie P, Asmer R, Gautier I, Laloux B, Guize L, Ducimetiere P, Benetos A. Aortic stiffness is an independent predictor of all-cause and cardiovascular mortality in hypertensive patients. Hypertension. 2001; 37: 1236-1241.

7) Blacher J, Asmer R, Djane S, London GM, Safar ME. Aortic pulse wave velocity as a marker of cardiovascular risk in hypertensive patients. Hypertension. 1999;33: 1111-1117.

8) Shimizu K, Takahashi M, Shirai K. A huge earthquake hardened arterial stiffness monitored with cardio-ankle vascular index. J Atheroscler Thromb. 2013; 20: 503-511.

9) Shimizu K, Takahashi M, Sato S et al. Rapid rise of cardio-ankle vascular index may be a trigger of cerebro-cardiovascular events: Proposal of smooth muscle cell contraction theory for plaque rupture. Vasc Health Risk Manag. 2021; 17:37-47.

PART 9

How to improve CAVI

WAON Therapy

Kazuhiro Shimizu[1], Keiichi Hirano[1,2], Hajime Kiyokawa[1], Masahiro Iwakawa[1] and Takahiro Nakagami[1]

Introduction

The rapid increase in heart failure (HF) patients is a major problem in recent years.

Symptomatic heart failure deteriorated patient's quality of daily life. Warming the body had been recommended as one of the non- invasive treatment for HF. Finnish Kuopio Ischemic Heart Disease Risk Factor Study reported that habitual sauna bathing (traditional Finnish sauna: 80°C to 100°C at the face) had associated with low mortality in a long term observation[1]. In Japan, Tei proposed Waon therapy, in which warming the patients with dry sauna at 60 degrees for 15 min, followed by bed rest in a warm blanket for 30 min[2]. Waon therapy was reported to be efficient for intractable HF patients taking maximum medical therapy by multicenter prospective randomized study[3]. However, the precise mechanism by which Waon therapy improved HF was not fully clear. We have been focusing on the "cardiac-vascular interaction" in the daily cardiovascular management. Zhang C and Ohira M reported that CAVI was negatively correlated with left ventricular ejection fraction (EF) in patients with heart failure. And, after treatment of heart failure, improvement of EF was correlated significantly with a decrease in CAVI. These results might be consistent with the idea that CAVI could play an afterload for the left ventricle, and adversely affect EF during heart failure[4].

Repeated sauna treatment was thought to be the improvement of endothelial function in patients with HF evaluated by Flow Mediated Dilation (FMD)[5]. We hypothesized that improvement in vascular endothelial function in heart failure patients would be expressed as a reduction in CAVI. We measured CAVI before and after the treatment of Waon therapy, and the role of CAVI was investigated.

Waon theapy

As shown in Fig. 1, Waon therapy uses a far infrared-ray dry sauna (Waon therapy equipment: CTW-5000, Fukuda Denshi, Tokyo, Japan), which is uniformly maintained at 60°C. Patients remained seated for 15 min, and then rested supine while covered with a warm blanket for an additional 30 min. Body weight was measured before and after the Waon therapy, and oral hydration with cold water was provided to compensate for the weight loss from perspiration. Waon therapy was performed once daily, 5 days each week[3]. Waon therapy is noninvasive and is supposed to reduce preload and afterload of the heart by

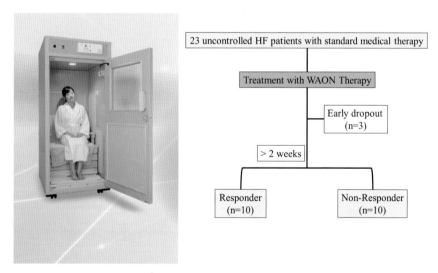

CTW-5000
Fukuda Denshi Co., Ltd. (Tokyo, Japan).

Fig. 1.   Waon therapy equipment: CTW-5000 and disposition of patients.
Waon therapy equipment is maintained at 60°C and warmed the body at 15 minutes in it. After out of the waon equipment, kept with a warm blanket for 30 minutes.

[1]Department of Internal Medicine, Toho University Sakura Medical Center, 564-1 Shimoshizu, Sakura City, Chiba 285-8741, Japan.
[2]Hirano clinic.

relaxing peripheral arterial tree[6-8].

CAVI during WAON therapy for HF patients
Case reports

We experienced a case who did not respond to Waon therapy and was subsequently converted to Left Venticular Assist Device (LVAD). This patient was 61 years old. His EF was worsened and CAVI was markedly increased after Waon therapy (EF; 20% to 13%, CAVI; 7.8 to 13.4). On the other hand, we experienced a very successful case. This patient was 35 years old. And he was weaned from the continuous inotropic infusion with dobutamine. This patient's EF was improved and CAVI was decreased after Waon therapy (EF; 24% to 36%, CAVI; 9.3 to 6.2). Therefore, we thought there would be two groups; one is response-type to Waon therapy, and the other is unresponsive type. To clarify the features of both types, the patients taking Waon therapy were divided according to the BNP-improving type and not improved type. And the changes of CAVI values of both groups were compared.

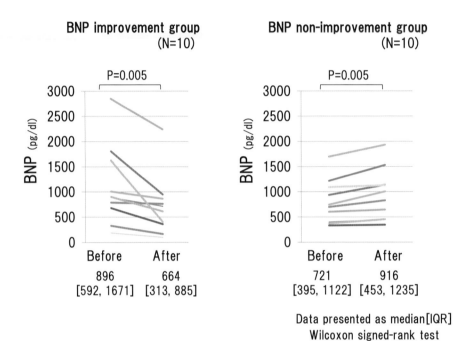

Fig. 2. The Changes of serum BNP during WAON therapy.
Abbreviation: BNP; brain natriuretic peptide.

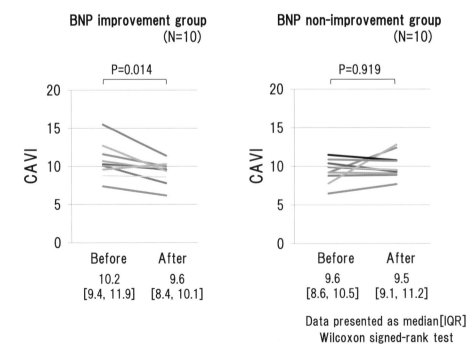

Fig. 3. The Changes of serum BNP level and CAVI during WAON therapy.
Abbreviation: BNP; brain natriuretic peptide. CAVI; cardio ankle vascular index.

CAVI changes in BNP improved group and not improved group

As shown in Fig. 1, from July 2011 to January 2021, 23 consecutive patients who took Waon therapy.

The patients were intractable HF patients (n = 23,) who had standard medical therapy for heart failure, but their symptoms could not be relieved. After 2 weeks of Waon therapy, some patients (n = 10) recovered efficiently with a decrease in BNP levels, while others (n = 10) did not recover from HF without a decrease in BNP levels. During Waon therapy the patients without improvement of BNP were not able to feel comfortableness for this therapy. The changes of BNP in both groups were shown in Fig. 2. And, The changes of CAVI of both groups were shown in Fig. 3. The initial CAVI values were higher in BNP-improving group. After Waon therapy, BNP improving group showed decreased CAVI significantly (10.2 to 9.6, p = 0.014). Whereas, BNP not-improving group did not decrease CAVI (9.6 to 9.5, p = 0.919).

Discussion:

We studied the effects of Waon therapy on the intactable HF patients. Depending on the response of BNP to Waon therapy, there were responsive type and non-responsive type. And responsive type showed rather higher CAVI before taking Waon therapy, and showed significantly decreased CAVI after Waon therapy. Recently it is known that CAVI reflected contraction of smooth muscle cells in the arterial tree[9,10] and works afterload for left ventricle. Considering those, above results suggested that there might be two type of intractable HF; one is mainly due to the overload by afterload, and the other is due to cardiac muscle dysfunction dominantly. And the former's symptoms of heart failure might be improved by decreasing the afterload through Waon therapy.

Conclusion:

Waon therapy improved the intractable HF patients whose CAVI was improved during Waon therapy. These results suggested that Waon therapy might relieve HF partly by reducing after-road to left ventricle and this was reflected to a decrease of CAVI.

References

1) Tei C., et al. Acute hemodynamic improvement by thermal vasodilation in congestive heart failure. Circulation. 1995; 91, 2582-2590.
2) Laukkanen T, Khan H, Zaccardi F, Laukkanen JA. JAMA Intern Med. 2015; 175: 542-548.
3) Tei C. WAON-CHF Study Investigators. Waon Therapy for Managing Chronic Heart Failure – Results From a Multicenter Prospective Randomized WAON-CHF Study-. Circ J. 2016; 80: 827-834.
4) Zhang C, Ohira M, Tomaru T, WANG H, Noike H, Shirai K, et al. Cardio-ankle vascular index relates to left ventricular ejection fraction in patients with heart failure. A retrospective study. Int Heart J. 2013; 54: 216-221.
5) Kihara T, Biro S, Tei C, et al. Repeated Sauna Treatment Improves Vascular Endothelial and Cardiac Function in Patients With Chronic Heart Failure. J Am Coll Cardiol. 2002; 39: 754-759.
6) Tei C. Waon therapy: Soothing warmth therapy. J Cardiol 2007; 49: 301-304.
7) Miyata M, Kihara T, Kubozono T, Ikeda Y, Shinsato T, Izumi T, et al. Beneficial effects of Waon therapy on patients with chronic heart failure: Results of a prospective multicenter study. J Cardiol 2008; 52: 79-85.
8) Fujita S, Ikeda Y, Miyata M, Shinsato T, Kubozono T, Kuwahata S, et al. Effect of Waon therapy on oxidative stress in chronic heart failure. Circ J 2011; 75: 348-356.
9) Shimizu K, Yamamoto T, Takahashi M, Sato S, Noike H, Shirai K. Effect of nitroglycerin administration on cardio-ankle vascular index. Vasc Health Risk Manag. 2016; 12: 313–319.
10) Yamamoto T, Shimizu K, Takahashi M, Tatsuno I, Shirai K. The effect of nitroglycerin on arterial stiffness of the aorta and the femoral-tibial arteries. J Atheroscler Thromb. 2017; 24: 1048–1057.

Weight control

Daiji Nagayama

Summary

1. Reduction of body weight in obese patients with metabolic and/or sleep apnea syndrome decreased the CAVI.
2. Reduction of accumulated visceral fat was associated with the rate of decrease of the CAVI.
3. Partial use of protein-sparing modified fasting (PSMF) using a formula diet is effective for decreasing the CAVI and visceral fat.
4. Patients with morbid obesity sometimes showed a low CAVI, and an increase in the CAVI after marked weight loss by bariatric surgery was reported. Considering that the CAVI was negatively associated with subcutaneous adipose tissue (SAT), this might be interpreted as that the low CAVI induced by massive SAT in morbid obesity returned to a near normal range with the reduction of SAT. Further prospective studies are needed in this regard.

Introduction

Generally, metabolic syndrome (MetS) patients and obese diabetic patients show a high CAVI. On the other hand, the "obesity paradox of the CAVI" exists, as described in **Chapter 19**. In short, the CAVI is negatively related to body mass index (BMI) but positively related to the visceral fat area (VFA) or the body shape index (ABSI), which is an index of visceral fat accumulation. In other words, the CAVI might differentiate between benign obesity and malignant obesity in terms of the vascular toxicity brought about by regional fat accumulations. This raises the question as to whether weight reduction therapy would contribute to an improvement in the CAVI.

In this chapter, the effects of weight reduction therapy on the CAVI are discussed.

1. Three patients whose diabetes control was linked to the CAVI

Among obese diabetic patients, the CAVI is often increased along with the deterioration of blood glucose control induced by an increase in body weight, and is decreased along with improvement of the diabetic condition by a body weight decrease.

Fig. 1 shows a diabetic patient whose CAVI increased with increasing body weight and HbA1c.

Fig. 2 shows a case whose transient increase in both body weight and HbA1c was also synchronized with CAVI variability.

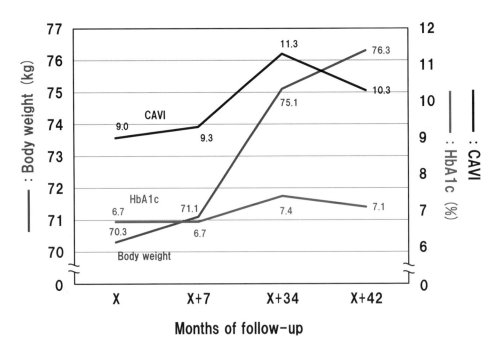

Fig. 1.   A 68-year-old man with type 2 diabetes mellitus who showed an increased in HbA1c and the CAVI with weight gain. (unpublished)

Nagayama Clinic, 2-12-22, Tenjin-Cho, Oyama-City, Tochigi 323-0032, Japan.

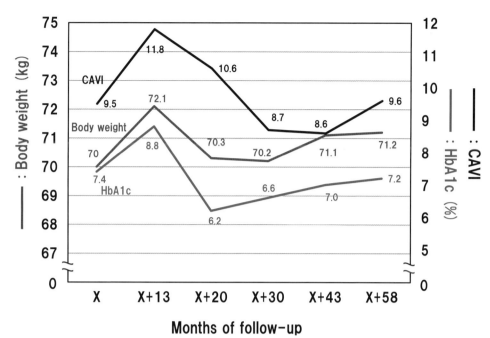

Fig. 2.   A 57-year-old man with type 2 diabetes mellitus whose diabetes mellitus status was consistent with his CAVI. (unpublished)

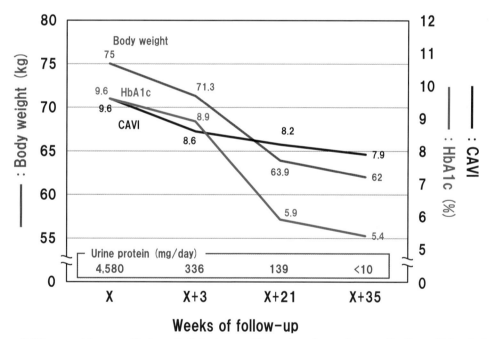

Fig. 3.   A 37-year-old man with type 2 diabetes mellitus who showed normalization of blood glucose, negative urine protein, and decreased CAVI with dose reduction. (unpublished)

Fig. 3 shows a diabetic patient who reduced body weight using a protein-sparing modified formula diet (PSMF) during hospitalization and showed a decrease in the CAVI as well as in urinary protein and HbA1c levels accompanying body weight reduction.

Body weight reduction in obese diabetic patients is clearly an effective way to improve the CAVI, as well as to control diabetes and improve renal function. These results indicated that the CAVI is useful for evaluating the vascular injury in obese diabetic patients in routine clinical practice.

2. Weight reduction improves obstructive sleep apnea, associated with an improvement in the CAVI

Obesity-induced obstructive sleep apnea (OSA) is known to contribute to arterial stiffening. Iguchi et al. reported that the severity of OSA was significantly correlated with the severity of MetS and the CAVI in obese patients[1]. Additionally, short-term weight reduction therapy for obese patients (mean age: 51.0 years, mean BMI: 31.0 kg/m^2) improved not only OSA, but also metabolic disorders and the CAVI. The change in the apnea–hypopnea index was an independent predictor of change in the CAVI.

3. Weight reduction therapy using a protein-sparing modified formula diet improves the CAVI in obese patients with metabolic disorder

We reported that weight reduction therapy using Protein-Sparing Modified Fasting (PSMF), the precise is written in next section, for obese patients with metabolic disorders improved the CAVI[2]. Shortly, we assessed the change in the CAVI in 47 obese Japanese subjects (mean age: 46 years, mean HbA1c: 8.4%, mean BMI: 33.3 kg/m^2, mean VFA: 180 cm^2) who underwent a 12-week weight reduction program consisting of a calorie restriction diet (20–25 kcal/day) using PSMF and exercise therapy. At baseline, the CAVI correlated positively with age (R = 0.70), blood pressure (R = 0.23), VFA measured by computed tomography (R = 0.26), and HbA1c (R = 0.39). After 12 weeks of weight reduction, the mean BMI decreased from 33.3 to 30.7 kg/m^2, and the mean CAVI decreased from 8.2 to 7.9 (**Table 1**). In subjects with a decrease in the CAVI, ΔVFA correlated positively with ΔCAVI (R = 0.47) (**Table 2**). No significant correlation was observed between changes in the CAVI and clinical variables, such as BMI, HbA1c, and lipid parameters; however, ΔVFA was a significant predictor of ΔCAVI. These findings are consistent with the concept that visceral fat exerts vascular toxicity effects, and the CAVI may be a sensitive indicator for these effects.

4. The effects of a protein-sparing modified formula diet on weight reduction and metabolic variables

A PSMF is comprised of high protein (20 g), low fat, low carbohydrate, and the necessary vitamins/minerals in a 170–260 kcal/pack. It is dissolved in 200–400 ml water and is taken as one meal. Usually, one regular meal is replaced by this formula diet (Microdiet®, Sunny Health Co., Ltd.; and Obecure®, USCure Co., Ltd. are available in Japan). It is possible to take this formula diet three times per day. Saiki et al. reported that weight reduction therapy using PSMF improved the renal function and proteinuria in obese patients with diabetic nephropathy[3]. In this study, decreases in BMI (from 30.4 to 28.2 kg/m^2) and urinary protein (from 3.27 to 1.50 g/day) were observed during 4 weeks of weight reduction therapy, even though no significant changes in creatinine clearance and serum albumin level occurred. This finding suggested that a protein-sparing low-calorie diet is effective for patients with obese diabetic nephropathy.

Furthermore, Yamaguchi et al. studied the effect of PSMF on epididymal fat accumulation, and glucose and lipid metabolism in the Zucker Diabetic Fatty rat, which is a model animal of obesity and insulin resistance[4]. Expressions of PPAR-gamma, adiponectin, and lipoprotein lipase in the subcutaneous adipose tissue were enhanced by administration of the formula diet (52 kcal/kg, protein: fat: carbohydrate ratio = 50:13:37) for 4 weeks, with decreases in body weight (-6%) and epidydimal fat (-22%).

Table 1. Participant characteristics at baseline and after weight reduction.
Data are presented as mean S.D, Paired *t*-test
Adapted from Ref. (2). 【with permission of Elsevier】

	Baseline	After treatment	P value
N (Male/Female)	47 (23/24)	-	-
Diabetes: N (%)	34 (72)	-	-
Age (years)	46 ± 13	-	-
Height (m)	1.69 ± 0.10	-	-
Body weight (kg)	90.1 ± 24.9	83.0 ± 21.7	<0.001
BMI (kg/m^2)	33.3 ± 7.5	30.7 ± 6.4	<0.001
CAVI	8.2 ± 1.3	7.9 ± 1.2	<0.01
Systolic BP (mmHg)	135 ± 17	132 ± 21	0.19
Diastolic BP (mmHg)	81 ± 9	80 ± 11	0.17
Visceral fat area (cm^2)	180 ±47	154 ± 49	<0.001
Subcutaneous fat area (cm^2)	345 ± 163	312 ± 142	<0.001
Total cholesterol (mg/dl)	209 ± 63	174 ± 48	<0.001
Triglyceride (mg/dl)	165 ± 101	109 ± 48	<0.001
HDL cholesterol (mg/dl)	47 ± 14	45 ± 13	<0.05
FPG (mg/dl)	160 ± 101	113 ± 38	<0.001
HbA1c (%)	8.4 ± 2.4	7.4 ± 1.8	<0.001
IRI (μU/ml)	12.0 ± 7.5	8.1 ± 4.8	<0.05
HOMA-IR	5.3 ± 3.5	2.2 ± 1.2	<0.01
Medication: N (%)			
Oral hypoglycemic agents	20 (43)	-	-
Statins	13 (28)	-	-
Calcium channel blocker	14 (30)	-	-
ARB/ACE-I	13 (28)	-	-

Table 2. Simple regression analysis of the correlation between change in the CAVI and clinical variables (CAVI decrease group, n = 30).
Adapted from Ref. (2). 【with permission of Elsevier】

ΔCAVI vs.	R	P value
ΔBMI	0.14	0.46
ΔSystolic BP	0.19	0.32
ΔDiastolic BP	0.23	0.22
ΔVisceral fat area	0.47	<0.01
ΔSubcutaneous fat area	0.22	0.25
ΔTotal cholesterol	0.21	0.26
ΔTriglyceride	0.19	0.31
ΔHDL cholesterol	0.16	0.39
ΔFPG	0.12	0.53
ΔHbA1c	0.07	0.71

Based on these results, diet therapy using a formula diet for obesity with metabolic disorder could restore insulin sensitivity and might relieve the vascular toxicity of insulin resistance.

5. Changes in the CAVI in morbid obese patients who have undergone bariatric surgery

Several studies have reported a significant increase in the CAVI after bariatric surgery, particularly in non-diabetic patients, even though favorable changes were observed in cardiometabolic parameters, such as the BMI, heart rate, and blood pressure[5,6]. Wang et al. reported that, in morbidly obese patients (mean age: 44.5 years), the CAVI increased 12 months after bariatric surgery (BMI: from 47.1 to 34.8 kg/m^2, CAVI: from 6 to 6.8)[6]. Considering that the mean CAVI in healthy Japanese subjects of the same age is about 7.5–7.8[7], a presurgical CAVI of 6 in morbidly obese patients was very low, and an increase in the CAVI to 6.8 after surgery might be interpreted as restoration of arterial stiffness by the large weight reduction achieved with bariatric surgery. The mechanism is unclear, but the obesity paradox of the CAVI, in which the CAVI is increased with visceral fat mass but decreased with subcutaneous fat mass, might be involved. This phenomenon suggests that subcutaneous adipose tissue might play some role in decreasing the CAVI. From this point of view, it might be possible that a low CAVI in morbid obesity is due to the vast amount of subcutaneous fat tissue, and an increase in the CAVI might be due to a reduction of such subcutaneous adipose tissue by bariatric surgery. The increase in the CAVI after bariatric surgery is not likely to contribute to adverse effects, since the efficacy of bariatric surgery on increasing life expectancy is certain. Nevertheless, this apparently contradictory finding is interesting and important for the diagnosis of obesity in terms of body shape. Further studies into this issue are required.

6. The future of weight control to improve the CAVI

The obesity paradox of the CAVI implies that the CAVI can distinguish between malignant obesity and benign obesity in terms of obesity-related vascular toxicity. During obesity treatment, monitoring the CAVI in addition to the metabolic and physiological states may help to confirm the appropriateness of various methods for weight reduction. Furthermore, using the CAVI, it needs to be elucidated which endogenous vasorelaxant substances may be expressed in obese patients.

References

1) Iguchi A, Yamakage H, Tochiya M, Muranaka K, Sasaki Y, Kono S, Shimatsu A, Satoh-Asahara N. Effects of weight reduction therapy on obstructive sleep apnea syndrome and arterial stiffness in patients with obesity and metabolic syndrome. J Atheroscler Thromb. 2013;20:807-820.

2) Nagayama D, Endo K, Ohira M, Yamaguchi T, Ban N, Kawana H, Nagumo A, Saiki A, Oyama T, Miyashita Y, Shirai K. Effects of body weight reduction on cardio-ankle vascular index (CAVI). Obes Res Clin Pract. 2013; 7: e139-e145. https://doi.org/10.1016/j.orcp.2011.08.154

3) Saiki A, Nagayama D, Ohira M, Endo K, Ohtsuka M, Koide N, Oyama T, Miyashita Y, Shirai K. Effect of weight loss using formula diet on renal function in obese patients with diabetic nephropathy. Int J Obes. 2005;29:1115-20.

4) Yamaguchi T, Miyashita Y, Saiki A, Watanabe F, Watanabe H, Shirai K. Formula diet is effective for the reduction and differentiation of visceral adipose tissue in Zucker fatty rats. J Atheroscler Thromb. 2012;19:127-136.

5) Galkine A, Dzenkeviciute V, Sapoka V, Urbanavicius V, Petrulioniene Z, Brimas G, Laucevicius A. Effects of body weight reduction on arterial stiffness and endothelial function after bariatric surgery in morbidly obese patients: a 4-year clinical study. Acta Endocrinol (Buchar). 2018;14:491-497.

6) Wang FM, Yang C, Tanaka H, Coresh J, Ndumele CE, Matsushita K. Increase in arterial stiffness measures after bariatric surgery. Atherosclerosis. 2021;320:19-23.

7) Saiki A, Sato Y, Watanabe R, Watanabe Y, Imamura H, Yamaguchi T, Ban N, Kawana H, Nagumo A, Nagayama D, Ohira M, Endo K, Tatsuno I. The role of a novel arterial stiffness parameter, cardio-ankle vascular index (CAVI), as a surrogate marker for cardiovascular diseases. J Atheroscler Thromb. 2016;23:155-168.

Anti-aging supplements and foods

Atsuhito Saiki

Summary

- The CAVI is known to increase linearly with age and may be appropriate for assessing ageing and anti-aging.
- Anti-aging supplements are designed to reduce the effects of aging but have not been proven to have any beneficial effects.
- Supplements such as resveratrol and S-equol, which are expected to have anti-aging effects, have been reported to have a CAVI-lowering effect.

Introduction—the concept of early vascular ageing

A large number of studies have verified that numerous factors, including arteriosclerotic diseases and coronary risk factors, affect the cardio-ankle vascular index (CAVI) value. Among these factors, the CAVI is known to increase linearly with age[1]. This age dependence of the CAVI may be useful in the field of geriatric medicine. With increasing age, cardiovascular risk and frailty increases with negative health consequences, such as cardiovascular diseases (CVDs) and dementia. However, this aging process seems to take a more rapid course in some individuals. Nilsson[2] proposed the new concept of the early vascular ageing (EVA) syndrome, which was first described in 2008. EVA is defined by measuring the carotid–femoral pulse wave velocity (cfPWV) in European countries (Fig. 1). However, the definition of EVA has recently been argued, and no conclusive definition has been established to date[3]. Furthermore, PWV is dependent on blood pressure at the measuring time-point, making it unsuitable as an index of aging. The CAVI might be appropriate in this respect, as the CAVI is independent of blood pressure.

Aging is a natural process that involves normal biological changes. Anti-aging supplements are designed to reduce the effects of aging. However, many of these supplements have not been proven to have beneficial effects. The lack of good indicators for assessing anti-aging effectiveness may be another reason for the lack of development in this field. On the other hand, several anti-aging supplements, such as an activator of sirtuin 1 (SIRT1), resveratrol[4], have been reported to lower the CAVI. Thus, the CAVI may be used to evaluate the effects of anti-aging supplements on vascular aging. The opposite phenotype of EVA is super-normal vascular aging (SUPERNOVA). The use of the CAVI may contribute to searches for protective mechanisms or new therapeutic targets against the aging process.

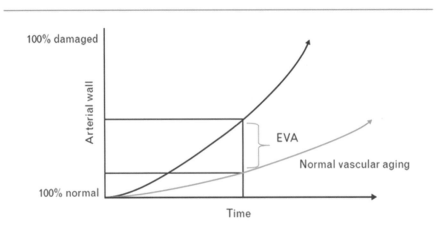

Early vascular aging. EVA, early vascular aging.

Fig. 1. The concept of early vascular aging (EVA). Cited from ref.25 [with permission from Wolters Kluwer Health, Inc.]

Center of Diabetes, Endocrine, and Metabolism, Toho University Sakura Medical Center 564-1, Shimoshizu, Sakura-City, Chiba, 285-8741, Japan.

Resveratrol and *Kaempferia parviflora*, activators of SIRT1

Resveratrol is a polyphenolic flavonoid found in the seeds and skins of grapes, red wine, mulberries, and peanuts. The effects of polyphenols are the same as those activated by calorie restriction, an intervention long known to enhance health and prolong lifespan[5]. An early target of resveratrol is the sirtuin class of nicotinamide adenine dinucleotide (NAD)-dependent deacetylases. Seven sirtuins have been identified in mammals, of which SIRT1 is believed to mediate the beneficial effects on health and longevity of both calorie restriction and resveratrol[6]. A number of intracellular pathways are activated by SIRT1. SIRT1 activates or suppresses specific genes, leading to a decrease in apoptosis, an increase in antioxidant activities, DNA protection, and anti-inflammatory effects[7]. The extent to which the sirtuin-activating actions of resveratrol are direct or indirect are not yet fully resolved[8]. Recently, Imamura et al. reported that resveratrol attenuated triglyceride accumulation associated with upregulation of SIRT1 and lipoprotein lipase in cultured 3T3-L1 adipocytes[9]. The study suggest that resveratrol may augment synthesis and oxidation of fatty acids, and possibly increases energy utilization efficiency in adipocytes through activation of SIRT1, supporting its efficacy in the treatment of obesity. Recently, resveratrol has become available in tablet form and is recommended as a dietary supplement. The results of research on the effects of resveratrol in humans are accumulating.

Several reports have demonstrated the effects of resveratrol on atherosclerosis. Jeon et al.[10] reported that 12-week supplementation of resveratrol suppressed high-fat diet-induced lipid accumulation in the aorta, with improvement in obesity and dyslipidemia in Apo E-knockout mice. Regarding the effect on arterial stiffness, Mattison et al.[11] reported that 2-year supplementation of resveratrol decreased PWV in rhesus macaques. Imamura et al. reported the effect of supplement of a 100-mg resveratrol tablet on the CAVI in patients with type 2 diabetes[4]. This was the first study that assessed the effect of resveratrol on arterial stiffness in humans in a double-blind, randomized, placebo-controlled study of 50 patients with type 2 diabetes, who received resveratrol or placebo daily for 12 weeks. Resveratrol supplementation decreased systolic blood pressure, diacron-reactive oxygen metabolites (d-ROMs; an oxidative stress marker) and the CAVI, and decreased the body mass index (Table 1). Multivariate logistic regression analysis identified resveratrol supplementation as an independent predictor of a CAVI decrease (Table 2).

Furthermore, *Kaempferia parviflora* is a plant belonging to the family Zingiberaceae. It also enhances the activity of SIRT1. Shimada et al. performed a randomized double-blind, placebo-controlled, crossover clinical study of 27 healthy volunteers given either a test product containing 100 mg of *Kaempferia parviflora* extract (SIRTMAX®, TOKIWA Phytochemical Co., Ltd., Chiba, Japan) or a

Table 1. Patient Characteristics in the Resveratrol and Placebo Groups at Baseline and After 12 Weeks of Treatment. Cited from ref.4

	Resveratrol		Placebo	
	Baseline	12 weeks	Baseline	12 weeks
n (Male/Female)	25 (15/10)	-	25 (11/14)	-
Age (years)	57.4 ± 10.6	-	58.2 ± 10.1	-
Height (cm)	163.3 ± 8.8	-	161.6 ± 10.2	-
BW (kg)	69.5 ± 13.0	68.7 ± 13.1	63.4 ± 13.9	63.3 ± 13.7
BMI (kg/m^2)	26.1 ± 4.2	25.7 ± 4.2	24.1 ± 4.0	24.1 ± 4.1
sBP (mmHg)	137.1 ± 18.7	131.6 ± 16.5*	137.1 ± 25.0	133.2 ± 26.5
dBP (mmHg)	82.0 ± 9.5	80.5 ± 11.2	80.8 ± 11.5	79.9 ± 11.5
Hypertension (%)	10/25 (40%)	-	9/25 (36%)	-
FPG (mg/dL)	152.0 ± 44.7	157.1 ± 50.9	138.1 ± 46.8	143.6 ± 73.2
HbA1c (%)	7.4 ± 1.1	7.3 ± 1.3	7.1 ± 1.4	7.1 ± 1.4
TC (mg/dL)	187.0 ± 24.4	189.8 ± 32.3	205.9 ± 44.7	207.6 ± 38.7
TG (mg/dL)	123.3 ± 67.6	126.7 ± 66.8	139.0 ± 66.7	136.5 ± 77.7
HDL-C (mg/dL)	56.2 ± 17.0	58.6 ± 18.4	56.1 ± 13.8	56.8 ± 10.6
Dyslipidemia (%)	8/25 (32%)	-	13/25 (52%)	-
CAVI	9.1 ± 1.1	8.6 ± 1.0**	8.9 ± 1.4	9.0 ± 1.3
d-ROMs (U.CARR)	379.9 ± 64.4	354.3 ± 50.6**	350.4 ± 72.8	351.5 ± 79.0
Medication (% of patients)				
Insulin	16.0	-	8.0	-
Oral hypoglycemic agent	72.0	-	64.0	-
Lipid lowering agent	40.0	-	40.0	-
Calcium channel blocker	4.0	-	16.0	-
ARB/ACE-I	20.0	-	12.0	-

Date are presented as the mean ± SD, or percent of patients. NS: not significant. *$P < 0.05$, **$P < 0.01$ versus baseline, paired t-test. BW indicates body weight; BMI, body-mass index; sBP, systolic blood pressure; dBP, diastolic blood pressure; HbA1c, hemoglobin A1c; FPG, fasting plasma glucose; TC, total cholesterol; TG, triglycerides; HDL-C, high density lipoprotein-cholesterol; CAVI, cardio-ankle vascular index; d-ROMs, derivatives of reactive oxygen metabolites; ARB, angiotensin II receptor blocker; and ACE-I, angiotensin enzyme inhibitor.

Table 2. Multivariate logistic regression analysis identified resveratrol supplementation as an independent predictor of a CAVI decrease. Cited from ref.4

Variable	Odds ratio	95% confidence interval	P
Gender (Male; 1, Female; 0)	1.24	0.216-7.14	0.808
Elderly (Age ≥ 65; 1, < 65; 0)	0.186	0.0211-1.63	0.129
High CAVI (≥ 9.0; 1, < 9.0; 0)	16.5	1.91-143	0.0109
Obesity (BMI ≥ 25; 1, < 25; 0)	1.92	0.261-14.1	0.522
Hypertension (+; 1, -; 0)	2.09	0.328-13.3	0.435
Dyslipidemia (+; 1, -; 0)	1.37	0.218-8.60	0.737
Resveratrol administration (+; 1, -; 0)	16.4	2.18-124	0.00664

AIC = 52.533, $P < 0.0001$.

placebo by oral administration for 7 weeks[12]. The CAVI tended to improve only in the SIRTMAX® group, and there was a slight increase in the production of advanced glycation end products (AGEs) in the SIRTMAX® group, as compared to a significant increase in the placebo group.

Oxidative stress is a potent promoter of vascular aging. These findings suggest that resveratrol and Kaempferia parviflora may inhibit vascular aging by suppressing oxidative stress through activation of SIRT1. The CAVI is considered to be a marker that sensitively reflects the effect of supplements on vascular aging.

S-equol, a non-steroidal estrogen

Epidemiological studies have indicated that a higher intake of soy and soy products is associated with a lower prevalence of CVD, osteoporosis, hormone-dependent cancer, and menopausal syndrome[13]. Isoflavonoids, phyto-estrogens that are present in soybeans, structurally and functionally resemble estradiol[14]. Daidzein, the principal isoflavone contained in soy, is converted to S-equol by intestinal bacteria. Not all individuals, however, can produce S-equol, which is considered the most biologically active metabolite.

Usui et al. reported the frequency of equol producers among overweight patients, and the effects of natural S-equol supplements for preventing overweight or obesity, features of metabolic syndrome, and CVD risk in a single-center, double-blinded, placebo-controlled, randomized, 2-period crossover design study[13]. Placebo or natural S-equol tablets containing 10 mg S-equol were orally ingested each day for 12 weeks. Fifty-four overweight or obese Japanese outpatients were enrolled. Equol non-producers accounted for 67.9% of the overweight or obese subjects. This percentage was higher than the previously reported percentage of non-producers in the general population, which was approximately 50%. Compared to the placebo group, the natural S-equol resulted in significant reductions in HbA1c, serum low-density lipoprotein cholesterol (LDL-C) levels, and CAVI. This effect was more pronounced in the subgroup of female equol non-producers (Fig. 2). These findings suggested that natural S-equol has a role in the prevention of diabetes and cardiovascular disease by suppressing the CAVI as well as HbA1c and LDL-C in overweight or obese individuals, based on sex

and equol-producing capability.

Furthermore, Ohkura et al. reported that S-equol supplementation improved nitric oxide-related endothelial function in ovariectomized rats[15]. Zhang et al. reported that S-equol had beneficial effects of cytoprotective antioxidant gene activation in human umbilical vein endothelial cells[16]. These findings suggest that S-equol supplementation improves vascular function and may suppress vascular aging in individuals with reduced equol production.

Standardized olive fruit extract, phenolic phytochemicals in olive fruit

Phenolic phytochemicals found in olive fruit are potent inhibitors of LDL oxidation, which is an important mechanism in the development of atherosclerosis[17]. Pais et al. reported a double-blind, placebo-controlled study investigating the impact of a proprietary standardized olive fruit extract (SOFE) on arterial stiffness using the CAVI[18]. Twelve of 36 subjects were assigned to each of the following groups: Group 1: SOFE 250 mg; Group 2: SOFE 500 mg; and Group 3: placebo. All three groups showed a decrease in th CAVI, although Group 2 had the largest reduction, with mean CAVI scores decreasing from 11.02 to 8.91 (Fig. 3). This report suggests that SOFE may inhibit vascular aging through the suppression of LDL oxidation.

Chlorogenic acid-enriched green coffee bean extract

Chlorogenic acids are phenolic compounds abundant in coffee beans. Chlorogenic acids are ester compounds of cinnamic acid derivatives (caffeic acid and ferulic acid) and quinic acid, and are mixtures of caffeoylquinic acids, feruloylquinic acids, and dicaffeoylquinic acids. Chlorogenic acid-enriched green coffee bean extract is reported to be effective against lifestyle-related diseases, such as hypertension, diabetes, and obesity, and exhibits antioxidant activity[19]. Matsui et al. reported the identification of 11 molecules (caffeoylquinic acids, feruloylquinic acids, dicaffeoylquinic acids, caffeic acid, and ferulic acid) after oral ingestion of chlorogenic acid-enriched green coffee bean extract in human plasma[20]. Among these molecules, ferulic acid enhances endothelium-dependent vasodilation by acetylcholine, a reaction that is attenuated by ROS[21]. Suzuki et al. reported a placebo-controlled double-blind

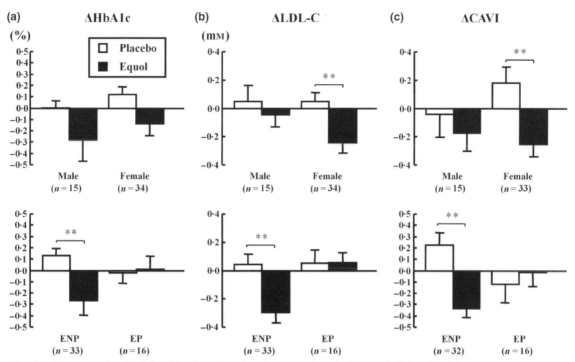

Fig. 2. Changes in HbA1c (a), low-density lipoprotein cholesterol (LDL-C) (b), and cardio-ankle vascular index (CAVI) (c) after natural S-equol supplementation. Cited from ref.13 [by permission of Oxford University Press]

Lower panel showed the changes from baseline in equol-producing capability. Natural S-equol supplementation significantly reduced HbA1c, LDL-C and CAVI values compared to placebo in equol non-producers (ENP). EP, equol producers. Data are shown as mean ± SE. *P < 0·05 vs placebo.

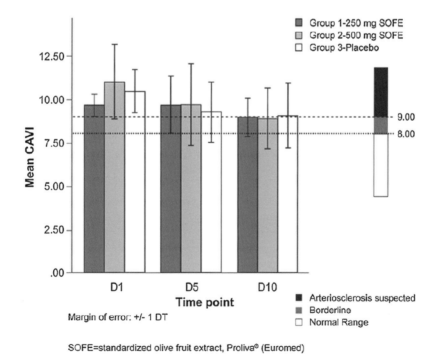

SOFE=standardized olive fruit extract, Proliva® (Euromed)

P=0.272 G1/G2; P=0.496 G2/P; P=0.674 G1/P; Day 10; Kruskal Wallis test

Fig. 3. Changes in cardio-ankle vascular index (CAVI) after standardized olive fruit extract (SOFE) administration. Cited from ref.18 [by permission from Springer Nature]

pilot study that investigated the effect of chlorogenic acid-enriched green coffee bean extract on arterial stiffness, based on the CAVI, in healthy Japanese men[19]. Subjects were divided into two groups and consumed beverages containing either chlorogenic acid-enriched green coffee bean extract or placebo daily for 2 weeks. The CAVI change

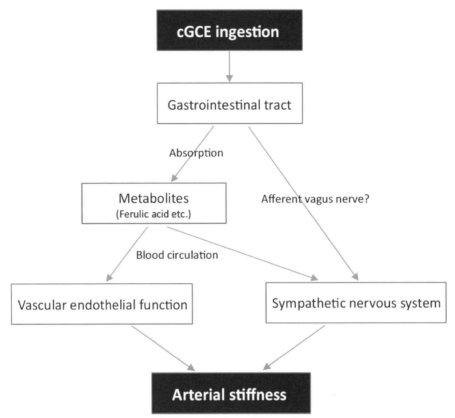

Fig. 4. Proposed mechanism for chlorogenic acid-enriched green coffee bean extract (cGCE) effects on arterial stiffness assessed by the cardio-ankle vascular index (CAVI). Cited from ref.19 [by permission of Taylor & Francis Ltd.]

was significantly greater in the chlorogenic acid-enriched green coffee bean extract group than in the placebo group. In addition, endothelium-dependent flow-mediated dilation increased and sympathetic nervous activity decreased in the chlorogenic acid-enriched green coffee bean extract group. These findings suggest that chlorogenic acid-enriched green coffee bean extract may improve arterial stiffness with enhanced endothelium-dependent vasodilation and reduced sympathetic tone (Fig. 4).

Cistanche deserticola extract

Cistanche deserticola extract (Koubakunikujuyou in Japanese) is widely used as a herbal medicine and has been reported to improve immunity and quality of life among senior citizens. The principal ingredient in *Cistanche deserticola* is phenylethyanoid, which is reported to have antioxidant action[22]. Aging mice treated with phenylethyanoid showed a reduction in malondialdehyde in blood serum and the liver[23]. Yonei et al. reported the effects of *Cistanche deserticola* extract on the CAVI in elderly persons for 12 weeks[24]. The CAVI significantly decreased by 10.9% in the right side and by 12.6% in the left side.

Conclusions

Many supplements have been claimed to have anti-aging effects, and it is becoming clear that some of them can improve the CAVI. The CAVI has been established as an indicator of vascular aging, and future studies are expected to determine whether long-term administration of

supplements has an anti-aging effect.

Future Perspective

- It is expected that true anti-aging supplements will be selected or developed using the CAVI as an aging indicator.

References

1) Takaki A, Ogawa H, Wakeyama T, et al. Cardioankle vascular index is a new noninvasive parameter of arterial stiffness. Circ J, 2007; 71: 1710-1714.
2) Nilsson PM. Early vascular aging in hypertension. Front Cardiovasc Med, 2020; 7: 6.
3) Cunha PG, Boutouyrie P, Nilsson PM, Laurent S. Early vascular ageing (EVA): definitions and clinical applicability. Curr Hypertens Rev, 2017; 13: 8-15.
4) Imamura H, Yamaguchi T, Nagayama D, et al. Resveratrol ameliorates arterial stiffness assessed by cardio-ankle vascular index in patients with type 2 diabetes mellitus. Int Heart J, 2017; 58: 577-583. https://doi.org/10.1536/ihj.16-373
5) Wood JG, RB, S Lavu, et al. Sirtuin activators mimic caloric restriction and delay ageing in metazoans. Nature, 2004; 430: 686-689.
6) Guarente L, Picard F. Calorie restriction—The SIR2 connection. Cell, 2005; 120: 473–82.
7) Morris BJ. Climate not cultivars in the NO-ing of red wines. J Hypertens, 2007; 25: 501-503.
8) Denu JM. The Sir 2 family of protein deacetylases. Curr Opin Chem Biol, 2005; 9: 431-440.

9) Imamura H, Nagayama D, Ishihara N, et al. Resveratrol attenuates triglyceride accumulation associated with upregulation of Sirt1 and lipoprotein lipase in 3T3-L1 adipocytes. Mol Genet Metab Rep. 2017; 12: 44-50.

10) Jeon SM, Lee SA, Choi MS. Antiobesity and vasoprotective effects of resveratrol in apoE-deficient mice. J Med Food 2014; 17: 310-316.

11) Mattison JA, Wang M, Bernier M, et al. Resveratrol prevents high fat/sucrose diet-induced central arterial wall inflammation and stiffening in nonhuman primates. Cell Metab 2014; 20: 183-90.

12) N Shimada, A Nakata, J Yang, et al. Evaluation of the safety and efficacy of *Kaempferia parviflora* extract (SIRTMAX®) in human—A randomized double-blind, placebo-controlled crossover clinical study. Jpn J Pharmacol Ther 2015; 43:997-1005.

13) Usui T, Tochiya M, Sasaki Y, et al. Effects of natural S-equol supplements on overweight or obesity and metabolic syndrome in the Japanese, based on sex and equol status. Clin Endocrinol (Oxf). 2013; 78 : 365-372. https://doi.org/10.1111/j.1365-2265.2012.04400.x

14) Bhathena SJ, Velasquez MT. Beneficial role of dietary phytoestrogens in obesity and diabetes. Am J Clin Nutr 2002; 76: 1191–1201.

15) Ohkura Y, Obayashi S, Yamada K, et al. S-equol partially restored endothelial nitric oxide production in isoflavone-deficient ovariectomized rats. J Cardiovasc Pharmacol 2015; 65: 500-507.

16) Zhang T, Liang X, Shi L, et al. Estrogen receptor and PI3K/Akt signaling pathway involvement in S-(-)equol-induced activation of Nrf2/ARE in endothelial cells. PLoS One 2013;8: e79075.

17) Aviram M, Dornfeld L, Rosenblat M, et al. Pomegranate juice consumption reduces oxidative stress, atherogenic modifications to LDL, and platelet aggregation: studies in humans and in atherosclerotic apolipoprotein E-deficient mice. Am J Clin Nutr 2000; 71: 1062-1076. https://doi.org/10.1093/ajcn/71.5.1062

18) Pais P, Villar A, Rull S. Impact of a poprietary standardized olive fruit extract (SOFE) on cardio-ankle vascular index, visual analog scale and C-reactive protein assessments in subjects with arterial stiffness risk. Drugs R D 2016; 16: 355-368. http://dx.doi.org/10.1007/s40268-016-0147-7

19) Suzuki A, Nomura T, Jokura H, et al. Chlorogenic acid-enriched green coffee bean extract affects arterial stiffness assessed by the cardio-ankle vascular index in healthy men: a pilot study. Int J Food Sci Nutr 2019;70: 901-908. https://doi.org/10.1080/09637486.2019.1585763, http://www.tandfonline.com

20) Matsui Y, Nakamura S, Kondou N, et al. Liquid chromatography-electrospray ionization-tandem mass spectrometry for simultaneous analysis of chlorogenic acids and their metabolites in human plasma. J Chromatogr B Analyt Technol Biomed Life Sci 2007; 858: 96-105.

21) Suzuki A, Yamamoto M, Jokura H, et al. Ferulic acid restores endotheliumdependent vasodilation in aortas of spontaneously hypertensive rats. Am J Hypertens 2007; 20: 508-513.

22) Xiong Q, Kadota S, Tani T, et al: Antioxidative effects of phenylethanoids from Cistanche deserticola. Biol Pharm Bull 1996;19: 1580-1585.

23) Xuan GD, Liu CQ: Research on the effect of phenylethanoid glycosides (PEG) of the Cistanche deserticola on anti-aging in aged mice induced by D-galactose. Zhong Yao Cai 2008; 31: 1385-1388, (in Chinese).

24) Y Yonei, T Kitano, M Ogura, et al. Effects of health food containing *Cistanche deserticola* extract on QOL and safety in elderly: An open pilot study of 12-week oral treatment. Anti-aging Med 2011; 8: 7-14.

25) Kotsis V, Stabouli S, Karafillis I, Nilsson P. Early vascular aging and the role of central blood pressure. J Hypertens. 2011; 29: 1847-53. https://doi.org/10.1097/hjh.0b013e32834a4d9f, https://journals.lww.com/jhypertension/pages/default.aspx

Summary: Methods for improving CAVI

Atsuhito Saiki[1] and Kohji Shirai[2,3]

The improvement methods in case of high CAVI were summarized in the table and Figure.

The efficacy of those methods was classified as follows

A: Definite, recommended; more than one paper, another paper

B: Probable; one paper, enough sample number

C: possible: need more study; one paper, small sample number

Next question is whether improved CAVI prevent future cerevro-cardiovascular evens. Those was discussed in next session.

	Improving factors	Drugs or Treatments	Ref	Efficacy
1.	Weight reduction in metabolic syndrome and obesity with diabetes	Formula diet	1,2	A
2.	Controlling hyperglycemia	Pioglitazone	3	B
		Glimepiride	4	B
		Rapid-acting insulin analog	5,6	A
		Sodium-glucose Cotransporter-2 Inhibitors	7	C
		α-glucosidase inhibitor	8	B
		Dipeptidyl peptidase 4 inhibitors	9	C
3.	Controlling hypertension	Renin-angiotensin-aldosterone system inhibitors	10-14	A
		T-type calcium channel blocker	15	B
		Mineralocorticoid receptor blocker	16	B
		Direct renin inhibitor	17,18	A
		α-blocker	19	A
		Nitroglycerin	20,21	A
4.	Controlling dyslipidemia	Pitavastatin	22,23	A
		Bezafibrate	24	B
		Ezetimibe	25	B
		Eicosapentaenoic acid	26	B
5.	Smoking cessation		27	A
6.	Continuous positive airway pressure		28	A
7.	WAON therapy	60° for 15 min and rest in a blanket for 30 min (in preparation for submission)		C
8.	Exercise		29	A
9.	Supplements	S-equal	30	B
		Resveratrol	31	B
		Olive fruit extract	32	B
		Chlorogenic acid-enriched green coffee bean extract	33	B
		Cistanche deserticola extract	34	C

[1]Center of Diabetes, Endocrine, and Metabolism, Toho University Sakura Medical Center, 564-1, Shimoshizu, Sakura-City, Chiba, 285-8741, Japan.
[2]Emeritus professor, Medical School, Toho university.
[3]Director, Seijinkai Mihama Hospital, 1-1-5 Utase, Mihama-ku, Chiba-shi, Chiba 261-0013, Japan.

Deteriorating Factors and Treatments for CAVI

1. **Aging, male**

2. **Arteriosclerosis**
   Coronary artery disease
   Cerebral artery disease
   Chronic kidney disease
   Carotid artery sclerosis
   Cognitive impairment

3. **Metabolic disorders**
   Diabetes mellitus(+Microangiopathy)
   Hypertension, Dyslipidemia
   Metabolic syndrome, Sarcopenia,
   Nonalcoholic fatty liver disease

4. **Smoking**

5. **Sleep apnea syndrome**

6. **Vasculitis**
   SLE, Polymyalgia rheumatica,
   Rheumatic arthritis, Chemotherapy

7. **Mental stress**
   Natural disasters, Mental shock

CAVI

1. **Weight reduction of Metabolic syndrome**   Formula diet

2. **Control of hyperglycemia**
   Pioglitazone, Glimepiride, Rapid-acting insulin analog, SGLT2 inhibitor, α-glucosidase inhibitor, DPP-4 inhibitor

3. **Controlling hypertension**
   ARB、Ca-blocker(L-type and T-type), Mineralocorticoid receptor blocker, Direct renin inhibitor, α-blocker, Nitroglycerin

4. **Controlling dyslipidemia**
   Statin (Pitavastatin), Bezafibrate, Ezetimibe, Eicosapentaenoic acid

5. **Smoking cessation**

6. **Continuous positive airway pressure**

7. **Waon therapy**

8. **Exercise**

9. **Suppliments** : S-equal, Resveratrol, Olive fruit extract, Green bean extract, Cistanche deserticola

References

1) Satoh N, Shimatsu A, Kato Y, Araki K, Koyama K, Okajima T, Tanabe M, Ooishi M, Kotani K, Ogawa Y: Evaluation of the cardio-ankle vascular index, a new indicator of arterial stiffness independent of blood pressure, in obese and metabolic syndrome. Hypertens Res, 2008; 31: 1921–1930.

2) Nagayama D, Endo K, Ohira M, Yamaguchi T, Ban N, Kawana H, Nagumo A, Saiki A, Oyama T, Miyashita Y, Shirai K: Effects of body weight reduction on cardio-ankle vascular index (CAVI). Obes Res Clin Pract, 2013; 7: e139-e145.

3) Ohira M, Yamaguchi T, Saiki A, Ban N, Kawana H, Nagumo A, Murano T, Shirai K, Tatsuno I: Pioglitazone improves the cardio-ankle vascular index in patients with type 2 diabetes mellitus treated with metformin. Diabetes Metab Syndr Obes, 2014; 7: 313-319.

4) Nagayama D, Saiki A, Endo K, Yamaguchi T, Ban N, Kawana H, Ohira M, Oyama T, Miyashita Y, Shirai K: Improvement of cardio-vascular vascular index by glimepiride in type 2 diabetic patients. Int J Clin Pract, 2010; 64: 1796–1801.

5) Ohira M, Endo K, Oyama T, Yamaguchi T, Ban N, Kawana H, Nagayama D, Nagumo A, Ohira M, Oyama T, Murano T, Miyashita Y, Yamamura S, Suzuki Y, Shirai K, Tatsuno I: Improvement of postprandial hyperglycemia and arterial stiffness upon switching from premixed human insulin 30/70 to biphasic insulin aspart 30/70. Metabolism, 2011; 60: 78–85.

6) Akahori H: Clinical evaluation of thrice-daily lispro 50/50 versus twice-daily aspart 70/30 on blood glucose fluctuation and postprandial hyperglycemia in patients with type 2 diabetes mellitus. Diabetology International, 2015; 6, 275–283.

7) Bekki M, Tahara N, Tahara A, Igata S, Honda A, Sugiyama Y, Nakamura T, Sun J, Kumashiro Y, Matsui T, Fukumoto Y, Yamagish SI: Switching dipeptidyl peptidase-4 inhibitors to tofogliflozin, a selective inhibitor of sodium-glucose cotransporter 2 improves arterial stiffness evaluated by cardio-ankle vascular index in patients with type 2 diabetes: a pilot study. Current Vascular Pharmacology, 2018; 16, 1-10.

8) Uzui H, Nakano A, Mitsuke Y, Geshi T, Sakata J, Sarazawa K, Morishita T, Satou T, Ishida K, Lee JD: Acarbose treatments improve arterial stiffness in patients with type 2 diabetes mellitus. J Diabetes Investig, 2011; 2: 148-153.

9) Shigiyama F, Kumashiro N, Miyagi M, Iga R, Kobayashi Y, Kanda E, Uchino H, Hirose T: Linagliptin improves endothelial function in patients with type 2 diabetes: A randomized study of linagliptin effectiveness on endothelial function. J Diabetes Investig, 2017; 8: 330-340.

10) Miyashita Y, Saiki A, Endo K, Ban N, Yamaguchi T, Kawana H, Nagayama D, Ohira M, Oyama T, Shirai K: Effects of olmesartan, an angiotensin II receptor blocker, and amlodipine, a calcium channel blocker, on cardio-ankle vascular index (CAVI) in type 2 diabetic patients with hypertension. J Atheroscler Thromb, 2009; 16: 621–626.

11) Bokuda K, Ichihara A, Sakoda M, Mito A, Kinouchi K, Itoh H: Blood pressure-independent effect of candesartan on cardio-ankle vascular index in hypertensive patients with metabolic syndrome. Vasc Health Risk Manag, 2010; 6: 571–578.

12) Ogihara T, Fujimoto A, Nakao K, Saruta T: ARB candesartan and CCB amlodipine in hypertensive patients: the CASE-J trial. Exert Rev Cardiovasc Ther, 2008; 6: 1195–1201.

13) Miyoshi T, Suetsuna R, Tokunaga N, Kusaka M, Tsuzaki R, Koten K, Kunihisa K, Ito H: Effect of azilsartan on day-to-day variability in home blood pressure: a prospective multicenter clinical trial. J Clin Med Res, 2017; 9: 618-623.

14) Kiuchi S, Hisatake S, Kawasaki M, Hirashima O, Kabuki T, Yamazaki J, Ikeda T: Addition of a Renin-Angiotensin-Aldosterone System Inhibitor to a Calcium Channel Blocker Ameliorates Arterial Stiffness. Clin Pharmacol, 2015; 7: 97-102.

15) Sasaki H, Saiki A, Endo K, Ban N, Yamaguchi T, Kawana H, Nagayama D, Ohhira M, Oyama T, Miyashita Y, Shirai K: Protective effects of efonidipine, a T- and L-type calcium channel blocker, on renal function and arterial stiffness in type 2 diabetic patients with hypertension and nephropathy. J Atheroscler Thromb, 2009; 16: 568–575.

16) Shibata T, Tsutsumi J, Hasegawa J, Sato N, Murashima E, Mori C, Hongo K, Yoshimura M: Effects of add-on therapy consisting of a selective mineralocorticoid receptor blocker. Intern Med, 2015; 54: 1583-1589.

17) Bokuda K, Morimoto S, Seki Y, Yatabe M, Watanabe

D, Yatabe J, Ando T, Shimizu S, Itoh H, Ichihara A: Greater reductions in plasma aldosterone with aliskiren in hypertensive patients with higher soluble (Pro)renin receptor level. Hypertens Res, 2018; 41: 435-443.

18) Miyoshi T, Murakami T, Sakuragi S, Doi M, Nanba S, Mima A, Tominaga Y, Oka T, Kajikawa Y, Nakamura K, Ito H: Comparable effect of aliskiren or a diuretic added on an angiotensin II receptor blocker on augmentation index in hypertension: a multicentre, prospective, randomised study. Open Heart, 2017; 4: e000591.

19) Shirai K, Song M, Suzuki J, Kurosu T, Oyama T, Nagayama D, Miyashita Y, Yamamura S, Takahashi M: Contradictory effects of b1- and a1-aderenergic receptor blockers on cardio-ankle vascular stiffness index (CAVI): the independency of CAVI from blood pressure. J Atheroscler Thromb, 2011; 18: 49–55.

20) Shimizu K, Yamamoto T, Takahashi M, Sato S, Noike H, Shirai K: Effect of nitroglycerin administration on cardio-ankle vascular index. Vasc Health Risk Manag, 2016;12:313-9.

21) Yamamoto T, Shimizu K, Takahashi M, Tatsuno I, Shirai K. The effect of nitroglycerin on arterial stiffness of the aorta and the femoral-tibial arteries. J Atheroscler Thromb, 2017; 24: 1048-1057.

22) Miyashita Y, Endo K, Saiki A, Ban N, Yamaguchi T, Kawana H, Nagayama D, Ohira M, Oyama T, Shirai K: Effects of pitavastatin, a 3-hydroxy-3-methylglutaryl coenzyme a reductase inhibitor, on cardio-ankle vascular index in type 2 diabetic patients. J Atheroscler Thromb, 2009; 16: 539–545.

23) Saiki A, Watanabe Y, Yamaguchi T, Ohira M, Nagayama D, Sato N, Kanayama M, Takahashi M, Shimizu K, Moroi M, Miyashita Y, Shirai K, Tatsuno I. CAVI-Lowering Effect of Pitavastatin May Be Involved in the Prevention of Cardiovascular Disease: Subgroup Analysis of the TOHO-LIP. J Atheroscler Thromb. 2020. Online ahead of print.

24) Yamaguchi T, Shirai K, Nagayama D, Nakamura S, Oka R, Tanaka S, Watanabe Y, Imamura H, Sato Y, Kawana H, Ohira M, Saiki A, Shimizu N, Tatsuno I: Bezafibrate ameliorates arterial stiffness assessed by cardio-ankle vascular index in hypertriglyceridemic patients with type 2 diabetes mellitus. J Atheroscler Thromb, 2019; 26: 659-669.

25) Miyashita Y, Endo K, Saiki A, Ban N, Nagumo A, Yamaguchi T, Kawana H, Nagayama D, Ohira M, Oyama T, Shirai K. Effect of ezetimibe monotherapy on lipid metabolism and arterial stiffness assessed by cardio-ankle vascular index in type 2 diabetic patients. J Atheroscler Thromb. 2010 Oct 27;17:1070-6.

26) Satoh N, Shimatsu A, Kotani K, Himeno A, Majima T, Yamada K, Suganami T, Ogawa Y: Highly purified eicosapentaenoic acid reduces cardio-ankle vascular index in association with decreased serum amyloid A-LDL in metabolic syndrome. Hypertens Res, 2009; 32: 1004–1008.

27) Noike H, Nakamura K, Sugiyama Y, Iizuka T, Shimizu K, Takahashi M, Hirano K, Suzuki M, Mikamo H, Nakagami T, Shirai K: Changes in cardio-ankle vascular index in smoking cessation. J Atheroscler Thromb, 2010; 17: 517–525.

28) Kasai T, Inoue K, Kumagai T, Kato M, Kawana F, Sagara M, Ishiwata S, Ohno M, Yamaguchi T, Momomura S, Narui K: Plasma pentraxin3 and arterial stiffness in men with obstructive sleep apnea. Am J Hypertens, 2011; 24: 401–407.

29) Alonso-Domínguez R, Recio-Rodríguez JI, Patino-Alonso MC, Sánchez-Aguadero N, García-Ortiz L, Gómez-Marcos MA: Acute effect of healthy walking on arterial stiffness in patients with type 2 diabetes and differences by age and sex: a pre-post intervention study. BMC Cardiovasc Disord, 2019; 19: 16.

30) Usui T, Tochiya M, Sasaki Y, Muranaka K, Yamakage H, Himeno A, Shimatsu A, Inaguma A, Ueno T, Uchiyama S, Satoh-Asahara N. Effects of natural S-equol supplements on overweight or obesity and metabolic syndrome in the Japanese, based on sex and equol status. Clin Endocrinol (Oxf). 2013 Mar;78:365-72.

31) Imamura H, Yamaguchi T, Nagayama D, Saiki A, Shirai K, Tatsuno I: Resveratrol ameliorates arterial stiffness assessed by cardio-ankle vascular index in patients with type 2 diabetes mellitus. Int Heart J, 2017; 58: 577-583.

32) Pais P, Villar A, Rull S. Impact of a Proprietary Standardized Olive Fruit Extract (SOFE) on Cardio-Ankle Vascular Index, Visual Analog Scale and C-Reactive Protein Assessments in Subjects with Arterial Stiffness Risk. Drugs R D. 2016 Dec;16:355-368.

33) Suzuki A, Nomura T, Jokura H, Kitamura N, Saiki A, Fujii A. Chlorogenic acid-enriched green coffee bean extract affects arterial stiffness assessed by the cardio-ankle vascular index in healthy men: a pilot study. Int J Food Sci Nutr. 2019 Nov;70:901-908.

34) Yonei Y, Kitano T, Ogura M, et al. Effects of Health Food Containing Cistanche Deserticola Extract on QOL and Safety in Elderly: An Open Pilot Study of 12-week Oral Treatment. ANTI-AGING MEDICINE 2011; 8, 7-14.

Does the improvement of CAVI lead to the improvement of prognosis?

Atsuhito Saiki[1] and Kohji Shirai[2,3]

Summary

- A high CAVI means the progression of arteriosclerosis and a potent risk for occurrence of cardiovascular diseases (CVD), but whether lowering CAVI improves morbidity and mortality is another problem.
- Based on several available follow-up studies, it could be considered that therapeutic interventions that lower CAVI may suppress future CV events.
- Even if the degree of improvement in risk factors is similar, the effect on CAVI may be different. Improving CAVI might be a better marker for various types of risk management.

Introduction

Cardio-ankle vascular index (CAVI) has been widely used in clinical medicine as an index for the evaluation of cardiovascular diseases (CVD) and risk factors. Most coronary risk factors such as hypertension, diabetes mellitus, and dyslipidemia increase CAVI and their improvement reduces CAVI. Additionally, several studies investigated the association between basal CAVI and future cardiovascular (CV) events, and concluded that baseline CAVI was a predictor of future CV events. In the meta-analysis of Matsushita et al., the pooled hazard ratio for composite CVD events per 1 standard deviation increment in CAVI was 1.20 in prospective studies[1]. Therefore, therapeutic interventions that lower CAVI would be expected to suppress future CV events. This chapter summarizes two articles suggesting that improvement of

CAVI during observation are associated with the decrease in CV events, and discusses the future prospects.

Impact of improved CAVI after management of risk factors on future CVD outcomes in patients with coronary artery disease

Otsuka et al. investigated the changes in CAVI after the management of atherosclerotic risk factors, and the impact of these changes on future CVD outcomes in 211 patients with coronary artery disease (CAD)[2]. Two CAVI examinations were performed, the second six months after the first, and all patients were followed up for more than 1 years or until the occurrence of a CVD event. The mean follow-up period was 2.9 ± 1.0 years. CAVI improved in 50% of patients after 6 months, but remained high in 50% of patients. In the Kaplan-Meier analysis, there was no

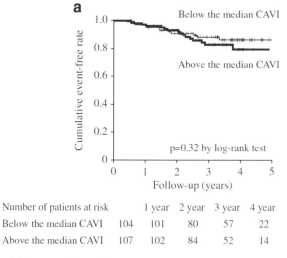
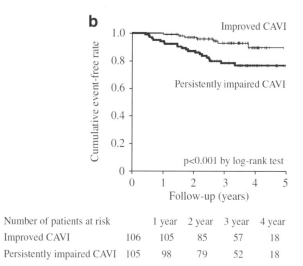

Number of patients at risk		1 year	2 year	3 year	4 year
Below the median CAVI	104	101	80	57	22
Above the median CAVI	107	102	84	52	14

Number of patients at risk		1 year	2 year	3 year	4 year
Improved CAVI	106	105	85	57	18
Persistently impaired CAVI	105	98	79	52	18

Fig. 1. (a) Comparison of Kaplan–Meier curves of event-free survival in patients above the median and below the median CAVI value in the first CAVI test. (b) Comparison of Kaplan–Meier curves of event-free survival in patients with persistently impaired CAVI and improved CAVI. CAVI, cardio ankle vascular index[2].

[1]Center of Diabetes, Endocrine and Metabolism, Toho University Sakura Medical Center, 564-1, Shimoshizu, Sakura-City, Chiba, 285-8741, Japan.
[2]Emeritus professor, Medical School, Toho university.
[3]Director, Seijinkai Mihama Hospital, 1-1-5 Utase, Mihama-ku, Chiba-shi, Chiba 261-0013, Japan.

significant prognostic difference between patients with CAVI values above or below the median in the first CAVI test, but significantly worse CVD outcomes for patients with persistently impaired CAVI group were observed when compared with the improved CAVI group as shown in the Kaplan–Meier analysis (Fig. 1). Additionally, a persistently high CAVI was an independent predictor of future CVD events. They concluded that the improved CAVI group had a better prognosis than the persistent CAVI group concerning future CVD events and maintained that serial measurements of CAVI provided important prognostic information on patients with CAD in clinical practice.

Interestingly, there was no difference in the usage of various medication in the two groups. However, HbA1c at second CAVI test in patients with improved CAVI was lower than that of the persistently impaired CAVI group. Diabetic control might be important when choosing among

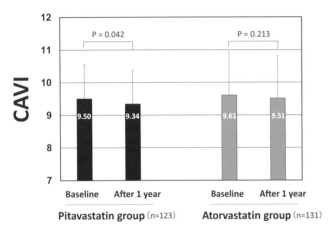

Fig. 2. Trend of CAVI in pitavastatin and atorvastatin groups during the 5-year study period (subgroup analysis of the TOHO-LIP). CAVI, cardio-ankle vascular index[4].

various types of treatments in terms of improving CAVI.

CAVI-Lowering effect of Pitavastatin may be involved in the prevention of cardiovascular disease (subgroup analysis of the TOHO-LIP)

We conducted a multicenter, open-label, randomized controlled, head-to-head trial, called the TOHO Lipid Intervention Trial Using Pitavastatin (TOHO-LIP), to compare the effects of pitavastatin (n = 332) with atorvastatin therapy (n = 332) for CV event prevention in patients with hypercholesterolemia at a high risk of CVD[3]. The primary end point was a composite of CV death, sudden death of unknown origin, nonfatal myocardial infarction (MI), nonfatal stroke, transient ischemic attack, and heart failure requiring hospitalization. Pitavastatin significantly reduced the risk of the primary end point compared to atorvastatin [pitavastatin, 2.9%; atorvastatin, 8.1%; hazard ratio (HR), 0.366], while there was no difference in the change in low-density lipoprotein cholesterol (LDL-C) level between the two groups.

To clarify the mechanism by which pitavastatin preferentially prevents CV events, we investigated the relationship between CV events and CAVI using the TOHO-LIP database[4]. In this subgroup analysis, 254 patients were enrolled after excluding those who had CV events at baseline or during the first year. The three-point major cardiac adverse events (3P-MACE) were added as a secondary end point. CAVI significantly decreased only in the pitavastatin group during the first year (Fig. 2), while the change in LDL-C did not differ between the two groups. The change in CAVI during the first year positively correlated with 3P-MACE and tended to be an independent predictor of 3P-MACE in the Cox proportional hazards model (Table 1). The annual change in CAVI throughout the observation period was significantly higher in subjects with CV events compared to those without (Fig. 3). Moreover,

Table 1. Cox proportional hazards regression analysis of the association between 3P-MACE and clinical variables (subgroup analysis of the TOHO-LIP). Cited from ref.4

(a) Model 1

Variables	Hazard Ratio	95% Confidential Interval	P-value
ΔLDL-C (Δmg/dl)	1.007	0.994 - 1.021	0.280
ΔCAVI	1.758	0.926 - 3.338	0.084
Group (Atorvastatin; 0, Pitavastatin; 1)	0.493	0.171 - 1.420	0.190

(b) Model 2

Variables	Hazard Ratio	95% Confidential Interval	P-value
Gender (male; 0, female; 1)	0.666	0.245 - 1.813	0.426
Age (years old)	1.039	0.978 - 1.104	0.215
ΔLDL-C (Δmg/dl)	1.006	0.993 - 1.020	0.363
ΔCAVI	1.736	0.938 - 3.213	0.079
Group (Atorvastatin; 0, Pitavastatin; 1)	0.501	0.172 - 1.461	0.206

Abbreviations: 3P-MACE, 3-point major cardiac adverse events; LDL-C, low-density lipoprotein cholesterol; CAVI, cardio-ankle vascular index.

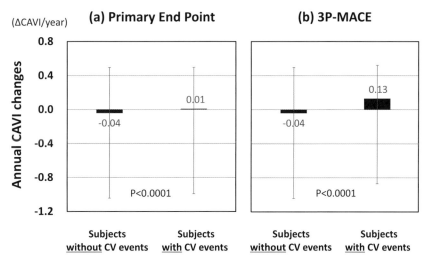

Fig. 3. Changes in CAVI during the first year in pitavastatin and atorvastatin groups. CAVI, cardio-
ankle vascular index (subgroup analysis of the TOHO-LIP)[4].

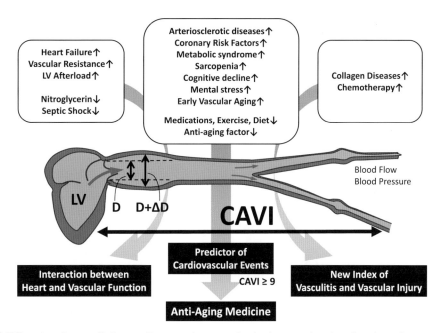

Fig. 4. CAVI not only predicts cardiovascular events, but may also be developed as a new index
for vascular functions.[15]

the baseline CAVI in the two groups was similar. Therefore, we concluded that the reduction in CV events tended to be associated with the CAVI-lowering effect of pitavastatin, which was independent of the LDL-C-lowering effect.

Miyashita et al.[5] reported that pitavastatin 2 mg/day significantly reduced CAVI together with serum markers of oxidative stress, malondialdehyde-LDL, and urinary 8-hydroxy-2'-deoxyguanosine in patients with type 2 diabetes. Furthermore, in the main TOHO-LIP study, C-reactive protein levels decreased after 1 year of pitavastatin therapy but did not change with atorvastatin therapy[3]. There is no doubt that LDL-C is an important risk factor; however, although the accumulation of LDL-C in blood vessels leads to lipidosis, the changes do not immediately affect the arterial stiffness[6]. These findings suggest that CAVI may increase after the development of

inflammation caused by oxidative stress, with the subsequent formation of a fibrous cap and a complicated lesion. In other words, pitavastatin may lower CAVI by improving the oxidative stress and inflammation, independent of the LDL-C-lowering effects. Furthermore, it is interesting to note that the change in CAVI during the first year was related to future CV events, which may be a type of legacy effect.

Conclusions

CAVI is high in patients with coronary risk factors. However, their effect on CAVI differs depending on the type of treatment, even when the degree of risk factor improvement is similar. For example, the response of CAVI to glucose-lowering treatment depends on the type of agent used[7]. Alpha-glucosidase inhibitors[8], rapid-acting insulin analogs[9,10], pioglitazone[11], and sodium-glucose cotransporter-2 inhibitors[12] reduce CAVI; however, dipeptidyl peptidase 4 inhibitors[13] and conventional sulfonylurea[14] do not improve CAVI. These findings suggest that postprandial hyperglycemia, insulin resistance and oxidative stress may influence CAVI in patients with diabetes. Rather than simply managing the conventional risk factors, CAVI should be used as a central indicator in routine practice to reduce future CV events (Fig. 4)[15].

Future Perspective

- Serial measurements of CAVI in clinical practice should be recommended to provide prognostic information.
- Further studies are needed to examine the effect of various therapeutic interventions on CAVI and their relationship with CV events.

References

1) Matsushita K, Ding N, Kim ED, Budoff M, Chirinos JA, Fernhall B, Hamburg NM, Kario K, Miyoshi T, Tanaka H, Townsend R: Cardio-ankle vascular index and cardiovascular disease: Systematic review and metaanalysis of prospective and cross-sectional studies. J Clin Hypertens, 2019; 21: 16-24.

2) Otsuka K, Fukuda S, Shimada K, Suzoshikawa J: Serial assessment of arterial stiffness by cardio-ankle vascular index for prediction of future cardiovascular events in patients with coronary artery disease. Hypertens Res, 2014; 37: 1014-1020. https://doi.org/10.1038/hr.2014.116

3) Moroi M, Nagayama D, Hara F, Saiki A, Shimizu K, Takahashi M, Sato N, Shiba T, Sugimoto H, Fujioka T, Chiba T, Nishizawa K, Usui S, Iwasaki Y, Tatsuno I, Sugi K, Yamasaki J, Yamamura S, Shirai K: Outcome of pitavastatin versus atorvastatin therapy in patients with hypercholesterolemia at high risk for atherosclerotic cardiovascular disease. Int J Cardiol, 2020; 305: 139-146.

4) Saiki A, Watanabe Y, Yamaguchi T, Ohira M, Nagayama D, Sato N, Kanayama M, Takahashi M, Shimizu K, Moroi M, Miyashita Y, Shirai K, Tatsuno I. CAVI-lowering Effect of Pitavastatin may be Involved in Prevention of Cardiovascular Disease: Subgroup Analysis of the TOHO-LIP. J Atheroscler Thromb. 2020 in press. https://doi.org/10.5551/jat.60343

5) Miyashita Y, Endo K, Saiki A, Ban N, Yamaguchi T, Kawana H, Nagayama D, Ohira M, Oyama T, Shirai K: Effects of pitavastatin, a 3-hydroxy-3-methylglutaryl coenzyme a reductase inhibitor, on cardio-ankle vascular index in type 2 diabetic patients. J Atheroscler Thromb, 2009; 16: 539–545.

6) Suzuki M, Takahashi M, Iizuka T, Terada H, Noike H, Shirai K: Frequency of coronary artery stenosis in patients with asymptomatic familial hypercholesterolemia and its association with carotid intimal thickness and cardio-ankle vascular index. Research Reports in Clinical Cardiology, 2016; 7; 83-90.

7) Ibata J, Sasaki H, Hanabusa T, Wakasaki H, Furuta H, Nishi M, Akamizu T, Nanjo K: Increased arterial stiffness is closely associated with hyperglycemia and improved by glycemic control in diabetic patients. J Diabetes Investig, 2013; 29; 4: 82-87.

8) Uzui H, Nakano A, Mitsuke Y, Geshi T, Sakata J, Sarazawa K, Morishita T, Satou T, Ishida K, Lee JD: Acarbose treatments improve arterial stiffness in patients with type 2 diabetes mellitus. J Diabetes Investig, 2011; 2: 148-153.

9) Ohira M, Endo K, Oyama T, Yamaguchi T, Ban N, Kawana H, Nagayama D, Nagumo A, Ohira M, Oyama T, Murano T, Miyashita Y, Yamamura S, Suzuki Y, Shirai K, Tatsuno I: Improvement of postprandial hyperglycemia and arterial stiffness upon switching from premixed human insulin 30/70 to biphasic insulin aspart 30/70. Metabolism, 2011; 60: 78-85.

10) Akahori H: Clinical evaluation of thrice-daily lispro 50/50 versus twice-daily aspart 70/30 on blood glucose fluctuation and postprandial hyperglycemia in patients with type 2 diabetes mellitus. Diabetology International, 2015; 6: 275-283.

11) Ohira M, Yamaguchi T, Saiki A, Ban N, Kawana H, Nagumo A, Murano T, Shirai K, Tatsuno I: Pioglitazone improves the cardio-ankle vascular index in patients with type 2 diabetes mellitus treated with metformin. Diabetes Metab Syndr Obes, 2014; 7: 313-319.

12) Bekki M, Tahara N, Tahara A, Igata S, Honda A, Sugiyama Y, Nakamura T, Sun J, Kumashiro Y, Matsui T, Fukumoto Y, Yamagish SI: Switching dipeptidyl peptidase-4 inhibitors to tofogliflozin, a selective inhibitor of sodium-glucose cotransporter 2 improves arterial stiffness evaluated by cardio-ankle vascular index in patients with type 2 diabetes: a pilot study. Current Vascular Pharmacology, 2018; 16, 1-10.

13) Shigiyama F, Kumashiro N, Miyagi M, Iga R, Kobayashi Y, Kanda E, Uchino H, Hirose T: Linagliptin improves endothelial function in patients with type 2 diabetes: A randomized study of linagliptin effectiveness on endothelial function. J Diabetes Investig, 2017; 8: 330-340.

14) Nagayama D, Saiki A, Endo K, Yamaguchi T, Ban N, Kawana H, Ohira M, Oyama T, Miyashita Y, Shirai K: Improvement of cardio-vascular vascular index by glimepiride in type 2 diabetic patients. Int J Clin Pract, 2010; 64: 1796-1801.

15) Saiki A, Ohira M, Yamaguchi T, Nagayama D, Shimizu N, Shirai K, Tatsuno I. New Horizons of Arterial Stiffness Developed Using Cardio-Ankle Vascular Index (CAVI). J Atheroscler Thromb. 2020; 27: 732-748.

PART 10

The meaning of rapid rise of CAVI just before cardiovascular events

Smooth muscle cell contraction theory for cardiovascular events

Kazuhiro Shimizu[1], Mao Takahashi[1], Shuji Sato[1], Atsuhito Saiki[1], Daiji Nagayama[1],
Masashi Harada[2], Chikao Miyazaki[2], Akira Takahara[3] and Kohji Shirai[1]

Introduction

An increased number of deaths due to atherosclerotic diseases have become a major concern not only in the developed countries but also in developing countries in recent times[1]. Various risk factors for the progression of atherosclerosis have been identified[2,3], and several hypotheses such as the cholesterol theory[4], response to injury hypothesis[5], and the plaque rupture theory for vulnerable plaque[6,7] have been proposed. However, those hypotheses are not always useful as an indicators of impending cardiovascular events. We know empirically that an increase in various risk factors does not necessarily lead to an immediate cardiovascular event. In the process of our daily clinical observations using cardio ankle vascular index (CAVI), an index that is independent of the blood pressure at the measurement time, we found that CAVI reflects the basal atherosclerotic state as an arterial stiffness[8-11]. However, when CAVI was measured sequentially in many patients, a rapid increase in CAVI was often observed. This phenomenon is due to the functional stiffness induced by the contraction of the smooth muscle cells (SMCs). In daily clinical practice, we experienced several cases in which the vascular events occurred after a few weeks or a few months after the rapid increase in CAVI.

Although these cases were not evaluated as part of any well-designed prospective mass study, we were obliged to consider that the cases indicate a suggestive sign that should not be overlooked. Many papers have reported a significant increase in the number of cardiovascular events immediately following natural calamities, sometimes accompanied by high blood pressure. However, an adequate explanation for such occurrences was not available until recently, although psychological stress or mental stress were considered as possible causes.

In recent times, pathological studies have shown the development of neovascularization in advanced atheromatous lesion, and these were derived from the vasa vasorum[12,13]. The vasa vasorum penetrates from the adventitia through the media layer and reaches the thickened atheromatous lesion in intima. Anatomically, the network of vasa vasorum runs through the medial SMC layer and supplies blood to the intimal atheromatous lesion, where many inflammatory reactions to cytotoxic substances such as oxysterols or other degenerated elements derived from infiltrated LDL occur[14]. During this stage, a rapid increase in the CAVI indicates contraction of the medial SMC, and this contraction of the medial SMC stifles the vasa vasorum in the medial layer and provokes ischemia in the intimal atheromatous lesion. During carotid endarterectomy, we confirmed that the blood to the intimal atheromatous lesion in the cervical artery was supplied by the vasa vasorum. This compelled us to consider the hypothesis of "SMC contraction theory" as a mechanism for the onset of vascular events.

In this chapter, the process to reach this new hypothesis "smooth muscle cell contraction theory for cardiovascular events" and the mechanism were discussed[15].

1. Background: Disaster and CAVI

It is known that the frequency of cardiovascular events increases just after a huge earthquake[16-19].

On March 11th, 2011, an earthquake of magnitude 9.0 occurred on the Pacific coast of Tohoku, Honshu Island, Japan, at 14:46 local time (the Great East Japan Earthquake). It was followed by a series of powerful aftershocks, with 31 earthquakes of magnitude larger than 6 in 3 days. Our institute (Toho University Sakura Medical Center Hospital) was situated about 300 km away from the epicenter. The building was strongly shaken and part of a wall collapsed. An unusual crisis occurred in our town. We started to investigate CAVI for healthy volunteers and the patients with cardiovascular risks just after the earthquake[19]. As shown in Fig. 1, we reported that CAVI was enhanced transiently just after the earthquake in healthy people and in CAD patients. Particularly in healthy people, CAVI increased even though blood pressure was not raised significantly. Furthermore, the number of deaths in our town increased in the year 2011 compared to 2009, 2010 and 2012 (Fig. 2A). We thought this increase in mortality in 2011 was primarily due to psychological stress caused by the huge earthquake[20]. Furthermore, patients suffering from

[1]Department of Internal Medicine, Toho University Sakura Medical Center, 564-1 Shimoshizu, Sakura City, Chiba 285-8741, Japan.
[2]Department of Neurosurgery, Toho University Omori Medical Center, 6-11-1 Omorinishi, Ota-ku, Tokyo 143-8541, Japan.
[3]Department of Pharmacology and Therapeutics, Faculty of Pharmaceutical Sciences, Toho University, 2-2-1 Miyama, Funabashi, Chiba 274-8510, Japan.

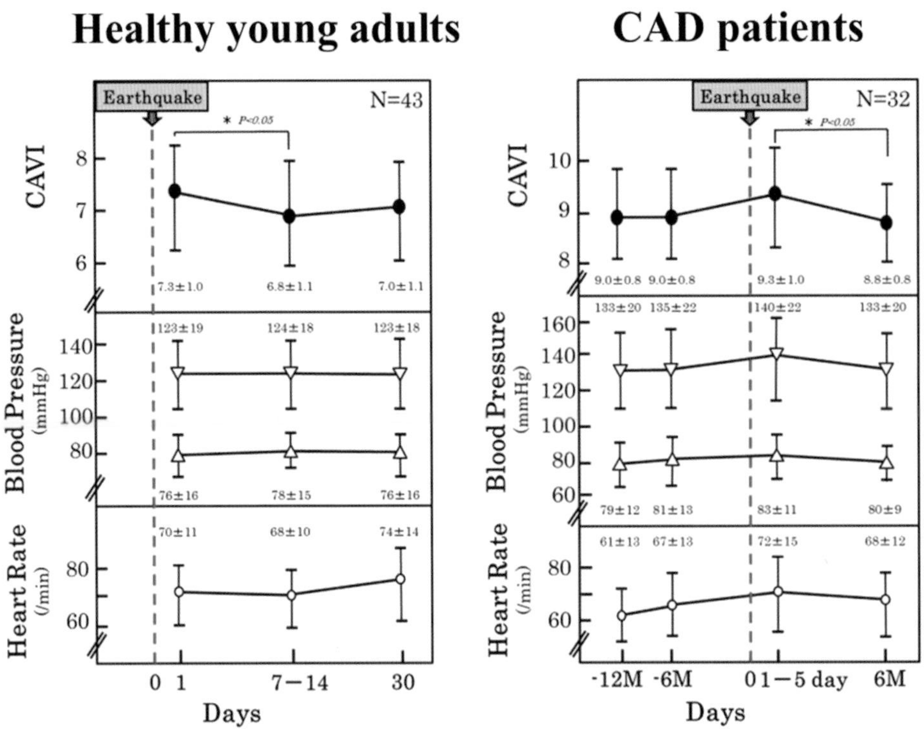

Healthy young adults

CAD patients

Data were expressed as mean ± SD. Comparisons of each measurements were evaluated by Tukey–Kramer test.

Fig. 1. Changes in CAVI damaged by huge earthquake. Adapted from ref.20

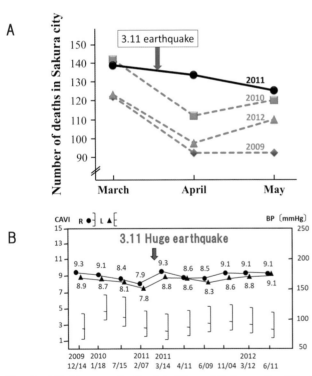

Fig. 2. (A) Changes in the fatalities of Sakura city. Cited from ref.20
(B) A case of increase in cardio-ankle vascular index (CAVI) just after the Great East Japan Earthquake (M9; March 11, 2011). Vascular Health and Risk Management 2021; 17:37-47; Originally published by and used with permission from Dove Medical Press Ltd[15)]

cerebral hemorrhage came to our hospital two times more than previous years. Fig. 2B shows the one case with metabolic disorders who had psychological damage by the huge earthquake and increased CAVI. He had been treated for diabetes mellitus, hypertension and dyslipidemia in our hospital. Because his hometown was damaged by the huge earthquake and subsequent nuclear power plant troubles caused by the ensuing tsunami, he felt deep stress and his CAVI increased considerably.

2. Several cases of Cerebro-Cardiovascular Events after a Rapid Rise in CAVI

We have observed the CAVI changes in several patients who suffered from myocardial infarction, cerebral hemorrhage and aortic dissection. These cases showed a rapid rise in CAVI before vascular events.

The case shown in Fig. 3A had acute myocardial infarction 4 months after a rapid rise in CAVI. He had gained body weight and worsened diabetic control. Fig. 3B shows a case who suffered from cerebral hemorrhage 7 days after a rapid rise in CAVI. She had suffered from domestic troubles. Fig. 3C showed the case who suffered from an aortic dissection 2 weeks after a rapid rise in CAVI. She had suffered from vertebral compression fracture. Fig. 3D shows the CAVI in an atherosclerotic patient who came to our hospital for 13 years. At the beginning, his baseline CAVI was already above nine. He developed unstable angina and cerebral infarction when his work was busy as a chef of his restaurant, and finally died of cerebral hemorrhage after a rapid rise in CAVI (11.5 to 12.8 in the last month). This case shows the gradual increase in CAVI with aging and the development of atherosclerotic diseases.

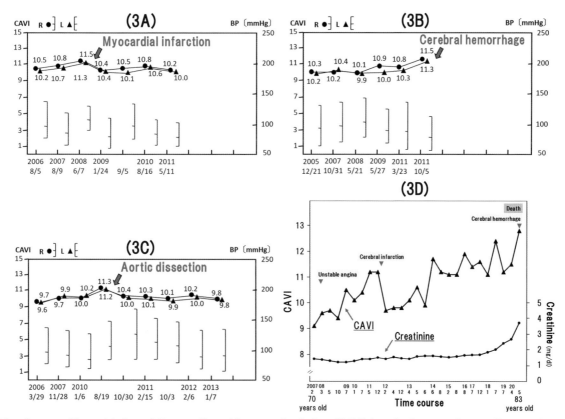

Fig. 3. **The Cases with rapid rise of the cardio-ankle vascular index (CAVI) just before cerebrocardiovascular events.**
3A: A case of acute myocardial infarction, **3B**: A case of cerebral hemorrhage, **3C**: A case of aortic dissection, **3D**: A case of cerebral hemorrhage

The above-mentioned cases might suffer from cardiovascular events simply by chance just after rapid rise of CAVI. And it might be very difficult to prove causal relationship directly or statistically. However, the possibility that a rapid rise in CAVI might be a prodrome of impending cerebrocardiovascular events could not completely denied. In following section, we tried to consider possible mechanism how those events would happen just after rapid rise of CAVI in a case having high CAVI.

3. Vasculature of atheromatous lesion: Vasa vasorum

To understand the rapid increase in the CAVI as a prodrome of a cardiovascular event, the structure of an atheromatous lesion and its vasculature needs to be reviewed. Arteries consist of three morphologically distinct layers: innermost layer, the intima; the middle layer, the media; and the external layer, the adventitia. The intima is bounded on the lumen side by a continuous layer of endothelial cells that form a protective barrier between the blood and arterial wall.

It is known that the advanced stage of intimal atheromatous lesions is rich in microvessels[12,13,21]. The vasa vasorum penetrates the medial smooth muscle cell layer from the adventitia to the intimal layer. The medial SMCs of the arterial wall can contract or relax, even in the advanced stage of arteriosclerosis. Yamamto showed that nigtroglycerin administration decreased CAVI at almost same rate among young people and in patients with

arteriosclerosis[22]. This indicates that medial SMCs layer is intact even in the advanced stages of arteriosclerotic changes in the artery. Osada et. al reported that most aortic dissections initially developed in the outer third of the media alongside the vasa vasorum. They suggested that dysfunction of the vasa vasorum might play a key role in prolonged ischemia or malnutrition of the aortic media, and that the resultant necrotic layer forms the dissecting aneurysm[23].

To confirm that the blood supply to the intimal lesion came from the adventitia, we observed carotid endarterectomy in a patient whose cervical artery had more than 90% stenosis caused by an atheromatous lesion (Fig. 4). During the surgery, when the intimal atheromatous layer of the carotid artery was separated, the medial smooth muscle layer was denuded. Just after separating the intimal layer, bleeding was immediately observed on the surface of the medial smooth muscle cell layer. However, when the surface of this medial smooth muscle layer was covered with gauze dipped in the noradrenaline; the bleeding was stopped. Such procedures are routinely performed during brain surgery. This phenomenon indicated that the blood supply of the intimal atheromatous lesion was mediated by the vasa vasorum, and this blood flow was interrupted by the contraction of the medial SMCs[15].

4. Smooth muscle cell contraction theory for vascular events

As shown in Fig. 5, we proposed "the smooth muscle

contraction hypothesis for cerebro-cardiovascular events" based on evidences described above[15].

First stage

The initial atheromatous lesions consist of an intimal thickness composed of proliferated synthetic type of SMCs, and fibrous components, such as collagen and elastin. These are arterial reactions to various stress injuries, such as infiltration of lipids, shear stress and endothelial injury, and others[5]. This stage is called the fibrous cap, which increases the arterial stiffness, which is reflected as an increase in the CAVI. Morphologically, this stage is recognized as vascular stenosis. This stage does not necessarily provoke acute coronary events, as mentioned by Fuster[6], and inflammatory reactions continue to occur[7]. However, this stage not only leads to vascular stenosis and/or a vulnerable plaque but also causes the vasa vasorum to reach the thickening layer

of the intima from the adventitia[24]. This neovascularization is induced by anoxia and/or inflammatory reactions in the cap. During this process, the developed microvessels begin to penetrate the medial SMC layer and supply blood into the intimal atheromatous lesion.

Second stage

When a person with an advanced stage of arteriosclerosis (basal CAVI > 10) encounters natural calamities such as a massive earthquake, natural disaster, and various other types of mental shock, the stress provokes contraction of medial SMCs of the arteries. This leads to a rapid increase in the CAVI. The contraction of the medial SMC layer "chokes" the micro vessels penetrating through the medial layer. As a result, the blood flow into the intimal layer is interrupted, making the plaque vulnerable to ischemia. This causes necrosis of the core of the intimal atheromatous lesion.

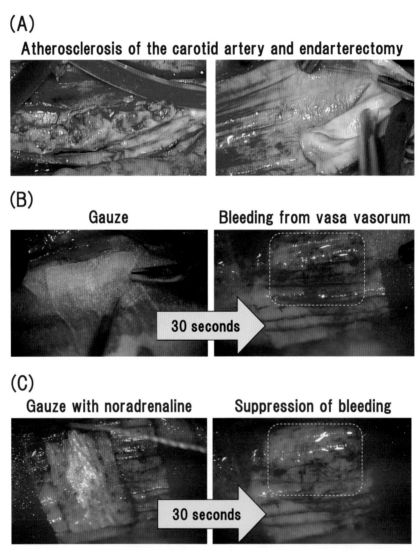

(A)

Atherosclerosis of the carotid artery and endarterectomy

(B)

Gauze   Bleeding from vasa vasorum

30 seconds

(C)

Gauze with noradrenaline   Suppression of bleeding

30 seconds

Fig. 4. Carotid endarterectomy of a patient with 90% stenosis of the cervical artery. (A) Atherosclerosis of the carotid artery and endarterectomy. (B) Gauze was applied for the bleeding which occurred after peeling off the intimal atheromatous layer of the carotid artery. (C) Gauze, dipped in the noradrenaline, was applied and inhibited the bleeding, indicating that the blood supply of the intimal atheromatous lesion was from the vasa vasorum and that it was stopped by contraction of the medial smooth muscle cells. Vascular Health and Risk Management 2021; 17:37-47; Originally published by and used with permission from Dove Medical Press Ltd[15]

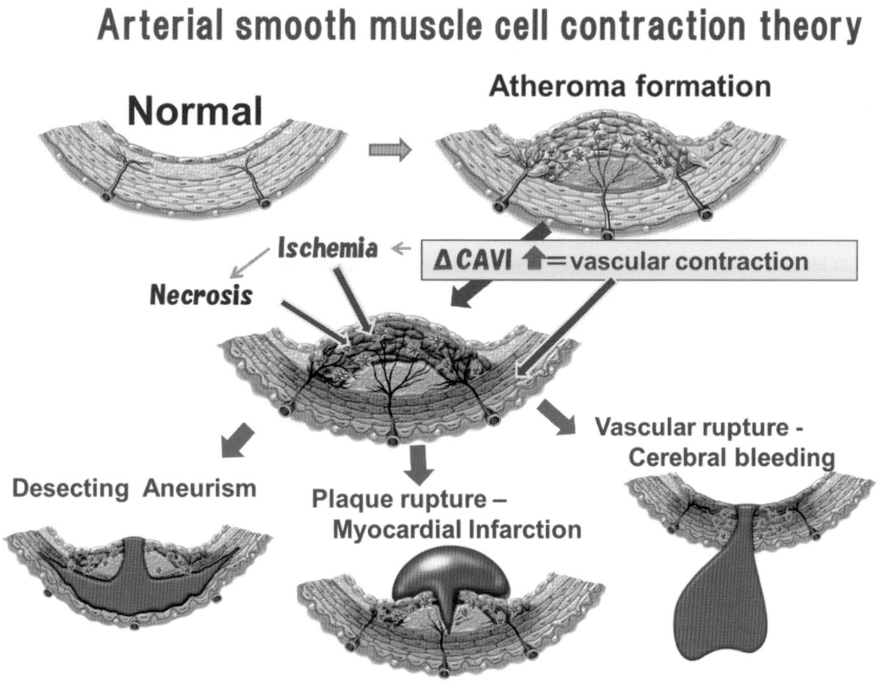

Arterial smooth muscle cell contraction theory

Fig. 5. Smooth muscle cell contraction hypothesis for plaque rupture. Vascular Health and Risk Management 2021; 17:37-47; Originally published by and used with permission from Dove Medical Press Ltd[15)]

Macrophages congregate around this necrotic core and start digesting the necrotic tissue. Thus, the cap of the vulnerable plaque becomes thin and triggers a rupture. In the case of the coronary artery, plaque rupture causes thrombus formation on the surface of the initial layer, leading to myocardial infarction. In the case of the aorta, the necrotic core in the wall could develop into a dissecting aneurysm. In the case of a cerebral artery, the thin arterial wall could be easily ruptured by necrosis of the SMC layer, resulting in brain hemorrhage.

5. Vascular health and risk management in our future life

To predict the looming vascular events, CAVI which detects rapid contraction of smooth muscle cells would be a distinctive indicator warning of conditions leading to cardiovascular events. Thus, we recommended to measure arterial stiffness with CAVI in short intervals.

Furthermore, we tentatively propose that a high basal value of CAVI is over 10 and enhanced ΔCAVI is over 0.7 for the sign of a looming cardiovascular event. Tentative basal value CAVI (= 10) was nearly mean CAVI (7.84) in Japanese + 2 x standard deviation (2x1.07). ΔCAVI (0.7) was correspondent to two times of coefficient variation (3.8%) of CAVI measurement[8, 25)].

Considering the mechanisms explained above, we proposed a "smooth muscle cell contraction" hypothesis of plaque rupture[15)]. According to this hypothesis, monitoring CAVI in daily life might be useful to predict the risk of occurrence of life-threatening cardiovascular events in the near future.

Summary

To prevent cardiovascular events, an attempt should be made to decrease or improve the CAVI using all methods mentioned in Chapter 56 to prevent the formation of an intimal atheromatous lesion. Furthermore, it is important to measure the CAVI frequently, and if an abrupt increase in the CAVI is noted, an immediate attempt to decrease the CAVI should be made by relieving mental stress, undertaking mild exercise, warming the body such as Waon therapy, and others.

Finally, we hope that monitoring arterial stiffness periodically, similar to measuring the blood pressure, would promote the vascular health of the people.

Acknowledgements

We express our deep thanks to the following colleagues for establishing this hypothesis.

Takahiro Nakagami[1], Keiichi Hirano[1], Hirofumi Noike[1], Yo Miyashita[1], Fusako Watanabe[1], Takumi Kurosu[2], Jun Suzuki[2], Kiyoshi Sakuma[3], Tatsuo Chiba[4], Yoshinobu Nagasawa[5], Tomoyuki Yamamoto[6]

[1]Department of Internal Medicine, Toho University Sakura Medical Center
[2]Department of Clinical Functional Physiology, Toho University Sakura Medical Center
[3]Department of Pharmacy, Toho University Sakura Medical Center
[4]Department of Pharmacy, Toho University Ohashi Medical Center
[5]Department of Pharmacology and Therapeutics, Faculty of Pharmaceutical Sciences, Toho University
[6]Fukuda Denshi Co., Ltd., Tokyo, Japan

References

1) Roth, G.A.; Johnson, C.; Abajobir, A.; Abd-Allah, F.; Abera, S.F.; Abyu, G.; Ahmed, M.; Aksut, B.; Alam, T.; Alam, K.; et al. Global, regional, and national burden of cardiovascular diseases for 10 causes, 1990 to 2015. J. Am. Coll. Cardiol. 2017, 70, 1–25.

2) Ralph B. D'Agostino, Ramachandran S. Vasan, Michael J. Pencina, Philip A. Wolf, Mark Cobain, Joseph M. Massaro, William B. Kannel. General Cardiovascular Risk Profile for Use in Primary Care. The Framingham Heart Study. Circulation. 2008; 117: 743-753.

3) Yandrapalli, S, Nabors, C, Goyal, A, et al. Modifiable risk factors in young adults with first myocardial infarction. J Am Coll Cardiol 2019; 73: 573-584.

4) E. H. AHRENS Jr. Drugs Spotlight Program: The Management of Hyperlipidemia: Whether, Rather than How. Annals of Internal Medicine 1976; 85: 87-93.

5) Ross R, Glomset J. The pathogenesis of atherosclerosis. N Engl J Med. 1976; 295:369–377, 420–425.

6) J E Muller, G H Tofler, and P H Stone. Circadian variation and triggers of onset of acute cardiovascular disease. Circulation. 1989; 79:733–743.

7) Peter Libby, Gerard Pasterkamp, Filippo Crea, Ik-Kyung Jang. Reassessing the Mechanisms of Acute Coronary Syndromes. The "Vulnerable Plaque" and Superficial Erosion. Circ Res. 2019; 124: 150-160.

8) Shirai K, Utino J, Otsuka K, Takata M. A noble blood pressure-independent arterial wall stiffness parameter; cardio-ankle vascular index (CAVI). J Atheroscler Thromb. 2006; 13: 101-107.

9) Namekata T, Suzuki K, Ishizuka N, Shirai K. Establishing baseline criteria of cardio-ankle vascular index as a new indicator of arteriosclerosis: a cross-sectional study. BMC Cardiovasc Disord. 2011;11:51.

10) Hayashi K, Yamamoto T, Takahara A, Shirai K. Clinical assessment of arterial stiffness with cardio-ankle vascular index: theory and applications. J Hypertens. 2015; 33: 1742–1757.

11) Saiki A, Ohira M, Yamaguchi T, Nagayama D, Shimizu N, Shirai K, Tatsuno I. New Horizons of Arterial Stiffness Developed Using Cardio-Ankle Vascular Index (CAVI). J Atheroscler Thromb. 2020; 27: 732-748.

12) Daniel G. Sedding, Erin C. Boyle, Jasper A. F. Demandt, Judith C. Sluimer, Jochen Dutzmann, Axel Haverich and Johann Bauersachs. Vasa Vasorum Angiogenesis: Key Player in the Initiation and Progression of Atherosclerosis and Potential Target for the Treatment of Cardiovascular Disease. Front Immunol. 2018;9:706. doi: 10.3389/fimmu.2018.00706. eCollection 2018.

13) Kume T, Okura H, Yamada R, et al. In vivo assessment of vasa vasorum neovascularization using intravascular ultrasound: A comparison between acute coronary syndrome and stable angina pectoris. Journal of Cardiology. 2017; 69: 601–605.

14) Ohtsuka M, Miyashita Y, Shirai K. Lipids deposited in human atheromatous lesions induce apoptosis of human vascular smooth muscle cells J Atheroscler Thromb. 2006;13:256-62. doi:10.5551/jat.13.256.

15) Shimizu K, Takahashi M, Sato S, et al. Rapid rise of cardio-ankle vascular index may be a trigger of cerebro-cardiovascular events: Proposal of smooth muscle cell contraction theory for plaque rupture. Vascular Health and Risk Management. Vascular Health and Risk Management. 2021; 17:37-47.

16) Trichopoulos D, Zavitsanos X, Katsouyanni K, Tzonou A, Dalla-Vorgia P. Psychological stress and fatal heart attack: the Athens (1981) earthquake natural experiment. Lancet. 1983; 321: 441–444.

17) Dobson AJ, Alexander HM, Malcolm JA, Steele PL, Miles TA. Heart attacks and the Newcastle earthquake. Med J Aust. 1991; 155: 757-761.

18) Leor J, Poole WK, Kloner RA. Sudden cardiac death triggered by an earthquake. N Engl J Med. 1996; 334: 413-419.

19) Kario K, Matsuo T, Kobayashi H, Yamamoto K, Shimada K. Earthquake-induced potentiation of acute risk factors in hypertensive elderly patients: Possible triggering of cardiovascular events after a major earthquake. J Am Coll Cardiol. 1997; 29: 926-933.

20) Shimizu K, Takahashi M, Shirai K. A huge earthquake hardened arterial stiffness monitored with cardio-ankle vascular index. J Atheroscler Thromb. 2013; 20: 503-511.

21) Doyle B, Caplice N. Plaque neovascularization and antiangiogenic therapy for atherosclerosis. J Am Coll Cardiol. 2007; 49: 2073–80.

22) Yamamoto T, Shimizu K, Takahashi M, Tatsuno I, Shirai K. The Effect of Nitroglycerin on Arterial Stiffness of the Aorta and the Femoral-Tibial Arteries. J Atheroscler Thromb. 2017; 24: 1048–1057.

23) Osada H, Kyogoku M, Ishidou M, Morishima M and Nakajima H. Aortic dissection in the outer third of the media: what is the role of the vasa vasorum in the triggering process? European Journal of Cardio-Thoracic Surgery. 2013; 43 e82-88.

24) Pedro R. Moreno, K. Raman Purushothaman, Valentin Fuster, Dario Echeverri, Helena TruszczynskaSamin K. Sharma, Juan J. Badimon, William N. O'Connor. Plaque Neovascularization Is Increased in Ruptured Atherosclerotic Lesions of Human Aorta Implications for Plaque Vulnerability. Circulation. 2004; 110:2032-2038.

25) Sato Y, Nagayama D, Saiki A, et al. Cardio-Ankle Vascular Index is Independently Associated with Future Cardiovascular Events in Outpatients with Metabolic Disorders. J Atheroscler Thromb. 2016; 23:596–605.

Afterword

Jitsuo Higaki

Blood vessels extend like a network in our bodies, enabling the supply of oxgen and nutrient-filled blood. Such a body fluid circulation system supports the vital activity in each perfusion region. According to the demand of the tissue at that time, delicate adjustments are performed by expanding and contracting the lumen at every moment under the complex interaction of the adjustment by the central nervous system, various organ correlations centered on the heart, and various bioactive substances generated by vascular cells. As has been said many times before, blood vessels are not just simple tubes, but are a living organ. There are various parameters for the evaluation of this vascular function, and several measurement systems have accordingly been devised. Among them, CAVI can be the ultimate vascular function measurement system that opens the door to new angiology.

As revealed in this book, CAVI can measure arterial stiffness in real time without the influent of blood pressure.

The so-called blood vessel stiffness consists of structural stiffness and functional tension. Not only can CAVI evaluate the long-term course by fixed-point observation, it can also evaluate the functional stress of blood vessels that change from moment to moment, mainly casused by increased sympathetic nerve conduction. As revealed in this book, CAVI can measure arterial stiffness in real time, so, not only can it evaluate the present arterioscletic status of hypertension, diabetes mellitus and dyslipidemia, but it also has evidence for their prognosis prediction, and shows the responsiveness of the blood vessels to drug interventions. Furthermore, CAVI may be applicable in anti-aging medicine, and the prediction of a just-approached heart attack or cerebral stroke.

Now, how will be the future led by CAVI change? The new evolution of CAVI devices and the corresponding fusion of artificial intelligence (AI) with it are expected. Various vascular function tests, combined with diagnostic imaging methods such as CT and MRI, may be combined by AI to monitor the dynamic qualitative and quantitative data of the bloodstream in the whole body, and discover supply and demand inbalance in the local area, and lead to the prevention and treatment of various diseases. Currently, biological information such as that for blood pressure, pulse, electrocardiography, blood sugar, oxygen concentration, etc. is incorporated into wearable equipment. This information will be integrated by ICT and AI, and will greatly contribute to the progress of precision medicine, such as the search for the cause of individual diseases and advances in predictive medicine. Since CAVI can accurately grasp the stress that triggers the onset of vascular disease, it is also expected to become a pre-onset warning similar to the emergency earthquake bulletin currently being carried out in Japan. CAVI has caused a new dawn to arise on the new science of angiology.

MD, PhD, Professor Emeritus, Ehime University
Director of Minami-Matsuyama Hospital, 1-3-10 Asodamachi, Matsuyama City, Ehime 790-8534, Japan.

CARDIO-ANKLE VASCULAR INDEX
OVERVIEW & CLINICAL APPLICATION

Kohji Shirai, Roland Asmar and Hajime Orimo

Japanese Society for Vascular Health (Specified Non-profit Organization)
NCK Bldg 5F, 3-3-11 Hongo, Bunkyo-ku, Tokyo 113-0033, Japan

@ Japanese Society for Vascular Health, 2021
Printed in Japan,
Oct. 24th 2021

COMPASS Co., Ltd.
NCK Bldg. 5F, 3-3-11 Hongo, Bunkyo-ku, Tokyo 113-0033, Japan

ISBN: 978-4-9912126-1-1